MANUAL OF

PREOPERATIVE and POSTOPERATIVE CARE

Second Edition

BY THE COMMITTEE ON
PRE AND POSTOPERATIVE CARE

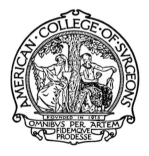

AMERICAN
COLLEGE
OF
SURGEONS

Editorial Subcommittee
JOHN M. KINNEY, M.D., *Chairman*
RICHARD H. EGDAHL, M.D.
GEORGE D. ZUIDEMA, M.D.

1971
W. B. SAUNDERS COMPANY · PHILADELPHIA · LONDON · TORONTO

W. B. Saunders Company: West Washington Square
Philadelphia, Pa.   19105

12 Dyott Street
London, WC1A   1DB

1835 Yonge Street
Toronto 7, Ontario

Manual of Preoperative and Postoperative Care   ISBN 0-7216-5440-1

Print No.:   9   8   7   6   5   4   3   2   1

COMMITTEE ON
PRE AND POSTOPERATIVE CARE

Contributors

CURTIS P. ARTZ, M.D., F.A.C.S. Professor of Surgery and Chairman of Department, Medical University of South Carolina. Chief of Surgery, Medical University Hospital, Charleston, South Carolina.

W. GERALD AUSTEN, M.D., F.A.C.S. Professor of Surgery, Harvard Medical School. Chief of Surgery, Massachusetts General Hospital, Boston, Massachusetts.

WALTER F. BALLINGER, M.D. Bixby Professor of Surgery and Head of the Department, Washington University School of Medicine. Surgeon-in-Chief, Barnes and Allied Hospitals, St. Louis, Missouri.

MARSHALL K. BARTLETT, M.D. Clinical Professor of Surgery Emeritus, Harvard Medical School. Board of Consultation, Massachusetts General Hospital, Boston, Massachusetts.

OLIVER COPE, M.D., (D. Hon. Causa), F.A.C.S. Professor of Surgery Emeritus, Harvard Medical School. Board of Consultation, Massachusetts General Hospital, Boston, Massachusetts.

STANLEY J. DUDRICK, M.D. Associate Professor of Surgery, University of Pennsylvania School of Medicine. Attending Surgeon, Hospital of the University of Pennsylvania; Chief of Surgery, University of Pennsylvania Division, Philadelphia Veterans Administration Hospital; Assistant Attending Surgeon, Philadelphia General Hospital, Philadelphia, Pennsylvania.

STANLEY R. FRIESEN, M.D., Ph.D. Professor of Surgery, University of Kansas School of Medicine. Staff, Department of Surgery, University of Kansas Medical Center, Kansas City, Kansas.

DAVID V. HABIF, M.D. Professor of Surgery, Columbia University College of Physicians and Surgeons. Attending Surgeon, Presbyterian Hospital, New York, New York.

JAMES D. HARDY, M.D. Professor and Chairman of Department of Surgery, The University of Mississippi Medical Center. Surgeon-in-Chief, University Hospital, University of Mississippi Medical Center, Jackson, Mississippi.

DAVID M. HUME, M.D., F.A.C.S. Professor and Chairman, Department of Surgery, Medical College of Virginia, Richmond, Virginia.

WILLIAM B. KIESEWETTER, M.D., F.A.C.S. Professor of Pediatric Surgery, University of Pittsburgh School of Medicine. Surgeon-in-Chief, Children's Hospital of Pittsburgh, Pittsburgh, Pennsylvania.

JOHN M. KINNEY, M.D., F.A.C.S. Professor of Surgery, Columbia University College of Physicians and Surgeons. Attending in Surgery, Presbyterian Hospital, New York, New York.

JOHN W. KIRKLIN, M.D., F.A.C.S. Professor and Chairman, Department of Surgery, School of Medicine, University of Alabama in Birmingham. Surgeon-in-Chief, University of Alabama Hospitals and Clinics, Birmingham, Alabama.

LLOYD D. MacLEAN, M.D., F.A.C.S. Professor and Chairman, Department of Surgery, McGill University. Surgeon-in-Chief, Royal Victoria Hospital, Montreal, Quebec, Canada.

FRANCIS D. MOORE, M.D., F.R.C.S. (Hon.), F.A.C.S. Moseley Professor of Surgery, Harvard Medical School, Surgeon-in-Chief, Peter Bent Brigham Hospital, Boston, Massachusetts.

GEORGE L. NARDI, M.D., F.A.C.S. Associate Clinical Professor of Surgery, Harvard Medical School. Visiting Surgeon, Massachusetts General Hospital, Boston, Massachusetts.

ERLE E. PEACOCK, JR., M.D., F.A.C.S. Professor and Chairman, Department of Surgery, University of Arizona College of Medicine. Chief of Surgery, University of Arizona Medical Center, Tuscon, Arizona.

SAMUEL R. POWERS, JR., M.D., D.Sc. (Med.) Professor of Surgery, Albany Medical College. Attending Surgeon, Albany Medical Center Hospital; Consultant Surgeon, Veterans Administration Hospital, Albany, New York.

HENRY THOMAS RANDALL, M.D., M.Sc.D. Professor of Medical Science (Surgery), and Section Head, Section of Surgery, Division of Biological and Medical Sciences, Brown University. Surgeon-in-Chief, Rhode Island Hospital, Providence, Rhode Island.

PAUL S. RUSSELL, M.D. John Homans Professor of Surgery, Harvard Medical School. Visiting Surgeon, Massachusetts General Hospital, Boston, Massachusetts.

EDWIN W. SALZMAN, M.D. Associate Professor of Surgery, Harvard Medical School, and Senior Research Associate, Massachusetts Institute of Technology. Associate Director of the Surgical Service, Beth Israel Hospital, Boston, Massachusetts.

WILLIAM R. SANDUSKY, M.D., F.A.C.S. Professor of Surgery, University of Virginia School of Medicine. Surgeon, University of Virginia Hospital, Charlottesville, Virginia.

SEYMOUR I. SCHWARTZ, M.D. Professor of Surgery, University of Rochester School of Medicine and Dentistry. Surgeon, Strong Memorial Hospital, Rochester, New York.

G. TOM SHIRES, M.D. Professor and Chairman, Department of Surgery, The University of Texas Southwestern Medical School at Dallas. Surgeon-in-Chief, Surgical Services, Parkland Memorial Hospital; Consultant Surgeon, St. Paul Hospital, Methodist Hospital, Baylor University Medical Center, Children's Medical Center, Dallas Veterans Administration Hospital, Gaston Episcopal Hospital, and Presbyterian Hospital of Dallas, Dallas, Texas.

D. EMERICK SZILAGYI, M.D., F.A.C.S. Clinical Professor of Surgery, University of Michigan. Chairman, Department of Surgery, Henry Ford Hospital, Detroit, Michigan.

RUPERT B. TURNBULL, JR., F.A.C.S. Head, Department of Colon and Rectal Surgery, Cleveland Clinic Foundation, Cleveland, Ohio.

HOWARD ULFELDER, M.D., F.A.C.S. Joe V. Meigs Professor of Gynecology, Harvard Medical School. Chief of Staff, Vincent Memorial Hospital, Boston, Massachusetts.

CARL W. WALTER, M.D., F.A.C.S. Clinical Professor of Surgery, Harvard Medical School. Surgeon, Peter Bent Brigham Hospital, Boston, Massachusetts.

W. DEAN WARREN, M.D., F.A.C.S. Professor of Surgery, University of Miami School of Medicine. Surgeon, Jackson Memorial Hospital, Miami, Florida.

CLAUDE E. WELCH, M.D., F.A.C.S. Clinical Professor of Surgery, Harvard Medical School. Visiting Surgeon, Massachusetts General Hospital, Boston, Massachusetts.

EDWARD R. WOODWARD, M.D., F.A.C.S. Professor and Chairman, Department of Surgery, University of Florida College of Medicine, Gainesville, Florida.

Preface

The purpose of this manual is to provide the busy clinical surgeon and surgical resident with quick and concise access to recent advances in surgical metabolism, nutrition, fluid and electrolyte balance, clotting disorders, infection and shock, together with cardiac, ventilatory and renal pathophysiology. It is intended to provide a useful outline of the modern management of problems of pre- and postoperative patients undergoing both elective and emergency operation. The authors have, in the latter chapters of this book, described the approaches to the handling of pre- and postoperative care of patients undergoing operation on particular body systems, including the management of related complications. Other chapters include the management of multiple injuries and the treatment of burns. The appendix includes a table of normal laboratory values, a list of selected tests of various organ systems and a brief discussion of acid-base balance.

The manual does not attempt to be a text, and so technical details of operations have usually been omitted in the interest of maintaining a volume of modest size and cost. References to standard texts and important articles will be found at the end of most chapters, and from them additional information can be obtained. It is hoped that such a manual may serve as a ready reference for the surgeon who lacks the time to read more extensive material on a given subject, or who might appreciate an abbreviated discussion prior to a more extensive review of the literature.

The manual has been prepared as an activity of the Committee on Pre and Postoperative Care of the American College of Surgeons with the approval of the Regents of the College. Since the Committee's formation in 1959 under the chairmanship of Dr. Francis D. Moore of Boston, a major activity has been the sponsoring of teaching sessions in pre- and postoperative care. The manual is an outgrowth of the course in pre- and postoperative care given annually at the Clinical Congress of the American College of Surgeons.

The selection of the material for the second edition reflects certain changes from the previous volume. There are fewer chapters, of some-what longer length, new illustrative material and additional references. This editorial committee does not contend that methods or approaches other than the ones presented in this volume may not be successful in the management of surgical patients. What we have endeavored to do is provide a useful guide for the management of surgical patients, based upon the description of the metabolic and physiologic principles that must underlie successful treatment.

We wish to acknowledge the unusual time and effort that was spent by the members of the first edition's editorial committee in translating the multiple wishes of the parent committee into initial book form. Our appreciation for this goes to Dr. Henry T. Randall, Chairman, Dr. James D. Hardy and Dr. Francis D. Moore. The success of the first edition confirmed the need for such a volume and contributed greatly to the preparation of this second edition.

Particular thanks are due to Dr. William Adams of the American College of Surgeons and Mr. Robert Rowan of W. B. Saunders Company for continuing advice and encouragement. In addition, we wish to thank the many secretaries whose patient and careful work contributed to the preparation of this volume.

RICHARD EGDAHL
GEORGE ZUIDEMA
JOHN M. KINNEY, *Chairman*
Editorial Subcommittee

Contents

Part I
GENERAL PRINCIPLES

Part II
SURGICAL CARE OF
ORGANS AND SYSTEMS

Part I

GENERAL PRINCIPLES

CHAPTER 1

WOUND HEALING AND CARE OF THE WOUND

Erle E. Peacock, Jr., M.D., F.A.C.S.

Healing—the most fundamental biological phenomenon in surgical biology—is affected significantly by pre- and postoperative care. Although most problems in wound healing are the result of local factors within the wound and immediate surrounding area, systemic factors are occasionally responsible for failure to heal, and some of these factors are amenable to pre- and postoperative manipulation. It is a good idea to remember, however, that the healing wound is dynamically very similar to a fetus, and like a developing embryo appears to have high priority when calling for the resources required for protein synthesis. Moreover, even though the entire body may be rather severely depleted of some fundamental building block, the relative amount of such a substance needed to heal a surgical incision is so small compared to the general body pool that it should not come as a surprise to learn that wound healing progresses remarkably well. Uremia, carcinomatosis, anemia, protein depletion, corticosteroid excess, and poorly controlled diabetes are but a few of the general metabolic disorders which have been implicated in the past as significantly retarding the gain of tensile strength in a healing wound. Of these, corticosteroid excess is the only one which has been shown so far to affect wound healing significantly in human beings, and then only to the extent of delaying gain in tensile strength—not preventing collagen synthesis and deposition. Other influences can be shown to inhibit gain of tensile strength in the wounds of laboratory animals, but the severity of the disorder and the clinical insignificance of the measured inhibition are of such an order that they are seldom important during management of a human patient. Addition of cartilage powder and zinc, for example, increases the rate of gain of burst strength to a mathematically significant degree in the healing wound of a laboratory animal; the effect of these agents is not great enough to be clinically significant in most patients, however.

An exception to the statement that systemic conditions are seldom responsible for severe inhibition of wound healing is depletion of specific catalysts, such as trace metals or ascorbic acid, which are needed in small amounts to catalyze important reactions, such as hydroxylation of proline. Serious deficiencies of these substances are extremely rare, however, and, in most patients, can be easily recognized. Variations in oxygen tension appear to be one of the most important factors responsible for failure to heal; measurement of oxygen tension in tissue is still extremely difficult, however, and much of our knowledge about the effect of oxygen tension is speculative.

Thus the surgeon can best control the healing phenomenon in 1971 by what he does to the wound, not by what he does to the entire patient. Principles of pre- and postoperative care of wounds are limited primarily, therefore, to care of wounds.

PREOPERATIVE CARE

Incisions. Recommendation by some surgeons that the skin of the abdomen or chest should be prepared for a surgical operation in exactly the same manner as the surgeon's hands are prepared is theoretically sound. Practically, however, it is often not possible and usually not necessary to prepare skin before making an incision in the abdomen or the thorax in exactly the same manner as the surgeon's hands. The hands carry organisms not commonly found on the remainder of the body, perspire profusely when encased in rubber gloves, and are prepared to enter and work within body cavities. Normally the skin of the abdomen and thorax has a pH below that which common pathogens can tolerate; accurate draping of the skin should prevent gross contamination of a body cavity by the wound edges. Operating room time is valuable, and the effect on the patient of a prolonged preparation of the skin in the operating room may have local as well as general effects. It is simply not always practical, therefore, to scrub the skin of the abdomen with a brush and medicated soap for ten minutes, as is usually done for the surgeon's hands.

The objectives of preparation of the skin for an abdominal or thoracic incision are to remove hair so that an incision can be made without introducing keratin and to remove any pathogens which might be on the skin because of unusual contact or failure of normal skin defense mechanisms. No better way to remove surface organisms has ever been found than application of a surface bactericidal agent. Two per cent iodine in alcohol has had recurring cycles of popularity followed by replacement with other agents. The few excellent studies which have been done, however, reveal that no other topical agent is more effective in reducing the number of pathogens on the surface of the skin than 2 per cent iodine and alcohol.

It is frequently stated that application of a surface bactericidal agent does not constitute complete preparation of the skin because it merely coagulates surface bacteria without reaching organisms in the depth of hair follicles and glands. From a theoretical bacteriological standpoint, the statement cannot be refuted; in practical experience, however, superiority of various preparations or regimens claming to sterilize the depths of skin appendages has not been established. Satisfactory control of body temperature, adequate draping, precise surgical technique (particularly guarding against soaking drapes with blood or other fluids), and completing the procedure in a reasonable length of time are probably more effective in preventing contamination of the wound from bacteria deep within the recesses of skin appendages than is scrubbing the skin with a detergent for a prolonged period of time. Detergents used for long periods with the objective of saponifying surface fats and cleansing the depths of skin appendages can change the bacterial flora differently from simple utilization of a surface bactericidal agent. However, clinical studies have not shown that such bacteriological changes have resulted in a significant reduction in the incidence of wound infections caused by topical bacteria. For those who want the best of two approaches, preliminary cleansing with soap and water to remove lipids and surface contaminants is recommended, followed by application of a bactericidal agent just before the incision is made. The preoperative use of soap and water, however, is a mechanical and chemical measure and should not be confused with the bactericidal effect of an agent included with soap. Actually, application of some bactericidal agents will inactivate the bacteriostatic agent included with some soap preparations. In the judgment of the author, there is no scientific basis at this time for spending ten minutes in the operating room scrubbing the abdomen or chest of an anesthetized patient in exactly the same manner as the surgeon is preparing his hands. Mechanical cleansing with soap and water and removal of hair the evening before an operation, followed by application of a topical bactericidal agent immediately prior to making the incision, is bacteriologically sound, practically effective, and provides the most efficient utilization of anesthetic and operating room time.

Shaving usually should be done late in the evening before the day the incision is made. Superficial abrasions or lacerations caused by shaving should not be allowed to become inflamed or infected. Experienced plastic and neurosurgeons make it a policy, however, not to shave hair on the scalp before a patient is taken to the operating room. Actually, extensive shaving of the scalp is best done after the patient is anesthetized. The reasons are mostly esthetic. The thoughtful surgeon does not force his patient to appear before other patients in the ward or visitors who may be present the evening or morning before an operation with an area of exposed scalp or a stocking cap. Loss of hair is associated with loss of dignity, and the few extra minutes required to prepare the scalp after the patient is asleep is a thoughtful gesture that most surgeons can afford to make in the interest of preventing embarrassment. Of course, the hair should always be saved when a serious intracranial procedure is contemplated. Again, however, this is a maneuver that neither the patient nor the family should be made aware of during preoperative preparation.

Preoperative use of antibiotics to prevent wound infection during elective procedures has been shown to be ineffective except when it is known that a contaminant is going to be introduced. Again, however, surgical technique is probably more important than preoperative preparation in preventing wound healing complications resulting from infection produced during an elective operation. Actually, indiscriminate administration of antibiotics prior to elective surgery has been shown to be detrimental; complications of such therapy outweigh theoretical advantages in most reported studies.

Preoperative Preparation of Traumatic Wounds for Primary Closure. The major objectives in the preoperative management of a traumatic wound are to prevent further contamination, reduce surface contamination before surgical debridement, and correct general metabolic and circulatory disorders caused by blood loss. Treatment of shock and general metabolic disorders is covered elsewhere in this manual. Prevention of further contamination is achieved by aseptic technique from the time the patient first comes under professional care. The knowledge that most major infections are traceable to the nose, throat, and hands of attendants after a patient reaches the hospital is a sobering reflection which demands that masks and gloves be worn and the best surgical technique be instituted from the time the patient is first seen in the emergency room. If several hours must elapse before surgical debridement of a contaminated wound can be performed, hydrodynamic flushing of the wound should be done early. The key principles of adequate hydrodynamic debridement are volume and force. A large volume of isotonic solution injected forcibly onto the surface or into the cavity of a wound can flush away a large number of bacteria and other contaminants. Of course, one would not use such a measure in a wound in which serious hemorrhage had occurred unless the hemorrhage had been stopped with hemostats or temporary ligatures. Hydrodynamic debridement of a wound can significantly lower the number of bacteria on the wound surface and make a significant difference in the ultimate ability of a surgeon to prevent contamination from becoming converted to infection. Of course, if the patient can be taken directly to the operating room, irrigation should be part of the surgical procedure and not considered as preoperative care. In many instances, however, it is not possible to take a patient with a massive wound directly to the operating room, either because of other conditions which have to be corrected or because of limited space and personnel. In such instances, the wound should not be disregarded during the waiting period. Hydrodynamic debridement to reduce the number of bacteria, institution of proper antibiotic therapy so that a high level of the proper agent is present at the time debridement is performed, and application of an accurate dressing to prevent further contamination can make it possible to delay surgery without wound healing complications much longer than if no attention is given to the wound while shock or other conditions are being treated. In addition to the mechanical cleansing effect of a jet of isotonic fluid, additional mechanical foaming effect can be produced by the use of a small amount of hydrogen peroxide. Hydrogen peroxide does cause dissolution of clot, however, and probably should not be used if the wound is extensive or hemorrhage has been a problem.

Bactericidal agents should not be placed within a wound. A good rule is that no chemical agent should be placed in a wound which cannot be tolerated in the conjunctival sac. In the first place, bacteria which cannot be removed by surface hydrodynamic action are probably not going to be affected by casual application of a topical bactericidal agent. Moreover, cells which are important in the control of infection and progression of healing are damaged by bactericidal agents; such agents, therefore, should never be introduced directly into a wound. After irrigation has been accomplished and before a dressing is applied, the surrounding intact skin can be prepared with soap and water to remove grease and dirt and with a topical bactericidal agent to destroy surface pathogens. Proper preparation of the surrounding skin is an important step in the preoperative preparation of a traumatic wound.

Of course, preparing the skin, irrigating the wound, and immobilizing the area are of small importance when compared to establishing an airway or treating shock. Care of the wound is a task that can be delegated to a member of a team, however. Even though the wound may not be of major importance at the time resuscitative therapy is being administered, it should not be forgotten, for complications caused by inadequate preoperative care can be extremely serious during the postoperative period. It is particularly necessary to provide expert preoperative care of a traumatic wound when a delay in providing definitive surgical care is unavoidable.

Even though cultures and sensitivity studies are not possible, antibiotics should be administered as part of preoperative care in a badly contaminated wound. Such use of antibiotics should not be considered as prophylactic therapy. When massive contamination has occurred, the situation is entirely different from that of considering precautionary antibiotics for elective surgery. A broad spectrum antibiotic, including adequate protection against clostridial organisms, should be instituted as part of preoperative management. A high level of antibiotic in blood and tissue is desirable before surgical manipulation begins as well as during the immediate postoperative phase. Specific measures for control of tetanus infection are presented in Chapter 5.

Secondary Healing Wounds. Preoperative care of a secondary healing wound is usually directed toward preparing the wound surface for secondary closure. In most instances, secondary closure will be by means of a free split thickness skin graft. If the operative manipulation involves exposure of bone without periosteum or some other tissue which will not support a free graft, closure will usually be obtained by a pedicle flap. Some wounds, however, can be allowed to close by natural processes of wound contraction, collagen synthesis, and epithelial proliferation. In these patients wound care is directed primarily toward preventing retardation of these processes.

Secondary healing wounds should be covered with either a natural or an artificial dressing. Natural dressings can be used effectively, provided the surgeon realizes all the biological implications of utilizing an eschar or scab and takes just as good care of these dressings as he would of artificial ones. A scab, of course, is the least efficient biological dressing, as it is primarily a film of crenated red cells. Although a scab provides superb covering for an epithelizing wound, it should not be utilized for a full thickness wound of the dermis because it does not last long enough to provide satisfactory coverage during more prolonged contraction and fibrous protein synthesis. An eschar, however, can be cared for over a long period of time and can provide a superb biological dressing which prevents wound contracture, epithelization, and fibrous protein synthesis. Thus, eschar is utilized primarily in treating large wounds such as burns (when contraction and fibrous protein synthesis are undesirable) so that the wound can be closed in stages, allowing time for donor sites to re-epithelize.

Proper care of a scab involves exposure and drying. As epithelization progresses beneath a scab, the crenated red cells become detached and curl centralward. The detached portion of the scab should be accurately removed as epithelization progresses. Regular inspection of a scab to determine if pockets of pus are forming beneath it is mandatory. Of course, excision of that portion of the scab should be done immediately if purulence is detected. As long as a scab remains perfectly dry and the injured area is adequately immobilized, a scab can serve as a superb biological dressing for a wound which does not involve full thickness of the dermis. Thus, scabs are used primarily as biological dressings for wounds which require only epithelization to heal.

Preoperative care of an eschar is directed primarily toward prevention of infection. A topical antibiotic is mandatory to prevent invasion of the dead skin and subcutaneous fat. Several years ago 0.5 per cent silver nitrate was shown to be the topical agent of choice; presently, Sulfamylon and newer silver preparations appear to be superior to silver nitrate in several ways (see Chapter 31). Eschar, like scabs, must be inspected carefully for signs of deep infection. Any general systemic or local evidence of infection should prompt the surgeon to excise enough eschar to provide adequate drainage. Eschar, like any other dressing, must be changed when it is soiled. Thus, eschar is used only as long as it provides a suitable biological dressing without evidence of infection. Preoperative care is directed toward preventing infection, but once any sign of infection develops, the eschar must be excised in that area.

In addition to topical antibiotics, exposure of eschar and drying are helpful adjuvants. Exposure is used primarily for large numbers of extensive burns or when it may not be feasible to use topical antibiotics. The history of the exposure treatment of eschar is primarily military history; exposure methods have been utilized in catastrophic events when other methods simply were not available. It should be remembered, however, that evaporative water loss through exposed eschar is twenty times as rapid as through normal skin. The energy loss accompanying the exposure treatment of major burns, therefore, can be awesome.

Preoperative care of a wound which is not covered by a scab or eschar features the skillful use of an artificial dressing. The term "open treatment of burns" has caused a serious misunderstanding about the proper treatment of a secondary healing wound. Actually, no wound is ever treated "open." The more correct term—exposure treatment of a burn—implies the skillful utilization of a biological dressing of heat-tanned collagen to close the wound; the term in no way implies that a wound with exposed fat or granulation tissue would ever be left without covering of some type. As soon as eschar is digested or surgically removed, an artificial dressing must be applied. Exposed fat or fascia in a fresh wound or granulation tissue in an older wound must be protected from surface contamination, trauma, and mechanical and chemical irritants. This is usually accomplished with a layer of fine mesh gauze so that granulation tissue cannot grow into the interstices of the dressing. Gauze can be medicated with some material which preferably is water soluble and bacteriostatic. Of the two, solubility is the more important, however. Dressings impregnated with bacteriostatic agents may reduce the number of bacteria on the surface, but they usually do not have a significant effect on the number of bacteria within tissues. Solubility is an important feature of a drug-impregnated dressing, however, as insoluble substances tend to coat the wound and reduce the effectiveness of subsequent dressing changes.

Presently, we do not have any substance to place on a dressing which has biologically proven epithelial stimulating or wound contraction accelerating properties. Many claims have been made for various dressings, but none have withstood critical evaluation. Scarlet red ointment, a by-product of the azo dye industry, is so similar structurally to some chemical carcinogens that it was hoped it would have epithelial stimulating powers. Scarlet red ointment, however, like all other ointments commonly used to impregnate dressing material, is useful only in that it is a water-soluble dressing with very mild bacteriostatic properties. Actually, the only reason for using any medication on the first layer of dressing is so that the dressing can be removed gently without disturbing fragile epithelial cells. A dry dressing is an excellent way to treat a re-epithelizing wound, however, provided the wound is clean and the dressing does not require changing often. Frequent changes of a dry dressing are very effective in removing surface debris, but often remove epithelial cells as well.

After the surface is covered, it is usual practice to utilize cotton waste or fluffed gauze as a conformer. Such material does not convey "pressure" to the surface of the wound, as it packs easily. A large bolus of cotton surrounded by a non-yielding circular gauze outer covering may place pressure momentarily on the surface of the wound, but manometers inserted in such a dressing reveal that within 30 minutes the gauze has become packed and pressure has become dissipated. It is helpful to use a bolus of dressing material, however, for immobilization effect and as a conformer in cavitary wounds. The next layer can be a stretchable type of gauze, but if an accurate dressing is required, the final layer should consist of non-yielding gauze and adhesive tape. Properly applied, such a dressing immobilizes an injured extremity almost as effectively as a plaster cast.

A dressing of the type just described can be left in place for several days over a clean wound which is healing normally. If the purpose of the dressing is to prepare the wound for grafting, however, it should be changed as often as necessary to prevent accumulation of surface drainage and necrotic material. Such a dressing prevents granulation tissue from becoming exuberant and will result in a fine granular surface with very little drainage. In the case of a secondarily healing incision, it is important not to pack the wound so as to mechanically inhibit wound contracture. In an open wound being prepared for grafting or being protected during wound contracture and epithelization, however, the dressing may be applied as accurately and snugly as desired without producing circulatory embarrassment.

Wet dressings are frequently misused because of failure to understand the biological implications of placing water on a wound. There is certainly nothing beneficial about the effect of water on the healing process. Water can make two contributions, however, and when specific needs exist, wet dressings are useful. A wet dressing tends to promote drainage in that capillary attraction is enhanced and drying of a viscous exudate on the surface is prevented. Thus, a wet dressing is helpful in wounds which have highly viscous but relatively small amounts of drainage. A wound which is draining profusely is much better treated with a dry dressing; a dry mop will absorb more water than a wet one. When exudate is very viscous and relatively small in amount, however, it tends to coagulate on the surface and interferes with subsequent drainage. Under these conditions, a wet dressing prevents surface coagulation and promotes drainage.

A second reason for utilizing a wet dressing is to conduct heat to tissue. Particularly in early infections, local heat appears to assist in promoting inflammation. Wet heat is much more penetrating than dry heat; thus, a warm, wet dressing may be more beneficial in promoting inflammation than a cool, wet dressing. One should never use a warm, wet dressing on a fresh graft or flap, as these tissues are unable to respond to temperature changes because of deficient circulation and absent neurological control. When damage from heat is not a problem, however, a wet dressing with external heat continually applied can promote surface drainage and be beneficial in localizing the inflammatory process. Obviously, such a dressing should be changed regularly and heat must be applied continually if the objectives outlined above are to be achieved. A cold wet dressing which is not changed often merely macerates the wound and may actually inhibit the healing process.

In summary, there is no known catalyst to accelerate normal growth of epithelial tissue, speed up the process of wound contraction, or increase the rate of collagen synthesis and deposition in a secondarily healing wound. Preoperative care is directed primarily toward prevention and correction of complications such as infection and protecting the wound from external influences which inhibit contraction, epithelization, and collagen synthesis. Mechanical, chemical, and bacteriological trauma are best prevented by skillful application and continuing care of a dressing. These objectives can be achieved by utilizing a natural dressing such as a scab for secondary wounds healing primarily by epithelization or by taking care of an eschar over a third degree wound where contraction and epithelization should be prevented. Artificial dressings should be selected specifically to promote drainage, prepare a granulating surface for grafting, or protect a wound surface during natural closure. Selection of the proper dressing material requires unerring diagnostic accuracy in assessing what is occurring in the wound as well as a clear-cut idea of what the objectives of wound healing are. Selection of the proper dressing, whether natural or artificial, should be followed by skillful care so that the dressing itself does not become an impediment to achieving preoperative objectives.

POSTOPERATIVE CARE

Incisions. It is customary to cover an incision in which the skin edges have been sutured with a small dry dressing. The main reason for doing so is that many patients prefer to have their incisions covered and state that they are more comfortable with some protection from contact with bed linen. Some surgeons do not apply a dressing to sutured wounds, however; there is no measurable effect on wound healing from exposure. Special wounds, such as that following the repair of a cleft lip, must be exposed, because it is impossible to keep an accurate dressing on the lip of an infant and an inaccurate dressing may result in a wound healing complication. Whenever it is impossible to apply an accurate dressing to maintain a clean surface beneath the dressing, exposure is better than an inaccurate or soiled dressing. On the face, where suture marks are to be meticulously avoided, collection of blood or serum around a suture as it passes out of the skin may actually cause a small stitch abscess beneath the blood clot. It is very important, therefore, that these sutures be cleansed frequently and that blood not be allowed to coagulate around them. Such suture lines should be mechanically cleansed frequently and, if secretions prevent adequate cleansing, a light or water-soluble ointment should be applied.

The most frequently asked question about postoperative care of incisions is, "When will the sutures be removed?" A wry but also penetratingly accurate answer is, "When they have done the job they were put in to do." The lesson, of course, is that sutures should never be removed as a function of time. Sutures are placed in a wound to provide tensile strength until natural phenomena provide the same function. They should not be removed, therefore, until the wound has adequate tensile strength to resist tissue tension and normal activity; in most instances, sutures should be removed as soon as that function has been achieved. One of the most fundamental truths in wound healing biology is that healing does not occur at the same rate in all tissues, in all people, or at all times. Careful inspection of a wound and accurate diagnosis of the state of healing are important prerequisites to removing sutures. Occasionally, the diagnosis may not be obvious and removal of one or two sutures followed by testing the strength of the wound is advisable.

Sutures which pass through epidermis and into dermal and subcutaneous tissues produce an epithelial-lined tract with undesirable consequences. Moreover, natural fiber sutures cause an inflammatory reaction which may augment scarring in the suture tract. Extruded monofilament sutures and metallic sutures do not cause significant tissue reaction but do provide a tract for epithelization and possible infection. Ideally, therefore, sutures should be removed as soon as the wound is strong enough to withstand normal stress. In wounds in which secondary widening of the scar would produce an unacceptable cosmetic result, it is helpful to splint the wound with small adhesive strips for an additional six weeks. Tension should be relieved by placing strips of adhesive tape transversely across the scar while the skin is held in a redundant position. Such strips can be removed to cleanse the area but should be reapplied for at least six to eight weeks if maximum protection against widening of the scar is desired.

Excessive scar formation is disappointing to both patient and surgeon but secondary revision or abrasion should not be considered until the full effect of remodeling has been realized. In some patients scars may continue to change by secondary remodeling of collagen for two years. Not until a scar has remained perfectly stable by actual measurements for at least three months should secondary revision or abrasion be attempted. Not every hypertrophic scar can be improved by secondary revision. Time is the most important factor in controlling the final appearance of a scar; there is no substitute for patience while remodeling of dense connective tissue is occurring.

Grafts. Free skin grafts are managed during the postoperative period by the application of an occlusive dressing or by the "open" technique. An occlusive dressing is used primarily to maintain a graft in close approximation to an irregular surface and to protect it from mechanical trauma. The combination of "stent" fixation of the dressing to skin and the application of external restraints should provide complete immobilization in most patients. Because the interface between graft and underlying tissue has the least resistance to shearing force of any of the layers of dressing and graft, weight of the dressing should be kept as small as possible. A heavy dressing is not as likely to move with the underlying bed and thus will cause a shearing effect between graft and recipient tissue. Following this reasoning, most experienced surgeons do not use a plaster cast to immobilize an extremity following application of a split thickness skin graft. A single anterior or posterior plaster splint will accomplish adequate immobilization without also acting as a heavy pendulum which could cause a shearing force between graft and bed if tissue movement occurs. Moreover, it is impossible to apply a circular plaster cast as accurately as a soft dressing reinforced with a plaster splint. Such a dressing can be reinforced continually to adjust for changes in circumference of the extremity, whereas the cast becomes a loose cylinder as disappearance of edema or development of muscular atrophy reduces the size of an extremity.

Dressings over grafts are changed for the purpose of removing sutures after capillary circulation has been re-established. It is usual to change the dressing and remove the sutures from most grafts between the fourth and seventh postoperative days. It should be remembered that even though a graft may have "taken" as evidenced by return of capillary circulation, it is not able to carry out all the functions of normal skin for some time. Resistance to infection, secretion of seborrheic material, keratinization, and so forth will not return in a free graft for some weeks. During this period, it is wise to protect the graft by placing a water-soluble emollient against the surface. Such a dressing prevents excessive drying and subsequent cracking of the graft in addition to protecting it from bacterial invasion and mechanical trauma. It is customary to change such a dressing in four or five days and to remove it permanently at the end of three weeks. Free grafts should be protected from exposure to sunlight for nine months; they tend to pigment more than surrounding skin if exposed to radiant energy during the first year after transplantation.

At each dressing, circumferential contacts between graft and surrounding skin should be inspected for small abscesses, hematomas, or devitalized skin overlapping normal epidermis. Such areas should be treated individually to prevent involvement of a larger area of the graft. Application of 20 per cent Mercurochrome around the circumference of a graft at its junction with normal tissue is occasionally done to coagulate devitalized protein which can be peeled away cleanly at a subsequent dressing. Mercurochrome (or any other medication except a water-soluble, bland emollient) should not be applied to the entire graft.

Free split thickness skin grafts sometimes are applied to infected wounds or moving wounds by the open technique. A wound of the chest wall is an example of an area of the body which cannot be immobilized completely. To apply a dressing over a graft of the anterior lower thorax either restricts the chest wall, causing dangerous pulmonary complications, or restrains the graft so that it cannot move with the underlying bed. Both situations are undesirable. A properly prepared wound of the chest wall can be grafted successfully by placing large sheets of split thickness skin directly on granulation tissue. No sutures or dressings are utilized. A plasma seal develops quickly and no further treatment other than protection by an external splint or continual observation is required. Bed linen should be suspended over a frame and not allowed to touch the graft. Graft and chest wall will move simultaneously while capillary circulation is being re-established.

Another use for open grafting is in wounds which continue to drain in spite of concentrated efforts to reduce infection. In these wounds, small patches of split thickness skin can be interspersed with open areas for exudate to escape. If bubbles of gas collect beneath the graft, they can be expressed with a moist swab; if they reappear, a hole should be made in the graft to allow continuous drainage. Application of moist sponges to such areas will increase capillary drainage between the grafts and will help maintain them in close approximation to the wound surface. It should be emphasized that open grafting should not be done on a freshly exicsed wound. Open grafting should be reserved for superbly prepared granulating surfaces, because fresh surgically prepared surfaces will invariably have capillary oozing and plasma transudation greater than desirable for formation of a seal between the graft and the wound bed.

In summary, the major objective in postoperative care for an open graft is to protect it in such a way that bed linen and attendants do not "wipe it off" during the time required for capillary circulation to be re-established and fibrous protein to be synthesized. Ingenuity in developing cages or splints and expert general nursing care without touching the grafted area are required. Early recognition of deep infection beneath the graft should be followed by accurate drainage and application of moist dressings to promote drainage between or through the center of the grafted area. The objective in a moving wound is to assure that the graft and the wound move together; the objective in an infected wound is to establish accurate drainage of some areas while providing coverage for others.

Flaps.   The most important objective in the postoperative care of a wound closed by a flap is to insure that proper circulation through the pedicle continues until circumferential vascular connections are re-established. Arterial insufficiency is usually a complication of operative technique and is obvious before the patient leaves the operating room. The major concern in the postoperative period, therefore, is venous return. It is normal for a flap to be generally dusky following transplantation to a new site; spasm in veins as well as a relative venous insufficiency compared to arterial input is responsible. The most important sign of serious venous insufficiency is a line of demarcation on one side of which the venous return is adequate whereas on the other side it is clearly inadequate. Diffuse gradual change in color is not necessarily significant; a sharp line between normal color and cyanosis is very significant. Unless something is done to erase a sharp color line, the flap will usually be lost by venous thrombosis within 30 to 45 minutes. Quite frequently removal of a suture is all that is required to restore adequate circulation. Gentle massage in the direction of the pedicle base following removal of a suture may aid venous drainage temporarily. If a line of demarcation cannot be removed by adjusting a dressing, removing a suture, or manually assisting venous return, the flap should be returned to the original site. The slightest torsion produced by rotation of a flap can be the cause of inadequate venous return and, rather than run the risk of losing the entire flap, it is better to return it to the original bed if a sharp color change cannot be erased by other means.

Obviously, flaps must be inspected regularly if the state of circulation is in doubt. Flaps which have no evidence of compromised circulation can be dressed as any other wound. Flaps which have a seriously restricted circulation and which are in danger from the time they are transferred should be left exposed; or if an occlusive dressing is needed, the distal end of the flap should be inspected regularly through a window in the dressing. Administration of heparin is theoretically sound but has not yet been proved to be practically useful; dextran has a measurable effect on blood viscosity and is probably of some value during the period of sluggish circulation following transfer of a composite tissue graft.

Drains and Tubes.   As every thoughtful surgeon recognizes, there is an almost irresistible urge to place tubes in every body cavity and orifice during performance of a surgical procedure. The wisdom or lack of wisdom in placing various tubes and drains in the human body will not be discussed in this chapter, but the need to take care of tubes and drains after they leave the operating room is an important item in postoperative care of the wound. Small wounds made for the purpose of inserting a venous pressure line or an arterial catheter can become major complications if they are the site of introduction of bacteria. It should be remembered that quite often catheters in major veins are inserted under emergency conditions; the initial insult usually can be handled, but chronic contamination is a real danger. In all probability, any intravenous or intra-arterial line placed in the circulation in an emergency room under crisis conditions should be removed within 24 hours. Certainly the entrance through the skin must be carefully inspected and protected during sophisticated postoperative care.

Patients with tubes coming out of wounds and attached to stationary devices do not move in bed as freely as those without connections to wall suction and other equipment. It is mandatory, therefore, that patients with extensive connections to stationary devices be especially watched for lack of movement, lack of satisfactory respiratory tract toiletry, and signs of venous thrombosis. Even more important, drains and tubes should be removed as soon as there is evidence that they are no longer needed or that they are not accomplishing their objective. There is a known morbidity and mortality from inserting any foreign object through a wound into a body cavity. Unless there is positive evidence that drains and tubes are performing a necessary function, they should be removed at the earliest possible moment. This statement is made not only from the standpoint of insuring uncomplicated wound healing but in preventing more serious complications caused by immobility, entrance of bacteria, and erosion of vital structures. Injudicious placement and retention of drains, internal splints, and indwelling tubes of all types undoubtedly account for strictures, infections (such as cholangitis), and erosion of vital structures. Thus, the postoperative care of a wound which is traversed by a rigid drain must include careful attention to the drain while it is functioning and removal as soon as it is no longer needed.

Many surgeons feel that drains placed in an incision increase the likelihood of postoperative dehiscence There are few data to support this notion, but careful inspection of all wounds for signs of early dehiscence is a part of good postoperative care. Dehiscence, alone, is an annoying, though not especially dangerous, complication. Evisceration is an extremely dangerous complication and should not be allowed to occur, if possible.

Escape of brown or blood-tinged fluid from an incision is a certain sign of partial or impending dehiscence and should be followed by exploration of the wound in the operating room. Emergency measures to prevent evisceration should be utilized until the patient can be transferred to the operating room. Avoidance of severe distention and respiratory effort is probably helpful in preventing dehiscence. Most dehiscences, however, are the result of complications in the wound such as infection, hematoma, or necrosis in the suture line.

Wound drainage should be carefully investigated. Viscosity, pH, enzyme content, and accurate identification of the source are important. Protection of the surrounding tissue is important when drainage contains proteolytic enzymes or other caustic substances. Sump removal of drainage, protection of the skin, and pharmacological control of secretions are effective in preventing more serious wound complications caused by digestion of surrounding tissues. As a general rule, gastrointestinal fistulas will close spontaneously unless there is distal obstruction, carcinoma, or a foreign body. It should be remembered, however, that distal obstruction can be physiological as well as mechanical and, as far as the fistula is concerned, there is very little difference. Postoperative care of gastrointestinal fistulas involves an accurate diagnosis of the cause of obstruction, accurate localization of the fistula, defunctionalizing the bowel as much as possible, and adequate replacement therapy. If all these measures are carried out satisfactorily, the normal healing process, consisting primarily of contraction and fibrous protein synthesis, will usually result in closure. A notable exception is a serious condition characterized by multiple fistulas of the small bowel and intraperitoneal infection which usually requires aggressive surgical management, including resection of segments of the bowel. A single fistula, however, properly managed by accurate diagnosis, reduction of function, protection of the surrounding tissue, and hyperalimentation will usually close unless there is an impediment to wound healing.

A common error in judgment is to plunge into a secondary healing wound (when there is no real danger to the patient from a fistula) without giving natural wound healing mechanisms an opportunity to solve the problem. A duodenal fistula is, of course, an extremely serious complication which tests the ability of a surgical house staff to keep a patient in proper metabolic balance. If distal obstruction or a foreign body is not present, however, postoperative care should be directed primarily toward protecting the surrounding tissues and adequate replacement therapy; closure is certain if normal wound healing mechanisms are not inhibited. Of course, fistulas which produce a generalized peritonitis are entirely different, and these usually require emergency operative therapy, including drainage of the peritoneal cavity and either exteriorization or repair of the involved bowel. Fistulas which are the result of a secondary healing wound and are excluded from the general peritoneal cavity by normal defense mechanisms can be treated as a complication of wound healing and can usually be successfully managed without operative intervention.

Summary. The major objectives of postoperative care of wounds are re-establishment of surface continuity and development of tensile strength sufficient to withstand normal stress. Complications which retard the achievement of these objectives are usually local, and postoperative therapy should be directed toward removing factors that impede normal wound contraction, epithelization and fibrous protein synthesis. Although systemic factors are occasionally involved in a wound healing complication, local complications such as infection, hematoma, necrosis of tissue, and fistula formation are the result of local miscues and can usually be cared for by taking care of the wound in such a way as not to inhibit the normal healing process.

REFERENCES

Alexander, H. C., and Pruden, J. F.: The causes of abdominal wound disruption. Surg., Gynec. & Obst. *122*:1223, 1966.

Ballinger, W. F., II, Gravens, D. L., Margraf, H. W., and Butcher, H. R., Jr.: Silver allantoinate as an inhibitor of cutaneous bacteria upon the hands of operating room personnel. Ann. Surg. *171*:836, 1970.

Bangham, A. D.: The effect of cortisone on wound healing. Brit. J. Exper. Path. *32*:77, 1951.

Creditor, M. C., Bevans, M., Mundy, W. L., and Ragan, C.: Effect of ACTH on wound healing in humans. Proc. Soc. Exper. Biol. Med. *74*:245, 1950.

Dudrick, S. J., Wilmore, D. W., Steiger, E., Mackie, J. A., and Fitts, W. T.: Spontaneous closure of traumatic pancreatoduodenal fistulas with total intravenous nutrition. J. Trauma *10*:542, 1970.

Dunphy, J. E., and Van Winkle, H. W., Jr.: Repair and Regeneration (337 pages). New York, McGraw-Hill Book Co., 1969.

Edlich, R. F., Rogers, W., Kasper, G., Kaufman, D., Tsung, M.S., and Wangensteen, O. H.: Studies in the management of the contaminated wound. I. Optimal time for closure of contaminated open wounds. II. Comparison of resistance to infection of open and closed wounds during healing. Amer. J. Surg. *117*:323, 1969.

Forrester, J. C., Zederfeldt, B. H., and Hunt, T. K.: A bioengineering approach to the healing wound. J. Surg. Res. 9:207, 1969.

Forrester, J. C., Zederfeldt, B. H., and Hunt, T. K.: The tape-closed wound—a bioengineering analysis. J. Surg. Res. 9:537, 1969.

Green, J. P.: Steroid therapy and wound healing in surgical patients. Brit. J. Surg. *52*:523, 1965.

Guiney, E. J., Morris, P. J., and Donaldson, G. A.: Wound dehiscence. A continuing problem in abdominal surgery. Arch. Surg. *92*:47, 1966.

Halasz, N. A.: Dehiscence of laparotomy wounds. Amer. J. Surg. *116*:210, 1968.

Higgins, G. A., Jr., Antkowiak, J. G., and Esterkyn, S. H.: A Clinical and Laboratory Study of Abdominal Wound Closure and Dehiscence. Arch. Surg. *98*:421, 1969.

Larsen, J. S., and Ulin, A. W.: Tensile strength advantage of the far-and-near suture technique. Surg., Gynec., & Obst. *131*:123, 1970.

Lehman, J. A., Jr., Cross, F. S., and Partington, P. F.: Prevention of abdominal wound disruption. Surg., Gynec. & Obst. *126*:1235, 1968.

Maitland, A. I. L., and Mathieson, A. J. M.: Suction drainage. A study of wound healing. Brit. J. Surg. *57*:193, 1970.

Peacock, E. E., Jr., and Van Winkle, W.: Surgery and Biology of Repair (640 pages). Philadelphia, W. B. Saunders Co., 1970.

Postlethwait, R. W.: Long-term comparative study of nonabsorbable sutures. Ann. Surg. *171*:892, 1970.

Sussman, M. D.: Effect of increased tissue traction upon tensile strength of cutaneous incisions in rats. Proc. Soc. Exper. Biol. Med. *123*:38, 1966.

White, J. J., Wallace, C. K., and Burnett, L. S.: Drug letter. Skin disinfection. Hopkins Med. J. *126*:169, 1970.

CHAPTER 2

CONVALESCENCE: THE METABOLIC SEQUENCE AFTER INJURY

Francis D. Moore, M.D., F.A.C.S.

PURPOSE AND CONTENT

Convalescence, like pregnancy, is initiated by a single event. An integrated endocrine and metabolic sequence runs its course in both, resulting in the one case in the birth of a full-term infant, and in the other in the return of a healed person to the main stream of society. This normal bodily sequence after injury is known as convalescence. It is complete when the body has returned to its normal functions: physical prowess or occupation appropriate to age and sex, eating, excreting, and reproducing.

The purpose of this chapter is to outline the main features of this sequence as initiated by injury or operation. The metabolic changes have clinical significance, and the humoral activators have scientific and evolutionary interest as central features of human survival. Complications, side effects, or detours of the main highway of convalescence can only be understood as departures from the normal route to recovery.

METABOLISM IN CONVALESCENCE: GENERAL CHARACTERISTICS AND CLINICAL APPEARANCES

1. The Early Phase: Injury

Bodily changes in metabolism observed in the initial period after injury may be characterized under three headings:

1. Loss of body cell mass — a lysis of cell protoplasm and protein,

19

with release of protein split-products and some whole protein as enzymes, with cell water and electrolyte, into the extracellular fluid.

2. *Volume conservation* — protection of the volume and composition of extracellular fluid (and therefore of the plasma) by renal and extrarenal mechanisms: conserving water, sodium, chloride, and bicarbonate, and excreting urea, xanthines, potassium, phosphate, and hydrogen ions.

3. *Change in energy source* — a shift of oxidative substrate for muscular contraction (the work of the heart and diaphragm, and external performance) from exogenous to endogenous sources. This is accomplished by the mobilization and combustion of fatty acids from neutral triglycerides and the combustion of amino acids as carbohydrate (i.e., gluconeogenesis) with the excretion of the nitrogen as urea.

These three basic metabolic changes are considered in greater detail below:

Loss of Body Cell Mass. Following severe injury, with or without superimposed infection (and despite the total absence of exogenous nitrogen intake) there is a gross increase in urinary nitrogen excretion, mounting over the course of two or three days to levels as high as 15 to 25 gm. a day, most of which appears in the urine as urea. Associated with this is a slight increase in the alpha-amino-nitrogen content of plasma and urine. These changes indicate that body cells are hydrolyzing proteins, some of the carbon residues being combusted and most of the nitrogen being excreted in the urine. There is a sudden increase in urinary creatinine, and in the male (in whom creatine is an abnormal urinary constituent) there is an associated increase in creatine lasting a day or two. This leaves little doubt that the source of much of this increased urinary nitrogen is the lysis of skeletal muscle proteins. If the post-traumatic period is prolonged, or if there is a delay in the resumption of intake, the wasting of skeletal muscle is quite evident by changes in the diameter of the thigh, leg, upper and lower arms. By contrast, other potential donors of cellular material, such as skin, bones, heart, lung, liver, intestine, brain, and glands, show little evidence of wasting or atrophy. In fact, they increase in relative size.

After extensive tissue trauma, there are other sources for these cellular materials lost to the extracellular fluid and into the urine, in addition to the undamaged muscles of the body. These are the tissues directly injured or rendered ischemic by the injury itself or blood lost into the tissues (within fascial planes or serous cavities). It is not a simple matter to distinguish the cell products appearing in the extracellular fluid and excreted in the urine, as between these two sources: normal muscle or traumatized tissue and blood. Hemoglobin and myoglobin (and high levels of lactic dehydrogenase) in blood or urine suggest the latter source, creatine and creatinine the former.

The potassium released to the extracellular fluid totals 100 to 300 mEq. in the first week (in an adult), depending a little on the severity of the injury. This potassium is released at a high ratio relative to the nitrogen lost (up to 10 to 15 mEq./gm.), indicating that cell water and salt are lost more rapidly than cell matrix as represented by protein. If renal function is normal, there is but a minor increase in plasma potassium concentration.

Aside from those tissues directly injured, there is little evidence for cell death or necrosis as a feature of this generalized proteolysis. The essentially complete reconstitution of muscular function, weeks or months later, leaves little doubt that the full complement of muscular cells, initially present in any muscle belly, has somehow maintained its integrity and its central neurological connections despite the acute post-traumatic change. Enzymes of cellular origin, such as the transaminases and lactic dehydrogenase, are not elevated in the blood unless large amounts of tissue have been rendered directly necrotic by the trauma.

Volume Conservation. The preservation of the effective volume of circulating blood appears to be an objective, or at least a result, of many of the metabolic changes occurring after injury. The plasma volume is directly supported by the interstitial fluid which refills the plasma volume after hemorrhage by a process known as transcapillary refill. This refill cannot take place unless the interstitial component of the extracellular volume is maintained at normal. This "sodium area" of body water (plasma and interstitial fluid) is maintained intact after trauma by a variety of mechanisms that conserve body water and its principal extracellular osmotic solutes: sodium, chloride, and bicarbonate.

The key to an understanding of this aspect of convalescence is the transcapillary support of the plasma volume by interstitial fluid, the nature of the refill, its relation to venous pressure, and the autoregulatory mechanisms which maintain an effective and functionally normal blood volume.

The retention of water and extracellular salts is clearly manifested in untreated unanesthetized injury, after which urinary volume, free water clearance, and sodium excretion are all drastically reduced. If no water or sodium salts are given immediately after the injury (even though there is no compromise of glomerular filtration), a reduction in free water clearance and of sodium bicarbonate excretion is evident, together with an increased excretion of hydrogen ion, potassium and urea. If modest infusions of water and salt are given, some dilution of protein will be produced in the plasma and extracellular fluid because clearances are impaired. If all these substances are given freely, the renal tendency to volume conservation is much less marked, and a freer diuresis is maintained although positive balance is clearly evident. Finally, if extracellular salts and water are given in huge excess during or immediately after the traumatic episode, the tendency to dilution of red cells and protein, and to water-logging with generalized, pulmonary and cerebral edema, is more marked than it is in the uninjured individual.

A reduction in free water clearance produces a urine of rising osmolality. After trauma it is often fixed in the region of 750 mO./liter because the conservation of sodium and bicarbonate (and to a lesser extent, chloride) produces a urinary sodium concentration of 10 mEq./liter or less in an acid urine. The urine solute is thus virtually confined to urea. A mild tendency to metabolic alkalosis will result from this situation, and the urinary sodium : potassium ratio reaches extremely low levels between the first and third days. All this is typical of an aldosterone-mediated response. As will be noted below, this effect on renal tubular cell function is most marked and prolonged if circulating blood volume has been restricted by the trauma. This same effect is potentiated by reduction in glomerular filtration rate if a low flow state supervenes. In the latter case, a mounting azotemia and hyperkalemia with acidosis will become evident.

If post-traumatic renal insufficiency supervenes, then the sodium concentration rises to a high fixed level between 80 and 100 mEq./liter (despite an evident need for sodium conservation), urea clearance drops, and the urine osmolality falls to that of plasma ultrafiltrate, or about 300 mO./liter. Most of the solute is now electrolyte. For these reasons, it is possible by studying the urine to differentiate between a normal response to trauma, the changes with volume-reduction, the response to marked restriction of glomerular filtration in a low-flow state and the onset of post-traumatic renal insufficiency.

The severely injured person, who has not been in a prolonged low-flow state (or "shock"), is typically quite alkalotic for several days. This is a mixed respiratory and metabolic alkalosis resulting from a combination of any or all of the following factors:

1. The oxidation of the citrate component of transfused blood to sodium bicarbonate.

2. Inability to excrete this sodium bicarbonate normally, owing to a persistent aldosterone effect engendered by an initial or lingering deficiency in circulating blood volume; this produces the "paradoxical aciduria" of post-traumatic alkalosis.

3. Nasogastric tube suction with removal of gastric acid.

4. Hyperventilation with hypocapnia.

This post-traumatic alkalosis shifts the oxyhemoglobin dissociation curve to the left (lowering the p50 to 23 mm. Hg or so, depending on pH), with an increased affinity of hemoglobin for oxygen and a decreased delivery of oxygen to the tissues. To this is added the left-shift induced by the transfusion of stored blood which is deficient in 2,3-diphosphoglycerate (see below). The net effect is tissue hypoxia quite aside from any deficiency in blood flow. The normal response to this defect in oxygen release is a marked elevation in cardiac output.

If a low-flow state supervenes, then a severe metabolic acidosis predominates, as the incomplete combustion of carbohydrate and the accumulation of lactic acid in the tissue far outweigh the alkalotic vectors described above.

These two factors — post-traumatic alkalosis and low-flow acidosis — compete for dominance of neutrality regulation after injury, entirely depending upon the clinical circumstances: the nature of the injury and its treatment.

Change in Energy Source. The injured person has an obvious need for energy-rich substrates to maintain his body temperature, contraction of diaphragm and heart, cerebral function, and the energy requirements of peripheral muscular activity and visceral function. If continued motion or muscular activity is required for retreat or escape, then the energy impost is even greater. Body temperature may be elevated owing to infection. Any loss of body surface water through the intact or burned skin adds an additional caloric load to support the evaporation of water and at the same time maintain body temperature.

In the absence of exogenous intake, this caloric requirement can be met from three endogenous sources: glycogenolysis with oxidation of preformed carbohydrate, proteolysis with gluconeogenesis from amino acid residues, and the hydrolysis of stored triglycerides to fatty acids.

The carbohydrate pathway, starting at glycogen, passing through glucose, the phosphorylated compounds, to the three-carbon stage of pyruvate and lactate, then to the Krebs cycle and finally mitochondrial oxidation through the cytochromes to CO_2 and water, provides a small and rapidly exhausted energy source. Liver glycogen is quickly gone. It has been estimated that not more than 1600 calories are available from this source; glycogenolysis and gluconeogenesis often exceed the rate that glucose can be burned, and hyperglycemia and glycosuria are regularly observed after severe injury.

The lysis of body protein is an expensive source of calories. Loss of muscular bulk and respiratory strength is a high price to pay for the relatively small yield in calories by combustion of the carbon chains; this is also inefficient since the carbon atoms excreted with nitrogen in the urea molecule are not fully oxidized and their energy not yet fully realized. For each gram of nitrogen excreted in the urine only 20 calories have been gained by the body, and much has been lost: 30 grams of wet muscle and 6.25 grams of muscle protein.

Recent research has been concerned with the teleology of this proteolytic process. There is evidence to suggest that certain amino acids such as alanine provide a source for the three-carbon fragments required for gluconeogenesis. Certain special tissues require glucose in the starving or post-traumatic patient. These special tissues are represented chiefly by the central nervous system (whose preferential oxidative substrate is glucose) and by the "healing process tissues" such as leukocytes and fibroblasts which likewise insist on a carbohydrate source. Certainly the proteolytic process is intensified by trauma as compared with starvation.

The oxidation of body fat stored in the neutral triglycerides of adipose tissue satisfies the major share of this caloric need. Although not peculiar to the human being, it is at least characteristic of our species that very large amounts of fat can easily be stored in the body (even up to 50 per cent of the body weight) and that this fat can be burned efficiently and rapidly during periods of starvation, including the post-traumatic state. The precise mechanism whereby neutral fats are hydrolyzed to free fatty acids, the latter transported in the blood, phosphorylated, hydrolyzed to two carbon fragments, and either combusted or recycled to glycerol, has been elucidated with increased clarity in the last ten years. Suffice it here to say that cortisol, epinephrine, insulin, glucagon, lipases, inorganic phosphates, potassium and blood flow are all importantly involved in activating this remarkable internal combustion engine employed by the body after operation and injury.

The mobilization of endogenous fat as the principal source of calories is unfortunately and inevitably accompanied by cell lysis and a negative nitrogen balance. This is true even in the resting, dieting individual. The metabolic association between these two forms of tissue lysis is a matter of importance whether one is a dieting housewife or a wounded soldier. The patient cannot get his money's worth of energy from fat without paying for it in muscle wastage. Only during athletic training is this combination possible: fat loss with muscle gain.

Whatever the precise details, the rate of endogenous fat oxidation after severe surgical trauma with super-added infection approaches 300 to 500 gm./day, equivalent to 2700 to 4500 calories per day. Former estimates of excessive caloric requirements by the injured patient have generally been downgraded by recent evidence. Body temperature is probably the most important single factor. For the normally built adult male after operation a caloric supply of around 2200 calories per day is probably adequate. This corresponds to about 230 gm. of fat. Each kilogram of fat oxidized yields to the internal environment slightly more than 1 liter of water. Each kilogram of muscle tissue that undergoes lysis yields about 730 ml. of water, 270 gm. of protein, the latter yielding approximately 1000 calories as gluconeogenesis, and 30 gm. of nitrogen excreted as 60 gm. of urea. For the normal adult male after operation about one third of this amount is lost daily for two or three days before the turning point is reached.

The water of oxidation and cell lysis provides not only calories to the starving patient, but water to the thirsting patient like the camel's hump in a drought. Indeed, the camel's hump is largely fat and the legend that it contains water is not in error. This endogenous water production by post-traumatic catabolism, although adequate to avoid dehydration under ideal conditions, is totally inadequate if there are excessive water losses caused by open wounds, ambient dryness, fever, or prolonged absence of intake.

During this period of tissue catabolism, conservation of extracellular fluid and rapid mobilization of fat, the patient is usually free of any desire to move about. He is often in pain from his incision; there is subnormal appetite, and little thought of food. Peristalsis is quiet, although not completely absent. Temperature and pulse are slightly elevated according to the extent of volume reduction and superimposed infection.

This remarkable series of events in post-traumatic catabolism yields then to diuresis and anabolism, the latter requiring the resumption of intake, which then becomes the key to recovery. These events are best viewed as features of the normal sequence of clinical convalescence.

2. THE TURNING POINT

This clear-cut clinical event in clean elective civilian surgery is often masked in military surgery and accidental injury, though still evident in metabolic terms. It is characterized by a sudden release and opening up of water and salt diuresis; there is a resumption of appetite; interest in surroundings is renewed; thoughts of food occur, with associated gastrointestinal peristalsis and expulsion of flatus; the patient again shows an interest in other people around him; the pulse and temperature return to normal; and the wound rapidly gains tensile strength. This phase, long recognized as the omen of early recovery, demonstrates a nice association between metabolic reversal and clinical behavior.

A return to normal excretion of sodium bicarbonate is associated with the restoration of positive potassium and nitrogen balance. The absolute rate of urinary nitrogen excretion decreases sharply to levels as low as 3 gm./70 kg./day even prior to the onset of caloric intake. As soon as nitrogen intake begins during the turning point phase, nitrogen metabolism becomes very efficient (i.e., positive balances are readily attained on lower intakes). The calorie : nitrogen ratio of oral intake during the turning point is important, with 200 calories per gram of nitrogen optimal, but positive balances are exhibited on ratios as low as 100 calories per gram of nitrogen.

3. THE ANABOLIC PHASE

This long and immensely important period lasts from three to ten or twelve weeks, depending upon the severity of the trauma and the duration of the injury phase. This is the phase formerly referred to as "convalescence" by those concerned solely with physical rehabilitation. It is a time when the patient eats with rapidly increasing appetite;

he wants to be up and around and rapidly recovers muscular strength. Just as the loss of nitrogen in the catabolic period of injury is mostly from skeletal muscle, so the restoration of this body protein returns muscular strength and vigor. The wound regains tensile integrity independent of the return to positive nitrogen balance (see below).

Whereas the conservation and replenishment of the plasma volume is a relatively rapid process (its most important rate-limiting factor being albumin synthesis), the re-establishment of a deficient red cell mass is far slower. A prolonged reticulocytosis and gradually rising hematocrit indicate that an increasing fraction of the blood volume is being occupied by red cells.

This long anabolic phase occurs at rates which peak at 3 to 5 gm. of nitrogen/70 kg./day. This is the normal growth rate of surgical convalescence and is associated with the resumption of weight and strength, with only a minimum deposition of fat. The diuresis of the turning point phase cannot be attained unless plasma volume and body water have been returned to normal. By the same token, nitrogen anabolism in the anabolic phase cannot be attained unless there is good intake of macronutrients (carbohydrate, fat, protein, and calories) at a high calorie : nitrogen ratio (about 200 calories per gram of nitrogen), and an adequate supply of micronutrients (vitamins and minerals). The termination of this period is marked by the reduction of nitrogen anabolism toward a normal zero balance and the final redeposition of fat.

4. The Fat Gain Phase

This is the final period of convalescence and may last from a few weeks to many months or even years after severe injury. It is a time of resumption of the storage of body lipid, and since this is a result of a balance between caloric intake and external work requirements, this period can only be exhibited if caloric intake is grossly in excess of caloric expenditure. Fat gain is often spectacular if some residual immobilization or paralysis results from the injury. It is for this reason that some patients after burns, fractures or paralyzing injury frequently become excessively overweight and quite obese. For the normal person engaged in normal pursuits, returning to work or play, the fat gain phase is one of return to normal body weight and habitus. Clothes fit again.

During the nitrogen anabolic or third phase, referred to above, nitrogen is being gained at 3 to 5 gm./70 kg./day, as noted. This represents only 18 to 30 gm. of protein and only 90 to 150 gm. of tissue. It is thus evident that during a week (with the gain of 1 kg. or less) weight gain will not be spectacular during this phase even at its peak rate. If during this same time, additional water and salt are being excreted, weight changes during nitrogen anabolism may be downward and are most deceptive.

In sharp contrast, the fat gain phase is associated with a clear increase in body weight. A daily weight chart will show this to be the final phase, rounding out the metabolism of convalescence, although local wound changes proceed for many years.

After major surgery in healthy young adults, most patients are back to work during the fat gain phase; if there has been severe compound injury as in an automobile accident, the problem of post-traumatic obesity, referred to above, may be particularly irksome if the patient's work is sedentary.

LOCAL HEALING IN INJURED TISSUE

Coincident with the convalescent sequence is a series of changes in the wound which are common to all tissue trauma, but vary in some details according to the nature of the tissue injured. In the initial phase, the wound coagulum gradually accumulates mucopolysaccharides, followed by the transmutation of these substances to procollagen, and then to collagen under the influence of ascorbic acid. All this occurs during the initial or catabolic phase of most surgical injury. The rapid increase in tensile strength of soft tissue wounds between the fifth and seventh days is usually coincident with the turning point phase and the onset of anabolism. Most surgical incisions achieve tensile integrity, permitting the resumption of normal soft tissue function and the removal of sutures before the patient passes into positive nitrogen balance.

The later phases of wound evolution occur during the prolonged later phases of convalescence. These include the thickening of deposited collagen, the laying down of bone matrix, its calcification and ossification (in the case of fractures), and the increase in cicatrix in some cases of soft tissue injury, to the point of keloid production or excessive cicatricial contracture. Then, for many years or decades the wound demonstrates a special need for ascorbic acid as evidenced by its disruption during the early phases of subclinical scurvy.

It is appealing to consider that these sequential changes in the wound are causally related to the over-all metabolism of the organism. The body places a very high priority on the wound and appears to disrupt muscular tissue to make amino acid substrates available for protein synthesis in the wound, as well as for gluconeogenesis to support fibroblasts and leukocytes. Muscles' loss is fibroblasts' gain. The same is evidently true of ascorbic acid because, in animals rendered mildly scorbutic, the wound heals but there are diffuse evidences of ascorbic acid deficiency. Despite these logical sequences in the bodily economy, a detailed activation link between the wound and general metabolism has yet to be established. Is there a "wound hormone" – or is the activation link merely the release to extracellular fluid of substances from directly damaged muscle tissue?

Despite this uncertainty about the precise mechanism whereby the wound activates diffuse bodily changes, there are several identifiable components in the traumatic experience that "trigger" or "drive" the metabolic and endocrine changes.

DRIVING FORCES: THE ACTIVATORS OF POST-TRAUMATIC METABOLISM

It is appropriate now to review briefly those mechanisms that activate, trigger, or drive the bodily responses of convalescence, as well as their endocrine accompaniments which act in some instances as mediators from the local injury to the diffuse bodily changes that ensue.

Volume Reduction. "Volume reduction" is an intentionally vague term that refers to the most important activating stimulus of all. It implies reduction in the effective volume of circulating blood. The precise area of body water initially lost (that brings reduced blood volume in its train) depends upon the nature of the injury, its sequelae and its treatment. In any event, the important challenge to the organism lies in the reduction in effective circulating volume of the blood. This, at its least, produces a decreased oxygen carrying capacity of the blood with subsequent transcapillary refill and an "anemia." At its most, volume reduction produces a low flow state with decreased perfusion of the three most critical areas of the arterial tree: the circle of Willis, the coronary arteries, and the renal vasculature.

A critical decrease in total blood volume may be brought about by a decrease in total body water, as is seen in desiccation-dehydration; by a specific reduction of extracellular volumes (losses of the type seen in vomiting, intestinal obstruction, or traumatic edema—the "third space" effect); or by frank hemorrhage varying in rate all the way from a liter per minute from an open arterial bleed downward to ordinary wound hemorrhage.

Whatever its cause, volume reduction is the primary activator of the metabolic response to injury. It is the only acute traumatic activator that can trigger a diffuse bodily response with virtually no tissue injury at all (as, for example, in massive hemorrhage from a small peripheral laceration). Acute volume reduction activates changes in renal function already discussed in some detail, a variety of endocrine changes, and, if continued, a low flow state with diffuse anaerobiosis. In addition, its treatment by large amounts of whole blood introduced directly into the venous side of the circulation produces a large load of foreign protein, cellular detritus, and immunologically competent cells directly into the lungs without any peripheral filtration or processing. This appears to be one of the underlying factors in acute pulmonary insufficiency after massive injury. From an evolutionary point of view, the ability of the animal to tolerate or compensate for various forms of reduction in effective blood volume has become progressively more efficient as one progresses up the phylogenetic scale. Darwinian "survival of the fittest" has evolved vertebrate species able to tolerate and compensate for volume reduction, at least for a long enough time to achieve volume restoration from endogenous sources.

Infection. Sepsis constitutes the second most potent activator of the metabolic response to injury; infection itself without injury produces a series of metabolic changes very similar to those of trauma. If the infection arises rather suddenly, as seen in spreading cellulitis, the tendency to tissue catabolism and extracellular fluid sequestration is very marked. When infection supervenes following injury (as seen in burns, in severe compound injuries, such as fractures and military wounds, and all too frequently in elective civilian surgery), the septic process becomes superimposed on the traumatic stimulus itself to produce a deepening and prolongation of the initial catabolic phase.

The catabolic trigger of a septic process occurs by at least three different mechanisms: first, increase in body temperature; second, direct loss of protein, water and salt into the exudate; and third, toxic products of the growth of the microorganisms themselves. The pyrogenicity of septic products is poorly understood. It is evident that several types of microorganisms can activate a diffuse cellular response closely resembling severe injury. Of these, the endotoxins of the gram-negative bacilli are most familiar. Exotoxins of gram-positive cocci and the exotoxins of clostridial spore-formers are equally important. Protein split-products from the infected tissue as well as cellular enzymes add to the catabolic stimulus.

Cross-Sectional Tissue Trauma and the Wound. It has long been evident that when a small amount of tissue is traumatized, there is much less tendency for post-traumatic metabolism to reach a deep catabolic trough than when extensive injury occurs. The surgeon intuitively senses that the cross-sectional area of tissue crushed, lacerated, traumatized or infected must somehow be a semiquantitative governor of the extent of the ensuing metabolic defect. This concept is extremely difficult to prove; there are strong evidences that secondary effects such as the extent of volume reduction and bacterial colonization are actually responsible for whatever linear relationship is observed between the extent of trauma and the depth of the catabolic response. Beyond these factors is the release into the circulation of the products of cells directly destroyed by injury, crush, bullet track or fracture.

Neural Stimuli, Emotions, Drugs. Pain, anger, hunger, fear and rage were the stimuli considered by Dr. Walter Cannon as the primary activators of the adrenal medullary system. They are important in unanesthetized trauma, and their understanding requires humanity as well as science. The patient who rests confident in her surgeon, without fear or apprehension, certainly has a different sort of convalescence from one roughly handled, whose apprehensions have been poorly ministered to, or whose fear of cancer is little assuaged by a hurried surgeon.

Almost all the drugs used in association with surgery, including anesthetics, analgesics, sedatives, and antibiotics, carry in their wake metabolic changes which alter the contours of normal convalescence. Morphine, for example, interferes with free water clearance. Ether is a potent stimulus to the release of epinephrine from the adrenal medulla. Spinal anesthesia produces diffuse vasodilatation often associated with hypotension. The effect of high oxygen tensions in the airway, the potassium load of banked blood or of extensive penicillin administration, the solute diuresis of glucose or mannitol administration — all these and many others demonstrate the obvious fact that steps taken by the anesthetist or the surgeon will modify the metabolic changes seen in the patient.

ENDOCRINE ACCOMPANIMENTS

Serial changes in the secretory rates of the endocrine glands, concentrations of hormones in the blood, and appropriate alterations in their conjugation, inactivation, or excretion, accompany the foregoing activators of post-traumatic metabolism. Direct one-to-one correlation is not always established between the activators, the endocrine changes, and the metabolic consequences, nor is a direct line of mediation always clearly evident. These endocrine changes are a part of the bodily response to injury, and if blunted, absent, or exaggerated, produce severe and potentially lethal distortions of the recovery process.

Adrenal Cortex—Glucocorticoids. A rise in free blood cortisol is one of the earliest changes observable after injury of any sort. This is characteristically seen in operations and unanesthetized injury; it is much less evident after simple volume reduction. The increase in free blood cortisol is quickly followed by binding, conjugation and reduction in ring-A with the accumulation in the blood of tetrahydro compounds, glucuronides, sulfonates, and protein-bound cortisol. This mixture of cortisol metabolites is excreted via the liver and in the urine. These, measured in the urine as the total 17-hydroxycorticosteroids, show a marked increase after injury, rising from normal levels of 10 to 15 mg./day to levels as high as 50 to 100 mg./day for several days. When infection supervenes, in burns or in other such continuing injuries, these levels are maintained at very high values for many weeks or even months.

There is good evidence that this rise in glucocorticoids is the result of a sudden outpouring of large amounts of adrenocorticotropic hormone (ACTH) from the pituitary, and that this, in turn, is the result of a variety of activating pathways, including a neurologic message from the injury itself to the supraoptic nuclei in the midbrain.

Long considered but never proved as activators of gluconeogenesis from protein, the glucocorticoids have a unique survival-significance.

In their absence even the mildest form of trauma or volume reduction is quickly lethal—as in Addison's disease or adrenal insufficiency. If glucocorticoid stimulation is excessive or excessively prolonged, there is an increased tendency to ulceration of the upper gastrointestinal tract (as in myocardial infarction and in burns). The normal functioning of muscles such as diaphragm and heart, the normal accommodation to antigen-antibody interaction, the combustion of carbohydrate, and the mobilization of fat are all, likewise, affected by the concentration of free cortisol in blood and extracellular fluid.

Adrenal Cortex—Aldosterone. Isotonic volume reduction (as in simple hemorrhage) is a most potent stimulus to increased secretion, blood level, and urinary excretion of aldosterone from the zona glomerulosa of the adrenal. The activation pathways here are several. First, ACTH itself, resulting from the stress of injury, produces a large increase in aldosterone secretion. Second, there appear to be extrapituitary central nervous system sites, in the midbrain, that are associated with the production of an aldosterone-increasing hormone known as glomerulotropin. And third, there is a local renal response to decreased renal blood flow and to changes in the concentration of sodium in the distal renal tubule. This stimulates the juxtaglomerular cells and the macula densa region of the kidney. From this area, renin is produced, then converted to angiotensin which in turn directly stimulates the adrenal cortex to produce aldosterone without the necessary intermediacy either of neural pathways, the central nervous system, or the pituitary. Aldosterone is, *par excellence*, the volume-regulatory hormone without which interstitial fluid volume and blood pressure are poorly maintained after injury.

The result of this complex activation is an increased aldosterone secretory rate with reduced urinary excretion of sodium bicarbonate, an acid urine, increased excretion of potassium and hydrogen ion, and a pressor effect on vascular smooth muscle that involves both the hormone itself and the altered ionic equilibrium and action-potentials across muscle cells. Prolonged excessive secretion of aldosterone is associated with metabolic alkalosis, hypernatremia, hypokalemia, and hypertension. Mild hyperaldosteronism is characteristic of the post-traumatic state. Prolonged activation of the aldosterone mechanism by trauma is in part responsible for the induction of post-traumatic alkalosis with its associated left-shift of the oxyhemoglobin dissociation curve and decreased oxygen delivery to the tissues. Both the glucocorticoids and aldosterone must be present in body fluids to permit survival after injury, to support transcapillary refilling of the blood volume and to enable the normal action of catecholamines.

Adrenal Medulla. The catecholamines, including epinephrine, norepinephrine, their precursors and breakdown products, are part of the emergency mechanism so easily activated by both psychic stimuli and tissue trauma.

Acute volume reduction is here, as in the case of aldosterone, a most potent stimulus; tissue injury, prolonged low flow, anoxia, hypercarbia, pain, anger, fear, rage, ether anesthesia, and infection are also potent stimuli to catecholamine production. Norepinephrine, stimulator of the alpha-adrenergic receptors in vascular smooth muscle, is produced throughout the body at neural synapses as well as in the adrenal medulla. Epinephrine, a mild vasoconstrictor but a potent beta receptor stimulator, important in gluconeogenesis and in the mobilization of glycerol and fatty acids from neutral triglycerides, is produced solely in the adrenal medulla. Of all the basic "stress hormones," epinephrine appears to be the most completely dispensable despite these many actions. After bilateral total adrenalectomy, epinephrine is completely absent from the body, and yet most forms of stress and injury are well borne so long as glucocorticoids and aldosterone are provided. Diffuse norepinephrine block, as by alpha-adrenergic blockade, is, however, poorly tolerated unless volume is added to the system.

Antidiuretic Hormone. Acute isotonic volume reduction is also a potent stimulus to the release of antidiuretic hormone (vasopressin) from the supra-optic nuclei and the posterior pituitary. The result is decreased free water clearance in the distal renal tubule and, in the absence of a solute load, decreased total urine volume at increased specific gravity or osmolality. This is of basic importance in surgical care because of its obvious volume-conserving significance, and because, while active, continued loads of solute-free water will produce sudden and drastic dilution of all serum constituents, most notably the serum sodium concentration. The severe hyponatremia often seen after injury, particularly in the presence of diffuse visceral disease, is usually a result of continued antidiuretic hormone secretion (resulting from either unrestored volume reduction or continued stress itself), plus excessive water administration and the retention of endogenously produced water.

Because simple hemorrhage—an almost inevitable feature of any bodily trauma—even in small amounts (as little as 50 ml.) activates the production of aldosterone, catecholamines, and antidiuretic hormone, one may consider that volume maintenance and the conservation of the sodium-containing area of body water are basic endocrine messages from injury. It is conceivable, though unproved, that many of the other changes that we see are secondary by-products of this primal response: maintenance of the circulation.

Erythropoietin. Chronic anemia or a reduction in the red cell mass is followed by the production of a hormone that has as its principal effect an increase of red cell synthesis in the bone marrow as manifested by reticulocytosis and increased radioiron uptake. This hormone (or hormones) appears to be produced in the kidney, secondarily modified in the liver, and of key significance in the gradual restoration of the hematocrit to normal.

Gonadal Steroids.   Cessation of menses in the female and loss of libido in the male are characteristics of the post-traumatic state. Precise endocrine measurements reflecting these changes have but rarely been recorded. The most common observation is the reduction in the urinary secretion of total 17-ketosteroids, a reduction which is continued until the termination of catabolism and well into the anabolic phase. The achievement of nitrogen anabolism is later associated with the restoration of menses and reproductive vigor. Prolonged starvation has these same effects and likewise is associated with a reduction in urinary 17-ketosteroids.

Growth Hormone.   The principal effect of growth hormone is the routing of substrates toward protein synthesis. This protein synthesis may be manifested by skeletal growth, by muscular growth or by other types of protein synthesis, of which milk production is most noteworthy, giving rise to the many similarities between growth hormone and the other lactogenic hormones of the pituitary. Systematic changes have not been demonstrated after injury.

The Energy-Converting Hormones: Glucagon, Insulin, and Thyroid Hormone.   The mobilization and combustion of carbon fuels from body fat, the production of 6-carbon sugars for the brain, the conversion of alternate amino acids to alanine and its subsequent recycling to either glucose or glycogen, the mobilization of glycogen itself, and the permeability of body cells to glucose are all affected by a complex interaction involving glucocorticoids, epinephrine, glucagon, and insulin. The gradual elucidation of the mechanism by which these various hormones maintain bodily function in the injured starving vertebrate has provided many insights into the post-traumatic metabolism. The reader is referred to the bibliography for some recent data on this important aspect.

Though important as a long-term regulator of the rate of combustion of body fuels, the thyroglobulins (slow to change in any case) do not undergo any systematic changes after injury, nor has it been possible to implicate them in the integration of altered energy cycles after trauma. Normal thyroid function is a necessary prerequisite for the metabolic sequences after convalescence just as it is in any other patient. As with so many other homeostatic endocrine mechanisms, the surgical patient gets along very poorly if thyroid hormones are absent; frank myxedema or even borderline hypothyroidism makes the patient remarkably sensitive to injury, drugs, and anesthesia.

Finally, the role of the *liver* must be mentioned in any outline of post-traumatic endocrinology. When liver function is compromised, the inactivation of hormones is altered. The most prominent result in the surgical patient is a prolonged and inappropriate activity of aldosterone and antidiuretic hormone; hypokalemia, alkalosis, and serum dilution are all characteristic of liver disease itself or of trauma superimposed on liver disease.

VARIATIONS ON A THEME

This basic sequence of endocrine activation and metabolic change after injury is prone to wide variation and extensive modification according to the nature of the injury, subsequent infection, or visceral impairment (brain, lungs, liver, kidney). A few of these variations on the theme of normal convalescence will be discussed here. In the interest of brevity this will include only those few that alter either the metabolic or biochemical sequences observed after injury.

Unanesthetized Trauma Versus Elective Surgery: The Role of Operation Itself. In unanesthetized bodily injury (e.g., the combat casualty, automobile accidents, homicidal and suicidal attempts), a series of changes is initiated which produces deterioration of organ function by continued blood loss, severe pain, mobile fractures, the onset of infection, or a severe low flow state. Here the role of operation is to restore continuity of tissues so that tensile integrity can later be regained, to drain infection, to exteriorize holed hollow viscera, and to restore the integrity of serous cavities or immobilize fractures. The operation — wound surgery — *terminates* a continuing injury initiated by the trauma and persisting, often with increased severity, until put to rest by this definitive operation. Trauma-termination is the role of wound surgery in the military, and of urgent surgery in the trauma of civilian life.

By contrast, in an elective clean operation, the totally uninjured organism first senses tissue injury through the induction of anesthesia and operation; the period of dissection and distortion is short (one to six hours), and the completion of the operation is marked by the restoration of tissues immediately to a posture from which healing can commence.

In a word, surgical operation puts an end to many hours of trauma in cases of unanesthetized injury while it both begins and ends that injury in civilian elective surgery. Everything that is done to support the patient before, during, or after the tissue dissection itself is a part of the surgical process and (whether pharmacologic, psychiatric, or anatomic) must be considered the responsibility of the surgeon.

Minor Injury. Minor injury without infection (such as a lesser fracture or second degree burn, or an elective clean soft tissue operation such as laparotomy, simple mastectomy or cholecystectomy) produces a metabolic response which is attenuated. Several features are less prominent. Nitrogen effects are scarcely distinguishable from those seen after starvation, and increased urinary excretion of creatinine and creatine is a rarity. Reductions in sodium excretion and in the sodium : potassium ratio in the urine are related solely to volume reduction, the period of fat mobilization is short, and the amount of fat lost is negligible.

Very Severe Trauma with a Low Flow State. In very severe injury such as is seen in crushing injury with multiple fractures, late perforations of the gastrointestinal tract, pressure pneumothorax, and severe head injury, or in extensive multivisceral ablative operations, the metabolic response to injury is greatly accentuated and prolonged. Total nitrogen loss rates may reach 15 to 20 gm./70 kg./day at the height of the catabolism. Acute volume reduction may be persistent despite many transfusions, and the restoration of flow requires the infusion of far more blood than can be recorded as lost to the exterior.

Such injury is associated with deficiency of blood flow and tissue perfusion which, if sepsis supervenes or blood transfusion is inadequate, is prolonged and dangerous. If prolonged, this low flow state ("shock") brings in its train a variety of characteristic biochemical and metabolic changes not to be considered as inevitable features of the metabolic response to injury; these are the metabolic and biochemical consequences of tissue ischemia and anaerobiosis. This is the precursor of tissue death. Most particular among these are prolonged oliguria (often progressing to acute tubular necrosis), hypoxic acidosis (with lacticacidemia at a high lactate : pyruvate ratio), and the release into the bloodstream of intracellular enzymes (such as the transaminases and lactic dehydrogenase).

If acute loss of blood volume results in immediate loss of blood pressure, then flow ceases at the circle of Willis and coronary ostia. This is the mechanism of death in massive hemorrhage. If the reduction in volume, pressure and flow is less drastic but more prolonged, then the characteristic sequence of the low flow state ensues, with all the changes so often enumerated in discussions of "shock." Prompt and appropriate restoration of effective blood volume is usually specific.

If the patient is now treated with sudden massive transfusions of chilled banked blood, a whole series of secondary alterations is produced which, although resulting from treatment, may produce a further variation in the metabolic consequences of injury. These transfusion-induced changes can be prevented by the use of fresh warm whole blood and the neutralization of excess citrate with calcium. In elective surgery, citrate excess is a rarity; in the treatment of massive trauma, burns, and shock it is a commonplace. Metabolic changes produced by the sudden massive infusion of cold banked blood include the following:

Hypothermia

Acidosis

Citrate accumulation with EKG changes and/or tetany

Left shift of the oxyhemoglobin dissociation curve owing to the accumulation of 2,3-DPG-deficient red cells (increased affinity of hemoglobin for oxygen and decreased delivery to tissues)

Hemoglobin load with hemoglobinuria and jaundice

Potassium loading and elevation of lactic dehydrogenase

Prolongation of the clotting process owing to low temperature effect on clotting enzymes and the dilution of platelets

This particular metabolic result of sudden massive transfusion of cold banked blood is mentioned here because it can too easily be confused with the metabolic response to low flow states themselves. In point of fact it is a pharmacologic reaction to the improper use of a poorly preserved biological product.

If recovery ensues from this low flow state, the changes of diffuse tissue anaerobiosis are quickly reversible in all areas save the kidney. If the kidneys escape damage, the patient will progress to a normal metabolic and endocrine recovery a few days later. Water and salt diuresis, the assumption of nitrogen anabolism, and the restoration of body fat are long-term evidences of the essential reversibility of low flow states when treatment has been prompt and accurate. Lingering visceral damage is prominent only in relation to the kidneys.

Post-Traumatic Renal Insufficiency. The cause of post-traumatic renal insufficiency is a combination of prolonged reduction in effective renal blood flow, together with the presentation to the kidney at that time of nephrotoxic substances, most commonly hemoglobin or myoglobin breakdown products. Post-traumatic renal insufficiency introduces a significant variant in the metabolic response to injury because the renal excretory pathway is denied to the products of proteolysis and cellular release. When this occurs, the upward course of blood urea, creatinine, and potassium is much more rapid than when renal function ceases in the resting and non-traumatized state. The rapidity of rise becomes in itself a measure of the rate of release from the body cell mass to the extracellular fluid of those compounds usually observed in the urine rather than in the blood. Just as in the case of low flow states as a group, the essential reversibility of acute tubular necrosis is one of its cardinal features. If the patient is properly managed so as to avoid overloading of water and salt and if toxic products of cellular lysis can be removed by dialysis, the outlook for recovery is improved. And yet, where very severe tissue injury is accompanied by renal failure, as in severe wounds or burns, the recovery rate is still extremely low despite the experience of the past twenty years in methods of hemodialysis (see Chapter 11).

Post-Traumatic Pulmonary Insufficiency. Progressive respiratory insufficiency is another specific organ defect which modifies the metabolic response to injury. Since this is a common cause of death and the most common terminal pathway for patients with severe injury, it must be regarded as an important variant of the normal metabolic sequence.

When progressive respiratory insufficiency occurs without initial pulmonary pathology, it is associated with several prior management components: massive blood transfusion, high oxygen tensions with low humidity in the airway and machine-driven respiratory assistance. Some of the steps taken to treat presumed respiratory tract injury aggravate the pulmonary pathology. Massive blood transfusion introduces antigens, antibodies, cellular debris, and small platelet thrombi directly into large veins and the right heart where they can lodge in the lung with no previous tissue filtration. High oxygen tensions at low humidity are injurious to the alveolar membrane and involve loss of pulmonary surfactant and of lung compliance. As pulmonary insufficiency progresses after severe injury, increasing airway pressures are required to achieve mechanical ventilation, and these in themselves accentuate the defect. Hyaline membrane is found in such lungs. This is a thin proteinaceous membrane on the inner lining of alveoli that can be produced by a wide variety of agencies harmful to the lungs. In this instance it appears to be the result of dehydration of proteinaceous alveolar edema. Positive pressure ventilation facilitates the evaporation of water from alveolar edema, leaving behind the protein component, later viewed under the microscope as hyaline membrane. Although an evidence of pulmonary injury, hyaline membrane has not been shown to constitute a significant barrier to gas diffusion.

Most important of all the steps taken early after injury that can produce pulmonary insufficiency is massive overload of water and salt solution. When water and sodium salts are given in excess, interstitial pulmonary edema results without any change in the central venous pressure. It is this edema of the interalveolar septa which is the first discernible change in experimental post-traumatic pulmonary insufficiency. Although the young patient is remarkably resistant to flooding with saline fluids, older people are sensitive to this misuse of intravenous fluids, and if there has been any primary pulmonary injury (burns, explosion, inhalation, peritoneal sepsis), saline flooding is uniquely hazardous.

The biochemical and metabolic reflections of post-traumatic pulmonary insufficiency are to be found in a progressive diminution in the arterial oxygen tension; this becomes refractory to the administration of high oxygen tensions in the airway. Calculations of pulmonary shunting, based on the arterial oxygen tension achieved at given airway oxygen tensions, will demonstrate progressive shunting of large amounts of blood through the lung without ventilation. This is due to the continued perfusion of unventilated alveoli in pulmonary segments occupied either by interstitial edema, alveolar edema, or atelectasis.

This progressive pulmonary defect is most difficult to reverse in its later stages and is inevitably associated with pulmonary colonization with microorganisms, frequently the same ones found in the wound, the bloodstream, or the upper airway.

Heart Disease. Prior to the advent of cardiac surgery, the effect of heart disease on the metabolic response to injury was of little more than academic interest since it only applied to those rare individuals with advanced heart disease who required emergency operations or who were accidentally injured. With the advent of cardiac surgery, it has become evident that heart disease introduces a variety of important metabolic variants. In addition, such patients cannot respond to an oxygenation defect by elevating cardiac output normally.

There are two cardinal changes in the surgical patient with chronic heart disease and borderline congestive failure. First, there is a persistent and pernicious tendency to retain water and extracellular salt to a far greater extent than normal, and second, a tendency to increased pressure in either the right or left atrium or both, with, appropriately, either pulmonary congestion or peripheral venous congestion, or both.

In the former case, pulmonary insufficiency supervenes even more rapidly than in the normal individual, and in the latter case edema of the liver and the periphery appears. Treatment requires an understanding of those modifications of normal surgical metabolism introduced by heart disease and, whenever possible, specific repair of the cardiac defect. In patients who have not previously been digitalized, medicinal management with digitalis and diuretics will produce a remarkable improvement prior to operation. In patients with acute pericardial effusion, hemopericardium, pneumothorax or massive pulmonary embolism, an operation itself may be necessary to enable the establishment of normal cardiac output.

Burns and Traumatic Edema. The metabolic response to burns has two metabolic characteristics which separate it from other types of trauma. First, the diffuse thermal injury to a large capillary bed produces an obligatory edema which is parasitic on the extracellular fluid volume. An area of fluid is accumulated under the burn, containing water, salt and protein in quantities approximating those in normal extracellular fluid. This enlarging third space reduces the volume of the plasma. Sufficient fluid must be infused intravenously to maintain plasma volume, normal blood flow and cardiac output despite this accumulation of nonfunctional fluid in the burned area.

Secondly, in burns, there is the inevitable development of sepsis in the region of thermal necrosis. This necrotic-septic sequence is seen in other forms of tissue injury, but its large size, surface location and inevitability are peculiar to burns (see Chapter 31).

Understanding of the disordered physiology of burns has called attention to a variety of other pathologic states in which the accumulation of an area of traumatic or septic edema reduces the plasma volume and mimics the burn physiology. Prominent among these states are venous thrombosis, peritonitis, pancreatitis, and tourniquet injury.

Prolonged Starvation. Finally, the patient who cannot or will not eat for many days or weeks after injury suffers an important variant in the metabolic response. During the early course of the injury itself and even through the turning point phase, he appears no different from his normal counterpart who is not expected to take food by mouth. But when, after the turning point is passed, the patient still cannot eat or absorb food, the upward swing of anabolism is blocked. In the normal sequence of convalescence, the patient reduces his urinary nitrogen excretion rate to values in the neighborhood of 3 to 5 gm./70 kg./day, and when appetite and food taking are resumed, he swings upward into his anabolic period, regains muscular strength, and gets well. *Without intake, this anabolism cannot occur,* and the patient settles down to a prolonged and chronic state of post-traumatic starvation; this continued slow catabolism and combustion of body fuels is superimposed upon the loss of body components already drained by the early post-traumatic catabolism. The end result is failure to respire and cough; broncho-pneumonia is the terminal event in starvation.

In such patients, the continuous intravenous provision of a caloric intake adequate to support both muscular work and protein synthesis will reduce nitrogen loss to very low levels. Such prolonged intravenous caloric supply can be either in the form of fat emulsions, glucose, or alcohol, or in some combination of the three. When to this is added an appropriate mix of amino acids or polypeptides, protein synthesis is supported and recovery of muscular strength and normal growth occurs. The central consideration in such prolonged intravenous alimentation is the simultaneous provision of nitrogen intermediates and caloric substrates at an adequate calorie : nitrogen ratio. This topic is discussed in full in the next chapter. Increasing logistical ability to provide high caloric nourishment intravenously has been a major advance in the metabolic care of those relatively few surgical patients who cannot pass into anabolism without it. While needed only in a small group of patients, especially in gastrointestinal surgery, the availability of high calorie parenteral feeding has remarkably improved their management.

SUMMARY

This chapter began with an analogy between convalescence and pregnancy. Both are initiated by a single event at a finite point in time. Both pursue a predictable course, based on normal metabolism and endocrinology. Both terminate with a happy issue: a full-term infant or a healed active person. In both situations the ideal understanding and successful management of complications are based on an elucidation of the normal sequence. But there, possibly, our analogy ends.

Unlike pregnancy, physical injury can occur in both sexes and to all age groups. Pregnancy does not vary in degree; there is no such thing as being "slightly pregnant." Fortunately, minor injury is a commonplace. Another difference lies in the fact that no amount of wisdom or intervention (short of abortion) can diminish or reduce pregnancy, whereas good surgical technique and intelligent treatment can both shorten and diminish the magnitude of physical injury and its bodily response.

Finally, there is an appealing addition to the analogy: that both in pregnancy and in injury one should avoid meddlesome treatment. Much of the bodily sequence is normal and healthy. Both processes are firmly rooted in evolution and have been running their course without the help of physicians for millennia. Now that the physician is here and the surgeon at the bedside, he should not confuse the availability of his armamentarium with the necessity for its employment. Simplicity in all things, most especially in the treatment of surgical injury!

REFERENCES

Albright, F.: Cushing's syndrome: its pathological physiology, its relationship to the adreno-genital syndrome and its connection with the problem of the reaction of the body to injurious agents ("alarm reaction" of Selye). Harvey Lect. Ser. 38:123, 1943.

Anrep, G. V., and Cannan, R. K.: The concentration of lactic acid in the blood in experimental alkalemia and acidemia. J. Physiol. 58:244, 1923.

Bartlett, R. H., and Yahia, C.: Management of septic chemical abortion with renal failure. N. Eng. J. Med. 281:747, 1969.

Cannon, W. B.: Bodily Changes in Pain, Hunger, Fear and Rage. An Account of Recent Researches into the Function of Emotional Excitement. 2nd Ed. Boston, C. T. Bradford Company, 1953.

Clowes, G. H. A., Jr., Vucinic, M., and Weidner, M. G.: Circulatory and metabolic alterations associated with survival or death in peritonitis: clinical analysis of 25 cases. Ann. Surg. 163:866, 1966.

Felig, P., Owen, O. E., Morgan, A. P., and Cahill, G. F., Jr.: Utilization of metabolic fuels in obese subjects. Amer. J. Clin. Nutr. 21:1429, 1968.

Huckabee, W. E.: Relationships of pyruvate and lactate during anaerobic metabolism. I. Effects of infusion of pyruvate or glucose and of hyperventilation. J. Clin. Invest. 37:244, 1958.

Huckabee, W. E.: Metabolic consequences of chronic hypoxia. Ann. N.Y. Acad. Sci. 121:723, 1965.

Kinney, J. M.: A consideration of energy exchange in human trauma. Bull. N.Y. Acad. Med. 36:617, 1960.

Lemieux, M. D., Smith, R. N., and Couch, N. P.: Electrometric surface pH of skeletal muscle in hypovolemia. Amer. J. Surg. 117:627, 1969.

Litwin, M. S., Smith, L. L., and Moore, F. D.: Metabolic alkalosis following massive transfusion. Surgery 45:805, 1959.

Lyons, J. H., Jr., and Moore, F. D.: Posttraumatic alkalosis: incidence and pathophysiology of alkalosis in surgery. Surgery 60:93, 1966.

McNamara, J. J., Molot, M. D., and Stremple, J. F.: Screen filtration pressure in combat casualties. Ann. Surg. 172:334, 1970.

Moore, F. D.: Bodily changes in surgical convalescence. I. The normal sequence — observations and interpretations. Ann. Surg. 137:289, 1953.

Moore, F. D.: Hormones and stress — endocrine changes after anesthesia, surgery and unanesthetized trauma in man. Rec. Prog. Hormone Res. 13:511, 1957.

Moore, F. D.: Metabolism in trauma: the meaning of definitive surgery — the wound, the endocrine glands and metabolism. The Harvey Lectures 1956-1957. New York, Academic Press, Inc., 1958.

Moore, F. D.: Systemic mediators of surgical injury. (Lister Lecture delivered at the 19th Annual Meeting of the Canadian Medical Association, Edmonton, Alberta, June 20, 1956.) Canad. M. A. J. 78:85, 1958.

Moore, F. D., Lyons, J. H., Pierce, E. C., Jr., Morgan, A. P., Jr., Drinker, P. A., MacArthur, J. D., and Dammin, G. J.: Post-Traumatic Pulmonary Insufficiency. Philadelphia, W. B. Saunders Company, 1969.

Morgan, A. P.: The pulmonary toxicity of oxygen. Anesthesiology 29:570, 1968.

Owen, O. E., Felig, P., Morgan, A. P., Wahren, A. J., Jr., and Cahill, G. F., Jr.: Liver and kidney metabolism during prolonged starvation. J. Clin. Invest. 48:574, 1969.

Owen, O. E., Morgan, A. P., Kemp, H. G., Sullivan, J. M., Herrera, M. G., and Cahill, G. F., Jr.: Brain metabolism during fasting. J. Clin. Invest. 46:1589, 1967.

Skillman, J. J., Awaad, H. K., and Moore, F. D.: Plasma protein kinetics of the early transcapillary refill after hemorrhage in man. Surg. Gynec. & Obst. 125:983, 1967.

Skillman, J. J., Eltringham, W. K., Zollinger, R. M., Jr., Lauler, D. P., and Moore, F. D.: Phenoxybenzamine-induced vasodilatation: A stimulus to increased plasma volume with reduced central venous pressure and aldosterone hypersecretion in man. Surgery 64:368, 1968.

Skillman, J. J., Lauler, D. P., Hickler, R. B., Lyons, J. H., Olson, J. E., Ball, M. R., and Moore, F. D.: Hemorrhage in normal man: effect on renin, cortisol, aldosterone, and urine composition. Ann. Surg. 166:865, 1967.

Skillman, J. J., Olson, J. E., Lyons, J. H., and Moore, F. D.: The hemodynamic effect of acute blood loss in normal man, with observations on the effect of the Valsalva maneuver and breath holding. Ann. Surg. 166:713, 1967.

Smith, L. L., and Moore, F. D.: Refractory hypotension in man — is this irreversible shock? N. Eng. J. Med. 267:733, 1962.

Smith, R. N., Lemieux, M. D., and Couch, N. P.: Effects of acidosis and alkalosis on surface skeletal muscle hydrogen ion activity. Surg. Gynec. & Obst. 128:533, 1969.

Spencer, F. C., Bosomworth, P., and Ritcher, W.: Fatal pulmonary injury from prolonged inhalation of oxygen in high concentration; in Brown, I. W., Jr., and Cox, B. G. (eds.): Proceedings of the Third International Conference on Hyperbaric Medicine, National Research Council Publication no. 1404. Washington, D.C., National Academy of Sciences-National Research Council, 1966, p. 189.

Walker, W. F., Shoemaker, W. C., Kaalstad, A. J., and Moore, F. D.: Influence of blood volume restoration and tissue trauma on corticosteroid secretion in dogs. Amer. J. Physiol. 197:781, 1959.

Walker, W. F., Zileli, M. S., Reutter, F. W., Shoemaker, W. C., Friend, D., and Moore, F. D.: Adrenal medullary secretion in hemorrhagic shock. Amer. J. Physiol. 197:773, 1959.

Walker, W. F., Zileli, M. S., Reutter, F. W., Shoemaker, W. C., and Moore, F. D.: Factors influencing the 'resting' secretion of the adrenal medulla. Amer. J. Physiol. 197:765, 1959.

CHAPTER 3

FLUID AND ELECTROLYTE THERAPY

G. Tom Shires, M.D.

Recognition and management of fluid and electrolyte problems in the surgical patient are among the more important aspects of surgical care. Operative trauma imposes a great impact on body physiology and involves changes far beyond that caused by simple lack of alimentation. A thorough understanding of the metabolism of water, salt, and other electrolytes will result in prevention of many fluid disorders and early diagnosis and successful therapy when such disorders develop.

An attempt will be made in this chapter to present a logical approach to the management of fluid therapy in the surgical patient and to present a usable concept or classification which has both physiologic and therapeutic meaning. Knowledge of the anatomy of body fluids, of the physiologic principles governing both gains and losses, and of the movement of water as well as salt and other electrolytes between body compartments is necessary.

ANATOMY OF BODY FLUIDS

A prerequisite to the understanding of fluid and electrolyte management is a knowledge of the extent and composition of the various body fluid compartments. Early attempts to define these compartments were relatively accurate, but a more precise definition has been obtained recently by many investigators through the use of isotope tracer techniques. The wide range of normal values is a function of body size, weight, and sex, but these compartments are relatively constant in size in the individual patient in the normal steady state. The figures used in this section, therefore, are approximate and are presented as a percentage of body weight.

Total Body Water. Water constitutes between 50 and 70 per cent of total body weight. Using deuterium oxide (D_2O) or tritiated water (THO) for measurement of total body water (TBW), the average normal value for young males is 60 per cent of body weight and for young females 50 per cent. A normal variation of ± 15 per cent applies to both groups. The actual figure in a given healthy individual is remarkably constant and is a function of several variables, including lean body mass and age. Leanness is association with a high body water and obesity with a low total body water. The lower percentage of total body water in females correlates well with a relatively large amount of subcutaneous adipose tissue. Moore and others have shown that total body water, as a percentage of total body weight, decreases steadily and significantly with age to a low of 52 per cent and 47 per cent in males and females respectively. Conversely, the highest proportion of total body water to body weight is found in newborn infants with a maximum of 80 per cent.

The water of the body is divided into three functional compartments (See Appendix, Fig. 1). The fluid within the body's diverse cell population, intracellular water, represents between 30 and 40 per cent of the body weight. The extracellular water represents 20 per cent of the body weight and is divided between the intravascular fluid, or plasma (50 per cent of body weight), and the interstitial or extravascular, extracellular fluid (15 per cent of body weight).

Intracellular Fluid. Measurement of intracellular fluid is determined indirectly by subtraction of the measured extracellular fluid from the measured total body water. The intracellular water is between 30 and 40 per cent of the body weight, with the largest proportion in the skeletal muscle mass. Because of the smaller muscle mass in the female, the percentage of intracellular water is less than in the male.

The chemical composition of the intracellular fluid is shown in the Appendix (Fig. 2), with potassium and magnesium the principal cations and phosphates and proteins the principal anions. This composition is an approximation because so few data concerning the intracellular fluid are available.

Extracellular Fluid. The total extracellular fluid volume represents approximately 20 per cent of the body weight. The extracellular fluid compartment has two major subdivisions. The plasma volume comprises approximately 5 per cent of the body weight in the normal adult. The interstitial or extravascular, extracellular fluid volume, obtained by subtracting the plasma volume from the measured total extracellular fluid volume, comprises approximatley 15 per cent of the body weight.

The interstitial fluid is further complicated by having, normally, a rapidly equilibrating or functional component as well as several slower equilibrating or relatively nonfunctioning components. The nonfunctioning components include connective tissue water, as well as water that has been termed transcellular and includes cerebrospinal and joint fluids. This nonfunctional component normally represents only 10 per cent of the interstitial fluid volume (1 to 2 per cent of body weight) and is not to be confused with the relatively nonfunctional extracellular fluid, often called a "third space," found in burns and soft tissue injuries.

The normal constituents of the extracellular fluid are shown in Figure 2 of the Appendix, with sodium the principal cation and chloride and bicarbonate the principal anions. There are minor differences in ionic composition between the plasma and interstitial fluid occasioned by the difference in protein concentration. Because of the higher protein content (organic anions) of the plasma, the total concentration of cations is high and the concentration of inorganic anions is somewhat lower than in the interstitial fluid, as explained by the Gibbs-Donnan equilibrium equation.* For practical consideration, however, they may be considered equal. The total concentration of intracellular ions exceeds that of the extracellular compartment and would seem to violate the concept of osmolar equilibrium between the two compartments. This apparent discrepancy is due to the fact that the concentration of ions is expressed in milliequivalents without regard to osmotic activity. In addition, some of the intracellular cations probably exist in undissociated form.

OSMOTIC PRESSURE

Relative to a discussion of the complicated interactions between the various body fluid compartments is the definition of commonly used terms. The physiologic and chemical activity of electrolytes depends on (1) the number of particles present per unit volume (mols or millimols per liter), (2) the number of electric charges per unit volume (equivalents or milliequivalents per liter), and (3) the number of osmotically active particles or ions per unit volume (osmols or milliosmols per liter).

A mol of a substance is the molecular weight of that substance in grams, and millimol (mM.) is that figure expressed in milligrams. For example, a mol of sodium chloride is 58 gm. (Na, 23; Cl, 35) and a mM. is 58 mg. This expression, however, gives no direct information as to the number of osmotically active ions in solution or the electric charges that they carry.

The electrolytes of the body fluids may then be expressed in terms of chemical combining activity or "equivalents." An equivalent of an

---

*The product of the concentrations of any pair of diffusible cations and anions on one side of a semipermeable membrane will equal the product of the same pair of ions on the other side.

ion is its atomic weight expressed in grams divided by the valence, whereas a milliequivalent of an ion is that figure expressed in milligrams. In the case of univalent ions, a milliequivalent is the same as a millimol. However, in the case of divalent ions, such as calcium or magnesium, one millimol equals two milliequivalents. The importance of this expression is that a milliequivalent of any substance will combine chemically with a milliequivalent of any other substance, and in any given solution, the number of milliequivalents of cations present is balanced by precisely the same number of milliequivalents of anions.

When the osmotic pressure of a solution is considered, it is more descriptive to employ the terms osmol or milliosmol. These terms refer to the actual number of osmotically active particles present in solution, but is not dependent on the chemical combining capacities of the substances. Thus, a millimol of sodium chloride which dissociates nearly completely into sodium and chloride contributes two milliosmols, and one millimol of sodium sulfate which dissociates into three particles contributes three milliosmols. One millimol of an un-ionized substance such as glucose is equal to one milliosmol of the substance.

The differences in ionic composition between intracellular and extracellular fluid are maintained by the cell wall, which functions as a semipermeable membrane. The total number of osmotically active particles is 290 to 310 milliosmols in each compartment. Although the total osmotic pressure of a fluid is the sum of the partial pressure contributed by each of the solutes in the fluid, the effective osmotic pressure is dependent on those substances that fail to pass through the pores of the semipermeable membrane. The dissolved proteins in the plasma, thus, are primarily responsible for effective osmotic pressure between the plasma and the interstitial fluid compartments. This is frequently referred to as the colloid osmotic pressure. The effective osmotic pressure between the extracellular and intracellular fluid compartments would be contributed to by any substance that does not traverse the cell membranes freely. Thus sodium, which is the principal cation of the extracellular fluid, contributes a major portion of the osmotic pressure, but substances that fail to penetrate the cell membrane freely, such as glucose, also increase the effective osmotic pressure.

Since the cell membranes are completely permeable to water, the effective osmotic pressure in the two compartments is considered to be equal. Any condition that alters the effective osmotic pressure in either compartment will result in a redistribution of water between the compartments. Thus, an increase in effective osmotic pressure in the extracellular fluid, which would occur most frequently as a result of increased sodium salts, would cause a net transfer of water from the intracellular to the extracellular fluid compartment. Conversely, a decrease of sodium salts in the extracellular fluid will cause a transfer of water from the extracellular to the intracellular fluid compartment. Depletion of the extracellular fluid volume without a change in the concentration of ions will not result in transfer of free water from the intracellular space.

Thus, the intracellular fluid shares in losses that involve a change in concentration or composition of the extracellular fluid, but shares slowly in changes involving loss of isotonic volume alone. For practical consideration, most losses and gains of body fluid are directly from the extracellular fluid volume phase.

CLASSIFICATION OF BODY FLUID CHANGES

The disorders in fluid balance may be classified into three general categories: disturbances of (1) volume, (2) concentration, and (3) composition. Of primary importance is the concept that although these disturbances are interrelated, each is a separate entity.

If an isotonic salt solution is added to or lost from the body fluids, only the volume of the extracellular fluid is changed. The acute loss of an isotonic extracellular solution, such as intestinal juice, is followed by a significant decrease in the extracellular fluid volume and little, if any, change in the intracellular fluid volume. Fluid will not be transferred from the intracellular space to refill the depleted extracellular space so long as the osmolarity remains the same in the two compartments.

If water alone is added to or lost from the extracellular fluid, the concentration of osmotically active particles will change. Sodium ion accounts for 90 per cent of the osmotically active particles in the extracellular fluid, and these principally determine tonicity of body fluid compartments. If the extracellular fluid is depleted of sodium, water will pass into the intracellular space until osmolarity is again equal in the two compartments.

The concentration of all other ions within the extracellular fluid compartment can be altered without significant change in the total number of osmotically active particles, thus producing only a compositional change. Normally functioning kidneys minimize these changes considerably, particularly if the addition or loss of solute or water is gradual.

An internal loss of extracellular fluid into a nonfunctional space, such as the sequestration of isotonic fluid in a burn, peritonitis, ascites, or muscle trauma, is termed a distributional change. The transfer or functional loss of extracellular fluid internally may be extracellular (e.g., peritonitis) or intracellular (e.g., as probably occurs in hemorrhagic shock). In any event, all distributional shifts or losses result in a contraction of the functional extracellular fluid space.

VOLUME CHANGES

Volume deficit or excess generally must be diagnosed by clinical examination of the patient. There are no readily available laboratory tests of benefit in the acute phase except measurement of the plasma volume. Changes secondary to longstanding derangements in volume may be discernible, however. For example, the blood urea nitrogen level slowly rises with a longstanding extracellular fluid deficit of sufficient magnitude to reduce the glomerular filtration. The concentration of serum sodium is not related to the volume status of extracellular fluid. A severe volume deficit may exist with a normal, low, or high serum sodium.

Volume Deficit. Extracellular fluid volume deficit is by far the most common fluid disorder in the surgical patient. The signs and symptoms of this state are easily recognized and are listed in Table 3-1. The CNS and cardiovascular signs occur early with acute rapid losses, whereas tissue signs may be absent until the deficit has existed for at least 24 hours. The CNS signs are similar to barbiturate intoxication, and those of the cardiovascular system are secondary to a deficit in plasma volume with varying degrees of hypotension. Skin turgor may

Table 3-1. EXTRACELLULAR FLUID VOLUME

	DEFICIT		EXCESS	
	Moderate	*Severe*	*Moderate*	*Severe*
CNS	Sleepiness Apathy Slow responses Anorexia Cessation of usual activity	Decreased tendon reflexes Anesthesia of distal extremities Stupor Coma	None	None
Gastrointestinal	Progressive decrease in food consumption	Nausea, vomiting Refusal to eat Silent ileus and distention	At surgery: Edema of stomach, colon, lesser and greater omenta and small bowel mesentery.	
Cardiovascular	Orthostatic hypotension Tachycardia Collapsed veins Collapsing pulse	Cutaneous lividity Hypotension Distant heart sounds Cold extremities Absent peripheral pulses	Elevated venous pressure Distention of peripheral veins Increased cardiac output Loud heart sounds Functional murmurs Bounding pulse High pulse pressure Increased pulmonary 2nd sound Gallop	Pulmonary edema
Tissue Signs	Soft, small tongue with longitudinal wrinkling Decreased skin turgor	Atonic muscles Sunken eyes	Subcutaneous pitting edema Basilar râles	Anasarca Moist râles Vomiting Diarrhea
Metabolism	Mild decrease in temperature (97–99°)	Marked decrease in temperature (95–98°)	None	None

be difficult to assess in the elderly patient or in the patient with recent loss of weight and is not diagnostic in the absence of other confirmatory signs. The body temperature tends to vary with the environmental temperature. In a cool room, the patient may be slightly hypothermic, and the febrile response to injury may be obscured.

Volume Excess. Extracellular fluid volume excess is generally iatrogenic or secondary to renal insufficiency. In the healthy young adult, the signs are generally those of circulatory overload manifested primarily in the pulmonary circulation and of excessive fluid in other tissue. In the elderly patient, congestive heart failure with pulmonary edema may develop rather quickly with a moderate volume excess.

CONCENTRATION

Since the sodium ion is primarily responsible for the osmolarity of the extracellular fluid space, determination of the serum concentration of sodium generally indicates the tonicity of body fluids. Hyponatremia and hypernatremia may be diagnosed on clinical examination (Table 3-2), but in contrast to volume changes, laboratory confirmation is available.

Hyponatremia. *Acute* hyponatremia (sodium less than 130 mEq. per liter) clinically is characterized by CNS signs of increased intracranial pressure and tissue signs of excessive intracellular water. There are no cardiovascular signs per se. The hypertension is probably induced

Table 3-2. ACUTE CHANGES IN OSMOLAR CONCENTRATION

	HYPONATREMIA (Water Intoxication)		HYPERNATREMIA (Water Deficit)	
CNS	Moderate: Muscle twitching Hyperactive tendon reflexes Increased intra- cranial pressure (compensated phase)	Severe: Convulsions Loss of reflexes Increased intra- cranial pressure (decompensated phase)	Moderate: Restlessness Weakness	Severe: Delirium Maniacal behavior
Cardiovascular	Changes in blood pressure and pulse secondary to increased intracranial pressure		Tachycardia Hypotension (if severe)	
Tissue Signs	Salivation, lacrimation, watery diarrhea "Finger printing" of skin (sign of intracellular volume excess)		Decrease saliva and tears Dry and sticky mucous membranes Red, swollen tongue Skin flushed	
Renal	Oliguria progressing to anuria		Oliguria	
Metabolic	None		Fever	

by the rise in intracranial pressure, for it returns to normal with the administration of hypertonic solutions of sodium salts. Of importance with severe hyponatremia is the relatively rapid development of oliguric renal failure, which may not be reversible if therapy is delayed.

Hypernatremia. Central nervous system and tissue signs, as listed in Table 3-2, characterize acute symptomatic hypernatremia. This is the only state in which dry sticky mucous membranes are characteristic. This sign does not occur with pure extracellular fluid volume deficit alone, and may be misleading in the patient who breathes through his mouth. Body temperature is generally elevated and may approach a lethal level as in the patient with heat stroke.

Although volume changes occur frequently without a change in serum sodium, the reverse is not true. The disease states that cause a significant *acute* alteration in the serum sodium frequently produce a concomitant change in the extracellular fluid volume.

COMPOSITION

Compositional abnormalities of importance include changes in acid-base balance and concentration changes of potassium, calcium, and magnesium.

Acid-Base Balance. The pH (the negative logarithm of the hydrogen ion concentration) of the body fluids is normally maintained within narrow limits in spite of the rather large load of acid produced endogenously as a byproduct of body metabolism. The acids are neutralized efficiently by several buffer systems and are subsequently excreted by the lungs and kidneys. Frequently, no clinical signs appear if the change in concentration of serum sodium occurs slowly as, for example, with congestive heart failure.

The important buffers include proteins and phosphates, which are of primary importance in maintaining intracellular pH, and the bicarbonate—carbonic acid system, which operates primarily in the extracellular fluid space and is quantitatively the largest in the body. The proteins and hemoglobin are of only minor importance in the extracellular fluid space, but the latter is of prime importance as a buffer in the red cell.

The buffer systems consist of a weak acid or base and the salt of that acid or base. The buffering effect is the result of the formation of an amount of weak acid equivalent to the amount of strong acid added to the fluid. The resultant change in pH is considerably less than if the substance had been added to water alone. The function of the buffer systems is expressed in the Henderson-Hasselbalch equation, which defines the pH in terms of the ratio of the salt and acid.

The pH of the extracellular fluid is defined primarily by the ratio of the amount of base bicarbonate (majority as sodium bicarbonate) to the amount of carbonic acid (related to the CO_2 content of alveolar air) present in the blood:

$$pH = pK + \log \frac{BHCO_3}{H_2CO_3} = \frac{27 \text{ mEq./L.}}{1.33 \text{ mEq./L.}} = \frac{20}{1} = 7.4$$

pK represents the dissociation constant of carbonic acid in the presence of base bicarbonate and by measurement is 6.1. At a body pH of 7.4, the ratio must be 20 to 1 as depicted. From a chemical standpoint, this is an inefficient buffer system, but the unusual property of CO_2 to behave as an acid or change to a neutral gas with subsequent excretion by the lungs makes it quite efficient biologically.

As long as the 20 to 1 ratio is maintained, regardless of the absolute values, the pH will remain at 7.4. If an acid is added to the system, the concentration of bicarbonate (the numerator in the Henderson-Hasselbalch equation) will decrease. Ventilation will immediately increase to eliminate larger quantities of CO_2 with a subsequent decrease in the carbonic acid (the denominator in the Henderson-Hasselbalch equation) until the 20 to 1 ratio is re-established. Slower, more complete compensation is effected by the kidneys with increased excretion of acid salts and retention of bicarbonate. The reverse would occur if an alkali were added to the system. Respiratory acidosis and alkalosis are produced by disturbances of ventilation, with an increase or decrease in the denominator and resultant change of the 20 to 1 ratio. Compensation is primarily renal, with a retention of bicarbonate and increased excretion of acid salts in respiratory acidosis and the reverse process in respiratory alkalosis.

The four types of acid-base disturbances are listed in Table 3–3. Use of the CO_2 combining power (approximates the plasma bicarbonate) or CO_2 content (includes bicarbonate, carbonic acid and dissolved CO_2) and knowledge of the patient's disease will generally allow an accurate diagnosis in the uncomplicated case. However, since CO_2 combining power is elevated with respiratory acidosis and metabolic alkalosis and depressed with respiratory alkalosis and metabolic acidosis, measurement of pH and pCO_2 is necessary for confirmation. Determination of the acidity or alkalinity of the urine is helpful but may be misleading. In renal tubular acidosis, for instance, systemic acidosis is present with alkaline urine owing to the inability of the renal tubule to conserve base bicarbonate.

Unfortunately, more complex acid-base disturbances are frequently encountered. Partially compensated states can be particularly misleading because primary respiratory disturbances cause compensatory changes in plasma bicarbonate and metabolic disturbances will secondarily affect the level of pCO_2. Combinations of the four acid-base states may also occur, such as respiratory acidosis complicated by a metabolic acidosis or alkalosis. Measurements of pH, pCO_2, pO_2, and

Table 3-3. ACIDOSIS-ALKALOSIS

	DEFECT	COMMON CAUSES	$\dfrac{BHCO_3}{H_2CO_3} = \dfrac{20}{1}$	COMPENSATION
Respiratory acidosis	Retention of CO_2 (decreased alveolar ventilation)	Depression of respiratory center—morphine, CNS injury. Pulmonary disease—emphysema, pneumonia	↑ Denominator Ratio less than 20:1 ↑ CO_2-combining power	Renal Retention of bicarbonate, excretion of acid salts, increased ammonia formation Chloride shift into red cells
Respiratory alkalosis	Excessive loss of CO_2 (increased alveolar ventilation)	Hyperventilation: emotional, severe pain, assisted ventilation, encephalitis	↓ Denominator Ratio greater than 20:1 ↓ CO_2-combining power	Renal Excretion of bicarbonate, retention of acid salts, decreased ammonia formation
Metabolic acidosis	Retention of fixed acids or loss of base bicarbonate	Diabetes, azotemia, lactic acid accumulation, starvation Diarrhea, small bowel fistulae	↓ Numerator Ratio less than 20:1 ↓ CO_2-combining power	Pulmonary (rapid) Increase rate and depth of breathing Renal (slow) As in respiratory acidosis
Metabolic alkalosis	Loss of fixed acids Gain of base bicarbonate Potassium depletion	Vomiting or gastric suction with pyloric obstruction Excessive intake of bicarbonate Diuretics	↑ Numerator Ratio greater than 20:1 ↑ CO_2-combining power	Pulmonary (rapid) Decrease rate and depth of breathing Renal (slow) As in respiratory alkalosis

CO_2 combining power concomitant with a review of the clinical situation will generally clarify the situation. In addition, the determination of "whole blood buffer base" or "base excess" may be of value.

Potassium Abnormalities. Ninety-eight per cent of the potassium in the body is located within the intracellular compartment, and it is the major cation of intracellular water. Although the total extracellular potassium is only 56 mEq. in a 70-kg. man (4 mEq./L. times 14 L.), this small amount is critical to cardiac and neuromuscular function. In addition, the turnover rate in the extracellular fluid compartment may be extremely rapid.

The intracellular and extracellular distribution of potassium is influenced by many factors. Significant quantities of intracellular potassium are released into the extracellular space in response to severe injury or surgical stress, acidosis, and the catabolic state. A significant rise in serum potassium may occur in these states in the presence of oliguric or anuric renal failure, but dangerous hyperkalemia (greater than 6mEq./L.) is rarely encountered if renal function is normal. After severe trauma, however, normal or excessive urinary volumes may not reflect the ability of the kidney to clear solutes or to excrete potassium. (See High Output Renal Failure.)

HYPERKALEMIA.   The signs of a significant hyperkalemia are limited to the cardiovascular and gastrointestinal systems. The gastrointestinal symptoms include nausea, vomiting, intermittent intestinal colic, and diarrhea. The cardiovascular signs are apparent on the electrocardiogram initially, with high T-waves and depressed S-T segments. Subsequent disappearance of T-waves, heart block, and diastolic cardiac arrest develop with increasing levels of potassium.

Treatment of hyperkalemia consists of immediate measures to reduce the serum potassium level, the withholding of exogenously administered potassium, and correction of the underlying cause if possible. Temporary suppression of the myocardial effect of a sudden rapid rise of potassium can be accomplished by the intravenous administration of a solution containing 80 mEq. of sodium lactate, 100 ml. of calcium gluconate, and 100 ml. of 50 per cent dextrose in water. The administration of insulin to these glycogen-depleted patients should be limited to 1 unit/5 gm. or more of glucose, because rebound hypoglycemia may be fatal. Administration of this solution over a two-hour period allows time for the preparations necessary for definitive removal of the excess potassium by hemodialysis or peritoneal dialysis. A slow rise of potassium (less than 1 mEq./L./day) can be controlled by the use of cation-exchange resins, preferably in the sodium cycle,* administered by rectum in doses of 25 gm. every 12 hours. To prevent rapid absorption of water from the colon, 200 ml. of 10 per cent dextrose in water is used as the vehicle.

HYPOKALEMIA.   The more common problem in the surgical patient is hypokalemia, which may occur as a result of (1) excessive renal excretion, (2) movement of potassium into cells, (3) prolonged administration of potassium-free parenteral fluids with continued obligatory renal loss of potassium (10 to 20 mEq. per day), or (4) loss in gastrointestinal secretions.

Potassium plays an important role in the regulation of acid-base balance. Increased renal excretion occurs with both respiratory and metabolic alkalosis. Potassium is in competition with hydrogen ion for renal tubular excretion in exchange for sodium ion. Thus, in alkalosis, the increased potassium ion excretion in exchange for sodium ion permits hydrogen ion conservation. Low serum potassium concentration may also produce metabolic alkalosis, because an increase in excretion of hydrogen ions occurs when potassium is not available in the tubular cell. In addition, the movement of hydrogen ions into the cells as a consequence of loss of potassium is in part responsible for the alkalosis. In metabolic acidosis, the reverse process occurs, and the excess hydrogen ion exchanges for sodium with retention of greater amounts of potassium.

---

*Kayexalate (Winthrop Laboratories).

Renal tubular excretion of potassium ion is increased when larger quantities of sodium are available for excretion. The more sodium ion available for reabsorption, the more potassium is exchanged for it in the lumen. Potassium requirements for prolonged or massive isotonic fluid volume replacement are increased probably on this basis. The same mechanism may also explain the increased potassium ion excretion with steroid administration.

The renal excretion of potassium may be small when compared to the potassium contained in gastrointestinal secretions. The amount per liter of various types of gastrointestinal fluids is shown in the Appendix. Although the average potassium concentration of some of these fluids is relatively low, significant hypokalemia will result if potassium-free fluids are used for replacement.

In summary, most of the factors that tend to influence potassium metabolism result in excess excretion, and a tendency toward hypokalemia is frequent in the surgical patient except when shock or acidosis interferes with the normal renal handling of potassium.

The signs of potassium deficit are related to failure of normal contractility of skeletal, smooth, and cardiac muscle and include weakness that may progress to flaccid paralysis, diminished to absent tendon reflexes, and paralytic ileus. Sensitivity to digitalis with cardiac arrhythmias and electrocardiographic signs of low voltage, flattening of T-waves, and depression of S-T segments are characteristic.

The signs of potassium deficit may be masked by those of a severe extracellular fluid volume deficit. The repletion of an extracellular fluid volume deficit may further aggravate the situation with a lowering of serum potassium secondary to dilution.

The treatment of hypokalemia involves, first, the prevention of this state. In replacement of gastrointestinal fluids, it is safe to replace the upper limits of loss, because an excess is readily handled by the normal kidney. Potassium is available in 20 mEq. and 40 mEq. ampules for addition to intravenous fluids. No more than 40 mEq. should be added to a liter for intravenous fluid. The rate of administration not only should include a prior assessment of urinary output, but, in addition, should be given intravenously no faster than 30 to 40 mEq. per hour. Potassium should not be given to the oliguric patient or for the first 24 hours following severe surgical trauma.

Calcium Abnormalities. The majority of the 1000 to 1200 gm. of body calcium is found in the bone in the form of phosphate and carbonate. Normal daily intake of calcium is between 1 and 3 gm. Most of this is excreted via the gastrointestinal tract and 200 mg. or less is excreted in the urine daily. The normal serum level is between 9 and 11 mg./100 ml. (depending on the individual laboratory's normal range), and approximately half of this is un-ionized and bound to plasma protein. An additional un-ionized fraction (5 per cent) is bound to other substances in the plasma and interstitial fluid, whereas the remaining 45 per cent is the ionized portion that is responsible for neuromuscular stability. Determination of the plasma protein level is, therefore, essential for proper analysis of the serum calcium level. The ratio of ionized to un-ionized calcium is also related to the pH; acidosis causes an increase in the ionized fraction, whereas alkalosis causes a decrease.

Disturbances of calcium metabolism are generally not a problem in the uncomplicated postoperative patient, with the exception of skeletal loss during prolonged immobilization. Routine administration of calcium to the surgical patient, therefore, is not needed in the absence of specific indications.

HYPOCALCEMIA. The symptoms of hypocalcemia (serum level less than 8 mg. per cent) are numbness and tingling of the circumoral region and the tips of the fingers and toes. The signs are of neuromuscular origin and include hyperactive tendon reflexes, muscle and abdominal cramps, tetany with carpopedal spasm, convulsions (with severe deficit), and a prolongation of the Q-T interval on the electrocardiogram.

The common causes include acute pancreatitis, massive soft tissue infections (necrotizing fasciitis), acute and chronic renal failure, pancreatic and small intestinal fistulas, and hypoparathyroidism. Transient hypocalcemia is a frequent occurrence in the hyperparathyroid patient following removal of a parathyroid adenoma owing to atrophy of the remaining glands. Asymptomatic hypocalcemia may occur with hypoproteinemia (normal ionized fraction), whereas symptoms may appear with a normal serum calcium level in a severely alkalotic patient. The latter is due to a decrease in the physiologically active or ionized fraction of total serum calcium. Calcium levels also may fall with a severe depletion of magnesium.

Treatment is directed toward correction of the underlying cause with a concomitant repletion of the deficit. Acute symptoms may be relieved by the intravenous administration of calcium gluconate or calcium chloride. Calcium lactate may be given orally, with or without supplemental vitamin D, in the patient requiring prolonged replacement. The routine administration of calcium during massive transfusions of blood in acid-citrate-dextrose solution is controversial. If the transfusions are administered slowly, the citrate binding of ionized calcium is generally compensated for by the mobilization of calcium from the bone. However, with rapid transfusion of blood, 1 gm. of calcium gluconate is given with every four or five units of blood infused.

HYPERCALCEMIA. The symptoms of hypercalcemia are rather vague and are of gastrointestinal, renal, musculoskeletal, and central nervous system origin. The early manifestations of acute hypercalcemic crisis include easy fatigue, lassitude, weakness of varying degree, anorexia, nausea, vomiting, and weight loss. With higher serum calcium levels, lassitude gives way to somnambulance, stupor, and finally coma. Other symptoms include severe headaches, pains in the back and extremities, thirst, polydypsia, and polyuria. The critical level for serum calcium is between 17 and 20 mg. per cent, and unless treatment is instituted promptly, the symptoms may rapidly progress to death.

The two major causes of hypercalcemia are hyperparathyroidism and cancer with bony metastasis. The latter is most frequently seen in the patient with metastatic breast cancer who is receiving estrogen therapy.

The treatment of acute hypercalcemic crisis is an emergency. Measures to lower the serum calcium are instituted immediately, while preparations are being made for more definitive treatment. Of particular importance is the rapid repletion of the associated extracellular fluid volume deficit, which will result in immediate lowering of the calcium by dilution. Other measures, which have been used and may be of temporary benefit, include the use of chelating agents (EDTA), steroids, sodium sulfate solution, and hemodialysis. The definitive treatment of acute hypercalcemic crisis in patients with hyperparathyroidism is immediate surgery.

The treatment of hypercalcemia in the patient with metastatic cancer is primarily that of prevention. The serum calcium level is checked frequently, and if it is elevated, the patient is placed on a low-calcium diet and measures to ensure adequate hydration are instituted.

Magnesium Deficiency. The importance of the magnesium ion in body metabolism and the recognition of the syndrome of magnesium deficiency is of current interest. The infrequent occurrence of magnesium deficiency and the previous lack of a rapid, precise technique for measurement of magnesium ion concentration accounts for the late appreciation of this entity.

The total body content of magnesium in the average adult is approximately 2000 mEq., about half of which is incorporated in bone and is only slowly exchangeable. The distribution of magnesium is similar to that of potassium, the major portion being intracellular. Plasma magnesium concentration normally ranges between 1.5 and 2.5 mEq./L.

The normal dietary intake of magnesium is approximately 20 mEq. (240 mg.) daily. The larger part is excreted in the feces and the remainder in the urine. The kidneys show a remarkable ability to conserve magnesium, and on a magnesium-free diet, renal excretion of this ion may be less than 1 mEq./day.

Magnesium deficiency is known to occur with starvation, malabsorption syndromes, protracted losses of gastrointestinal fluid, and prolonged parenteral fluid therapy with magnesium-free solutions. Other causes include acute pancreatitis, diabetic acidosis during treatment, primary aldosteronism, and chronic alcoholism.

The magnesium ion is essential for proper function of most enzyme systems, and a depletion is characterized by neuromuscular and central nervous system hyperactivity. The signs and symptoms are quite similar to those of calcium deficiency and include hyperactive tendon reflexes, muscle tremors, and tetany with a positive Chvostek sign. Progression to delirium and convulsions may occur with a severe deficit. A concomitant calcium deficiency is occasionally noted in these patients, particularly in those with clinical signs of tetany.

The diagnosis of magnesium deficiency depends on an awareness of the syndrome and clinical recognition of the symptoms. Laboratory confirmation is available but not reliable as the syndrome may exist in the presence of a normal serum magnesium level.

Treatment of magnesium deficiency is by the parenteral administration of magnesium sulfate or magnesium chloride solution. Magnesium sulfate (50 per cent solution contains approximately 4 mEq. of magnesium ion per milliliter) may be given intravenously or intramuscularly. The intravenous route is preferable for the initial treatment of a severe deficit and can be safely accomplished by the addition of 80 mEq. of magnesium sulfate (20 ml. of 50 per cent solution) to 1000 ml. of intravenous fluids administered over a two- to four-hour period. When large doses are given, the heart rate, blood pressure, respiration, and electrocardiogram should be monitored closely for signs of magnesium toxicity which could lead to cardiac arrect. Partial or complete relief of symptoms may follow this infusion as a result of increased concentration of magnesium ion in the extracellular fluid compartment, although continued replacement over a one- to three-week period is necessary to replenish the intracellular compartment. For this purpose, and for the asymptomatic patient who is likely to have significant magnesium depletion, 10 to 20 mEq. of 50 per cent magnesium sulfate solution is given daily intramuscularly, in divided doses. Multiple injection sites are used because the intramuscular injection of this solution is painful. Following complete repletion of intracellular magnesium and in the absence of abnormal loss, balance may be maintained by the administration of as little as 4 mEq. of magnesium ion daily.

Magnesium ion should not be given to the oliguric patient or in the presence of severe volume deficit unless actual magnesium depletion is demonstrated. If given to a patient with renal insufficiency, considerably smaller doses are used and the patient is carefully observed for signs or symptoms of toxicity.

NORMAL EXCHANGE OF FLUID AND ELECTROLYTES

Knowledge of the basic principles governing both the internal and external exchanges of water and salt is mandatory for care of the patient undergoing major operative surgery. The wide range of physiologic compensations in maintaining a constant internal fluid environment, which is accomplished by the kidney, brain, lung, skin, and gastrointestinal tract, may be compromised by severe surgical stress or direct damage to any of these organs.

Normal Water Exchange. The normal individual consumes roughly 2000 to 2500 ml. of water per day; approximately 1500 ml. of water is taken by mouth and the rest is extracted from solid food, either from water it contains or water of oxidation (Table 3-4). The daily water losses normally equal the amount gained. Normal losses include 250 ml. in stools, 800 to 1500 ml. as urine, and approximately 600 to 900 ml. as insensible loss. A patient deprived of all external access to water must still excrete a minimum of 500 to 800 ml. of urine per day in order to excrete the products of catabolism in addition to the mandatory insensible loss through the skin and lungs.

Insensible loss of water occurs through the skin (75 per cent) and the lungs (25 per cent) and is increased by hypermetabolism, hyperventilation, and fever. The insensible water loss through the skin is not from evaporation of water from sweat glands, but water vapor formed within the body and lost through the skin. With excessive heat production (or excessive environmental heat), the capacity for insensible loss through the skin is exceeded and sweating occurs. These losses may, but seldom do, exceed 250 ml. per day per degree of fever. An unhumidified tracheostomy with hyperventilation increases the loss through the lungs and results in a total insensible loss up to 1.5 L. per day.

A frequently overlooked source of gain is the water of solution, which is the water that holds carbohydrates and proteins in solution in the cell. Normally, gain of water from this source is zero, but after four to five days without food intake, the postoperative patient may begin to gain significant quantities of water (maximum 500 ml. daily) from ex-

Table 3-4. WATER EXCHANGE (60–80 Kg. Man)

H₂O GAIN–ROUTES	AVERAGE DAILY VOLUME (ml.)	MINIMAL (ml.)	MAXIMAL (ml.)
Sensible			
Oral fluids	800–1500	0	1500/hr.
Solid foods	500– 700	0	1500
Insensible			
Water of oxidation	250	125	800
Water of solution	0	0	500
H₂O LOSS–ROUTES			
Sensible			
Urine	800–1500	300	1400/hr. (diabetes insipidus)
Intestinal	0– 250	0	2500/hr.
Sweat	0	0	4000/hr.
Insensible			
Lungs and skin	600– 900	600–900	1500

Table 3–5.   Sodium (Salt) Exchange (60–80 Kg. Man)

Sodium exchange	Average	Minimal	Maximal
Sodium gain			
Diet	50–90 mEq./day	0	75–100 mEq./hr. (oral)
Sodium loss			
Skin (sweat)	10–60 mEq./day°	0	300 mEq./hr.
Urine	10–80 mEq./day	<1 mEq./day†	110–200 mEq./L.‡
Intestines	0–20 mEq./day	0	300 mEq./hr.

°Depending on the degree of acclimatization of the individual.
†With normal renal function.
‡With renal salt washing.

cessive cellular catabolism. The amount depends on the degree of trauma and the complications occurring postoperatively.

Salt Gain and Losses.   In the normal individual, the salt intake per day varies between 50 and 90 mEq. (3 to 5 gm.) as sodium chloride (Table 3–5). Balance is maintained primarily by the normal kidneys that excrete the excess salt. Under conditions of reduced intake or extrarenal losses, the normal kidney can reduce sodium excretion to less than 1 mEq./day within 24 hours after restriction. In the patient with salt-wasting kidneys, however, the loss may exceed 200 mEq./L. of urine. Sweat represents a hypotonic loss of fluids with an average sodium concentration of 15 mEq./L. in the acclimatized patient. In the unacclimatized individual, the sodium concentration in sweat may be 60 mEq./L. or more. Insensible fluid lost from the skin and lungs by definition is pure water. For practical considerations then, normal losses are relatively free of salt in a previously healthy individual.

The volume and composition of various types of gastrointestinal secretions fluid are shown in the Appendix. Gastrointestinal losses are usually isotonic or slightly hypotonic, although there is considerable variation in the composition. Their replacement should be by an essentially isotonic salt solution. It is also important to reiterate that distributional or sequestration losses at any point in the operative or postoperative course also represent isotonic losses of salt and water.

TYPES OF PARENTERAL SOLUTIONS

The composition of various parenteral fluids available for administration is shown in the Appendix. This list is of sufficient variety to manage the majority of fluid requirements in the surgical patient. The proper choice of parenteral fluid in a given situation will correct the abnormalities present while imposing minimal demands on the kidneys.

A good available isotonic salt solution for replacement of gastrointestinal losses and repair of pre-existing volume deficits, in the absence of gross abnormalities of concentration and composition, is lactated Ringer's solution. This solution is "physiologic" and contains 130 mEq. of sodium balanced by 109 mEq. of chloride and 28 mEq. of lactate. This fluid has minimal effects on normal body fluid composition and pH even when infused in large quantities. The chief disadvantage of lactated Ringer's solution is the slight hypo-osmolarity with respect to sodium. Each liter of lactated Ringer's solution furnishes approximately 100 to 150 ml. of free water. This represents little or no clinical problem if this fact is considered in calculating the water loss replacement.

The remainder of the solutions listed in the Appendix are used for correction of specific defects. The choice of a particular fluid depends on the volume status of the patient and the type of concentration or compositional abnormality present.

Isotonic sodium chloride contains 154 mEq. of sodium and 154 mEq. of chloride per liter. The high concentration of chloride above the normal serum concentration of 103 mEq./L imposes on the kidneys an appreciable load of excess chloride which cannot be rapidly excreted. Thus, a dilutional acidosis may develop.* This solution is ideal, however, for the initial correction of an extracellular fluid volume deficit in the presence of hyponatremia, hypochloremia, and metabolic alkalosis. In a similar situation with moderate metabolic acidosis, one-sixth molar sodium lactate (167 mEq. per liter each of sodium and lactate) may be given. Another solution for this purpose can be made by the addition of one ampule of sodium bicarbonate (40 ml. solution containing 40 mEq. each of sodium and bicarbonate) to 1000 ml. lactated Ringer's solution.

Molar sodium lactate or 3 or 5 per cent sodium chloride may be used for correction of symptomatic hyponatremic states. The choice of anion (lactate or chloride) is determined by the accompanying acid-base derangement.

The need for ammonium chloride solutions in the treatment of an uncompensated metabolic alkalosis is extremely rare. Indications for their use include very shallow or slow breathing with cyanosis or severe tetany.

Following the correction of concentration or compositional abnormalities using specific repair solutions, a balanced salt solution is used for repletion of the remaining volume deficit.

PREOPERATIVE FLUID THERAPY

Preoperative evaluation and correction of existing fluid disorders are integral parts of surgical care. An orderly approach to these prob-

---

*Infusion of a large volume of isotonic sodium chloride solution may induce or aggravate a pre-existing acidosis by reducing the amount of base bicarbonate in the body relative to the carbonic acid content.

lems requires an understanding of the common fluid disturbances associated with surgical illness and adherence to a few simple guidelines.

Changes in the volume of extracellular fluid are the most frequent
and important abnormalities encountered in the surgical patient. Depletion of the extracellular fluid compartment without changes in concentration or composition is the more common problem. The diagnosis
of volume changes is made almost entirely on clinical grounds as
alluded to previously. The signs that will be present in an individual
patient depend not only on the relative or absolute quantity of extracellular fluid which has been lost, but also on the rapidity with which it is
lost and the presence or absence of the signs of associated disease.

Volume deficits encountered in the surgical patient may occur as a
result of external loss of fluids or as a result of an internal redistribution
of extracellular fluid into a nonfunctional compartment. Generally, it
involves a combination of the two, but the internal redistribution is
frequently overlooked.

The phenomenon of internal redistribution or translocation of extracellular fluid is peculiar to many surgical diseases, and in the individual patient the loss may be quite large. Although the concept of a
"third space" is not new, it is generally thought of only in relation to
patients with massive ascites, burns, or crush injuries. Of more importance, however, is the "third space" loss into the peritoneum, the
bowel wall, and other tissues with inflammatory lesions of the intra-
abdominal organs. The magnitude of these losses may not be fully
appreciated without realization of the fact that the peritoneum alone is
approximately 1 square meter in surface area. A slight increase in
thickness from sequestration of fluid, which would not be appreciated
on casual observation, may result in a functional loss of several liters of
fluid. Swelling of the bowel wall and mesentery and secretion of fluid
into the lumen of the bowel will cause even larger losses. Similar
deficits may occur with massive infection of the subcutaneous tissues
(necrotizing fasciitis) or with severe crush injury.

These "parasitic" losses remain a part of the extracellular fluid
space and may be measured as a slowly equilibrating volume. The term
nonfunctional is used because the fluid is no longer able to participate
in the normal functions of the extracellular fluid compartment and may
just as well have been lost externally. Any transfer of intracellular fluid
to the extracellular compartment for replenishment of the loss is insignificant in the acute phase. The patient with ascites may have an
enormous total extracellular fluid volume, although the functional component is severely depleted. The same is true of extensive inflammatory or obstructive lesions of the gastrointestinal tract, although the loss
is not as obvious. These losses will evoke the signs and symptoms of an
extracellular fluid volume deficit with or without the concomitant external loss of fluids.

Exact quantitation of these deficits is both quantitatively impossible and, at the present time, probably unnecessary. An estimate of the defect can be made based on the severity of the clinical signs. A mild deficit represents a loss of approximately 4 per cent of body weight; a moderate deficit, 6 to 8 per cent of body weight; and a severe deficit, approximately 10 per cent of body weight. It is important to re-emphasize the fact that cardiovascular signs predominate, with acute rapid loss of fluid from the extracellular fluid compartment and few to no tissue signs.

Fluid replacement should be started and changes made depending on the response of the patient as noted by frequent clinical observation. The reliance on a single clinical sign to determine adequacy of resuscitation is fraught with danger. Rather, reversal of the signs of the volume deficit combined with stabilization of the blood pressure and pulse and an hourly urine volume of 30 to 50 ml. is used as a general guideline. Reliance on only a good hourly urine output, although usually a good index of volume replacement, may be totally misleading. The excessive administration of glucose (over 50 gm. in a two- to three-hour period) may result in osmotic diuresis, whereas an osmotic agent such as mannitol tends to produce urine at the expense of the vascular volume. Patients with chronic renal disease of incipient acute renal damage occurring from shock and injury may also have inappropriately high urinary volumes. In addition, the rapid administration of salt solutions may transiently expand the intravascular volume and result in an immediate outpouring of urine, although the total extracellular fluid space is still quite depleted.

The choice of the proper fluid for replacement depends on the existence of concomitant concentration or compositional abnormalities. With pure extracellular fluid volume loss or when only minimal concentration or compositional abnormalities are present, the use of a balanced salt solution, such as lactated Ringer's, is desirable.

If severe symptomatic hyponatremia or hypernatremia complicates the volume loss, prompt correction of the concentration abnormality to the extent that symptoms are relieved is necessary. Replenishment of volume should then be accomplished with slower correction of the remaining concentration abnormality. For immediate correction of severe hyponatremia, 5 per cent sodium chloride solution or molar sodium lactate solution should be used, depending on the patient's acid-base status. In any case, the sodium deficit should be estimated by multiplying the decrease in serum sodium below normal times the liters of extracellular water, taken as 20 per cent of the body weight. Half this amount of sodium should be administered slowly, followed by clinical and chemical re-evaluation of the patient before further administration of sodium.

In the treatment of moderate hyponatremia with an associated volume deficit, volume replacement can be started immediately with concomitant correction of the serum sodium. Isotonic sodium chloride solution (normal saline) is used initially in the presence of metabolic alkalosis, whereas one-sixth molar sodium lactate is used to correct associated acidosis. Only 1 to 2 L. of these solutions may be necessary to correct the serum sodium concentration, and the remainder of the volume deficit may be repaired with lactated Ringer's solution. Treatment of hyponatremia associated with volume excess is by restriction of water.

Correction of hypernatremia may be concomitant with replenishment of volume, using half-strength sodium chloride or half-strength lactated Ringer's solution.

The rate of administration of fluid varies considerably, depending on the severity and type of fluid disturbance, the presence of continuing losses, and the cardiac status of the patient. In general, severe volume deficits may be safely replaced initially at a rate of approximately 2000 ml./hour with a subsequent reduction as the fluid status improves. The fluids may be given more rapidly if necessary, but constant observation of the patient is mandatory in this situation. In addition, with rapid administration, a significant portion of the fluid may be lost as urinary output owing to a transient overexpansion of the plasma volume.

In the elderly patient, the existence of associated cardiovascular disorders does not preclude the correction of existing volume deficits. Rather, it requires slower, more careful correction with constant monitoring of all functions, including the central venous pressure.

Hypertonic salt solutions should be given under close supervision, and the rate of administration should not exceed 200 ml./hour.

Correction of existing potassium deficits should be instituted after an adequate urine output is obtained, particularly in the patient with metabolic alkalosis, because the alkalosis may be secondary to, or aggravated by, a potassium depletion. Potassium chloride is available in 20-mEq. and 40-mEg. ampules for addition to intravenous fluids. A maximum of 40 mEq. of potassium chloride per hour may be safely administered to the adult of average size who is not severely depleted of extracellular fluid volume, in frank hypovolemic shock, or in established oliguric or high output renal failure. The concentration of potassium chloride should not exceed 40 mEq./L. of intravenous fluids, with rare exceptions, such as the treatment of digitalis intoxication during which constant monitoring of the electrocardiogram is essential.

Calcium and magnesium are rarely needed during preoperative resuscitation, but should be given if any doubt exists, particularly in patients with massive subcutaneous infections, those with acute pancreatitis, and those who have been chronically starved.

The existence of fluid abnormalities also must be considered in the patient for whom an elective procedure is planned. Chronic illness is frequently associated with extracellular fluid volume deficits, and concentration and compositional changes are not uncommon. Correction of anemia and recognition of the fact that a contracted blood volume may exist in the chronically debilitated patient are of obvious importance. The choice of whole blood versus packed cells for correction of anemia depends on the volume status. If there is any question, one unit of packed cells may be given with subsequent determination of the hemoglobin and hematocrit. The hemoglobin generally increases approximately 2 gm. following the infusion of 250 cc. of packed cells in the adult of average size. The increase will be significantly greater than 2 gm. per cent in the patient with a contracted intravascular volume, indicating the probable need for whole blood transfusions. If available, measurement of the blood volume is obviously more accurate.

Of additional importance is the prevention of volume depletion during the preoperative period. Prolonged periods of fluid restriction in preparation for various diagnostic procedures and the use of cathartics and enema for preparation of the bowel may cause a significant acute loss of extracellular fluid. Prompt recognition and treatment of these losses are necessary for prevention of complications during the operative period.

INTRAOPERATIVE MANAGEMENT OF FLUIDS

If replacement of extracellular fluid volume has been incomplete preoperatively, hypotension may develop promptly with the induction of anesthesia. This can be quite insidious as the awake patient can compensate for mild volume deficit which is revealed only when the compensatory mechanisms are abolished with anesthesia. This problem is prevented by maintenance of baseline requirements and replacement of abnormal losses of fluids and electrolytes by intravenous infusions in the preoperative period.

Blood loss during the operative procedure should be replaced as steadily as it is lost. It is probably unnecessary to replace blood loss of less than 500 cc., but after the loss has exceeded this, replacement should begin. The warnings against the use of a single transfusion during operation have been somewhat confusing. There is a very definite need for a single unit transfusion in the patient who loses between 500 and 1000 cc. of blood during operation.

In addition to blood losses that occur directly in operative surgery, there also appear to be losses of extracellular fluid during major operative procedures. Some of these losses, including edema from extensive dissection, collections within the lumen and wall of the small bowel, and accumulations of fluid in the peritoneal cavity, are clinically discernible and well recognized. Such losses are generally felt to represent distributional shifts, in that the functional volume of extracellular fluid is reduced but not externally lost from the body. These functional losses are often referred to as "a parasitic loss of extracellular fluid," a "third space edema," or "a sequestration" of extracellular fluid. Another source of loss of extracellular fluid during major operative trauma is the wound itself. This is a relatively smaller loss, and is very difficult to quantitate except in extensive and major operative procedures.

At the beginning of this century, surgeons became aware that many changes occurred in urinary output, blood volume, and fluid and electrolyte composition during and after operative surgery. Assessment of these changes, however, awaited the development of analytic techniques and their application to patient-studies. In the following 25 years, saline solutions were given in varying combinations to patients undergoing operative surgery. Often administration of such fluids was excessive. Work in the late 1930s and early 1940s by Dr. Carl Moyer, and by many others, indicated that during and after operative procedures, saline and water solutions should be withheld entirely, because if small amounts of water or saline solutions were given during or after a major operative procedure, most of the fluid administered was retained. The possibility existed that the operative and postoperative retention of salt and water, when administered in these relatively small amounts, might simply be physiologic retention to replace a deficit of salt and water incurred by the operative procedure. Subsequent studies have revealed that a decrease in functional extracellular fluid occurs with major abdominal operations. Preliminary data indicate that this loss is a sequestered loss into the operative site. Replacement of this extracellular fluid volume deficit can be accomplished with a balanced salt solution during the operative procedure. These data have led to the conclusion that the need for an extracellular "mimic" in the form of balanced salt solution during operation therefore would seem to approximate 500 ml./hour, unless there are other measurable losses.

Correction of the volume deficit during operation markedly reduces "postoperative salt intolerance." Salt administration during the procedure is not intended to be a substitute for blood replacement. It is felt rather to be a physiologic supplement, or adjunct.

The pendulum swung from indiscriminate use of salt solutions in the first quarter of this century, to almost total withholding of fluid and electrolytes from surgical patients in the second quarter of the century. Studies at present seem to indicate that the proper management lies somewhere between these two extremes.

Several qualifying remarks should be made about the intraoperative administration of saline solutions as a "mimic" for the extracellular fluid. Since the sequestration of extracellular fluid in patients undergoing operative surgery varies from an almost imperceptible minimum to a high of approximately 3 L. during an uncomplicated procedure, these losses are extremely difficult to quantitate with the presently available means of measuring functional extracellular fluid. Consequently, no accurate formula for administration of fluids during operative procedures can yet be derived. Several arbitrary clinically useful guidelines would include the following: (1) As mentioned previously, blood should be given as lost. This replacement of blood loss is irrespective of any additional fluid and electrolyte therapy that may be given. (2) The replacement of extracellular fluid should begin during the operative procedure and should not be delayed until the postoperative period. Recent data reveal that if the operative replacement of extracellular fluid is delayed until the adrenal compensatory mechanisms have already started to react to the operative trauma, dangerous overloads may be produced by delayed administration of fluids in the immediate postoperative period. (3) A recent series of 670 patients undergoing major aortoiliac reconstructive operation reported by Thompson shows a useful guideline regimen. In this group of patients, the average amount of Ringer's lactate administered was 3555 ml., giving an average intraoperative replacement of salt solution of 677 ml./hour of operative procedure. This was in addition to whole blood replacement. In the last six years of this study, there were two deaths in 298 operations, an operative mortality of 0.67 per cent. Among the entire 670 patients, only two patients died of renal failure, an incidence of 0.3 per cent. Most series in the literature report an incidence of renal failure of some degree, in this type of surgery, to as high as 36 per cent, with a mortality rate from renal failure as high as 12 per cent. (4) Utilizing the above regimen, results indicate an extremely low incidence of renal failure even in the presence of extensive operative trauma. In this series, none of the patients developed pulmonary edema or pulmonary failure, even though this was a series of patients with standardized, major operative trauma.

Balance studies reveal that the nonfunctional fluid volume which is sequestered into the operative site does become functional again in 24 hours to 5 days. If this deficit has been replaced during surgery, the resultant diuresis is so minimal, over the next 1 to 5 days, that it is hardly discernible without balance studies. Nevertheless, there is a slow reinfusion of extracellular fluid from this area of sequestration. As with all fluid replacement in the aged, or in patients with cardiovascular disease, care should be used to maintain slow rates of infusion with careful monitoring. This will include such parameters as central venous pressure, urinary output, and clinical signs of adequate cardiovascular function.

POSTOPERATIVE MANAGEMENT OF FLUIDS

Immediate Postoperative Period. Orders for postoperative fluid are not written until the patient is in the recovery room and the fluid status has been assessed. Evaluation at this point should include a review of preoperative fluid status, the amount of fluid loss and gain during operation, and clinical examination of the patient with assess-

ment of the vital signs and urinary output. Initial fluid orders are
written to correct any *existing* deficit followed by maintenance fluids
for the remainder of the day. In the patient with complications who has
received or lost large amounts of fluid, it is frequently difficult to
estimate the fluid requirements for the ensuing 24 hours. In this situation, intravenous fluids are ordered 1 liter at a time and the patient
checked frequently until the situation is clarified. Proper replacement
of fluids during this relatively short period will facilitate subsequent
fluid management.

Immediately after operation, extracellular fluid volume depletion
may occur as a result of continued losses of fluid at the site of injury or
operative trauma—for example, into the wall or lumen of the small
intestine. Several liters of extracellular fluid may be deposited in such
areas within a period of a few hours or more slowly in the first day or so
from the time of injury. Unrecognized deficits of extracellular fluid
volume during the early postoperative period are manifest primarily as
circulatory instability. The signs of volume deficiency in other organ
systems may be delayed for several hours in this type of fluid loss. The
presence of hypotension and tachycardia postoperatively requires
prompt investigation regarding the cause, followed by appropriate therapy. The generally accepted adequacy of blood pressure of 90 over 60
and a pulse of less than 120 in postoperative patients may not be
sufficient to prevent renal ischemia unless, in addition to lack of signs
of shock, urine flow is adequate. Evaluation of the level of consciousness, pupillary size, airway patency, breathing patterns, pulse rate and
volume, skin warmth, color, body temperature, and a 30- to 50-ml.
hourly urine output combined with a critical review of the operative
procedure and the operative fluid management is usually rewarding.
Since operative trauma frequently involves a loss or transfer of significant quantities of whole blood, plasma, or extracellular fluid which can
be only grossly estimated, circulatory instability is most commonly
caused by an underestimation of the initial losses or insidious, con-
cealed, continued losses. Operative blood loss is usually estimated by
the operating room surgeon to be 15 to 40 per cent less than the
isotopically measured blood loss from that patient. In addition, several
liters of extravascular, extracellular fluid can be sequestered in areas of
injury and be manifested only by oliguria and mild depression of the
blood pressure with a rapid pulse. In a patient with circulatory instability, further volume replacement of an additional 1000 cc. of isotonic
salt solution, while determining whether continuing losses or other
causes are present, often resolves the circulatory instability. Vigorous
pursuit of contributing causes with all diagnostic aids must be carried
out before excessive volumes of fluid have been administered.

It is unnecessary and probably unwise to administer potassium
during the first 24 hours postoperatively, unless a definite potassium
deficit exists. This is particularly important in the patient subjected to

prolonged operative trauma involving one or more episodes of hypotension and in the post-traumatic patient with hemorrhagic hypotension. Oliguric renal failure or the more insidious high-output renal failure may develop, and the administration of even a small quantity of potassium may be quite detrimental.

Later Postoperative Period. The problem of volume management during the postoperative convalescent phase is one of accurate measurement and replacement of all losses. In the otherwise healthy individual, this involves the replacement of measured sensible losses, which are generally of gastrointestinal origin, and the estimation and replacement of insensible losses. The insensible loss is relatively constant in the usual patient and will average 600 to 900 ml. daily. This loss may be increased by hypermetabolism, hyperventilation, and fever to a maximum of approximately 1500 ml. daily. The estimated loss is replaced with 5 per cent dextrose in water. As alluded to previously, this loss may be partially offset by an insensible gain of water from excessive tissue catabolism in the complicated postoperative patient, particularly if associated with oliguric renal failure.

Approximately 1 liter of fluid should be given to replace that volume of urine required to excrete the catabolic end products of metabolism (800 to 1000 cc. per day). In the individual with normal renal function, this may be given as 5 per cent dextrose in water because the kidneys are able to conserve sodium with excretion of less than 1 mEq. daily. It is probably unwise to stress the kidneys to this degree, however, and a modest amount of salt solution should be given to cover urinary loss. In the elderly patient with salt-losing kidneys or in patients with head injuries, an insidious hyponatremia may develop if urinary losses are replaced with water. Urinary sodium in these circumstances may exceed 100 mEq./L. and result in a daily loss of significant amounts of sodium. Measurement of urinary sodium will facilitate accurate replacement.

Urine volume is not replaced on a milliliter-for-milliliter basis. A urinary output of 2000 to 3000 ml. on a given day may simply represent diuresis of fluids given during surgery or may represent excessive administration of fluids. If these large losses are completely replaced, the urine output will progressively increase, and may logically progress to a unique situation resembling diabetes insipidus with urinary outputs in excess of 10 liters daily.

Sensible losses by definition can be measured or, as in the case of sweating, an estimate of the amount can be made. Gastrointestinal losses are usually isotonic, or slightly hypotonic, and their replacement is made with an essentially isotonic salt solution. When the estimated loss is slightly above or below isotonicity, appropriate corrections can be made in the daily water administration while isotonic salt solutions are used to replace these losses, volume for volume.

Sweating is not usually a problem except in the febrile patient in whom losses may, but seldom do, exceed 250 ml. per day per degree of fever. Excessive sweating may, in addition, represent a considerable loss of sodium in the unacclimatized individual.

Determination of serum electrolytes is generally unnecessary in the patient with an uncomplicated postoperative course maintained on parenteral fluids for two or three days. A more prolonged period requiring parenteral replacement or one complicated by excessive fluid losses requires frequent determinations of the serum sodium, potassium, chloride, and carbon dioxide combining power. Adjustments can then be made by the use of intravenous fluids of appropriate composition. For example, replacement of gastrointestinal losses with isotonic sodium chloride solution is indicated in a patient with hyponatremia, hypochloremia, and mild metabolic alkalosis, and should be continued until these abnormalities are corrected. In the hyponatremic patient with obvious overload, the amount of water given is restricted. In the presence of hyponatremia and mild metabolic acidosis one-sixth molar sodium lactate or lactated Ringer's solution with added sodium bicarbonate may be used. In this way, then, severe concentration and compositional changes can be avoided while an adequate extracellular fluid is maintained by administration of appropriate maintenance fluids.

Maintenance fluids are administered at a steady rate over an 18- to 24-hour period as the losses are incurred. If given over a shorter period of time, renal excretion of the excess salt and water may occur while the normal losses continue over the full 24-hour period. For the same reason, fluids of different composition are altered and additives to intravenous fluids (e.g., potassium chloride and antibiotics) are evenly distributed in the total volume of fluid given.

In summary, daily fluid orders should begin with an assessment of the patient's volume status and a check for possible concentration or compositional disorders as reflected by proper laboratory determinations. Replacement of all measured and insensible losses with fluids of appropriate composition is carried out with allowance made for any pre-existing deficit or excess.

Replacement of potassium includes 40 mEq. daily for renal excretion of potassium in addition to approximately 20 mEq./L. for replacement of gastrointestinal losses. Inadequate replacement may prolong the usual postoperative ileus and contribute to the insidious development of a resistant metabolic alkalosis.

Calcium and magnesium are replaced when needed as previously discussed.

SPECIAL CONSIDERATIONS IN THE POSTOPERATIVE PATIENT

Volume Excesses.   The administration of isotonic solutions in excess of volume losses (external or internal) will result in overexpansion of the extracellular fluid spaces. The otherwise normal person in a postoperative state tolerates an acute overexpansion extremely well. Excesses administered over a period of several days, however, will soon exceed the kidney's ability to excrete sodium; and since water losses continue, hypernatremia will ensue. Therefore, it is important to determine as accurately as possible from intake and output records and serum sodium concentrations the actual needs of the patient managed over several postoperative days.

Attention to the signs and symptoms of overload usually prevents this fluid abnormality. It arises most frequently in an attempt to meet excessive volume losses that are not measurable, such as those occurring from drainage of a fistula that is not totally controlled.

The earliest sign is a weight gain (when obtainable) during the catabolic period when the patient should be losing one-fourth to one-half pound per day. Heavy eyelids, hoarseness, or dyspnea on exertion may rapidly appear. Circulatory and pulmonary signs of overload are late in appearance and represent a rather massive overload. Peripheral edema may be a sign of, but does not necessarily indicate, volume excess. In the absence of additional evidence for volume overload, other causes of peripheral edema should be considered. Of particular importance is the fact that overexpansion of the *total* extracellular fluid may co-exist with a *depletion* of the functional extracellular fluid compartment.

The use of central venous pressure is of limited usefulness in following volume replacement. A rise in central venous pressure above normal is indicative of too rapid administration of fluid, but does not accurately establish volume status of the patient.

Hyponatremia. Significant postoperative changes in serum sodium concentration are not frequently observed if the fluid resuscitation during operation has included adequate volumes of isotonic salt solutions. The kidneys retain the ability to excrete moderate excesses of salt water administered in the early postoperative period if adequate replacement of functional extracellular fluid has been given during the operative or immediate postoperative period. Previous studies of sodium balance have revealed that patients do excrete sodium when replacement of a functional deficit incurred by the shift of extracellular fluid has been replaced. The normal capacity to excrete water postoperatively has been demonstrated by Wright and Gann when isotonic salt solutions are administered prior to a challenge with a water load. Thus, the commonly described hyponatremia associated with surgical procedures and traumatic injury is prevented by the replacement of extracellular fluid deficits. A daily maintenance of normal osmolarity is then simplified to the replacement of observable losses of known sodium content.

Hyponatremia may easily occur when water is given to replace losses of sodium-containing fluids or when water administration consistently exceeds the water losses. The latter may occur with oliguria or in association with decreased water loss through the skin and lungs, intracellular shifts of sodium, or the cellular release of excessive amounts of endogenous water. Severe or refractory hyponatremia, however, is difficult to produce if renal function remains normal.

REPLACEMENT OF SODIUM LOSSES WITH WATER. A common error is replacement of gastrointestinal losses with only water or a hypotonic solution. Patients with head injury or with pre-existing renal disease (loss of concentrating ability) may elaborate urine with a high salt concentration (50 to 200 mEq./L.). Progressive hyponatremia in the patient with head injury, despite adequate administration of salt, is believed to be due to excessive secretion of antidiuretic hormone with consequent water retention. Replacement of these urinary losses with water for a short time may result in hyponatremia, accompanied by symptoms of water intoxication.

DECREASES IN URINARY VOLUME. Oliguria, from whatever cause (prerenal or renal), reduces the daily water requirements if not corrected. The metabolic acidosis produced by the retention of nitrogenous waste products increases the cellular release of water. Therefore, the gain of endogenous water decreases the total water requirement beyond those expected when urinary volume is low.

DECREASED INSENSIBLE LOSS. Cutaneous vasoconstriction from any cause decreases both insensible and evaporative water loss by this route. This situation is most commonly encountered in the use of generalized hypothermia.

ENDOGENOUS WATER RELEASE. The patient maintained on intravenous fluids will, between the fifth and tenth days, release the intracellular water solutions as cells disrupt, thus decreasing the quantity of exogenous water required per day.

INTRACELLULAR SHIFTS. Systemic bacterial sepsis is often accompanied by a precipitous drop in serum sodium concentration. This sudden change in extracellular fluid sodium concentration is poorly understood, but usually accompanies loss of extracellular fluid volume as either interstitial or intracellular sequestrations. This can be treated by withholding water, restoring extracellular fluid volume, and initiating treatment of the sepsis.

Many hyponatremic states are asymptomatic until the serum sodium level falls below 120 mEq./L. The moderate asymptomatic hyponatremia, however, signifies inappropriate therapy or points to the diagnosis of the basic underlying condition. Symptomatic hyponatremia or water intoxication is difficult to produce if renal function is normal. Convulsions and apnea from uncorrected water excesses occur most often in children and elderly adults. Within the limits imposed by the circulatory apparatus, these deficits should be corrected by the administration of hypertonic salt solution to a serum sodium level above 130 mEq./L. Mild or moderate degrees of hyponatremia may be simply corrected by temporary restriction of the intake of water.

Hypernatremia. Hypernatremia (serum sodium concentration above 150 mEq./L.), although uncommon, is a dangerous abnormality. In contradistinction to decreased serum sodium concentration, hypernatremia is easily produced when renal function is normal.

The extracellular fluid hyperosmolarity results in a shift of intracellular water from within the cell to the extracellular fluid compartment; in this situation, the presence of a high serum sodium level may indicate a significant deficit of total body water.

In surgical patients hypernatremia arises most often from excessive or unexpected water losses, although it may occur as a result of use of salt-containing solutions to replace water losses. The following classification of water losses may be helpful in preventing and treating this abnormality.

EXCESSIVE EXTRARENAL WATER LOSSES. With increased metabolism from any cause, but particularly associated with fever, the water loss through evaporation of sweat may reach 200 to 300 ml./hour (3 to 3½ L./day). Patients with tracheostomy in dry environments can (with excessive minute volume air exchange) evaporate as much as 1 to 1.5 L. water per day by this route. The increased evaporation of water from a granulating surface is of significant magnitude in the thermally injured patient, and water losses may be as great as 3 to 5 L./day.

INCREASED RENAL WATER LOSSES. Extremely large volumes of solute-poor urine may occur from hypoxic damage to the distal tubules and collecting ducts or loss of antidiuretic hormone stimulation from damage to the central nervous system. In both instances, facultative water resorption is impaired. The former occurs in high-output renal failure, and in our experience this is the most common type of renal failure following severe injury or operative trauma. The latter occurs with extensive head injuries in which a temporary state of diabetes insipidus occurs.

SOLUTE LOADING. High protein intake may produce an increased osmotic load of urea which necessitates the excretion of large volumes of water. Hypernatremia, azotemia, and extracellular fluid volume deficits follow. In general, these can be prevented by furnishing 7 ml. water per gram of dietary protein.

Excessive glucose administration results in the need for a large volume of water for excretion. In this situation, hypernatremia occurs more rapidly.

In addition, all osmotic diuretics such as mannitol and urea result in the obligatory excretion of a large volume of water as well as increasing urinary sodium losses. Isotonic salt solutions, if used to replace pure water losses, rapidly produce hypernatremia.

Acid-Base Derangements. Significant problems of acid-base control are frequent in the postoperative period. Of particular importance are the derangements that occur in patients with pulmonary complications, hypoxic renal damage, and those conditions requiring prolonged parenteral fluid management.

RESPIRATORY ACIDOSIS. This problem is particularly serious in the patient with chronic pulmonary disease in whom pre-existing respiratory acidosis may be accentuated in the postoperative period. A number of conditions resulting in inadequate ventilation—airway obstruction, atelectasis, pneumonia, pleural effusion, hypoventilation caused by the pain of upper abdominal incisions, or abdominal distention limiting diaphragmatic excursion—may exist singly or in combination to produce respiratory acidosis. Although restlessness, hypertension, and tachycardia in the immediate postoperative period may be due to pain, similar signs are indicative of inadequate ventilation with hypercapnia. The use of narcotics in this situation will compound the problem by further depressing respiration.

Management involves prompt correction of the pulmonary defect when feasible and measures to ensure adequate ventilation. Tracheostomy and mechanical assistance to ventilation are occasionally necessary to achieve this objective.

RESPIRATORY ALKALOSIS. Respiratory alkalosis is a more common problem in the surgical patient than was previously recognized. Hyperventilation caused by apprehension, pain, and CNS injury, and hyperventilation produced by mechanical respirators, either inadvertently or in an attempt to raise the pO_2 in the hypoxic patient, are common causes.

Mild respiratory alkalosis is of little consequence in the majority of patients and requires no therapy. One important exception is the patient with impaired cerebral blood flow from obstructive arterial disease or during performance of carotid endarterectomy, in whom modest hypocapnia with cerebral vasoconstriction may cause irreparable damage. Correction of severe, persistent respiratory alkalosis is necessary but often difficult because of the underlying causes of hyperventilation.

METABOLIC ACIDOSIS. Renal damage may interfere with the important role of the kidneys in the regulation of acid-base control. The kidneys serve a vital function in the normal maintenance of acid-base equilibrium through the excretion of nitrogenous waste products and acid metabolites and the reabsorption of bicarbonates. If renal damage occurs and these functions are lost, a rapidly developing metabolic acidosis ensues. With normal kidneys, acidosis may develop when capacity of the kidneys in handling chlorides is exceeded.

Metabolic derangements of acid-base balance are common in patients maintained on parenteral fluid for several days. Metabolic derangements of acid-base balance are common in patients maintained on parenteral fluid for several days. Metabolic acidosis may develop when there is excessive loss of alkaline gastrointestinal fluids from the pancreas and lower intestinal tract. The administration of fluids with an inappropriate chloride-bicarbonate ratio, such as isotonic sodium chloride solution, will not correct the pH change, and the use of a balanced salt solution, such as lactated Ringer's, is indicated.

Acute circulatory failure often produces a profound metabolic acidosis owing to lactic acid accumulation. This is a reflection of tissue hypoxia caused by inadequate perfusion, although it is only one of the manifestations of cellular dysfunction. Severe acidosis per se will impair circulation by decreasing the responsiveness of the myocardium and vascular smooth muscle to epinephrine, but attempts to correct the acidosis by large amounts of sodium bicarbonate without restoration of flow are futile. Following restoration of adequate tissue perfusion in a patient with hemorrhagic hypotension of short duration, the lactic acid is quickly metabolized and pH returned to normal. The use of lactated Ringer's solution to replace the extracellular fluid deficit incurred with hemorrhagic shock concomitant with administration of whole blood does not accentuate the lactic acidosis. Instead, there is a rapid decrease of lactate and return of pH to normal, as opposed to the use of whole blood alone.

In the more protracted states of metabolic acidosis and following cardiac arrest, the adjunctive use of sodium bicarbonate is essential for proper resuscitation.

METABOLIC ALKALOSIS. Metabolic alkalosis occurs from uncompensated loss of acids or retention of bases and is closely related to potassium metabolism. The majority of patients with metabolic alkalosis have some degree of hypokalemia. Depletion of cellular potassium results in entry of hydrogen and sodium ions into the cell with a resultant lowering of intracellular pH and extracellular alkalosis. Metabolic alkalosis, in turn, results in excessive urinary potassium loss in exchange for sodium, which further accentuates the alkalosis. The dangers of metabolic alkalosis are those related to potassium depletion and include cardiac arrhythmias, tetany, sensitivity to digitalis, and paralytic ileus.

An interesting and not infrequent problem in the surgical patient is hypochloremic, hypokalemic metabolic alkalosis as a result of persistent vomiting or gastric suction in the patient with pyloric obstruction. Unlike vomiting with an open pylorus (involving a loss of gastric, pancreatic, biliary, and intestinal secretions), this situation results in a loss of fluid with high chloride and hydrogen ion concentration in relation to sodium. The loss of chloride causes an initial accelerated loss of sodium in the urine and partial compensation of the alkalosis. Subsequently, however, potassium and hydrogen ions are excreted into the urine in increasing quantities in an attempt to conserve sodium, resulting in an uncompensated alkalosis and hypokalemia. The initially alkaline urine becomes acid after a period of time owing to the hydrogen ion excretion ("paradoxic aciduria"). Proper management includes replacement of the volume deficit with isotonic sodium chloride solution in addition to replacement of potassium.

REFERENCES

Allen, K. G., Harkins, H. N., Moyer, C. A., and Rhoads, J. E.: Surgery: Principles and Practice. Philadelphia, J. B. Lippincott Company, 1961.

Bartlett, W. C.: Acute hyperparathyroid crisis. Amer. J. Surg. *114*:796, 1967.

Baxter, C. R., Zedlitz, W. H., and Shires, G. T.: High-output acute renal failure complicating traumatic injury. J. Trauma *4*:567, 1964.

Berliner, R. W., Kennedy, T. J., Jr., and Orloff, J.: Relationship between acidification of the urine and potassium metabolism. Amer. J. Med. *11*:274, 1951.

Berry, R. E. L.: The pathophysiology and management of complex problems of body fluid homeostasis attending surgical disease states. Surg. Clin. N. Amer. *149*:342, 1952.

DeCosse, J. J., Randall, H. T., Habif, D. V., and Roberts, K. E.: The mechanism of hyponatremia and hypotonicity after surgical trauma. Surgery *40*:27, 1956.

Henzel, J. H., DeWeese, M. S.. and Ridenhour, G.: Significance of magnesium and zinc metabolism in the surgical patient. I. Magnesium. Arch. Surg. *95*:974, 1967.

Jenkins, M. T., and Beck, G. P.: Differential diagnosis of hypotension occuring during anesthesia and surgery. Amer. J. Surg. *116*:669, 1968.

Latimer, R. G., Rees, V. L., and Peterson, C. N.: Hypercalcemic crisis treated with inorganic phosphate solution. Amer. J. Surg. *116*:669, 1968.

McClelland, R. N., et al.: Balanced salt solutions in the treatment of hemorrhagic shock. J.A.M.A. *199*:166, 1967.

Moncrief, J. A., and Mason, A. D.: Water vapor loss in the burned patient. Surg. Forum *13*:38, 1962.

Moore, F. D., et al.: Body Cell Mass and Its Supporting Environment: Body Composition in Health and Disease. Philadelphia, W. B. Saunders Company, 1963.

Moyer, C. A.: Fluid Balance. Chicago, Year Book Publishers, Inc., 1954.

Pitts, R. F.: Physiology of Kidney and Body Fluids. Chicago, Year Book Publishers, Inc., 1963.

Randall, H. T.: Fluid and electrolyte therapy in surgery; *In* Schwartz, S. I.: Principles of Surgery. New York, McGraw-Hill Book Company, 1969.

Randall, H. T., and Roberts, K. E.: The significance and treatment of acidosis and alkalosis in surgical patients. Surg. Clin. N. Amer., *36*:315, 1956.

Schwartz, W. B., and Relman, A. S.: A critique of the parameters used in the evaluation of acid-base disorders. N. Eng. J. Med. *268*:1382, 1963.

Shires, G. T.: What's new in surgery, shock, and metabolism. Surg. Gynec. & Obstet. *124*:284, 1967.

Shires, G. T., and Carrico, C. J.: Current status of the shock problem. Curr. Probl. Surg., March, 1966.

Shires, G. T., Coln, D., Carrico, J., and Lightfoot, S.: Fluid therapy in hemorrhagic shock. Arch. Surg. *88*:688, 1964.

Shires, G. T., and Holman, V.: Dilutional acidosis. Ann. Int. Med. *28*:551, 1948.

Shires, G. T., and Jackson, D. E.: Postoperative salt tolerance. Arch. Surg. *84*:703, 1962.

Shires, G. T., Williams, J., and Brown, F.: Acute changes in extracellular fluids associated with major surgical procedures. Ann. Surg. *154*:803, 1961.

Thompson, J. E., Vollman, R. W., Austin, D. J, and Kartchner, M. M.: Prevention of hypotensive and renal complications of aortic surgery using balanced salt solution. Ann. Surg. *167*:767, 1968.

Wright, H. K., and Gann, D. S.: Correction of defect in free water excretion in postoperative patients by extracellular fluid volume expansion. Ann. Surg. *158*:70, 1963.

Zimmerman, B.: Postoperative management of fluid volumes and electrolytes. Curr. Probl. Surg., Dec., 1965.

CHAPTER 4

SURGICAL NUTRITION: PARENTERAL AND ORAL

Henry T. Randall, M.D.

The purpose of this chapter is to discuss problems of nutrition in patients of interest to the surgeon. Its focus is on the types of patients for whom adequate nutrition is essential, or of great benefit, during stages of their illness when adequate oral intake of food is not possible. Such patients constitute a small but difficult and challenging part of surgical practice.

Recent advances in understanding of the requirements of seriously ill patients for calories, amino acids, electrolytes, vitamins, and trace elements, together with major improvements in available materials and methods of administering chemically defined mixtures of nutrients intravenously, or into segments of the gastrointestinal tract, permit reduction or even correction of depletion of body reserves. It is now possible to give the substrates necessary for normal metabolic needs, for wound healing, for assistance in control of sepsis, and even for normal growth, without a normally functioning gastrointestinal tract.

Most severely ill surgical patients are also starving, or nearly so, and many chronically ill patients who must undergo surgery have lost weight and depleted body reserves to a serious degree. It is for such patients that nutrition is of great importance.

BODY COMPOSITION AND FUEL RESERVES: ADAPTATION TO STARVATION

The ability of a patient to tolerate partial or complete starvation, and also to meet additional energy demands produced by sepsis, trauma, or major surgery, depends on body reserves of fuel, ability to mobilize these reserves, and the extent to which exogenous sources of essential fuels can be given to prevent depletion of limited reserves.

Cahill[1] has reviewed current knowledge of body composition and the rate of energy expenditure and fuel consumption in man. Fuel is accumulated in the form of neutral fat, protein, and carbohydrate stored as glycogen. Table 4–1 shows values in calories for the body of a 70-kg. man.

Glycogen storage in muscle and liver involves the inclusion per gram of 1 to 2 gm. of intracellular water, with appropriate electrolytes for isotonicity in intracellular fluid, and is therefore relatively inefficient, yielding only 1 to 2 calories per gram. The total amount available in muscle and liver is also limited, and is only partially used in starvation.

Protein, Cahill emphasized, is *not* stored merely as a nitrogen reservoir. Each molecule of protein serves another purpose, as a part of contractile protein in muscle, a part of the content or cell membrane of all cells, or perhaps as an enzyme. *Protein loss is therefore loss of essential function.* Skeletal muscle, which provides the largest part of protein lost in starvation, is a poor fuel source, with a yield of slightly less than 1 calorie per gram of muscle.

Fat is stored in cells without associated water. Human adipose tissue yields approximately 9 calories per gram, and, in patients from a well-fed population, usually provides a large and often an excessive caloric reserve.

In a 24-hour period, a normal man who consumes 1800 calories a day in a resting state, if fasting, will burn about 75 gm. of protein, largely from muscle, and about 160 gm. of triglyceride from adipose tissue.[1] He will excrete 12 to 15 gm. of nitrogen in his urine, largely in the form of urea, and will lose about 500 gm. in body weight.[2] Endogenous glucose production will be of the order of 180 gm., of which the nervous system, mainly brain, will use 144 gm., which is completely oxidized to carbon dioxide and water.[1] The remainder is used by other glycolytic tissues, erythrocytes, leukocytes, kidney medulla and bone marrow, and perhaps to some degree by skeletal muscle. This fraction of glucose is primarily converted to lactate and pyruvate, which is carried back to the liver, where it is resynthesized into glucose. This is the Cori cycle. The liver also converts glycerol and the glucogenic amino acids into glucose, and uses as its own energy source fatty acids derived from neutral fat.

In starvation the remainder of the body also uses either fatty acids derived directly from the circulation, or partially oxidized fatty acids released by the liver as acetoacetate or β-hydroxybutyrate. Since glucose cannot be directly synthesized from fatty acids, the effect of conversion of metabolism of most of the body tissues to the exclusive use of fatty acids and ketones is to spare protein as a gluconeogenic precursor by reducing glucose requirements.

Insulin appears to be the regulating mechanism in both deposition and mobilization of amino acids and of fats. Both are mobilized as insulin levels fall, and deposition is increased as insulin levels rise. Insulin levels, in turn, are exquisitely sensitive to small changes in levels of blood glucose, thus providing the feedback loop proposed by Cahill[1] to control mobilization of both protein and fat, and maintain blood glucose concentration within very narrow limits.

That administration of glucose in starvation both decreases nitrogen loss in urine and prevents ketosis has long been recognized. Gamble[3] advocated the use of glucose for these purposes in his famous monograph on body fluids. He showed that 100 gm. of glucose a day reduced fasting consumption of protein from 70 gm. to 40 gm. in young male volunteers, and in addition prevented ketone excretion in their urine. The infusion of 100 to 150 gm. of glucose as 5 or 10 per cent dextrose in water in starving adults will reduce the average urinary nitrogen losses by about one half.[2] Unfortunately, additional glucose administration results in relatively little additional reduction in nitrogen loss, and therefore in protein sparing, until total calories administered approach the total energy requirements of the patient. Even with this level, amino acids are also required to prevent a negative nitrogen balance.

Cahill postulated that the small amount of glucose administered is detected by the insulin-producing mechanism, and that the higher levels of insulin produced inhibit muscle proteolysis by as much as two thirds of the 75 gm. per day otherwise burned in starvation. Since many severely ill patients ultimately die of pulmonary complications related to ineffectual clearing of the airways and inability to ventilate adequately, and these conditions are brought about by muscle wasting, the importance of sparing protein by glucose administration is obvious.

Further steps in adaptation to starvation which conserve protein have been delineated by Cahill,[1] and an excellent illustrative study has been published by Morgan et al.[4] Major steps involve reduction of obligatory gluconeogenesis through adaptation of the brain to use of ketoacids instead of glucose, increasing gluconeogenesis by the kidney cortex as ammonia excretion increases with amino acid residues being synthesized to glucose, and a shift in blood amino acid concentrations, particularly a fall in alanine, which appears to decrease liver glucose production. All these processes combine to reduce daily nitrogen losses from an average of 12 to 15 gm. a day in early starvation, to about 4 gm. a day, representing 25 gm. of protein, or about 150 gm. of lean muscle. Even this level of loss, however, will result in death from protein loss and muscle weakness before most of the adipose tissue calories are depleted in many patients.

TOLERANCE LIMITS OF PROTEIN LOSS

What is the limit of protein loss compatible with survival, and to what extent are amount and rate of protein loss related to surgical complications, to prolonged convalescence, or to death? Answers to these questions are obviously the key to the importance and timing of providing nutrition. Unfortunately, precise answers are not available, and individual variations in patient response further complicate an already complex problem.

However, certain approximations, based on body composition studies and on clinical observations, are useful in clinical care. Rhoads[6] reported a much higher infection rate in hypoproteinemic patients than in normal patients subjected to the same types of operations. Lawson[7] has observed that an acute loss, within 30 days of 30 per cent of body weight in severely ill surgical patients, was uniformly fatal. Cahill[1] and Morgan[4] have both postulated that rapid loss of approximately one third of total body protein by previously normal individuals is lethal. Protein in man must be measured by indirect methods. Body composition studies as well as metabolic balance studies are clinical investigative procedures of considerable complexity. Both, however, have yielded important information which is useful in predicting the clinical course of patients, and in decision making with regard to nutritional requirements.

Table 4-1, based on composition studies, indicates that about 2 kg. of protein loss (one third of total protein) is the limit of tolerance for a previously normal average-sized male. Table 4-2, derived from body composition studies of Moore et al.,[5] shows the average exchangeable potassium, and nitrogen and protein content of 70-kg. males and 60-kg. females in three different age groups. Individual variance of at least 20 per cent must be considered, so such values are rough guides.

Another important factor is, of course, the amount of protein and fat calories that a patient has when surgery or acute illness occurs. Figure 4–1, also based on body composition studies by Moore et al.,[5]

Table 4–1. Fuel Composition in Normal Man[*]

Fuel		Kg.	Calories
Tissues:			
Fat (adipose triglyceride)		15	141,000
Protein (mainly muscle)		6	24,000
Glycogen (muscle)		0.150	600
Glycogen (liver)		0.075	300
	Total		165,900
Circulating fuels:			
Glucose (extracellular fluid)		0.020	80
Free fatty acids (plasma)		0.0003	3
Triglycerides (plasma)		0.003	30
	Total		113

[*]From Cahill.[1]

Table 4–2. ESTIMATES OF POTASSIUM, NITROGEN AND
PROTEIN CONTENT OF MAN BY SEX AND AGE

	AGE	EXCHANGEABLE POTASSIUM	NITROGEN	PROTEIN	BODY CELL MASS
Males, 70 kg.	16–30	3395 mEq.	1132 gm.	7.18 kg.	28.3 kg.
	31–60	3218 mEq.	1073 gm.	6.72 kg.	26.8 kg.
	61–90	2626 mEq.	875 gm.	5.46 kg.	21.9 kg.
Females, 60 kg.	16–30	2350 mEq.	783 gm.	4.90 kg.	19.6 kg.
	31–60	2194 mEq.	733 gm.	4.59 kg.	18.3 kg.
	61–90	1839 mEq.	613 gm.	3.82 kg.	15.3 kg.

Calculated for 70-kg. man and 60-kg. woman, based on studies of Moore et al.[5] Body cell mass = 8.33 × Ke.

All estimates are subject to normal variance among individuals of at least 20 per cent of the values shown.

shows body composition changes observed during one type of acute illness, and another more chronic. Body caloric values for a normal 60-kg. woman and for each of the two patients are shown in Table 4-3.

The patient with peritonitis (Fig. 4-1), previously perfectly well, had a subphrenic abscess, edema, ascites, pulmonary edema and bronchopneumonia as complications following a bowel resection. The body composition study, done on the fifteenth day of illness, shows a loss of

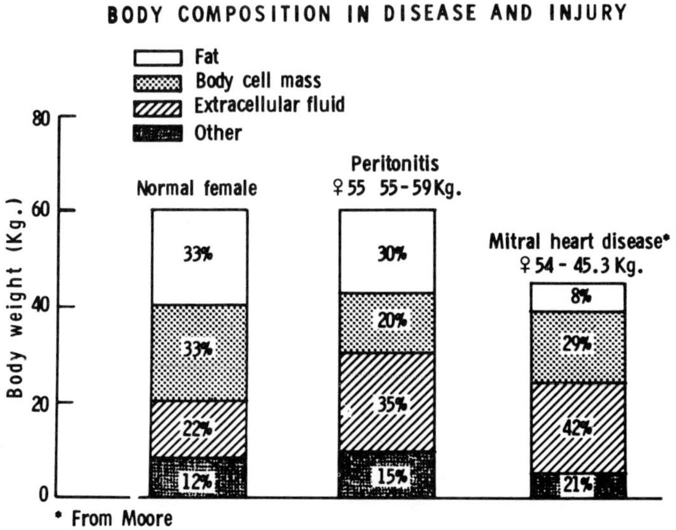

BODY COMPOSITION IN DISEASE AND INJURY

Figure 4–1. Body composition data from Moore et al.,[5] cases 61 and 96. Marked loss of body cell mass with nearly intact fat stores and expanded ECF are shown in the patient with peritonitis after 15 days of acute illness. These compare with marked loss of fat and considerable reduction in body cell mass in a patient with mitral stenosis and insufficiency who weighed 68 kg. seven years previously.

Table 4–3.   ESTIMATED BODY COMPOSITION OF PATIENTS,
FIGURE 4–1 AND TEXT*

	FUEL	KG.	CALORIES
Normal female, 60 kg.	Fat	20	180,000
	Protein	5	20,000
Peritonitis patient, 59 kg.	Fat	18	162,000
(Case 61)	Protein	3	12,000 2 days before death
Mitral patient, 45 kg.	Fat	3.6 (25.4)	32,400 (228,600)
(Case 96)	Protein	3.25 (5.2)	13,000 (20,800)

*Data from Moore et al.[5] Figures in parentheses are estimated normal for Case 96 prior to onset of cardiac decompensation.

more than one third of her body cell mass, with great overexpansion of the extracellular fluid space. The patient died two days later as the result of respiratory failure and sepsis, with most of her adipose tissue calories intact. Within two weeks she had had a loss of body cell mass of almost 40 per cent of her calculated total.

The patient with mitral heart disease (Fig. 4-1), had both mitral insufficiency and stenosis. She was studied during a phase of late congestive heart failure. She had lost weight, 22.7 kg. in seven years, and was edematous and orthopneic. The study was done four days after admission and following loss of 4 kg. of weight on treatment. This case demonstrates both extensive loss of fat calories, about 20 kg., or 180,000 calories, and a loss of body cell mass of 6.6 kg., representing 1.65 kg. of protein, or 36 per cent of the original value when compared with her original weight of 68 kg. and calculated composition seven years previously. Her extracellular fluid volume, expanded even for her original weight, represents more than 40 per cent of her weight at the time of study.

Although this patient was not subjected to surgery, such a patient would obviously be a severe risk because of her marked debility. Part of that risk would be due to very little remaining protein and total caloric reserve.

THE EFFECT OF TRAUMA, SEPSIS, AND MAJOR SURGERY ON ENERGY REQUIREMENTS

Surgery, trauma, or sepsis, singly or in combination, initiates a complex series of events in man, known as the metabolic response to injury (see Chapter 2). In patients so stressed, there is often an acute increase in metabolism at a time of decreased or absent food intake, and therefore a large demand on endogenous sources for energy. An increased secretion of urinary nitrogen beyond fasting levels indicates heightened protein catabolism. Most patients will not tolerate a high caloric diet and many cannot eat at all for periods of from a few days to weeks in complicated cases. As a result, there is an obligatory dependence on endogenous sources or on parenteral administration for the substrates required.

The hypermetabolic state accompanying trauma and sepsis deprives the body of two important defense mechanisms against reduced caloric intake. It cannot lower metabolic rate, as is the case in adaptation to simple starvation,[4] nor can it apparently readjust mixtures of endogenous fuel, as is the case in prolonged starvation, so that high energy-producing fatty acids and glycerol are used more effectively to spare calorically inefficient protein-containing lean muscle mass.

The severity of the catabolic phase of illness and its duration depend upon the extent or type of operation or injury, the presence of significant infection, the duration of immobilization of the patient, and the duration of inadequate ingestion or digestion of food. The severity of the catabolic phase of response to injury has also been shown to depend on age, sex, previous nutritional states, and the conditioning effects of chronic illness, and of previous surgery or other stress in the immediate past.

Figure 4-2 illustrates the average daily negative nitrogen balance of four groups of patients. Complete starvation in the first group is compared with the effect of 100 gm. of glucose a day intravenously in the second group without surgery. The third group of patients underwent

DAILY NITROGEN BALANCE WITH ZERO

OR MINIMAL N. INTAKE & < 10 CALORIES /Kg./DAY

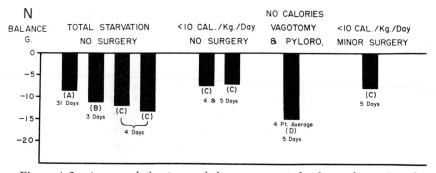

Figure 4–2. Average *daily* nitrogen balance over periods of time shown. Data from the literature: (A) Benedict[9]; (B) Howard et al.[10]; (C) Holden et al.[11] and (D) Johnston et al.[12] Nitrogen in grams per day average loss for the period shown is plotted from the zero balance line downward to indicate negative balance. (From Randall.[2])

vagotomy and pyloroplasty without any postoperative nutrition for five days, and had a somewhat larger daily nitrogen, and therefore protein, loss than was seen in simple starvation. The fourth group underwent herniorrhaphy or hemorrhoidectomy and received 100 gm. of glucose a day parenterally. Their nitrogen losses are less than expected from starvation alone.

Figure 4-3 illustrates daily nitrogen loss at the peak in a series of severely ill patients, contrasted with patients undergoing surgery of moderate degree. Losses of 20 to 35 gm. of nitrogen represent 125 to 220 gm. of protein a day, a rate that would result in death from protein depletion in ten days to two weeks in adult patients of average size and previously normal nutrition. All these patients received intravenous glucose, and some of Moore's cases received small amounts of protein (as plasma). The cases of J. E. Howard[10] illustrate negative nitrogen balance existing in young men with a long bone fracture, despite an intake of 19 gm. of nitrogen (120 gm. of protein) in diet. They also illustrate the point that although adequate nutrition cannot prevent nitrogen loss at the peak of catabolic response, *it can significantly reduce the net loss from the patient's protein reserve.*

This point is further substantiated in Figure 4-4, showing balance studies on four series of patients treated with high caloric parenteral

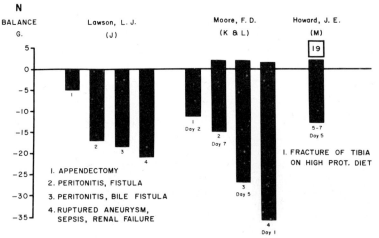

MAJOR COMPLICATED ILLNESS
PEAK DAILY LOSS

1. CLOSED ELECTIVE, MOD. SEVERITY (K)
2. TOTAL GASTRECTOMY, SPLEEN & PANCREAS (L)
3. SEVERE TRAUMA & SEPSIS (K)
4. ULCERATIVE COLITIS, FEVER, LAPAROTOMY (L)

Figure 4–3. Daily loss of nitrogen at peak of loss from two series (Lawson et al.,[7] and Moore et al.[5, 13]), compared with negative balance following a fractured tibia on day 5 despite 19 gm. nitrogen intake in food (Howard et al.[10]). (From Randall.[2])

ELECTIVE SURGERY — PARENTERAL NUTRITION

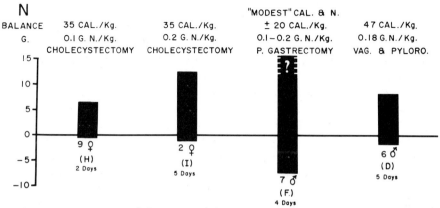

Figure 4–4. Average daily nitrogen balance postoperatively in four series of patients given high caloric intravenous nutrition in the immediate postoperative period. Nitrogen intake (as amino acids from protein hydrolysate) is plotted from the zero line upward, and then total nitrogen loss is plotted from the point representing total intake downward. Overall nitrogen balance extends below the zero line, indicating negative balance, in all four series. However, the amount of negative balance is small, and represents a much diminished *net* loss of protein from the patients, when compared to similar cases in Figure 4–2 without high caloric intake. (H. Waldstrom et al.;[14] I. Werner et al.;[15] F. Holden et al.;[11] D. Johnston et al.[12]) (From Randall.[2])

nutrition. Comparison of daily nitrogen losses in these patients with similar cases in Figure 4-2 and the moderately severe cases in Figure 4-3 reveals that nitrogen losses have been *reduced by 80 per cent or more* as the result of provision of adequate nutrition, even in the immediate postoperative period. This being the case, the question of clinical importance becomes: What types of patients should receive more than just baseline glucose as nutritional therapy, and how can the requirements for these patients best be met?

INDICATIONS FOR NUTRITIONAL SUPPORT OF SURGICAL PATIENTS

Clinical experience, now backed by substantial evidence from metabolic studies in man, indicates that the well-nourished and reasonably healthy patient who is subjected to a single and relatively uncomplicated major operation or who suffers moderately severe trauma, does well with a simple parenteral program designed to maintain adequate circulatory volume, and to provide enough water, salt, potassium, and glucose to prevent dehydration or electrolyte imbalance and spare body protein breakdown for glucogenesis.[8] Although a high caloric, high protein parenteral regimen can and will reduce the nitrogen deficit and weight loss that results from semi-starvation and the metabolic response to trauma, body reserves of protein and fat are sufficient to carry most patients for a week or more of inadequate intake without serious consequences. Oral intake should be resumed as soon as it can be tolerated to permit repletion in these, the large majority of general surgical patients. The risks of either high caloric parenteral therapy or the use of elemental diets probably outweigh their advantages in these patients.

On the other hand, a significant minority of surgical patients require that their nutritional program be planned as carefully as their operative procedure. These patients are of two types: those who preoperatively are severely debilitated as the result of chronic or subacute disease or chronic malnutrition, and those who, as the result of severe trauma, sepsis, or complications of surgery, are unable or unwilling to eat adequately for a prolonged period of time. Examples of major preoperative debility include patients with severe inflammatory disease of the large or small bowel, carcinoma of the stomach or colon, chronic pancreatitis, chronic infection, or some forms of liver, kidney, or heart disease. All have in common a substantial weight loss with severe reduction of their skeletal muscle mass and total body protein. Most have an increase in the relative proportion of extracellular fluid and total sodium despite quite common hyponatremia.[5]

More acute problems include patients with acute or subacute pancreatitis, unresolved peritonitis, small bowel fistulas, abdominal trauma, major wound sepsis, retroperitoneal hematoma, major burns, and particularly those with severe multiple injury trauma, including long bone or pelvic fractures. Many of these patients were healthy and well nourished before the onset of their acute problem, but because of major catabolic response to trauma or sepsis and simultaneous partial starvation, the demands on fat and particularly protein stores are so great that available reserves are exhausted within two to four weeks, and death will occur from muscle weakness, respiratory failure, and sepsis, unless they are provided with fuel in sufficient quantity and of proper qualities to spare essential body cell mass.

ESSENTIAL COMPONENTS OF CHEMICALLY DEFINED NUTRIENT SOLUTIONS

Calories.   Basal metabolism in man as the average of three large series of cases[16] shows a slowly declining metabolic rate from childhood to old age, and a consistently lower rate in females compared to males. Table 4-4 gives standard figures for basal metabolic rate per square meter by sex and age (A), a calculation of basal rate per day and basal +30 per cent for bed activity (B), and recently recommended daily allowances for calories and protein for moderate activity (C). These

Table 4–4. REFERENCE DATA FOR CALORIC REQUIREMENTS

A. Calories M.²/Hour by Age and Sex:

AGE IN YEARS	MALES	FEMALES
	Range	
5	56.3 (48.5–64.1)	53.0 (45.7–60.3)
10	47.7 (41.1–54.3)	44.9 (38.7–51.1)
15	43.7 (37.7–49.7)	38.3 (33.0–43.6)
20	39.8 (34.3–45.3)	35.3 (30.4–40.2)
30	37.6 (32.4–42.8)	35.0 (30.2–39.8)
40	36.5 (31.5–41.5)	34.3 (29.6–39.0)
50	36.0 (31.0–40.0)	33.4 (28.8–38.0)
60	34.8 (30.0–39.6)	32.4 (27.9–36.9)
70	33.1 (28.5–37.7)	31.3 (27.0–35.6)
75+	31.8 (27.4–36.2)	31.1 (26.8–35.4)

B. Basal and "Bed Activity" Caloric Requirements for "Standard" Male and Female Adults:

	AGE	BASAL CALORIES PER HOUR (24 hours)	BED ACTIVITY, BASAL + 30 PER CENT (24 hours)
Male, 70 kg., 175 cm.	20	73.6 (1770)	95.7 (2290)
154 lbs., 69 inches	40	67.5 (1620)	87.4 (2100)
1.85 M.²	60	64.4 (1545)	83.7 (2010)
	75+	58.8 (1410)	76.5 (1835)
Female, 58 kg., 163 cm.	20	56.5 (1355)	73.5 (1765)
128 lbs., 64 inches	40	54.9 (1320)	71.5 (1715)
1.6 M.²	60	51.8 (1245)	67.5 (1620)
	75+	49.8 (1195)	64.8 (1550)

C. Recommended Daily Dietary Allowances, Normal Activity and Temperate Climate:

	AGE	CALORIES	PROTEIN (Gm.)
Male, 70 kg., 175 cm.	18–35	2900	70
	35–55	2600	70
	55–75	2200	70
Female, 58 kg., 163 cm.	18–35	2100	58
	35–55	1900	58
	55–75	1600	58
	Pregnant	+200	+20
	Lactating	+1000	+40

A. From Basal Metabolism, Man.[16]
B. Calculated from A, with DuBois table for surface area.
C. Food and Nutrition Board, National Academy of Science, National Research Council, 1963 Revision.

figures serve as general guidelines in estimating patient requirements for average or "standard" men and women.

Trauma, sepsis, and, in particular, burns raise the basal metabolic expenditure substantially, and increase the breakdown of protein with resulting increased nitrogen excretion in the urine, largely as urea. Figure 4-5, from Kinney,[17] illustrates the effect of trauma on basal metabolic expenditure and nitrogen excretion. Patients with sepsis have similar energy requirements and nitrogen loss, as is shown in Figure 4-3.

Caloric requirements of seriously ill patients depend on the severity of trauma and the presence of complications such as sepsis. Although 35 calories per kilogram per day with 0.1 gm. of nitrogen per kilogram as amino acids has resulted in virtually no nitrogen loss following cholecystectomy in women,[15] patients with major sepsis or extensive burns may require 4000 calories or more and 20 gm. of nitrogen as amino acids a day, to meet their requirements and produce significant reduction in protein loss.

Protein.   Preparations used in surgical nutrition, either parenterally or in chemically defined diets, are usually either enzymatic or acid hydrolysis products of casein or plasma fibrin. Several types are commercially available in the United States, and are usually distributed in the form of a 5 per cent solution, often mixed with 5 per cent glucose or 5 or 10 per cent mixtures of glucose and fructose. Higher concentrations

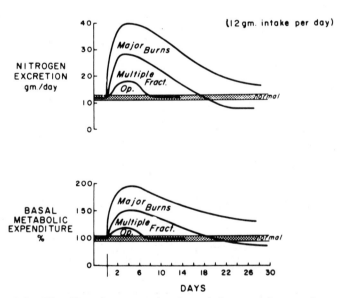

Figure 4–5.   The effect of trauma on basal metabolic expenditure and nitrogen excretion. Sepsis produces a similar pattern. (From Kinney[17].)

of carbohydrate tend to be unstable over prolonged storage in solution with amino acids. When high caloric mixtures of amino acids and sugars are required, they must be mixed or reconstituted from the dry state within a short time before use.

Pure amino acid mixtures, which have the advantages of fewer side reactions and more precise control over ratios of essential and nonessential amino acids, should be available before long for general clinical use.

Hydrolysates or other preparations of amino acids should be given slowly and continuously over 24 hours, and should be given *simultaneously with* nonprotein calories, usually as glucose or fructose. A ratio of 5 to 6 gm. of nonprotein nutrient per gram of amino acids is recommended, both for economy and to reduce utilization of amino acids for calories rather than for protein synthesis.

Carbohydrates. Dextrose, fructose and invert sugar (a mixture of dextrose and fructose) are the forms available for parenteral nutrition. In addition, sucrose, *which is not metabolized if given intravenously,* can be used in chemically defined diets, and has the advantage of lower osmolality per gram and calorie. Sorbitol and xylitol have been widely used in Japan and Europe, but are not presently available for general use in the United States.

Concentrations of glucose from 5 per cent to 50 per cent are available for parenteral use. The use of a long nonreactive catheter for infusion into the superior vena cava and the slow continuous infusion of mixtures of glucose in concentrations of 20 to 25 per cent, together with 5 per cent protein hydrolysates and necessary electrolytes and vitamins, as pioneered by Dudrick et al.,[18] have obviated the complications resulting from infusion of hypertonic mixtures into peripheral veins and permitted sustained nutrition, positive nitrogen balance, and even normal growth. A section on intravenous nutrition follows in this chapter. Similar experience has now been achieved with elemental diets as well, in situations in which the gastrointestinal tract is at least partially functional, but will not tolerate adequate amounts of normal foods.[19]

Fats. Fat, with the exception of linoleic acid in infants and children, does not appear essential either for growth or for significant repletion of protein and caloric stores in man. The fat-soluble vitamins, A and D, can be administered as water-soluble salts for parenteral use, or for solution in elemental diets. Parenteral administration of fat requires that it be in a very fine emulsion, and although such preparations are extensively and apparently successfully used in Europe,[24] no preparation is available for general use in the United States today.

Vitamins. Knowledge of exact vitamin requirements for parenteral nutrition or in chemically defined diets is largely lacking. However, vitamins of the B group are known to play an important role in amino acid, carbohydrate and fat metabolism, and presumably do so in parenteral or chemically defined oral feedings as well. Meng[20] recommends the following doses as daily requirements:

Thiamine	5-10 mg.
Riboflavin	4-5 mg.
Niacin	8-20 mg.
Pantothenate	20 mg.
Pyridoxine	15 mg.
Folacin	0.15-0.2 mg.
Vitamin B_{12}	15-30 mcg.
Biotin	150-300 mcg.
Vitamin C	300-500 mg.
Vitamin A	2500-4000 I.U.
Vitamin D	400 I.U.
Vitamin E	10 I.U.

Several commercial preparations available for intravenous use will supply these requirements.

In addition, *vitamin K is essential* for patients on either parenteral or defined elemental diets. Ten mg. given intramuscularly three times a week seems adequate in most cases. Patients on broad-spectrum antibiotics require particular attention to vitamin K needs, but hypoprothrombinemia can occur without antibiotics in patients on parenteral or chemically defined diets, and should be prevented.

Electrolytes and Water. Most formulas for either chemically defined diets or high caloric parenteral feedings contain baseline quantities of sodium, potassium, magnesium, and calcium, and diets contain zinc, iron, and some trace elements as well. Abnormal losses of electrolytes require additional provisions to prevent or correct depletion. Often these can be added to the mixture being given, or can be given as a supplement into the gastrointestinal tract, or intravenously.

Additional water beyond that contained in high caloric preparations may be necessary, either into the gastrointestinal tract if patients can tolerate it, or intravenously as 5 per cent dextrose in water. If the patient has a high urinary solute load, or is unable to concentrate urine beyond a glucose-free specific gravity of 1015, hyperosmolar dehydration will result if additional water is not given.

SURGICAL NUTRITION BY CHEMICALLY DEFINED, BULK-FREE DIETS

The use of chemically formulated bulk-free elemental diets for human nutrition is relatively new. However, extensive animal studies have demonstrated that these diets will support normal longevity, reproduction, growth and lactation in rats.[20] In 1965, 16 volunteer male inmates of the California Medical Facility, Vacaville, California, received between 2100 and 3700 calories per day of an elemental diet as their sole nutritional source for 19 weeks.[21] Blood studies during the entire test period failed to reveal abnormalities of any parameter tested except lowered cholesterol levels with glucose diets which returned to normal when sucrose was half the carbohydrate source. Fecal elimination in all individuals was strikingly reduced, with the subjects experiencing smaller than normal bowel movements at regular intervals of five to six days.

Elemental diets have several advantages over presently available high caloric, high protein food supplements. Their completely bulk-free, virtually fat-free composition requires minimal digestion, thereby bypassing the need for most pancreatic and biliary secretions.

Because of bulk-free composition, stool volume is reduced. Diarrhea has not been much of a problem when diets are administered slowly and continuously, probably because of rapid and almost total absorption. Adjustable concentration and increasing patient tolerance have permitted up to 5200 calories per day to be given over prolonged periods.

Stephens and Randall[19] have reported a series of surgical patients who were provided total nutrition by means of an elemental diet. Bury, Stephens and Randall[23] have reported the use of elemental diets in the management of a series of 13 patients with fistulas of the alimentary tract. Morgan et al.[4] have discussed elemental diets as a part of consideration of nutrition in surgical patients. Reports on use of elemental diets in nutritional support of patients with inflammatory disease of the small and large bowel, and in nutrition of premature and newborn infants with anatomic or functional disorders of the gastrointestinal tract, are in preparation. Clinical experience, although encouraging, still remains limited.

Elemental diets appear to have considerable value when at least a part of the small bowel is sufficiently functional to permit absorption of solutions of simple sugars and amino acids. Elemental diets, like high caloric parenteral mixtures, which they closely resemble except for added trace elements and the use of sucrose in some diets, permit physician control of caloric intake, as well as of water volume and electrolytes. They appear to be safer than high caloric parenteral nutrition, obviating the risk of infection caused by intravenous catheters, but have the limitation of requiring at least a functional segment of small bowel for absorption.

COMPOSITION OF ELEMENTAL DIETS

Elemental diets consist of mixtures of purified L-amino acids derived from acid hydrolysis of casein readjusted to restore tryptophan content, carbohydrate in the form of glucose, sucrose, or a mixture of glucose and partially hydrolyzed starch, electrolytes at a level calculated to meet baseline needs, water- and fat-soluble vitamins exclusive of vitamin K, and trace minerals found essential to growth and reproduction in the rat.

In some instances, particularly with Vivonex, efforts have been made to add flavoring material to disguise the rather strong organic taste and smell inherent in amino acid mixtures. This is quite successful at lower amino acid concentrations, at which oral tolerance is fair to good, and less so at therapeutic levels of protein administration of 35 to 40 gm. per 1000 calories. High protein diets presently available must be tube fed.

Table 4-5 gives the composition of two elemental diets used by one of the authors (H.T.R.) during the past three years. If should be noted that the formulas for high caloric intravenous nutrition, given in the next section, can be used quite effectively into the gastrointestinal tract by tube feeding. These preparations lack iron, zinc, and other trace elements present in mixtures prepared as diets. Such elements can be added if the mixture is to be used in the gastrointestinal tract.

INDICATIONS FOR USE OF ELEMENTAL DIETS

Elemental diets have been found useful in the following types of patients when there is sufficient function of the gastrointestinal tract to permit use.

Table 4–5. COMPOSITION OF DIETS PER 1000 CALORIES

	CODELID 62H	VIVONEX 100
Carbohydrate	197 gm. (Sucrose)	212 gm. (Glucose)
Nitrogen	6 gm.	3.3 gm.
Protein	37 gm.	20 gm.
Fat	0 gm.	0.87 gm.
Sodium	25 mEq.	55 mEq.
Potassium	24 mEq.	30 mEq.
Chloride	37 mEq.	76 mEq.
Magnesium	7.2 mEq.	7.1 mEq.
Calcium	24 mEq.	22 mEq.

Codelid 62H Diet—Schwarz BioResearch, Mountain View Avenue, Orangeburg, New York 10962.

Vivonex 100—Eaton Laboratories, Norwich, New York 13815.

Diets contain standard quantities of water and fat-soluble vitamins for normal daily requirements based on 2000 calories. Vitamins of the B group and vitamin C should be supplemented to therapeutic levels by addition of a standard high potency preparation either intravenously or into the gastrointestinal tract.

Both diets contain iron, copper, zinc, manganese and iodide, and Codelid contains molybdenum at normal dietary levels.

Diets do *not* contain vitamin K or cobalt.

1. Patients depleted of protein reserves owing to disease of the gastrointestinal tract:

> Ulcerative colitis, acute
> Granulomatous disease of small and large bowel
> Chronic infection
> Cancer of stomach or colon, preoperative preparation
> Intestinal atresia — infants
> Malabsorption syndrome, nonspecific, infants or adults
> Chronic malnutrition of various types

2. Patients with partial function of the gastrointestinal tract:

> Esophageal, gastric and duodenal fistulas — with feeding distal to the fistula
> Small bowel fistulas — feeding either proximal or distal, depending on level
> Colonic fistula (low bulk)
> Acute pancreatitis, after ileus has cleared
> Short gut syndrome

3. Patients with accelerated metabolic states who will not or cannot eat adequately:

> Fractures of the jaw
> Long bone fractures (as a supplement)
> Severe burns
> Multiple trauma

4. Incidental uses:

> As a preoperative bowel preparation, or preparation for x-rays of the colon, to avoid semistarvation or excessive catharsis
> As a virtually nonallergenic source of food
> As a dietary supplement (Vivonex 100)

METHODS OF ADMINISTRATION

Oral. Flavored preparations, such as Vivonex 100, made up as 25 per cent weight/volume solution, provide 1000 calories per liter. Served cool, and ingested in small amounts, 100 to 150 ml. at a time because of the high osmolality, 2000 or more ml. can be taken in 16 hours, providing in the process 2000 calories, including 40 gm. of protein.

Intragastric Tube Feeding. This can be accomplished either with a small, No. 8 French transnasal intragastric infant feeding tube which is well tolerated by most patients, or by gastrostomy, if one is present for other reasons or placed for the purpose. A Barron or other controlled volume flow pump has been found more reliable than a gravity drip to provide constant infusion rate, but either can be used.

Diet should be drawn from a small (500 to 1000 ml.) reservoir, preferably kept at ice temperature.

Initial concentration should be 12.5 or 15 per cent weight/volume, and should be administered at an initial rate of 40 to 50 ml./hour. If tolerated without nausea, vomiting or large gastric residue, the concentration can be increased to 25 per cent weight/volume in 24 hours. Volume can then be progressively increased by steps of 500 ml. or more each 24 hours until the desired caloric and protein intake is achieved. Diets containing 6 gm. of nitrogen per liter at 25 per cent weight/volume are recommended, either Codelid or high protein Vivonex, to give 37.5 gm. protein per liter.

With either nausea or diarrhea, the diet should be slowed or stopped entirely for 12 to 24 hours, and then re-started more slowly.

In elderly patients and unconscious patients, elevation of the head of the bed to an angle of 30 degrees may forestall aspiration. It is wise to discontinue feeding at night with elderly or very weak patients who may aspirate if supine.

Water ad lib. may be permitted if it can be drunk. At 25 per cent weight/volume and over 2500 ml. a day, most patients are neither thirsty nor hungry, unless they have abnormal external losses of water. Water via gastrostomy tube can be given for thirst on a demand basis as well.

Directly into Small Bowel. Feedings directly into the small bowel are given either through a jejunostomy, or through a long tube, such as a small Miller-Abbott tube or Baker tube, placed so that several feet of small bowel distal to the feeding point are available for absorption in adults.

Initial feedings should be nearly isotonic. Ten per cent weight/volume solutions at a rate of 40 to 60 ml. per hour are gradually increased, first in concentration to 25 per cent weight/volume, then in volume to the desired amount. Diarrhea is an indication to slow or stop the feeding, and begin again at a slower rate. Codeine, 15 to 30 mg. given by hypodermic injection every four to six hours, is quite helpful in controlling diarrhea, and sometimes excessive fistula output.

Abnormal Losses of Water and Electrolytes. Additional sodium as 5 per cent sodium chloride solution, or potassium as potassium chloride (40 mEq. in 20 ml.) can be added to the elemental diet, to a total of not more than 100 mEq. of sodium and potassium together per liter.

Additional water can be provided, either by diluting the diet below 25 per cent weight/volume and increasing the rate, or by adding 100 ml. units (at body temperature!) as a bolus in a tube.

COMPLICATIONS OF ELEMENTAL DIET USE

Gastrointestinal. Nausea, vomiting and diarrhea all are related to rate and concentration of administration. None have proved insurmountable.

Aspiration. This is a real risk in the elderly, very weak, or unconscious patient. It is preventable by elevating the head of the bed, by avoiding night feeding into the stomach in the elderly, and by careful attention to gastric retention.

Disturbances of Water Balance. Virtually all patients placed on a high carbohydrate intake will hold water, an average of 2 to 4 pounds in adults. Diuretics can be used to unload water excess, if necessary.

Hypertonic dehydration, and hypertonic nonketotic coma may occur if higher than 25 per cent weight/volume concentrations are used in adults, or above 10 to 12 per cent in infants. Extra water must be given if urine solute load is high, evaporative water loss is excessive, or relative renal insufficiency is present.

Hyperglycemia and glycosuria may occur in unsuspected diabetes and in severely stressed patients. Judicious use of insulin permits concentration of diet. Insulin is not necessary or indicated in most patients.

Hypoprothrombinemia will occur unless vitamin K is given supplementally. There is no vitamin K in available diets.

SUMMARY

Elemental diets represent an intermediate step in surgical nutrition between high caloric parenteral therapy and normal ingestion and digestion of food. They are indicated in patients who require nutritional support, who have at least a part of their small bowel available for absorption, and who are unable to eat and digest enough calories and protein to meet their energy demands.

REFERENCES

1. Cahill, G. F., Jr.: Starvation in man. N. Eng. J. Med. 282:668, 1970.
2. Randall, H. T.: Indications for parenteral nutrition; *In* Meng, H. C., and Law, D. H. (eds.): Parenteral Nutrition. Springfield, Ill., Charles C Thomas, Publisher, 1970, pp. 13-39.
3. Gamble, J. L.: Chemical Anatomy, Physiology and Pathology of Extracellular Fluids. 5th Ed. Cambridge, Harvard University Press, 1949.
4. Morgan, A., Filler, R. M., and Moore, F. E.: Surgical nutrition. Med. Clin. North Amer. 54:1367, 1970.
5. Moore, F. D., Olesen, K. H., McMorrey, J. D., Parker, H. J., Ball, M. R., and Boyden, C. M.: The Body Cell Mass and its Supporting Environment. Philadelphia, W. B. Saunders Co., 1963.
6. Rhoads, J. E.: Introduction; *In* Meng, H. C., and Law, D. S. (eds.): Parenteral Nutrition. Springfield, Ill., Charles C Thomas, Publisher, 1970, pp. 8-12.

7. Lawson, L. J.: Parenteral nutrition in surgery. Brit. J. Surg. 52:795, 1965.
8. Randall, H. T.: Fluid and Electrolyte Therapy in Surgery; *In* Schwartz, S. I. (ed.): Principles of Surgery. New York, Blakiston Division, McGraw-Hill Book Co., 1969.
9. Benedict, F. G.: Publication No. 280, Carnegie Institute, Washington, D.C., 1919.
10. Howard, J. E., Bigham, R. S., Jr., Eisenberg, H., Wagner, D., and Barley, E.: Studies on fracture convalescence: The influence of diet on post-traumatic nitrogen deficit exhibited by fracture patients. Bull. Johns Hopkins Hosp. 75:209, 1944.
11. Holden, W. D., Krieger, H., Levey, S., and Abbott, W. E.: The effect of nutrition on nitrogen metabolism in the surgical patient. Ann. Surg. 146:563, 1957.
12. Johnston, I. D., Marino, J. D., and Steven, J. Z.: The effect of intravenous feeding on the balances of nitrogen, sodium and potassium after operation. Brit. J. Surg. 53:885, 1966.
13. Moore, F. D.: Metabolic Care of the Surgical Patient. Philadelphia, W. B. Saunders Co., 1959.
14. Waldstrom, L. B., and Wiklund, P. E.: Effect of fat emulsions on nitrogen balance in the postoperative period. Acta Chir. Scand. 325:50, 1964.
15. Werner, S. C., Habif, D. V., Randall, H. T., and Lockwood, J. S.: Postoperative nitrogen loss: A comparison of the effect of trauma and of caloric readjustment. Ann. Surg. 130:688, 1949.
16. Handbook of Biologic Data, Table 239. Spector, W. S. (ed.). Philadelphia, W. B. Saunders Co., 1956, p. 259.
17. Kinney, J. M.: Proceedings of a Conference on Energy Metabolism and Body Fuel Utilization. Cambridge, Harvard University Press, 1966.
18. Dudrick, S. S., Wilmore, D. W., Vars, H. M., and Rhoads, J. E.: Long-term parenteral nutrition with growth, development, and positive nitrogen balance. Surgery 64:134, 1968.
19. Stephens, R. V., and Randall, H. T.: Use of a concentrated, balanced, liquid elemental diet for nutritional management of catabolic states. Ann. Surg. 170:642, 1969.
20. Meng, H. D.: Principles of parenteral nutrition. Hospital Medicine 1/71, 102–112.
21. Greenstein, J. P., Birnbaum, S. M., Winitz, M., and Otey, M. D.: Quantitative nutritional studies with water-soluble, chemically defined diets. 1. Growth, reproduction and lactation in rats. Arch. Biochem. Biophys. 72:396, 1957.
22. Winitz, M., Graff, J., Gallagher, N., Narkin, A., and Seedman, D. A.: Evaluation of chemical diets as nutrition for man-in-space. Nature 205:741, 1965.
23. Bury, K. D., Stephens, R. V., and Randall, H. T.: Use of a chemically defined, liquid, elemental diet for nutritional management of fistulae of the alimentary tract. Am. J. Surg. 121:174, 1971.
24. Section 4, Fat emulsions; *In* Parenteral Nutrition, Meng, H. C., and Law, D. H. (eds.). Springfield, Ill., Charles C Thomas, Publisher, 1970.

Parenteral Nutrition

STANLEY J. DUDRICK, M.D.

The establishment and maintenance of an adequate feeding regimen may be vital to the successful management of the critically ill surgical patient. However, it may be difficult, or at times impossible, to provide optimal enteral nutrition to the patient with a disorder or dysfunction of the alimentary tract. Not infrequently, periods of relative or complete anatomic or functional disruption of the gastrointestinal tract accompany or complicate the patient's primary pathologic process, further compounding any pre-existing nutritional problem by obviating adequate gastrointestinal nourishment. Accordingly, the patient must endure excessive morbidity and may eventually succumb, not from his primary disease, but rather from the complications of primary or secondary malnutrition. Thus, restoration and maintenance of nutritional and metabolic balance is desirable during all phases of diagnosis, therapy and convalescence in surgical patients. This may be achieved with thoughtful attention to dietary regimens, tailored to the specific needs and conditions of patients, and delivered to the alimentary tract orally or by various feeding tubes whenever possible and practical. However, when use of the gastrointestinal tract is inadequate, ill advised or impossible for prolonged periods of time, nourishment must be provided by parenteral means.

With the use of routine isotonic intravenous feeding regimens, parenteral alimentation can satisfy only a small fraction of the nutritional requirements of a debilitated patient. Peripheral infusion of 5 per cent dextrose solutions within the limits of water tolerance of 2500 to 3500 ml. per day in the average adult provides only 500 to 700 calories. In the average resting adult, functional basal caloric requirements are approximately three times this amount. Thus all peripherally infused nutrients are metabolized for heat and energy rather than for tissue synthesis, and additional energy requirements are met by the catabolism of the body stores of glycogen, fat and protein. If nutrient needs are further increased by pre-existing malnutrition, trauma, sepsis or other pathologic processes, the patient supported by the usual peripheral intravenous feeding regimen is receiving only one fifth to one third of his nutritional requirements and is clearly existing on a starvation diet.

Several approaches to increasing the efficacy of intravenous alimentation have achieved limited clinical success. (1) By infusing somewhat hypertonic (10 to 15 per cent) solutions of dextrose, fructose or invert sugar within limits of water tolerance, 2000 to 2400 calories per day have been administered by peripheral vein. However, long-term parenteral nutrition by this technique is complicated by a prohibitive incidence of thrombophlebitis. (2) Using intravenous diuretics as an adjunct to the infusion of 5 to 7 L. of isotonic or slightly hypertonic nutrient solutions has allowed the provision of up to 2600 calories per day, while facilitating renal excretion of the surplus vehicular water. However, the risk of water overload, electrolyte imbalance or cardiovascular decompensation has restricted the widespread use of this technique. (3) Energy substrates of high caloric density, such as ethyl alcohol (7 calories per gram) and fat (9 calories per gram) have also fallen short of expectations. The side effects of intoxication, obtundity and cellular damage have limited the range of clinical usefulness of ethyl alcohol as a nutrient, and a safe, effective and stable fat emulsion is currently not available for clinical use in this country. Thus, the only

universally applicable approach to providing adequate nutrition parenterally is to concentrate the nutrients known to be safe and efficacious
into the volume of water known to be safely tolerated.

Parenteral hyperalimentation is the intravenous administration of
suitable carbohydrates and protein moieties together with other necessary nutrients in quantities substantially greater than the requirements
for caloric and nitrogen equilibrium, in order to achieve positive nitrogen balance and tissue synthesis in patients who have increased nutritional needs. It requires the continuous infusion of highly concentrated
(25 to 30 per cent) nutrient solutions through an indwelling catheter
inserted into the superior vena cava.

INDICATIONS FOR HIGH CALORIE CENTRAL VENOUS ALIMENTATION

The primary aim of parenteral hyperalimentation is to provide
essential nutrients exclusively by vein for prolonged periods of time in
quantities as high as $2\frac{1}{2}$ times the basic requirements. Thereby positive nitrogen balance and an anabolic state can be achieved during
conditions usually associated with a catabolic response. In infants requiring total intravenous feeding, an additional goal is to promote
normal weight gain, growth and development until adequate enteral
feeding can be resumed.

The technique of total parenteral hyperalimentation has proved
efficacious in several hundred malnourished infant and adult patients
for periods of as long as 22 months at the University of Pennsylvania
Medical Center. Wound healing, weight gain, increased strength and
activity, and feeling of well-being have been observed in the vast
majority of adults; normal growth and development have been achieved
regularly in infants fed exclusively by vein. Enterocutaneous fistula
closure can be accomplished by a combination of suction, bowel rest
and adequate parenteral nutrition. Patients with granulomatous enterocolitis, ulcerative colitis and other inflammatory diseases of the gastrointestinal tract have experienced spontaneous remissions on this
regimen. If surgical procedures are eventually required, the patient who
has been fed adequately intravenously is in better condition to withstand the stresses of anesthesia and operation and to resist infection.
Infants with multiple or complex anomalies may grow and develop
while reconstruction procedures are staged. Adults with body wasting
and hypoproteinemia have restored serum and tissue proteins while
receiving all nourishment parenterally. Patients with renal failure or
impaired hepatic function have also been supported adequately by vein
with specially formulated solutions of L-amino acids and hypertonic
glucose, when feeding via the gastrointestinal tract was impossible or
inadequate.

In patients with major complicated burns, in whom nutrient requirements have been too great to meet by the enteral route alone, as
much as 6000 calories have been given by vein daily to supplement
oral or tube feedings of 4000 to 5000 calories. Following massive small
bowel resections, parenteral hyperalimentation has allowed provision
of sufficient nutrient substrates and time for wound healing and bowel
adaptation to occur. In patients receiving chemotherapy for gastrointestinal tract tumors, total intravenous feeding and bowel rest have reduced alimentary tract toxicity manifestations, thus allowing the administration of two to three times the usual 5-fluorouracil dose. Finally,
maintenance of the anabolic state in all patients requiring major operative procedures may allow a decreased incidence of complications, may
reduce duration and cost of hospitalization, and may achieve more
rapid patient rehabilitation. Since there is virtually no pathologic process which can be treated better in a malnourished patient than in a
well-nourished patient, it is no longer justifiable that critically ill patients be nutritionally deprived or subjected to the stresses of starvation
because they cannot eat.

PREPARATION OF HIGH CALORIE SOLUTIONS

The basic hypertonic nutrient solution consists of approximately 20
to 25 per cent dextrose and 4 to 5 per cent protein hydrolysate or
crystalline amino acids. It provides about 5.25 to 6.0 gm. of nitrogen
(32.5 to 37.5 gm. of protein equivalent), and 900 to 1000 calories per
liter. It can be prepared in bulk lots from commercially available products by a manufacturing pharmacist or technician, or in individual
units by a physician, pharmacist, nurse or technician using strict aseptic
mixing technique (Table 4-6). Recently, kits containing the basic solution components and transfer apparatus have increased the safety and
facility of this procedure.

In the bulk method of solution preparation, which requires a manufacturing pharmacy, anhydrous dextrose U.S.P. is dissolved in 5 per
cent protein hydrolysate in 5 per cent dextrose in the ratio of 165 gm. of
the former to 860 ml. of the latter. The resultant solution is sterilized
promptly after mixing by passage through a large 0.22 micron membrane filter into sterile liter bottles. Steam-autoclaving the concentrated
carbohydrate–amino acid solution is impossible because of the intense
browning (Maillard) reaction which occurs. Aliquots of the solution are
sent for bacterial, fungal and pyrogen testing, and each lot is quaran-
tined under refrigeration, pending receipt of negative results of these
tests.

Individual units of the base solution can be prepared from commercially available parenteral solutions immediately prior to infusion.
Using strictly aseptic mixing technique (ideally in a laminar-flow, fil-

Table 4–6. PREPARATION OF HIGH-CALORIE SOLUTIONS FOR ADULTS

BULK METHOD (Pharmacy)	SINGLE UNIT METHOD (Ward or Pharmacy)
165 gm. anhydrous dextrose U.S.P. PLUS 860 ml. 5% fibrin hydrolysate in 5% dextrose	350 ml. 50% dextrose PLUS 750 ml. 50% fibrin hydrolysate in 5% dextrose
Sterilization through 0.22 micron membrane filter under laminar-flow filtered-air hood.	Aseptic mixing technique under laminar-flow filtered-air hood.

Volume	1000	ml.	1100	ml.	
Calories	1000	Kcal.	1000	Kcal.	
Glucose	208	gm.	212	gm.	
Hydrolysates	43	gm.	37	gm.	
Nitrogen	6.0	gm.	5.25	gm.	
Sodium	8	mEq.	7	mEq.	
Potassium	14	mEq.	13	mEq.	

Additions to each unit of base solution
(average adult):
Sodium   (chloride and/or bicarbonate) 40–50 mEq.
Potassium (chloride)   30–40 mEq.

Additions to only one unit daily:

Vitamin A	5000–10,000 U.S.P. units	Magnesium (sulfate) 4–16 mEq.
Vitamin D	500–1000 U.S.P. units	
Vitamin E	2.5–5.0 I.U.	
Vitamin C	250–500 mg.	
Thiamine	25–50 mg.	
Riboflavin	5–10 mg.	
Pyridoxine	7.5–15 mg.	
Niacin	50–100 mg.	
Pantothenic acid	12.5–25 mg.	

Optional additions to daily ration:

Vitamin K	5–10 mg.	⎫ Alternatively may be given I.M. in daily or weekly dosages
Vitamin B$_{12}$	10–30 mcg.	
Folic acid	0.5–1.5 mg.	
Iron	2.0–3.0 mg.	⎭
Calcium (gluconate)	4.5–18 mEq.	
Phosphate (potassium acid salt)	4–18 mEq.	

Micronutrients such as cobalt, copper, iodine, manganese and zinc are present as contaminants in hydrolysate solutions, but may be given in plasma transfusion once or twice weekly if desired.

tered-air hood), 350 ml. of 50 per cent dextrose is added to 750 ml. of 5 per cent protein hydrolysate in 5 per cent dextrose. A unit of nutrient base solution prepared by this method provides 100 ml. more water and somewhat less nitrogen, dextrose and calories than a liter of solution prepared by the bulk method.

Although the base solutions contain small amounts of some electrolytes, the composition and concentrations of which vary from one hydrolysate to another, additives must be made prior to infusion in order to satisfy nutrient and metabolic requirements. For the average adult patient with no significant cardiovascular, renal or hepatic dysfunction, 40 to 50 mEq. of sodium (as chloride and/or bicarbonate) and 30 to 40 mEq. of potassium (as chloride and/or acid phosphate) are added to *each* liter of base solution. To base solutions formulated from crystalline amino acids, which usually contain 35 to 50 mEq. of chloride per liter, sodium should be added as the bicarbonate and not the chloride salt in order to avoid production of hyperchloremic acidosis. One ampule of parenteral fat- and water-soluble vitamins and 4 to 16 mEq. of magnesium sulfate are added to any *one* bottle of the solution daily. Vitamin B_{12}, vitamin K and folic acid can be either added to one bottle of base solution daily or given intramuscularly intermittently in required dosages. Calcium (as gluconate) and phosphorus (as potassium acid phosphate) are not given routinely to adults, but are added to the regimen as indicated by weekly serum levels of these ions. In general 4 to 5 mEq. of calcium and phosphorus are given simultaneously per 1000 calories when fibrin hydrolysate or crystalline amino acids are used to formulate the base solution. However, because commercially available casein (a phosphoprotein) hydrolysate solutions contain 25 to 35 mEq. of phosphate per liter, more than enough phosphate is present in base solutions prepared from casein hydrolysate, and additional phosphate is neither required nor advisable.

Iron can be added to the solution daily or weekly in appropriately calculated doses or given intramuscularly in depot form. In patients with less than 10 gm. of hemoglobin per 100 ml., it is advisable to restore blood volume by transfusion of whole blood or packed erythrocytes prior to initiating intravenous hyperalimentation. Trace elements such as cobalt, copper, iodine, manganese and zinc are present as contaminants in most parenteral solutions, particularly in protein hydrolysate solutions, and are therefore not added routinely to the hyperalimentation regimen. In infants and in severely malnourished adults, however, they may be infused intermittently as specially prepared additives, or provided alternatively by the administration of 10 ml. of plasma or albumin per kilogram of body weight per week.

To provide the nutrients necessary for normal growth and development in infants, more complete formulations are required for daily infusion. Bulk and individual unit methods of preparation of pediatric nutrient solutions are outlined in Tables 4-7 and 4-8.

Modification of the usual adult formula is required for treatment of patients with (1) congestive heart failure, liver disease, or massive nutritional edema, in whom sodium administration is reduced, (2) slightly compromised renal function, in whom potassium administration is reduced or omitted, and (3) renal or hepatic failure, in whom protein hydrolysates or racemic mixtures of crystalline amino acids are restricted. Special solutions for the treatment of renal or hepatic failure contain nitrogen of highest biological value in the form of essential L-amino acids in 50 to 70 per cent dextrose (Table 4-9), thus providing adequate nutrition while promoting reduction of urea nitrogen and ammonia. Solution modification is often necessary following the initiation of parenteral hyperalimentation, determined by the patient's metabolic response to his disease, trauma, operation, infection or other

Table 4–7. Unit Preparation of Pediatric High Calorie Solutions

Composition of base solution;

400 ml. 5% fibrin hydrolysate in 5% dextrose	160 kcal.	⎰ 20 gm. hydrolysates
250 ml. 50% dextrose	500 kcal.	⎱ 20 gm. dextrose
650 ml.	660 kcal.	

Additions to each unit of base solution:

Sodium	20 mEq.	Sodium chloride (2 mEq./ml.)	10 ml.
Potassium	25 mEq. ⎫		
	⎬	Potassium acid phosphate	13 ml.
Phosphorus	25 mEq. ⎭	(2 mEq./ml.)	
Calcium	20 mEq.	Calcium gluconate, 10% (0.45 mEq./ml.)	44 ml.
Magnesium	10 mEq.	Magnesium sulfate, 50% (8 mEq./ml.)	1.2 ml.
Multiple vitamin infusion			4 ml.
Vitamin K	⎫		
Vitamin B_{12}	⎬	Added to solution daily or weekly	1 ml.
Folic acid	⎭	or given intramuscularly	
Iron			
Trace elements		Added to solution daily or given as 10 ml./kg. plasma twice weekly	1 ml.
			75 ml.

Base solution	650 ml.	
Additives	75 ml.	
Final solution	725 ml.	(given at rate of 145 ml./kg./day= 130 Kcal./kg./day)

Table 4–8. Bulk Preparation of Basic Pediatric High Calorie Solution

Fibrin hydrolysate 5% in dextrose 5%	12,000	ml.
Anhydrous dextrose, U.S.P.	2200	gm.
Calcium gluconate 10%	150	ml.
Multiple vitamin infusion	100	ml.
Potassium acid phosphate (2 mEq./ml.)	30	ml.
Magnesium sulfate 50%	2.5	ml.
Phytonadione (10 mg./ml.)	1.5	ml.
Iron (20 mg./ml.)	1.5	ml.
Cyanocobalamin (100 mcg./ml.)	1.0	ml.
Folic acid (50 mg./ml.)	0.5	ml.
Trace elements (optional)	5	ml.
Total volume	14,000	ml.

(Final pH of 5.2 to 5.5 may be adjusted to neutrality with sodium bicarbonate or sodium hydroxide as desired.)

Table 4–9. PREPARATION AND COMPOSITION OF ESSENTIAL
L-AMINO ACID – DEXTROSE SOLUTION

ESSENTIAL AMINO ACIDS	MINIMUM DAILY REQUIREMENTS (Gm.)
L-Tryptophan	0.25
L-Threonine	0.50
L-Isoleucine	0.70
L-Lycine	0.80
L-Valine	0.80
L-Leucine	1.10
L-Methionine	1.10
L-Phenylalanine	1.10

Total 6.35 gm. per 100/ml.

PLUS

750–1000 ml. 50–70% dextrose

Volume	850–1110 ml.
Calories	1500–2500 Kcal.
Dextrose	375–500 gm.
Nitrogen	1.0 gm.

complications. It is essential to recognize that no single intravenous nutrient solution can be ideal for all conditions in all patients at all times or for the same patient during various phases of a single pathologic process. Individual metabolic requirements must be met appropriately as they arise in the course of therapy.

ADMINISTRATION OF HIGH CALORIE SOLUTIONS

The average daily ration of hypertonic nutrient solution is comprised of 25 to 30 per cent solute, which must be infused continuously over 24 hours at a constant rate in order to achieve maximum assimilation of the nutrients without exceeding the body's capability for water, dextrose or amino acid metabolism. Because of the necessary hyperosmolarity (1800 to 2400 milliosmoles per liter) of the solution, it must be delivered to the circulatory system through a large-diameter, high-flow blood vessel, ideally the superior vena cava. Starting at the usual levels of water metabolism (2000 to 2500 ml. per day in adults or 100 ml. per kilogram per day in infants) and dextrose utilization (0.4 to 1.2 gm. per kilogram per day), the daily intravenous nutrient ration is increased gradually to tolerance (3000 to 4000 ml. per day in adults or 130 to 150 ml. per kilogram per day in infants).

The basic guidelines for safe intravenous hyperalimentation include accurate daily measurements of body weight and water balance, fractional urine sugar concentration every six hours, serum electrolytes daily until stable and every two or three days thereafter, and hemogram, blood urea nitrogen and blood sugar weekly. It is also advisable to evaluate hepatic function, serium calcium, phosphorus, magnesium and proteins initially and every one to three weeks thereafter during high calorie intravenous therapy. Occasional determinations of serum osmolality and vitamin levels, and urine specific gravity, osmolality, acetone and electrolytes may be helpful in monitoring the metabolic status of certain patients. Periodic measurements of arterial and central venous pressure, blood gases and pH may also be necessary in the management of critically ill patients with significant cardiovascular, respiratory or metabolic derangements.

Occasional adjustment of water volume, sugar concentration, nitrogen source or electrolyte content may be necessary during the clinical course of the critically ill or traumatized patient. Relative glucose intolerance may occur with initiation of parenteral hyperalimentation therapy, immediately following trauma, during operation, in the immediate postoperative period, in premature or newborn infants, in the aged, in patients with pancreatic disorders or in the presence of sepsis. To avoid persistent excessive glycosuria, secondary osmotic diuresis, and increased urine electrolyte losses, the infusion is maintained at a rate which will not allow quantitative urinary glucose to exceed 2 gm. per cent (greater than 3+ reaction). Ideally, the patient does not excrete any sugar in the urine. However, trace to 2+ glucose in the urine does not represent a significant loss of the total sugar administered. Such small amounts of glycosuria will induce a mild diuresis which may actually be helpful in excreting any excess vehicular water, and it indicates that the limit of the patient's ability to metabolize dextrose has been reached.

In the average patient, dextrose infusion is gradually increased as the normal pancreas increases its output of endogenous insulin in response to the continuous carbohydrate infusion. In all patients with diabetes mellitus, crystalline insulin is given routinely either subcutaneously in evenly divided doses or equally distributed in the intravenous fluid. Occasionally, in nondiabetic patients with relative glucose intolerance, supplemental crystalline insulin must be added to the nutrient solution in amounts of 5 to 25 units per 1000 calories. The addition of insulin may be indicated in the presence of elevated blood sugar to encourage more rapid and efficient glucose utilization and positive nitrogen balance in elderly patients with borderline glucose tolerance, in patients with known pancreatic disorders, in the early post-trauma period, and in critically ill, nutritionally depleted patients whose survival appears to depend upon the expedient achievement of positive caloric and nitrogen balance.

In patients with marked hypoproteinemia or anemia, albumin or blood is sometimes given early in the course of intravenous hyperalimentation to restore colloid osmotic pressure and red cell mass to normal levels. In patients with borderline serum protein concentrations, judicious administration of the nutritional solutions alone is often sufficient to correct the deficiencies. When circulating blood volume is inadequate to maintain normal cardiovascular dynamics, prompt administration of colloid as blood or albumin is essential to establish homeostasis before instituting parenteral hyperalimentation. Colloid is not administered for nutritional purposes, because the half-life is too long for albumin to be an efficient nutrient. On the other hand, the amino acids are immediately available as substrates for protein synthesis, and should not be administered for the purpose of maintaining osmotic pressure.

INTRODUCTION AND MAINTENANCE OF CENTRAL VENOUS INFUSION CATHETER

Infusion of the hypertonic solution can be accomplished through catheters directed into the superior vena cava following percutaneous or cutdown insertion into the external or internal jugular veins, or the cephalic, basilic or saphenous veins. However, infraclavicular percutaneous subclavian vein puncture has been the safest and most effective technique for long-term catheterization of the superior vena cava in adults and in children weighing more than 10 pounds. Either subclavian vein may be used safely by this technique unless a specific contraindication is present, such as ipsilateral thoracotomy, radical neck dissection, clavicular fracture or radical mastectomy. Despite the theoretical possibility of thoracic duct injury, this complication has not been observed.

The patient is positioned head-down 15 degrees (Trendelenburg position) to allow dilatation of the subclavian vein, making it a larger target. The shoulders are thrown back maximally or hyperextended over a rolled sheet placed longitudinally under the thoracic spine. With the shoulders then depressed caudally and the head turned maximally to the opposite side, the subclavian vein becomes easily accessible for percutaneous catheterization.

The skin over the lower neck, shoulder and upper chest is shaved, cleansed with ether or acetone to remove skin oil and prepared with 2 per cent tincture of iodine or Merthiolate in a manner identical to preoperative skin preparation. Using strict aseptic technique with sterile surgical gloves and instruments, the area is draped with sterile towels and local anesthetic is infiltrated into the skin, subcutaneous tissue and periosteum at the inferior border of the midpoint of the clavicle. A 2-inch-long, 14-gauge needle attached to a 2- or 3-ml. syringe is inserted bevel down through the wheal and advanced beneath the inferior margin of the clavicle in a horizontal (frontal) plane with the needle tip aimed for the anterior margin of the trachea at the level of the suprasternal notch (Fig. 4-6, A). With the needle and syringe barrel in a frontal plane and adjacent to the anterior deltoid promi-

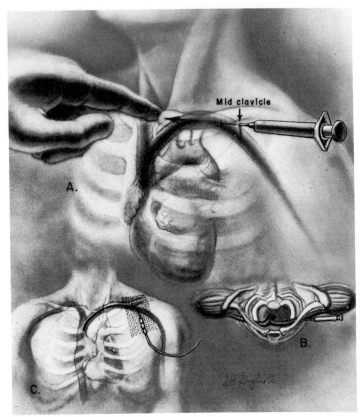

Figure 4-6. Landmarks for percutaneous infraclavicular subclavian vein catheterization.

nence, the needle enters the anterior wall of the subclavian vein (Fig. 4-6, *B*). As the needle is advanced beneath the clavicle, slight negative pressure applied through the syringe will help to ascertain accurate venipuncture with a flashback of blood. The needle is advanced a few millimeters further after blood first appears in the syringe to insure that the entire beveled tip is inside the vein. The patient is asked to perform a Valsalva maneuver, and the syringe is removed carefully while the needle is held firmly in place. A 16-gauge, 8-inch-long radiopaque catheter is introduced immediately through the needle and threaded its full length into the vein. The catheter should advance easily if the needle tip is entirely within the lumen of the vein and if the original direction of the needle has been maintained. The proximal end of the catheter is attached to the solution bottle by sterile intravenous administration tubing and flushed with fluid, the needle is withdrawn, and the catheter is secured by a 3-0 silk suture placed lateral to the skin puncture site. At this point, the solution bottle is momentarily lowered below bed level to insure free flow in both directions, an indication that proper placement of the catheter within the superior vena cava has been accomplished. A broad-spectrum antibiotic ointment is applied to the puncture site, and an occlusive sterile gauze dressing is fixed to the skin with tincture of benzoin and adhesive tape (Fig. 4-1, C). To prevent accidental disengagement of the intravenous tubing from the catheter and possible air embolism, the tubing-catheter connection is carefully reinforced with adhesive tape. A loop is made in the intravenous tubing and it is secured again with tape to guard against accidental traction on the catheter itself. Prior to beginning infusion of the hypertonic solution, a chest roentgenogram should be obtained to verify the position of the catheter in the superior vena cava.

The same basic technique may be used with commercially available 8-inch-long internal-needle-and-external-catheter combinations. The longer needle may be helpful in reaching the vein in large-framed or obese individuals. Catheters may also be placed percutaneously into the superior vena cava via an external or internal jugular vein, or by the supraclavicular approach to the subclavian vein. Because of the mobility of the neck and location of adjacent hair-growing areas, these puncture sites are less comfortable and are more difficult to keep sterile than is the infraclavicular subclavian route.

In infants weighing less than 10 pounds, the small subclavian vein and high apex of the lung can make percutaneous subclavian puncture very difficult and dangerous. Long-term intravenous catheterization in such patients is achieved more safely by inserting the catheter via external or internal jugular vein cut-down, using a 1 cm. incision at the base of the neck. After proper placement of its tip into the superior vena cava, the catheter is secured to the vein, and the proximal end is brought out through a subcutaneous tunnel to a stab wound in the parietal area of the scalp. The skin exit site is thereby removed to a point distant from the phlebotomy site, reducing the risks of infection and mechanical kinking, and making aseptic catheter maintenance easier. The neck wound is closed, and the catheter is sutured at the scalp exit site with 4-0 silk. An antibiotic ointment is applied, and the scalp is dressed in a fashion similar to the infraclavicular subclavian catheter site.

To achieve safe long-term intravenous catheterization, compulsive and meticulous care and maintenance of the catheter is just as important as proper insertion. Every two or three days, the intravenous tubing is changed, and the dressing over the puncture site is removed. Using aseptic technique and sterile gloves, the area is again defatted with acetone or ether and prepared with tincture of iodine or Merthiolate. Antibiotic ointment is re-applied and a sterile occlusive dressing is replaced. Withdrawal or administration of blood through the subclavian catheter should be avoided, because these practices significantly increase the possibility of contamination or clotting of the catheter.

Antibiotics, heparin or steroids are not added routinely to the solutions, but may be administered through a Y-tubing attached to the intravenous catheter if indicated or desired. Extreme care in adding medications or measuring central venous pressure should be practiced to prevent contamination of the solution or tubing.

INFUSION APPARATUS FOR CENTRAL VENOUS ALIMENTATION

In ambulatory adult patients, standard intravenous fluid bottles and infusion sets are used to deliver the nutrient solution continuously by gravity drip. Rolling intravenous poles allow ambulation and mobility which are essential for optimal nutrition and rehabilitation. Use of closed filtered infusion systems provides maximum safety against airborne contaminants which may gain entry into the solution or tubing. Lightweight AC/DC portable pumps attached to the intravenous pole or directly to the patient can be used to insure constant rate of infusion, allowing considerable freedom of position and activity.

In infants, the nutrient solution can be delivered continuously at a constant rate by means of a peristaltic pump with variable speed controls. Syringe pumps must never be used with nutrient solutions, as the risk of solution contamination with such pumps is too great. Between the pump and the catheter, the infusion tubing is attached to a 0.22 micron membrane filter. This in-line "final filter" protects against transmission of contaminants which may be introduced into the solution or tubing and prevents inadvertent air embolism, because air does not pass through the pores once the filter is moistened with the solution. In-line membrane filters may also be used in adult patients, but a larger pore size of 0.45 micron is necessary to permit an adequate rate of infusion. The larger pores theoretically permit passage of certain species of Pseudomonas organisms, but in practice these filters have been satisfactory bacterial barriers. The filter and administration set are replaced every three days or more often as required.

COMPLICATIONS OF CENTRAL VENOUS ALIMENTATION

Prevention of infection and sepsis is of utmost importance to the success of long-term intravenous hyperalimentation. The incidence of catheter sepsis is negligible if aseptic and antiseptic principles are conscientiously observed in insertion and maintenance of the intravenous cannula. Because the solutions are good culture media for many species of bacteria and fungi, meticulous asepsis must also be maintained in solution preparation, additive insertion and long-term infusion. Should fever occur without an obvious cause, the solution and tubing are promptly replaced, and specimens of the blood and the solution are cultured. If the fever persists following replacement of the solution and tubing, infusion is terminated. The subclavian catheter is removed, and the tip is immediately placed into thioglycolate broth and sent for culture. Depending upon the clinical situation, another catheter may be inserted into the opposite subclavian vein, or administration of isotonic dextrose may be started by peripheral vein. Broad-spectrum antibiotic therapy is rarely required. If desired, however, antibiotics may be started at this time and modified when specific sensitivity testing is completed.

The presence of fever or sepsis prior to the institution of intravenous hyperalimentation is not necessarily a contraindication to the use of the technique. In a traumatized or critically ill patient, sepsis actually accentuates the need for adequate nutrition. Antibiotic therapy has already been instituted in many such patients, and, although seeding of the indwelling catheter by circulating microorganisms is a distinct possibility, it has not been a significant problem, and resolution of systemic infections has occurred frequently during the period of intravenous hyperalimentation. Whenever the clinician is suspicious that the infectious course of the patient might be caused or aggravated by the superior vena cava catheter, the catheter should be removed and cultured promptly.

Although thrombophlebitis is theoretically a possibility with the use of long-term indwelling catheters and hypertonic solutions, superior vena cava thrombosis has not been observed clinically in over 1000 patients. The high blood flow in this vessel assures prompt dilution of the hypertonic fluid. Attention to sterility practically eliminates the threat of thrombophlebitis. Rare instances of thrombophlebitis have occurred, particularly in patients whose catheter tip was misdirected into an internal jugular, external jugular, or axillary vein.

Other complications such as inadvertent air embolism, catheter embolism and catheter clotting can be avoided readily by adherence to principles and techniques previously discussed. A thorough knowledge of the anatomy, coupled with common sense and strict adherence to the technique of percutaneous subclavian catheterization, should minimize the risk of accidental pneumothorax, hydrothorax, hemothorax, subclavian artery puncture, bleeding, or injury to the thoracic duct or brachial plexus.

Hyperosmolar nonketotic hyperglycemia can be precipitated acutely by infusion of the hypertonic fluid too rapidly, causing marked osmotic diuresis, serum and urine electrolyte aberrations, dehydration, and central nervous system irritability. The chronic form of this syndrome can occur insidiously when impaired glucose utilization is not recognized, particularly in the presence of diabetes mellitus, extensive burns or major trauma, or after intracranial operations. If blood and urine sugar concentrations are not conscientiously monitored in such patients, blood sugar can become markedly elevated, with accompanying weakness, listlessness and eventual coma. Treatment of hyperosmolar hyperglycemia consists of judicious infusion of isotonic or half-strength solutions of saline or glucose along with insulin, at the same time obtaining frequent measurements of fluid loss, central venous pressure, electrolytes and blood sugar. Thorough assessment and understanding of the patient's disease process, his metabolic status, and the established principles of the technique of intravenous hyperalimentation will prevent most of these complications.

CONCLUSION

Parenteral nutrition has been progressively improved in each decade, but rarely until now has a prolonged sustained and meaningful state of anabolism been achieved exclusively with intravenous feeding, particularly under conditions ordinarily associated with a catabolic response. The seriously ill patient requires increased nutritional support for restoration of body tissues and metabolism. Superimposed on this need are the increased energy and nitrogen requirements resulting from preoperative and intraoperative relative starvation, the postoperative catabolic response and the accelerated metabolism associated with postoperative complications. By the judicious intravenous administration of adequate basic nutrients, tissue synthesis, weight gain, growth and development can be achieved to the benefit of surgical patients who cannot or should not eat.

REFERENCES

Dudrick, S. J., Steiger, E., and Long, J. M.: Renal failure in surgical patients. Treatment with intravenous essential amino acids and hypertonic glucose. Surgery 68:180, 1970.

Dudrick, S. J., Steiger, E., Long, J. M., and Rhoads, J. E.: Role of parenteral hyperalimentation in management of multiple catastrophic complications. Surg. Clin. N. Amer. 50:1031, 1970.

Dudrick, S. J., Wilmore, D. W., Vars, H. M., and Rhoads, J. E.: Long term parenteral nutrition with growth, development and positive nitrogen balance. Surgery 64:134, 1968.

Dudrick, S. J., Wilmore, D. W., and Vars, H. M.: Long-term venous catheterization— an adjunct to surgical care and study. Current Topics Surg. Res. 1:325, 1969.

Filler, R. M., Eraklis, A. J., Rubin, V. G., and Das, J. B.: Long term parenteral nutrition in infants. N. Eng. J. Med. 11:589, 1969.

Geyer, R. P.: Parenteral nutrition. Physiol. Rev. 40:150, 1960.

Meng, H. C., and Law, D. H.: Parenteral nutrition. Springfield, Ill., Charles C Thomas, 1970.

Wilmore, D. W., and Dudrick, S. J.: Growth and development of an infant receiving all nutrients exclusively by vein. J.A.M.A. 203:860, 1968.

CHAPTER 5

INFECTION AND ANTIMICROBIAL AGENTS

WILLIAM R. SANDUSKY, M.D., F.A.C.S.

THE SIGNIFICANCE OF INFECTION IN SURGERY

The diagnosis, treatment, and prevention of infection are matters of singular importance in the preoperative and postoperative care of all surgical patients.

Infection is a response of the body to injury by microorganisms. It differs from contamination, a state in which organisms are present in the body or on its surfaces but are not multipying and excite no inflammatory reaction. There is another relationship between microbe and host which is neither infection nor contamination. In certain areas, such as the skin, respiratory passages, alimentary tract, and vagina, bacteria are normally present. They multiply and live in harmony with their host, and in this environment they produce no disease. Yet, if permitted access to tissue not protected by skin or mucous membrane, these same organisms may become the agents of sepsis.

The clinical response to microorganisms is varied. For example, *Clostridium tetani*, growing in human tissue and producing little or no local reaction, yields a powerful exotoxin which acts upon nerve cells remote from the site at which the toxin is elaborated. Other organisms grow in the blood stream and cause generalized manifestations such as typhoid fever. Still others produce a localized reaction from which secondary extension may occur. Moreover, the behavior of various parts of the body to the same microorganism may be different. Some organisms seem to have a predilection for certain tissues or organs, whereas other areas seem to possess natural resistance to the very same organism.

A significant characteristic of many surgical infections is local inflammatory response with destruction of tissue, usually requiring oper-

ative methods for the release of pus or elimination of necrotic material
or both. This is in contrast to nonsurgical infection, which produces
little or no tissue necrosis but excites systemic response.

COMMON POSTOPERATIVE INFECTIONS

The intensity of the pathophysiologic reaction to microbial injury
may vary greatly, ranging from scarcely recognizable symptoms and
signs to profound alterations capable of affecting multiple organ systems. Irrespective of the organ system involved, surgical infections
assume certain patterns by which they may be recognized clinically.
These are cellulitis, abscess, reticular and tubular lymphangitis, lymphadenitis, septic thrombophlebitis, septicemia, necrosis, ulcer, sinus,
and fistula. Any of these patterns, either singly or in combination, may
appear in the postoperative period in almost any location, but the sites
of infection commonly seen in surgical patients following operation are
the wound, the pulmonary tree, and the urinary tract.

Wound Infection. The terms redness, swelling, heat, and pain,
used by Celsus in his classic description of inflammation, cannot be
improved upon for depicting local wound sepsis. To complete the
description, the modern surgeon would add such manifestations as
malaise, tachycardia, fever, chills, leukocytosis, and increased sedimentation rate. In addition, he would be mindful of the presence and
character of any wound discharge and, in cases of doubt, he would
employ, judiciously and with asepsis, the exploring clamp or the trocar.
It is, of course, not necessary that all the descriptive criteria be present
to establish a diagnosis of postoperative wound infection. It is essential
to issue the warning that, in the patient who is receiving steroids or
antibacterial therapy, infection may exist in the operative incision or
elsewhere in forms so modified that one or more of the usual stigmata
of inflammation may be missing.

Pulmonary Infection. One of the common complications in the
postoperative period is pulmonary atelectasis which, if unrelieved,
usually leads to pneumonitis. Atelectasis is recognized by fever, tachycardia, sometimes tachypnea and, rarely, cyanosis, yet physical signs are
often absent. Obstruction of the tracheobronchial tree is followed by
absorption of trapped gases and collapse of pulmonary tissue, the extent
of which depends upon the site of obstruction. The obstruction is
caused by retained bronchial secretions which, in turn, are the result of
such factors as a change in the character of the normal secretions,
ineffective clearing of the tree, or reduction in its caliber. If collapse of
pulmonary tissue is unrelieved, infection inevitably ensues. Atelectasis
is more frequent after upper abdominal operations and prolonged anesthesia. Factors contributing significantly to atelectasis are pain, analgesics, and ineffectual coughing, all of which may lead to shallow respira-

tions and hypoventilation. Pulmonary sepsis, notably lung abscess, also may follow the aspiration of foreign materials such as blood and gastric content.

Urinary Tract Infection. In the postoperative state there may be factors that frequently predispose to urinary tract infection. Two of these are urinary stasis and foreign body. The inability to void, with resultant urinary retention, may be due to recumbency or to reflex disturbances in neuromuscular control caused by anesthesia, drugs, or operative manipulation, or it may be due to pre-existent obstruction, either congenital or acquired. The foreign body may have been intrinsic, but more often than not it takes the form of that exceedingly useful agent of postoperative care, the catheter, introduced and withdrawn on several occasions, or left *in situ* for considerable periods of time. Postoperative urinary infection may involve the urethra or its appendages, the bladder, or the upper tract. The offending microorganisms are usually enteric bacteria. They are rarely blood-borne but usually ascend. The urethral meatus in both male and female is laden with bacteria, some of which normally migrate into the distal urethra. They gain a foothold by trauma, or they may be pushed higher by the catheter.

MICROORGANISMS COMMONLY ASSOCIATED WITH SURGICAL INFECTIONS

It is possible for any microorganism to produce a lesion of surgical significance. Witness the rare occurrence of wound diphtheria or the now nearly extinct typhoidal cholecystitis. There are a few organisms, however, which cause the bulk of surgical infections. It is convenient to group them as follows:

Gram-Positive Cocci. The most common of these is the staphylococcus. Frequently this organism is carried on skin and in the nasal passages of healthy individuals. Pathogenic strains produce coagulase, liquefy gelatin, belong to a relatively few phage types, and yield antigenic exotoxin which is hemolytic and dermatonecrotic. In addition to coagulase, this organism elaborates the enzymes fibrinolysin, leukocidin, and hyaluronidase, but the relative importance of the individual enzymes in pathogenesis is not altogether understood. Staphylococcal disease may be acute, chronic, or recurrent and may range in seriousness from simple folliculitis to fulminating septicemia.

Another common pathogen is the streptococcus. There are many varieties: some hemolyze culture media; others produce a greenish pigment; some grow best in an environment low in oxygen. The most common offender so far as human infection is concerned is the group A hemolytic streptococcus. Its pathogenicity appears to be associated with an erythrogenic toxin and a mucoprotein responsible for resistance to phagocytosis. The role in pathogenesis of other streptococcal enzymes, such as streptokinase, proteinase, hyaluronidase, and hemolysins is not clear. Streptococci are noted for invasiveness; frequently, untreated streptococcal disease progresses from an insignificant lesion to overwhelming sepsis in a remarkably short time. The more common clinical manifestations of streptococcal infections are cellulitis, lymphangitis, lymphadenitis, and serous surface infection. *Streptococcus viridans,* although seen in subacute bacterial endocarditis, is not often the agent of surgical infection. Another aerobic streptococcus, the enterococcus, being a component of the fecal flora, may be associated with infections tracing their origin to the intestinal tract.

Occasionally, the pneumococcus assumes surgical significance by causing a pus-forming lesion such as empyema, peritonitis, or postoperative pneumonitis. This organism is unique in that it produces disease solely through its invasive properties and possesses no demonstrable toxin.

The facultative and the obligate anaerobes have a unique place as agents of surgical infection. Because of the cultural requirements of these organisms they are not always identified, and it is probable that their frequency is in fact greater than is evident. The microaerophilic hemolytic streptococcus produces a rare but characteristic lesion, the undermining, burrowing ulcer of skin and subcutaneous tissue. Strictly anaerobic streptococci are present as normal inhabitants of the oral cavity, the intestine, and the vagina, and occasionally produce sepsis, usually abscesses, in a variety of locations. Some anaerobic streptococci are nonhemolytic; others, hemolytic. One species of the latter, in symbiosis with the staphylococcus or infrequently with some other organism, gives rise to a rare lesion, progressive bacterial synergistic gangrene, which involves skin and subcutaneous tissue in a locally destructive process.

Gram-Negative Enteric Bacilli. Prior to the introduction of modern antimicrobic drugs, most infections that were seen by surgeons were those caused by gram-positive cocci. This is no longer true. The leading offenders are now the gram-negative enteric bacilli, and the one most commonly isolated from surgical lesions is *Escherichia coli.* Others frequently identified are *Enterobacter aerogenes, Pseudomonas aeruginosa,* the proteus group, *Klebsiella pneumoniae,* and *Alcaligenes faecalis.* The salmonella group and the shigella group cause typhoid and enteric fevers and bacillary dysentery, but rarely are they associated with surgical disease.

It is currently of considerable interest and importance that organisms formerly regarded as nonpathogens, *Serratia marcescens,* for example, are emerging as the causative agents of serious surgical infections including septicemia. The changing pattern of surgical bacteriology is further illustrated by the increasing frequency with which infections caused by members of the bacteroides group are being reported. Chief among these are *Bacteroides fragilis, Bacteroides funduliformis,* and *Bacteroides melaninogenicus.* These gram-negative organisms are obligate anaerobes, and it is likely that they outnumber the aerobic flora of the normal gut.

Excepting salmonella and shigella, the gram-negative enteric bacilli possess very little pathogenicity while they remain within the intestinal tract of man and lower animals. Yet, outside their normal habitat, these organisms have a definite potential for producing sepsis. Because of anatomic proximity, the site of infection is usually the peritoneal cavity, the appendix, the hepatobiliary system, and the urinary tract, but wound infection, burn sepsis, and septicemia are not infrequent. The lesion itself may assume any of the clinical patterns described in the previous section.

The ability of gram-negative bacilli to cause disease is probably related to an endotoxin, a lipopolysaccharide, which is liberated when the organism dies. As a rule, the flora of infections associated with enteric bacilli is polymicrobial. Although this may be a matter of chance, there is good reason to believe that in many circumstances the pathogenicity of the enteric bacilli is enhanced by symbiotic activity with other microbes. Among other factors which abet these opportunist pathogens are reduced local vascularity, obstruction to the lumen of a hollow organ, foreign body, and altered host resistance.

The Anaerobic Spore-Forming Bacilli.   The gram-positive, anaerobic, spore-forming bacilli known as the clostridia are organisms of considerable interest in surgery. Their bacterial cell contains a very hardy spore which remains viable under the most adverse physical conditions. All are common inhabitants of the gastrointestinal tract of man and other animals and because of their spores are able to survive for a long time in soil, in dust, and on clothing. This large family includes the causative agent of tetanus (*Cl. tetani*) and the several organisms (*Cl. welchii, Cl. septicum, Cl. novyi, Cl. sordellii*) which produce the clinical entity called gas gangrene (clostridial cellulitis, clostridial myositis). They frequently contaminate wounds resulting from trauma, particularly war wounds. *Cl. welchii*, the most commonly encountered member of this group, produces multiple enzymes among which are lethal, hemolyzing, and necrotizing toxins. *Cl. tetani*, a noninvasive organism, produces very little local reaction but elaborates a powerful neurotoxin.

Other Microorganisms.   Other microbes occasionally produce lesions requiring surgical attention. These include *Mycobacterium tuberculosis,* actinomycetes, spirochetes, fusiform organisms, candida, nocardia, aspergilli, sporotrichi, and blastomycetes. The place of the viruses in surgical sepsis is unknown.

THE PREVENTION OF INFECTION

General Considerations.   Sterilization means the destruction or removal of all living organisms. The basic methods available are thermal and chemical. Mechanical cleansing, for example, with soap or detergent and water, is an essential first step in all processes of degerming. Heat kills bacteria by coagulation, with wet heat being more effective than dry. An increase in pressure raises the temperature and shortens the time necessary for destruction of bacteria and their spores; as a result, steam under pressure is the most widely used method for sterilization. It is the method of choice for any object or material that will not be damaged by high temperature and water. The use of heat demands careful regulation relative to time, temperature, and wetness. Chemical sterilization, although having historic primacy, is utilized only when heat cannot be employed. Ethylene oxide, formaldehyde, or betapropiolactone, in closed chambers, is used to sterilize instruments and materials that would be injured by heat or by direct application of strong chemical solutions.

There are many surfaces and objects in the hospital, both movable and immovable, which become the reservoirs of dust, dirt, and microbes. They cannot be sterilized, but their threat to the environment can be reduced by simple cleanliness, reinforced, if necessary and when practical, by the application of germicidal chemicals such as alcohol, the phenols, the halogens, and aldehydes.

Air is one of the factors in the transmission of microorganisms. The reduction of dust, lint, and other particles and the physical activity that distributes them are of prime importance in controlling air contamination in all parts of the hospital. Special consideration should be given to the source of air and to the mechanical means by which it is cooled, heated, washed, filtered, humidified, and circulated. Although it is possible to reduce the bacterial content of air by ultraviolet irradiation, this method has not proved effective in lessening surgical sepsis.

The meticulous aseptic protocol of the surgical suite is aimed at reducing contamination from every source. Training develops and discipline enforces an awareness of what asepsis is and when it is violated and a sense of responsibility for the safety of the patient in every person connected with the operation.

Measures intended to prevent infection should not be limited to the surgical suite. Of signal importance is the attack on cross-contamination stemming from septic lesions and other reservoirs in the hospital environment. Elemental in this effort is good housekeeping in all parts of the hospital and intelligent and conscientious techniques in caring for wounds. Sterile instruments and supplies should be used when dressing wounds. The communal dressing carriage has outlived its usefulness and ought to be replaced by individual dressing trays and separately packaged instruments and other materials such as catheters, needles, and syringes.

Lesions that have septic discharges should be isolated and not touched by bare hands. Open denuded areas, such as burns, should be protected from cross contamination by isolation techniques involving the use of masks, gowns, and gloves. So-called minor procedures, such as venipuncture, spinal tap, and catheterization, should be performed under aseptic conditions. Great care must be exercised in the collection and disposal of soiled dressings, linens, and excreta from patients with infection lest they become a source for the dissemination of virulent microorganisms.

Prevention of Wound Infection.   No wound is free from microorganisms. Moreover, every wound offers an environment conducive to bacterial growth; namely, warmth, moisture, and pabulum. The sources of contamination of the clean operative incision are numerous: the skin of the patient; the noses and throats of all persons who enter the surgical suite; the hands of the surgeon and his assistants; air; the instruments and materials used during the procedure; remote or inapparent infection in the patient; and septic lesions, even small ones involving personnel attending the patient. The wound resulting from trauma is liable to contamination from any of these sources as well as others during injury, first aid, and transportation.

Contamination from the noses and throats of persons in the operating room is minimized by the use of masks. The removal of ordinary outside clothing and the wearing of scrub suits, caps, sterile gowns, and shoe covers affords additional protection of the wound from air-borne contamination. The importance of self-discipline in these matters, especially the exclusion from the operating suite of personnel with septic lesions, even small and apparently insignificant ones, needs to be emphasized and re-emphasized.

The skin cannot be sterilized completely, but its bacterial content can be reduced to a point at which operation is relatively safe. All hair should be removed from the operative site. Although chemical depilatory agents are recommended by some, careful shaving is the preferable method, and it should be done as near the time of operation as is feasible, lest unavoidable abrasions become colonized with bacteria. Grease, dirt, desquamated epithelium, and loose bacteria are removed from the skin by mechanical scrubbing with soap, detergents, or solvents. Except for operations on hands or feet, it is best not to scrub with stiff brushes but rather to cleanse vigorously with a soft cloth. The mechanical phase of preparation is followed by the application of a germicidal agent. The substance used should be bactericidal, harmless to skin, and capable of penetrating its crevices. Many preparations have been employed. None, however, is more effective in destroying microorganisms than iodine tincture (2 per cent iodine, 2.4 per cent sodium iodide in alcohol). Currently, the iodophors are enjoying popularity. They possess certain desirable features, but their germicidal qualities are derived from the iodine they make available; thus they are no better than a tincture of comparable strength.

Preparation of the hands and forearms of the surgical team is accomplished by thorough and systematic scrubbing, using a brush, hot water, and soap. Particular attention should be given to nails and natural skin crevices. It is probable that the number and character of brush strokes is more important than the length of the hand scrub but, in actual practice, a scrub protocol based upon time is the more practical. Undoubtedly, one of the most important factors in the effectiveness of the hand scrub is the care and conscientiousness with which it is performed. A soap and water scrub is followed by soaking or rinsing the hands in 70 per cent ethyl alcohol, a very effective germicide. Instead of plain soap, a soap or a detergent containing hexachlorophene may be preferred. In this event, the scrub should not be followed by alcohol lest the hexachlorophene be neutralized.

Additional protection of the wound from hand contamination is provided by rubber gloves, and contact of the patient's own skin with the deeper wound structures is reduced by the use of fabric drapes, or towels, or with materials that adhere to the skin.

No matter how careful the technique, some wound contamination results; yet relatively few contaminated wounds become infected. It is obvious that factors other than microorganisms influence the development and the persistence of infection. Among these are the inherent vascularity of the region involved, foreign bodies, anemia, undernutrition, hypoproteinemia, steroid therapy, and bone marrow suppression from causes such as drugs, irradiation, or blood dyscrasia. These are factors over which the surgeon exercises little or no control. Conversely, there are other factors of extreme importance which he can influence. These are concerned with proper wound management, the basic tenets of which are the removal of debris and devitalized tissue; exact hemostasis; scrupulous preservation of blood supply; gentle handling of tissue; careful layer to layer approximation without tension, and the avoidance of dead space.

Prevention of Pulmonary Infection. Atelectasis and aspiration are significant events predisposing to the development of postoperative pulmonary infection. Atelectasis may be prevented by relief of pain, deep breathing, coughing, changes in position, activity, suction (via nasotracheal catheter, endotracheal tube, or bronchoscopy), humidification of the atmosphere, bronchodilators, intermittent positive pressure breathing, respiratory exercises, avoidance of drugs which increase viscosity of secretions, and abstention from smoking prior to operation. Relief of pain needs to be balanced against the avoidance of heavy sedation and, on rare occasions, intercostal nerve block may be required. If atelectasis occurs, its treatment is the relief of obstruction by suction, followed by the maintenance of adequate pulmonary ventilation. Many of the measures utilized in prevention are applicable in therapy. Antimicrobic agents are not indicated unless pneumonia ensues. The aspiration of blood or gastric content may lead to pulmonary sepsis. Such mishaps can be prevented by emptying the stomach before operation, maintaining the head-down position during periods of unconsciousness, and using cuffed endotracheal tubes. If aspiration is recognized and relieved quickly, nothing results other than chemical irritation of the bronchopulmonary apparatus. Prophylactic antibacterial agents and corticosteroids are indicated.

Prevention of Urinary Tract Infection. The incidence of urinary tract infection is lessened by early walking, adequate fluid intake, and especially by discretion, gentleness, and asepsis in the use of the catheter. Recognizing the risk of the indwelling catheter, various precautionary measures against infection have been introduced. These include the use of closed systems for the collection of urine and the local application of antiseptic agents. There is no convincing evidence that routine systemic antimicrobic agents are of value in the prevention of urinary tract infection.

Antimicrobic Agents in the Prevention of Infection. The prophylaxis of infection with antimicrobic agents implies that the microorganisms are attacked during the period of contamination before colonization has occurred, or, if colonization has taken place, before invasive infection begins. The prophylactic use of the modern antibacterial drugs has been put to the test by controlled prospective clinical observation, by retrospective analyses, and by animal experimentation. Yet not all surgeons share a unanimity of opinion as to their effectiveness.

The routine use of these valuable drugs is to be avoided. This means that drug prophylaxis has no place in operative procedures which carry minimal risk relative to sepsis. Conversely, drug prophylaxis may reduce the incidence and severity of infection in certain conditions in which such risks are great. For example:

1. Wounds resulting from trauma which are heavily contaminated or for which thorough debridement and mechanical cleansing are not possible or are delayed.

2. Burns.

3. Operative sites associated with heavy contamination or established infection.

4. Preparation of the large intestine for operation.

5. Operations requiring the insertion of permanent prostheses.

6. Surgical procedures on patients prone to infection because of factors such as impoverished local blood supply, the carrier state, undernutrition, pre-existing infection remote from the operation site, or therapy which may alter host defense mechanisms.

The principles outlined for the therapeutic use of antimicrobial agents (see p. 121) are applicable to their prophylactic employment. Several additional considerations need emphasis. If prophylaxis is indicated, it is logical to expect the agent to be more effective if it is present at the time of contamination than if it is given later. This means administration prior to operation if the need for a drug can be anticipated; or, if the requirement is not apparent until the operative findings are known, the drug should be started before the operation is finished.

The agent should be given in sufficient amount and by a route that assures an effective concentration in the contaminated tissue.

The duration of administration in the postoperative period is an unresolved question. Although there is no convincing basis for its answer, it is reasonable to assume that unless the initial contamination is overwhelming or unless there is reason to expect continuing contamination, a 24-hour period of prophylaxis should be sufficient. Exceptions are Group 2 and 6 cases which may require longer protection. A short period of drug administration lessens the likelihood of adverse consequences such as toxic reactions or superinfection.

The common wound pathogens are staphylococci, gram-negative enteric bacilli, occasionally group A hemolytic streptococci and, in wounds resulting from trauma, clostridia. It is obvious that against this array of potential invaders there is no all-purpose preventive agent; however, one or the other of the following regimens is appropriate: (1) a combination of agents including penicillin G, since this is the drug of choice against nonpenicillinase-producing staphylococci, group A hemolytic streptococci, and the clostridia; in addition, there should be one of the penicillins not hydrolyzed by penicillinase (methicillin, nafcillin, oxacillin, cloxacillin, or dicloxacillin) plus an agent effective against the enteric bacteria, such as gentamicin or kanamycin; or (2) one of the cephalosporins.

Preparation of the Bowel for Operation. The preoperative preparation of the large intestine includes the use of antimicrobic drugs for prophylactic purposes, but it by no means involves only the simple administration of these agents. Rather, it is the application of all methods known to reduce the microbial flora in the intestinal tract. An essential first step is thorough mechanical cleansing. Moreover, preoperative preparation must not be relied on to the exclusion of other sound and well-established principles and practices in intestinal surgery. The use of drugs is not without risk or inconvenience. Drastic reduction of bacteria in the bowel may be followed by the overgrowth of fungi. In many instances diarrhea and perianal irritation result, but of far more consequence is the overgrowth of staphylococci and, in the case of certain enterotoxigenic strains, the development of pseudomembranous enterocolitis. It is to prevent these complications that some programs of intestinal preparation include antistaphylococcal and antifungal agents.

A variety of drugs have been employed for intestinal antisepsis. The two regimens used most frequently are (1) a neomycin-phthalylsulfathiazole (Sulfathalidine) combination administered as neomycin, 1 gm., and Sulfathalidine, 1.5 gm., every hour for 4 hours and every 4 hours thereafter; or (2) kanamycin, 1 gm. every hour for 4 hours and every 4 hours thereafter. In the unobstructed patient a purgative should be given a short time before the first dose of the antibacterial agent, and enemata should be administered following catharsis to evacuate colonic residue. Once the purgative has been given, diet should be restricted to clear liquids. There is some difference in opinion relative to the duration of preparation; authoritative recommendations range from 20 to 72 hours.

The Prevention of Tetanus. There are several acceptable programs for active immunization to protect against tetanus. They differ chiefly in the kind of tetanus toxoid used, the number of injections, and the interval between injections. The following program is recommended for immunization of adults: 0.5 ml. of precipitated toxoid (alum precipitated, aluminum hydroxide adsorbed or aluminum phosphate adsorbed), intramuscularly, on two occasions at an interval of 4 to 6 weeks, followed by another injection 6 to 12 months later. In the pediatric age group it is desirable to combine tetanus immunization with that for diphtheria and pertussis. The American Academy of Pediatrics has recommended a schedule essentially as follows: three 0.5 ml. intramuscular injections of DTP (alum precipitated, aluminum hydroxide adsorbed or aluminum phosphate adsorbed diphtheria and tetanus toxoids, and pertussis vaccine) at intervals of 1 month during early infancy, followed by a fourth injection a year later and by a fifth injection when the child enters school.

A person who has received active immunization with toxoid develops a measurable level of circulating tetanus antitoxin generally believed to be adequate for protection and keeps it for an indeterminate period, surely for at least 1 year, probably much longer. Beyond this period of active immunity, the individual possesses the ability to recall a protective level of antitoxin when toxoid is administered again. Although it is not known how long he retains this ability, one report indicates that a protective titer may be recalled after a lapse of 25 years. No information, either negative or positive, is available for longer periods. The U.S. Public Health Service Advisory Committee on Immunization Practices has recommended a booster every 10 years. This interval would appear to be well within the limits of safety, and there is no need for more frequent routine boosters.

Temporary and passive immunologic protection can be obtained by administering preformed antitoxin from a human, equine, or bovine source. Whenever human immune globulin is available, there is no excuse for subjecting the patient to the risks of foreign proteins. Two hundred fifty units of human immune globulin administered intramuscularly gives immediate and adequate protection which lasts well beyond the usual incubation period of *Cl. tetani.* Sensitivity testing is unnecessary when human immune globulin is used, but should it be necessary to administer antitoxin from another source sensitivity testing is mandatory. Whenever prophylactic antitoxin is given, one should begin active immunization with toxoid at the same time; however, the two must not be given in the same syringe or into the same injection site.

Any wound may be contaminated with tetanus organisms — either spores or vegetable forms. These organisms find an environment favorable for growth and toxin production in traumatized tissue. Consequently, prophylaxis of tetanus must be initiated by prompt and adequate surgical care of every potentially contaminated wound. This demands the excision of dead tissue, the removal of foreign material, and thorough mechanical cleansing. The objective is to eliminate or to reduce the number of microorganisms and the material on which they live and to make sure of the vascular integrity of the part, so that the entire wound surface is in contact with well-oxygenated arterial blood. In addition to careful wound surgery, the patient should receive the further protection afforded by appropriately administered toxoid or antitoxin.

Some of the antibacterial agents, notably penicillin and the tetracyclines, are effective in protecting against experimentally induced tetanus. Although their value in the prophylaxis of human tetanus has not been established, the use of antibiotics in addition to wound surgery should be considered in wound management whenever immunologic prophylaxis is not available, or when it is contraindicated. It is important to remember that the mode of action of the antibiotic differs from that of antitoxin. The latter has no effect on the microorganism but neutralizes the exotoxin, whereas the antibiotic acts on the microorganism but has no effect on exotoxin.

Sometimes tetanus occurs after trivial or even unrecognized injury. Nonetheless, certain wounds provide a more favorable environment for the growth of anaerobic microorganisms than do others. Such wounds may be recognized by their extent, particularly their depth, by the amount of devascularization of tissue, by the presence of foreign material, or by the fact that adequate surgical care has been delayed. These criteria are not infallible, but they do provide useful guides for planning prophylaxis. When there is doubt, even slight doubt, the safe option is to assume that the wound in question is "tetanus prone."

In addition to wound surgery, which is the *sine qua non* of tetanus prophylaxis, certain immunologic measures are recommended for specific situations as follows:

> Immunization completed previously; booster dose within 12 months:
> *No additional toxoid is required.*

> Immunization completed within the previous 10 years:
> *Administer 0.5 ml. fluid tetanus toxoid booster.*

> Immunization completed more than 10 years previously; last booster within the previous 10 years:
> *Administer 0.5 ml. fluid tetanus toxoid booster.*

> Immunization completed more than 10 years pre-

viously; no booster within the previous 10 years; wound relatively clean; treated promptly and adequately:

Administer 0.5 ml. fluid tetanus toxoid booster.

Immunization completed more than 10 years previously; no booster within the previous 10 years; wound "tetanus prone" (see above):

Administer 0.5 ml. fluid tetanus toxoid, and 250 units tetanus immune globulin (human).

No history or record of immunization; wound very clean; wound surgery prompt and adequate:

Begin immunization, using 0.5 ml. precipitated tetanus toxoid.

No history or record of immunization; wound other than very clean or not treated promptly or adequately:

Administer 250 units of tetanus immune globulin (human); begin immunization.

TREATMENT OF ESTABLISHED SURGICAL INFECTIONS

In essence, the treatment of established surgical infection consists of general measures which support the resistance of the host and the use of antimicrobial therapy which attacks the microorganism directly. The importance of early diagnosis as the first step in effective treatment must be emphasized.

General Measures. Support of the host's resistance is directed at the maintenance of normal fluid-electrolyte balance, blood volume, and nutrition; rest for the patient; immobilization of the region involved; the relief of pain; and elevation, if possible, to promote lymphatic and venous drainage and to relieve swelling, and with it pain. Moist heat is applied in certain cases to increase the local blood supply, promote comfort, facilitate the discharge of exudate, prevent the formation of crusts, and hasten the separation of sloughs. To these measures are added the employment of appropriate and properly timed surgical intervention when indicated.

Antimicrobial Therapy. Certain principles are inherent in the use of antimicrobial agents to treat established infection:

1. *The organism causing infection must be sensitive to the drug administered.* Identification of the offending microbe and the determination of its susceptibility to antimicrobic agents are the first steps in the planning of effective drug therapy. There are, however, significant exceptions. In certain infections, such as those due to the group A beta

hemolytic streptococcus, the pneumococcus, or *Hemophilus influenzae,* identification of the organism without testing for sensitivity is sufficient. Conversely, in other circumstances it may be more important to determine the drug spectrum of an organism than to name it. In rapidly developing serious infections, such as lymphangitis or cellulitis, from which recovery of organisms is not possible immediately, or while awaiting the results of a culture, it is not only permissible but even obligatory to administer drugs of low toxicity known to be effective against the organisms that tend to be associated with the particular clinical problem at hand.

Microscopic examination of the gram-stained direct smear is an often-neglected diagnostic method. This test is easy, inexpensive, and rapid, and gives immediate information that is valuable as a guide to therapy.

Re-evaluation is imperative if satisfactory response to drug therapy does not occur. Further laboratory surveillance is then necessary to determine whether or not the initial susceptibility to the drug may have changed, whether a new organism may have been introduced, or whether those organisms initially present in small numbers and insensitive to the agents being employed may have overgrown and become the predominant flora.

In placing emphasis on the very important role of the laboratory in planning therapy, one must not lose sight of the fact that often an accurate diagnosis can be made by clinical means. Although confirmation is desirable, it is equally important that reliance should not be put on the laboratory to the exclusion of careful clinical evaluation of the patient.

2. *The drug must come in contact with the organism.* An antibacterial agent applied locally must reach every part of the lesion. If the agent is used systemically, the blood supply to the area of infection must be adequate to permit transport of an effective concentration of the drug to the site of microbial activity. Moreover, the contact must be made at an appropriate time in the metabolic cycle of the microorganism. For example, penicillin which interferes with bacterial cell wall synthesis acts only on young cells multiplying actively.

In the acute unlocalized infection without tissue necrosis, such as lymphangitis and cellulitis, blood flow into the area of infection is usually abundant. Vascular contact with the site of bacterial activity is readily maintained, and drugs introduced by conventional routes can be expected to reach the area of inflammation. Conversely, there are lesions, such as pyogenic abscesses, which are not penetrated so readily. Another well-known factor interfering with contact is the foreign body which serves to ensconce the organism and place it beyond the reach of the agent.

3. *The drug should be relatively free from unfavorable side effects, and the clinician must be prepared to recognize and treat the adverse*

consequences of drug therapy. None of the available effective agents is free from the potentiality of producing an unfavorable side effect such as toxic action of the drug or hypersensitivity on the part of the patient. Such effects may range from simple fevers, minor skin rashes, or troublesome gastrointestinal symptoms to renal tubular necrosis, irreversible blood dyscrasias, or anaphylactic shock. The physician who prescribes any drug must be familiar with its adverse consequences and prepared, during the course of therapy, to monitor the patient for their appearance. The threat of a drug-induced complication is reason enough to condemn indiscriminate drug employment. Although toxicity has limited the use of certain very valuable agents, it must not be allowed to discourage the taking of carefully calculated risks in executing antimicrobic therapy in the face of overwhelming infections.

Superinfection is a well-known unfavorable side effect of antimicrobial therapy. Elimination of drug-susceptible organisms in a mixed microbial flora permits the overgrowth of more resistant forms. If the latter are pathogens, a new infection occurs caused by organisms unresponsive to the agent initially administered; or, as is sometimes the case, the equilibrium of a microbial population normally present in some part of the body is upset, and pathogens that were present previously in inconsequential numbers now assume significant proportions and produce disease.

4. *No substance should be present that will inhibit action of the drug where its effect is desired.* The nature of the inflammatory exudate may reduce or abolish antimicrobial activity of the drug. For example, the sulfonamides are not effective where there is suppuration and necrosis. The products of tissue breakdown, particularly para-aminobenzoic acid, prevent action by competing with the drug for the metabolic needs of the bacteria. Penicillinase, a specific enzyme which acts as a drug-inhibitive substance, is developed in lesions by staphylococci and coliform bacilli.

5. *The defense mechanisms of the host against infection must be active.* Some drugs are bacteriostatic and inhibit rather than destroy bacteria; thus, disappearance of the infection depends on the natural defenses of the body, and it follows that if effective drug therapy is to be expected, the usual defense mechanisms must be active. An exception to this requirement is found in the rationale for using bactericidal agents in those individuals whose defense reactions are altered by disease or by intentional medication.

OPERATIVE INTERVENTION AND ITS RELATION TO ANTIMICROBIAL THERAPY

The indications for and the timing of surgical intervention often pose one of the more difficult decisions associated with the use of drugs

in surgery. Patients are sometimes seen in whom indications for operation may have been overlooked or operative intervention may have
been postoponed, when important structures could have been saved if
operation had been performed at the optimal time. A clearer understanding of the relation between drug therapy for infections and the timing
and extent of surgical intervention may be gained if one utilizes some
form of grouping as a frame of reference. With this in mind, surgical
infections, based on pathologic physiology and therapeutic requirements, are categorized in four groups as follows:

Localized Infection. When localization and abscess have occurred, the general principle of surgical decompression is undisputed.
In the presence of suppuration, antimicrobial agents do not replace the
scalpel or the trocar. Here the surgical method is paramount, and, more
often than not, a drug is not required. When it is, its purpose is to
prevent invasive infection or extension to uninvolved tissue.

Unlocalized Infection Not Confined to an Anatomic Closed Space.
Before localization has occurred, drug therapy without operative intervention is sound, provided the tissues at the site of bacterial activity are
intact, well vascularized, and not threatened by pressure. Lymphangitis, lymphadenitis, cellulitis, and serous surface infections in their
early stages usually meet these requirements.

Unlocalized Infection Confined to Anatomic Closed Space. Unlocalized infection characterized by the building up of pressure within a
closed space lies between the extremes of localized abscess and diffuse
cellulitis. Infections of the tendon sheaths, fascial spaces, and hollow
viscera are examples of conditions which may result in pressure within
a closed space. In the early stages of these infections, the vascular
supply is intact, but rapidly developing pressure compromises the
blood supply and ultimately causes necrosis of tissue. The diminished
blood flow also prevents access of drug to the area of bacterial activity.
Prompt surgical intervention is necessary to relieve pressure or to
prevent its development. The aim of operation is single and clear:
restoration of effective local circulation to an area which is being asphyx-
iated by unreleased pressure. The surgical procedure should consist of
decompression, if vital structures are concerned, or removal of the
lesion if part or all of the involved organ, for example, the vermiform
appendix, can be spared. Operative treatment should, of course, be
supplemented by the appropriate antibacterial agent if the operation
does not remove all the infected tissue.

Late Infection. There are late infections typified by a dense,
relatively avascular barrier of scar tissue interposed between the site of
bacterial activity and the blood and lymph channels, thereby limiting
the contact of a systemically administered drug with the site of bacterial
activity. Examples of such lesions are cavities and sinuses with thick
scarred walls and ulcers with dense fibrotic bases. With few exceptions,
recovery is dependent on operative treatment which should be directed toward the re-establishment of vascular contact.

ANTIMICROBIAL AGENTS

There are literally hundreds of antibiotic and chemotherapeutic agents. Those which are currently or potentially useful in surgical practice will be described briefly, emphasizing microbial spectra and principal adverse reactions, and including a range of dosage (see Tables 5-1 and 5-2) which may be used for individuals with unimpaired ability to metabolize the drug and to excrete it. It is not practicable to include many important details concerning drug administration. Therefore it is essential that product information material be consulted when planning drug therapy.

Bacitracin. Bacitracin is a bactericidal drug which acts against streptococci, pneumococci, staphylococci, corynebacteria, clostridia, gonococci, meningococci, actinomycetes, and spirochetes. There is practically no absorption of bacitracin from the gastrointestinal tract and, therefore, if systemic distribution is desired, it must be given by a parenteral route.

Nephrotoxicity resulting from bacitracin is of sufficient severity to restrict its systemic employment except for infections that have failed to respond to other antibacterial agents and are so severe that the hazard of infection is greater than that of kidney damage. Topical application constitutes the only safe method of employment. Bacitracin may be used repeatedly without fear of developing hypersensitivity reactions. It is strikingly nontoxic when applied locally to the nervous system by intrathecal or intraventricular injection.

The usual systemic dose of bacitracin is 10,000 to 20,000 units every 8 hours. Up to 100,000 units daily may be administered if there is adequate intake and output of fluids. For topical use, concentrations of 500 units per milliliter of vehicle may be used.

Cephalosporin. There are several clinically useful semisynthetic antibiotics derived from the microorganism *Cephalosporium acremonium.* They are cephalothin, cephaloridine, cephaloglycin, and cephalexin. These agents are both bactericidal and bacteriostatic. Their spectrum includes gram-positive organisms, gram-negative cocci, actinomycetes, and some gram-negative bacilli. The antimicrobial activity of the cephalosporins is not interfered with by penicillinase, and therefore these drugs are effective against staphylococci which produce it. On the other hand, a number of strains of organisms produce an enzyme (cephalosporinase) which inactivates the cephalosporins.

Adverse reactions include fever, skin rashes, eosinophilia, and in rare instances, neutropenia. Cephaloridine is nephrotoxic. There is some evidence of partial cross-allergenicity of the pencillins and the cephalosporins. Cephalothin (Keflin) and cephaloridine (Loridine) are not absorbed from the gastrointestinal tract. Cephaloglycin (Kafocin) and cephalexin (Keflex) are suitable for oral administration. Both are excreted in high concentration in the urinary tract, but cephalexin gives higher blood levels than cephaloglycin.

(*Text continued on page 131*)

Table 5-1.   ANTIMICROBIAL AGENTS: DOSAGE FOR ADULTS

DRUG	ORAL DOSE	INTRAMUSCULAR DOSE	INTRAVENOUS DOSE
Bacitracin	See text	See text	See text
Cephalosporins			
Cephalexin	1-4 gm./d. ÷ 4	—	—
Cephaloglycin	1-2 mg./d. ÷ 4	—	—
Cephaloridine	—	1.5-4.0 gm./d. ÷ 3-4*	1.5-4.0 gm./d. ÷ 3-4*
Cephalothin	—	2-6 gm./d. ÷ 4-6†	2-6 gm./d. ÷ 4-6†
Chloramphenicol	50-100 mg./kg./d. ÷ 4	Not recommended	50-100 mg./kg./d. ÷ 4
Erythromycin	1-2 gm./d. ÷ 4	200-600 mg./d. ÷ 2-6	1-4 gm./d. ÷ 4-6
Gentamicin	—	3-7.5 mg./kg./d. ÷ 3†	Not recommended
Kanamycin	3-4 gm./d. ÷ 6§	1.0-1.5 gm./d. ÷ 2	Not recommended
Lincomycin	1.5-2.0 gm./d. ÷ 3-4	600 mg.-1.2 gm./d. ÷ 1-2	600 mg.-1.8 gm./d. ÷ 2-3
Neomycin	4-12 gm./d. ÷ 8-24§	Not recommended	Not recommended
Penicillins			
Ampicillin	1-2 gm./d. ÷ 4¶	1-2 gm./d. ÷ 4¶	1-2 gm./d. ÷ 4¶
Carbenicillin	—	20-40 gm./d. ÷ 4-6**	20-40 gm./d. ÷ 4-6**
Cloxacillin	1-2 gm./d. ÷ 4††	—	—
Dicloxacillin	0.5-1 gm./d. ÷ 4	—	—
Methicillin	—	4-6 gm./d. ÷ 4-6†	4-6 gm./d. ÷ 4-6†
Nafcillin	1-6 gm./d. ÷ 4-6††	2-6 gm./d. ÷ 4-6††	2-6 gm./d. ÷ 4-6††
Oxacillin	2-6 gm./d. ÷ 4-6††	2-6 gm./d. ÷ 4-6††	2-6 gm./d. ÷ 4-6††

Penicillin G	See text	See text	See text
Phenethicillin	375 mg.–1.5 gm./d. ÷ 3†	—	—
Phenoxymethyl penicillin	375 mg.–1.5 gm./d. ÷ 3†	—	—
Polymyxin B	—	1.5–2.5 mg./kg./d. ÷ 4	2.5 mg./kg./d. ÷ 2–3
Polymyxin E (colistin)	—	2.5–5.0 mg./kg./d. ÷ 2–4	2.5–5.0 mg./kg./d. ÷ 2–4
Streptomycin		2–4 gm./d. ÷ 2–4‡‡	Not recommended
Sulfonamides	See text	See text	See text
Tetracyclines			
Chlortetracycline	1–2 gm./d. ÷ 4	—	0.5–2 gm./d. ÷ 2
Demethylchlortetracycline	600–900 mg./d. ÷ 2–4	—	—
Doxycycline	100–200 mg./d. ÷ 1–2	—	—
Methacycline	600 mg./d. ÷ 2–4	200–400 mg./d. ÷ 2–4	0.5–2 gm./d. ÷ 2
Oxytetracycline	1–2 gm./d. ÷ 4	200–600 mg./d. ÷ 2–6	1–2 gm./d. ÷ 2–4
Tetracycline	1–2 gm./d. ÷ 4–6	Not recommended	2–3 gm./d. ÷ 2–3
Vancomycin	See text		

*Should not exceed 4 gm./d.
†Should not exceed 12 gm./d.
‡For urinary tract infection: 0.8–1.2 mg./kg./d.
§See text for use in bowel preparation.
‖Up to 12 gm./d. for severe infections.
**For urinary tract infection: 8 gm./d. ÷ 4.
††Should not exceed 6 gm./d.
‡‡See text for use in tuberculosis.

Table 5–2.   Antimicrobial Agents: Dosage for Children

Drug	Oral Dose	Intramuscular Dose	Intravenous Dose
Bacitracin	See text	See text	See text
Cephalosporins			
Cephalexin	25–50 mg./kg./d. ÷ 4	—	—
Cephaloglycin	25–50 mg./kg./d. ÷ 4	—	—
Cephaloridine	—	30–100 mg./kg./d. ÷ 3–4°	30–100 mg./kg./d. ÷ 3–4°
Cephalothin	—	40–80 mg./kg./d. ÷ 4	40–80 mg./kg./d. ÷ 4
Chloramphenicol	50–100 mg./kg./d. ÷ 4	Not recommended	50–100 mg./kg./d. ÷ 4
Erythromycin	25–40 mg./kg./d. ÷ 4	10–20 mg./kg./d. ÷ 3–4	40–70 mg./kg./d. ÷ 4
Gentamicin	—	3–7.5 mg./kg./d. ÷ 3†	Not recommended
Kanamycin	50 mg./kg./d. ÷ 4–6	15 mg./kg./d. ÷ 2	Not recommended
Lincomycin	30–60 mg./kg./d. ÷ 3–4	10–20 mg./kg./d. ÷ 2–3	10–12 mg./kg./d. ÷ 2–3
Neomycin	50–100 mg./kg./d. ÷ 4	Not recommended	Not recommended
Penicillins			
Ampicillin	50–200 mg./kg./d. ÷ 4	50–200 mg./kg./d. ÷ 4–6	50–200 mg./kg./d. ÷ 4–6
Carbenicillin	—	50–500 mg./kg./d. ÷ 4–6	50–500 mg./kg./d. ÷ 4–6
Cloxacillin	50 mg./kg./d. ÷ 4	—	—
Dicloxacillin	25 mg./kg./d. ÷ 4	—	—

Methicillin	—	25 mg./kg./d. ÷ 4	25 mg./kg./d. ÷ 4
Nafcillin	50–100 mg./kg./d. ÷ 4	50–100 mg./kg./d. ÷ 4	50–100 mg./kg./d. ÷ 4
Oxacillin	50–100 mg./kg./d. ÷ 4–6	50–100 mg./kg./d. ÷ 4	50–100 mg./kg./d. ÷ 4
Penicillin G	See text	See text	See text
Phenethicillin	25–40 mg./kg./d. ÷ 4	—	—
Phenoxymethyl penicillin	25–50 mg./kg./d. ÷ 4	—	—
Polymyxin B	—	2.5 mg./kg./d. ÷ 4	2.5 mg./kg./d. ÷ 4
Polymyxin E (colistin)	—	2.5–5.0 mg./kg./d. ÷ 2–4	2.5–5.0 mg./kg./d. ÷ 2–4
Streptomycin	—	20–40 mg./kg./d. ÷ 2–3†	Not recommended
Sulfonamides	See text	See text	See text
Tetracyclines			
Chlortetracycline	20–40 mg./kg./d. ÷ 4	—	10–20 mg./kg./d. ÷ 2
Demethylchlortetracycline	6–12 mg./kg./d. ÷ 2–4	—	—
Doxycycline	2–4 mg./kg./d. ÷ 2	—	—
Methacycline	6–12 mg./kg./d. ÷ 2–4		
Oxytetracycline	25–50 mg./kg./d. ÷ 4	6 mg./kg./d. ÷ 2	10–20 mg./kg./d. ÷ 2
Tetracycline	20–40 mg./kg./d. ÷ 4	12 mg./kg./d. ÷ 2	10–15 mg./kg./d. ÷ 2
Vancomycin	See text	Not recommended	20 mg./kg./d. ÷ 2–3

*Should not exceed 4 gm./d.
†For urinary tract infection: 0.8–1.2 mg./d.
‡See text for use in tuberculosis.

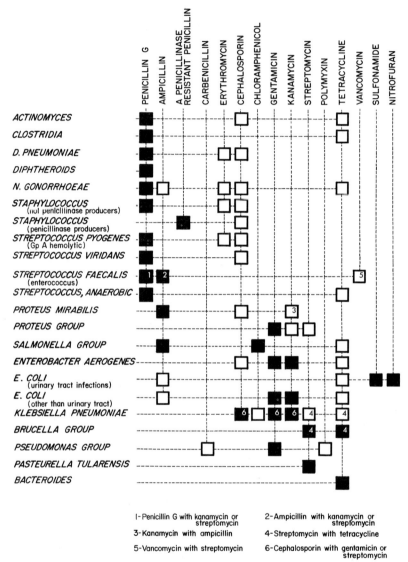

Figure 5–1. A guide to antimicrobial therapy in surgical infections when specific sensitivity determinations are not available. The microorganisms listed are those most commonly associated with surgical infections. An agent of choice is given for each microorganism. This is indicated by a solid square; alternative, but effective agents are indicated by open squares. Variation in drug sensitivity among different strains of the same species of microorganism is such that the most reliable guide to drug therapy is one based on isolation of the causative microorganism and, except in the case of the pneumococcus and group A hemolytic streptococcus, the testing for susceptibility to antimicrobial agents. In serious and rapidly developing infections from which recovery of organisms is not possible immediately, or while awaiting the result of a culture, drugs known to be effective against the organisms usually associated with the particular clinical problem at hand should be administered. This guide is based on this concept. The agents recommended should be used in accordance with the accepted principles of drug employment and sound surgery. (Service Vol. 5, 1965.)

Chloramphenicol. Chloramphenicol is a bacteriostatic, broad-spectrum antibiotic with a range of effectiveness essentially the same as that of the tetracyclines with relatively little cross-resistance. It is the drug of choice for the treatment of typhoid fever and other salmonella infections, other than gastroenteritis.

The drug may be given orally, parenterally, or topically. Absorption on oral administration is complete. Good distribution is attained in body tissues and fluids, and concentrations in the cerebrospinal fluid are significantly greater than those usually attained by other antibiotics. A serious toxic effect, which is not dose-related, is that of bone marrow depression which frequently terminates in fatal aplasia. This complication is rare and affects but a small proportion of the total number of patients receiving chloramphenicol. Nevertheless, chloramphenicol should be prescribed in the recommended dosage only for specific infection, and careful observation for hematopoietic damage should be maintained during drug therapy. Another complication caused by chloramphenicol, namely the "gray syndrome" in newborn infants, is characterized by rapidly developing hypothermia and circulatory collapse. In the newborn infant, the liver is unable to conjugate chloramphenicol, and the kidneys are unable to excrete it rapidly. As a result, toxic levels of the drug accumulate.

Erythromycin. Erythromycin belongs to a group of drugs known as the macrolides. It is effective against streptococci, staphylococci, pneumococci, clostridia, neisseria, hemophili, brucella, and corynebacteria. Erythromycin may be bactericidal or bacteriostatic, and its chief usefulness is for streptococcal and pneumococcal infections in patients who cannot take penicillin because of sensitivity or other reasons. Some strains of bacteria initially sensitive to erythromycin rapidly develop resistance to it. Following absorption, erythromycin is well distributed in body organs and tissues except in the cerebrospinal fluid where only low levels are obtained. Erythromycin is a safe drug, and only rare and minor gastrointestinal disturbances have been recorded. Hepatotoxicity, however, has been reported following the use of the mono-propionyl ester of erythromycin, which is one of the forms employed for oral administration.

Gentamicin. Gentamicin is an aminoglycoside antibiotic similar to neomycin, kanamycin, and streptomycin. It is bactericidal and active against most gram-negative bacteria, including *E. coli*, enterobacter, klebsiella, pseudomonas, proteus, salmonella, and shigella, and some gram-positive organisms, including staphylococcus. Gentamicin has been effective in a variety of infections such as pneumonitis, septicemia, meningitis, enteritis, burn sepsis, peritonitis, cellulitis, and urinary tract infections when these are due to sensitive organisms. It is nephrotoxic and should be used with caution in patients having impaired renal function. Occasional patients show transient proteinuria or transient elevation of blood urea nitrogen, both of which return to normal when the drug is stopped. A serious side effect may be loss of vestibular function which is irreversible and may be delayed in onset. The kinship of this drug to kanamycin and neomycin suggests the potential danger of respiratory arrest when it is used intravenously or intraperitoneally in the anesthetized patient (see Kanamycin and Neomycin, p. 133).

Isoniazid and Other Antituberculosis Drugs. The place of drug therapy in the management of tuberculosis is well established. There are many agents which exhibit either bactericidal or bacteriostatic activity *in vitro* or *in vivo* against *M. tuberculosis*; however, none has equaled the effectiveness and safety of isoniazid, ethambutol, streptomycin, and para-aminosalicylic acid. These four or their derivatives, in the order named, are the most important antituberculosis drugs. They must be employed with other supportive measures, including surgical intervention if indicated.

The treatment of tuberculosis is one of the areas in which drug combinations have proved superior to single agents. This is because of the well-known tendency of the tubercle bacillus to develop drug resistance. A combination of drugs delays and, in some instances, may prevent the emergence of drug-resistant organisms. In severe forms of tuberculosis more than one agent should be employed; in fact, most physicians now use multiple drug therapy for all but minimal disease. Isoniazid, being the most effective agent, should form part of every combination. Isoniazid alone may be used for prophylaxis or treatment of uncomplicated primary tuberculosis. Prolonged administration is a principle of utmost importance. One year is the minimal period of drug administration for prophylaxis. Eighteen months is the minimum period for treatment of active disease. In some individuals, these periods may be extended for an indefinite time. It is recommended that antituberculosis drugs be administered without interruption. This is to safeguard against exacerbation of activity of the process, and it is said to be of some value in preventing the development of bacterial resistance.

The administration of isoniazid to adults is based on a dosage of 300 to 400 mg. per day in one dose; infants and children tolerate proportionately larger daily amounts. In seriously ill patients, larger doses may be employed if accompanied by 50 mg. of pyridoxine per day to prevent peripheral neuritis. The recommended oral dose of ethambutol is 15 to 25 mg. per kg. per day. The dose of para-aminosalicylic acid for adults ranges from 9 to 15 gm. per day, and for children it is 200 mg. per kg. per day, and is divided into three or four equal doses that should be taken with meals because of untoward gastrointestinal symptoms.

The toxic manifestations of streptomycin limit, but by no means preclude, its usefulness in tuberculosis. The usual dose administered intramuscularly is 0.5 gm. per day, but it may be given in larger amounts for more severe forms of disease if limited to 60 to 90 days and if a certain amount of permanent damage to the eighth nerve can be accepted as a calculated risk.

If, during therapy, using the drugs of choice, drug complications or laboratory or clinical resistance develop, then another of the antituberculosis agents avoided initially because of toxicity or inferior effectiveness may need to be employed. These secondary agents are pyrazinamide, kanamycin, cycloserine, and viomycin. Rifampin, a new and still experimental drug, promises to rank with isoniazid, because of effectiveness and low toxicity.

Kanamycin. Kanamycin, one of the aminoglycocide antibiotics, is closely akin to streptomycin, gentamicin, and neomycin. It is effective against a large variety of gram-positive, gram-negative, and acid-fast organisms. It is, however, relatively inactive against streptococci, pneumococci, and clostridia. In contrast to gentamicin, it is not effective against pseudomonas. Organisms sensitive to kanamycin are usually sensitive to gentamicin, but the converse is not true, e.g., some organisms resistant to kanamycin are sensitive to gentamicin. It has been used to treat a wide variety of surgical infections, including peritonitis of fecal origin, and has been employed with considerable success as an intestinal antiseptic in preparation for operation and in hepatic coma.

Kanamycin, when given parenterally, causes damage to the kidneys and to the eighth nerve. Its excretion is largely urinary by glomerular filtration and, being nephrotoxic, it must be used with caution in patients who have altered kidney function. It is reported that kanamycin when used in conjunction with certain anesthetic agents acts to produce respiratory arrest. It is thought that neuromuscular blockade produced by kanamycin is potentiated by ether or succinylcholine. Yet Cohn, Cotlar, and Richard (Amer. Surg. 29:756, 1963) have been impressed with the safety of 1 gm. administered intraperitoneally during anesthesia. Nevertheless, when intraperitoneal administration is required in the anesthetized patient, the means for assisted ventilation must be at hand. When it is necessary to deliver this drug, or a similar one, into the peritoneal cavity, it is safer to do so in the fully conscious patient and to use for this purpose a tube or catheter placed at the time of operation.

Lincomycin. Lincomycin is chemically distinct from all other clinically available antibiotics. Its primary action is bacteriostatic, and it is effective against gram-positive organisms such as staphylococci, streptococci, pneumococci, and *C. diphtheriae*. Although its spectrum includes bacteroides, fusospirochetes, and actinomycetes, the usual gram-negative enteric bacilli are resistant. Bile is an important route of excretion. Adverse effects include pruritus, skin rash and urticaria, nausea, vomiting, and diarrhea. Lincomycin has not been used extensively and, at present, its chief usefulness appears to be that of substitute for penicillin in patients possessing penicillin hypersensitivity, as well as against penicillinase-producing staphylococci.

Neomycin. Neomycin is similar to streptomycin, kanamycin, and gentamicin. Its antibacterial spectrum covers a large variety of gram-negative organisms, including proteus and enterobacter, some strains of staphylococci, and the mycobacteria. It is particularly effective against the gram-negative organisms which inhabit the intestinal tract. On this property hangs its great usefulness in surgery. Being poorly absorbed from the gastrointestinal tract, it has found wide application in preparation of the bowel for operation as well as in the treatment of hepatic coma and certain enteric infections. Neomycin is both neurotoxic and nephrotoxic. This precludes its use parenterally, but it can be given by mouth with safety. Respiratory arrest has occurred subsequent to transperitoneal administration of neomycin in the anesthetized patient. Presumably the cause is neuromuscular blockade produced by this drug and potentiated by succinylcholine or ether. Neomycin, possessing the quality of low allergenicity, has proved an effective agent for topical application. It may be incorporated into various vehicles in the strength of 0.5 per cent and may be used alone or in combination with other bactericidal agents such as bacitracin and polymyxin.

Penicillin.   Penicillin, a bactericidal antibiotic, interferes with cell wall synthesis and is most effective against actively growing microorganisms. Its spectrum includes gram-positive cocci, clostridia, spirochetes, actinomycetes, and some gram-negative organisms, notably the gonococci and meningococci. It is the agent of choice against group A hemolytic streptococcal, pneumococcal, gonococcal, spirochetal, actinomycetic, and sensitive staphylococcal infections. Hundreds of penicillins are available. The most stable, the least toxic, and the most widely used is penicillin G (benzyl penicillin). An aqueous solution produces rapid, high tissue and blood levels of short duration. The procaine and benzathine salts of penicillin G are useful as long-acting repository forms.

One of the well-publicized problems in antimicrobial therapy has been the frequency with which staphylococci resistant to penicillin are encountered. Penicillinase, an enzyme produced by certain strains of staphylococci and gram-negative bacilli, destroys penicillin by hydrolysis before it can injure the microorganism. Some of the semi-synthetic penicillins possess a property not found in earlier penicillins; namely, resistance to hydrolysis by penicillinase. The prototype of the penicillinase-resistant penicillins is methicillin. Its intrinsic activity is low; therefore, high serum concentrations of methicillin are required for effective therapy. Thus, this agent is not as satisfactory as penicillin G against gram-positive cocci which do not produce penicillinase, and it should be used only for penicillin G resistant staphylococci. Other available penicillins which resist hydrolysis by penicillinase are nafcillin, oxacillin, cloxacillin, and dicloxacillin. Unlike methicillin, each of these is available in a form suitable for oral administration. Like methicillin, all these derivatives are less active than penicillin G against those gram-positive cocci which do not produce penicillinase.

There is another group of penicillins, the phenoxymethyl derivatives, which are stable in acid medium and, as a result, may be given orally without destruction in the stomach. To this group belong phenethicillin, propicillin, and phenoxymethyl penicillin (penicillin V), the last being the most widely used of the three. These derivatives are not penicillinase-resistant and are indicated only for oral use against organisms sensitive to penicillin G. Moreover, compared with penicillin G, acid-stability has been gained at the expense of decreased activity.

Ampicillin (alpha aminobenzyl penicillin) is another semisynthetic penicillin unique in its possession of a broad antimicrobial spectrum. Its activity is similar to that of penicillin G against gram-positive cocci. The major advantage lies in its greater activity against *H. influenzae, Str. faecalis,* some strains of *E. coli,* salmonella, shigella, and proteus. Ampicillin is not effective against penicillinase-producing organisms but is acid-resistant and well absorbed orally. Hetacillin is another penicillin with an alpha aminobenzyl side chain; the indications for its employment are similar to ampicillin. Another semisynthetic penicillin, carbenicillin, (alpha carboxybenzyl penicillin), possesses a broad spectrum and is effective against some strains of pseudomonas, but resistance develops rapidly.

A significant number of individuals who receive penicillin exhibit allergic manifestations of varied kind and degree. These may take the form of simple or complex dermatologic manifestations, fever alone or combined with malaise, painful and swollen joints, lymphadenopathy, or anaphylactic reactions, some of which terminate fatally.

The dosage of penicillin varies, depending on the site and the seriousness of the infection; for example, early uncomplicated streptococcal cellulitis may respond readily to as little as 50,000 units of penicillin G given intramuscularly every 4 hours. On the other hand, one is accustomed to thinking in terms of multimillion unit doses in the face of fulminating septicemia or bacterial endocarditis. One unit of penicillin is equal to 0.6 μg.; 1 mg. is equal to 1667 units. Dosages for the semisynthetic penicillins are indicated by weight.

Polymyxin. Several antibacterial agents produced by *B. polymyxa* are known as polymyxins. Only two, designated polymyxin B and polymyxin E (colistin), are available commercially, and their microbial spectra are closely parallel. Particularly important from the surgical standpoint is their effectiveness against *Ps. aeruginosa.* Polymyxin is also markedly effective against *E. coli,* salmonella, shigella, klebsiella, enterobacteriaceae, *H. influenzae,* and *H. pertussis.* It is moderately effective against brucella and certain strains of staphylococci. Proteus, hemolytic streptococci, *S. viridans,* and certain strains of staphylococci, however, are refractory to the polymyxins.

Polymyxin is bactericidal; the rapidity of its action *in vitro* suggests that it is not necessary for the bacteria to be dividing in order to be susceptible to the drug. There is no evidence that species of organisms readily develop resistance to polymyxin, nor is it allergenic or toxic when applied topically or taken orally. Diffusion in cerebrospinal and pleural fluids following parenteral administration is poor.

The chief deterrent to the use of polymyxin rests on the very high incidence of its renal and neural toxicity. Although the polymyxins are nephrotoxic, they may be used with caution if one looks closely for evidence of renal damage and discontinues the drug when such evidence appears. Neural toxicity takes the form of paresthesias and hyperesthesias, mild dizziness, and weakness. These symptoms disappear after withdrawal of the drug. Polymyxin also inhibits neuromuscular transmission.

Streptomycin. This bactericidal antibiotic has proved extremely effective against a large variety of gram-negative bacilli and some strains of staphylococci. Especially important is its effectiveness against the mycobacteria (see Isoniazid, p. 132). Streptomycin is not absorbed effectively from the alimentary canal; the only effective and safe routes are the intramuscular and the topical. When given parenterally, it diffuses rapidly into most body tissues with the notable exception of the brain.

Streptomycin possesses a serious limitation. Strains of organisms initially sensitive to this drug readily develop resistance both *in vitro* and *in vivo*. Within as short a time as a few days, a bacterial population which initially had been sensitive may become predominantly resistant. This is particularly true in the case of *E. coli*, in which resistance may develop in as short a time as 48 hours. Fortunately, with the tubercle bacillus, resistance develops more slowly. Because of this phenomenon, it is advisable to employ streptomycin in combination with another drug to which the organisms are sensitive. Another limitation of streptomycin is its reduced effectiveness in the presence of necrotic tissue.

Toxic reactions to streptomycin are not uncommon and may be evidenced by histamine-like headaches, flushing of the skin, neurologic disturbances, and hypersensitivity reactions such as fever, skin eruptions, and eosinophilia. By far the most significant changes are the selective disturbances of the eighth nerve that take the form of tinnitus, vertigo, and deafness which may be permanent. As much as 1 gm. per day can be given intramuscularly to adults for long periods without producing eighth nerve injury. Streptomycin is an aminoglycocide antibiotic and carries the same potential for respiratory arrest as do kanamycin and neomycin (see p. 133). Dihydrostreptomycin should never be used because it is likely to produce permanent deafness.

Sulfonamides. The sulfonamides are bacteriostatic and have a broad range of activity against gram-positive and gram-negative bacteria. They are of value in surgery primarily as intestinal antiseptics, for which phthalylsulfathiazole (Sulfathalidine) is employed; for bacillary urinary tract infections, for which sulfisoxazole (Gantrisin), sulfamethoxazole (Gantanol), and sulfisomidine (Elkosin) are used; and in combating burn sepsis, for which mafenide (Sulfamylon) applied topically has proved quite effective. The sulfonamides are the agents of choice in nocardia infections. With the exception of mafenide, the sulfonamides are inactivated by the products of tissue breakdown. This circumstance limits their effectiveness in surgical infections which are frequently characterized by pus, necrotic material, and devitalized tissue. An additional limitation to sulfonamide therapy is its toxicity, such as crystalluria, hematologic disorders, skin rash, and gastrointestinal disturbances. Other drugs that are less toxic and more effective restrict the indications for using the sulfonamides. The long-acting sulfonamides cannot be recommended, because their advantages over the short-acting ones do not outweigh potential toxic reactions.

For urinary tract infections, the initial oral dose of sulfisoxazole is 4 gm. followed by 1 to 2 gm. every 4 hours; sulfamethoxazole, 2 gm. initially followed by 1 gm. two or three times daily; sulfisomidine, 1 gm. initially and 1 gm. every 8 hours. The dose of sulfadiazine for systemic infections in adults is 4 to 6 gm. per day, and in children 25 to 50 mg. per kg. per day, divided into four to six doses. It may be given orally or intravenously.

Tetracycline. Although a number of tetracyclines have been described, only six have received clinical acceptance. They are chlortetracycline (Aureomycin), oxytetracycline (Terramycin), tetracycline, demethylchlortetracycline (Declomycin), methacycline (Rondomycin), and doxycycline (Vibramycin).

The tetracyclines provide a wide antimicrobial coverage, including generally those gram-positive organisms which are also sensitive to penicillin and such gram-negative bacteria as the escherichia, proteus, salmonella, aerogenes, and klebsiella groups and some species of pseudomonas. In addition, the tetracyclines are effective antagonists against the rickettsiae, the treponemata, and the actinomycetes. The tetracyclines are classified as bacteriostatic agents, but against some strains there is bactericidal activity. Since they are absorbed in both stomach and intestine, the tetracyclines can be administered orally; they diffuse into all body fluids and tissues and are capable of penetrating the blood-brain barrier. Bile is an important route of excretion. There is no evidence that the tetracyclines are allergenic. Associated with administration have been some minor gastrointestinal disturbances such as nausea, vomiting, and local irritation, but the major complicating effect is that of alteration of the normal intestinal flora with resultant overgrowth of yeasts and nonsensitive strains of staphylococci and gram-negative organisms. The results may range from nothing more than troublesome diarrhea to fatal staphylococcus enterocolitis. Demethylchlortetracycline may induce a photodynamic reaction to sunlight on exposed parts of the body, which is reversible on withdrawal of the drug.

Vancomycin. Vancomycin is active against gram-positive bacteria, but gram-negative organisms and fungi are resistant. It is a most effective agent in the treatment of staphylococcal infections; however, because of its toxicity and the availability of other drugs effective against gram-positive organisms, its use should be restricted to severe staphylococcal infections resistant to penicillin, cephalosporin or erythromycin, or in patients in whom none of these drugs can be used. Vancomycin is rapidly bactericidal. Irritation at the site of injection, hypersensitivity reactions, and skin rashes have been produced by vancomycin, but its most significant untoward reactions are ototoxicity and nephrotoxicity. Vancomycin can be used for staphylococcal enterocolitis because it is not absorbed in significant amounts after oral administration. The recommended oral dosage is 0.5 to 1.0 gm. every 6 hours.

REFERENCES

Meleney, F. L.: Clinical Aspects and Treatment of Surgical Infections. Philadelphia, W. B. Saunders Co., 1949.

Pulaski, E. J.: Common Bacterial Infections. Philadelphia, W. B. Saunders Co., 1964.

These two monographs were written by surgeons who were also bacteriologists with extensive clinical experience in the management of infection in surgery. In their laboratories they contributed significantly to the advancement of science. Meleney's book is a classic; Pulaski's includes current material on antimicrobial agents.

Altemeier, W. A., and Culbertson, W. R.: Applied surgical bacteriology and surgical infections; Chapters 3 and 4, *in* Rhoads, J. E., Allen, J. G., Harkins, H. N., and Moyer, C. A.: Surgery: Principles and Practice. 4th ed. Philadelphia, J. B. Lippincott Co., 1970.

Altemeier has made many distinguished contributions to the understanding of surgical infections and related microbiology. These chapters which he and his colleague, Culbertson, have written provide an excellent survey of the subject.

Rubbo, S. D., and Gardner, J. F.: A Review of Sterilization and Disinfection. Chicago, Year Book Medical Publishers, 1965.

Lawrence, C. A., and Block, S. S.: Disinfection, Sterilization and Preservation. Philadelphia, Lea & Febiger, 1968.

Comprehensive reference material on disinfection and sterilization is provided by these two monographs.

Kunin, C. M., and Finland, M.: Restrictions imposed on antibiotic therapy by renal failure. Arch. Int. Med. *104*:1030, 1959.

Not infrequently nephrotoxic drugs are indicated in patients with impaired renal function. This problem and its resolution are discussed in this excellent article.

Isolation Techniques for Use in Hospitals. Public Health Service Publication No. 2054. Washington, D.C., U.S. Government Printing Office, 1970.

This manual on isolation techniques for general use by all hospital personnel is highly recommended.

Sandusky, W. R.: Use of antibiotics and chemotherapeutics in surgery; *in* Current Problems in Surgery. Chicago, Year Book Medical Publishers, 1964.

Sandusky, W. R.: Antibiotics in surgery; *in* Cooper, Surgical Annual. New York, Appleton-Century-Crofts, 1969.

In the preparation of this chapter for the Manual of Preoperative and Postoperative Care, its author has drawn upon two articles published previously. The first of these contains a bibliography to which the interested reader is referred.

CHAPTER 6

BLOOD DONORS, BLOOD AND TRANSFUSION

CARL W. WALTER, M.D., F.A.C.S.

Safe and effective use of blood transfusion calls to account the judgment and skills of the surgeon. It requires timely and detailed definition of the recipient's needs, perception of what can be accomplished by transfusion, appraisal of the risk to the particular patient, conviction to choose the proper quality and quantity of blood and skill to infuse compatible blood at a beneficial rate. Hence, the surgeon must organize his knowledge of blood transfusion to permit its ready application as dictated by the divers problems of homeostasis seen in an array of patients. It is hoped that this chapter will advance the surgeon's attitude toward transfusion from the category of a standing order to that of a challenge to surgical judgment. The morbidity and mortality of transfusion exceed those of serious surgical illness or major surgical procedures; transfusion warrants personal participation and supervision (Walter). Recruitment of donors is an essential step in preparation for elective surgery. The crisis of emergency surgery is justifiably exploited to marshal donors. A depleted blood bank limits surgical treatment. Hospitals should organize to collect blood from concerned relatives and friends rather than to depend upon a central procurement agency.

SELECTION OF DONORS

Culling suspects is the chief safeguard against the transmission of disease. History alone discloses carriers of hepatitis, malaria and brucellosis. Potential donors suspected of drug addiction must be rejected, as must those who have been tattooed within the preceding six months. Similar quarantine applies to recipients of blood or its components unless the derivatives have been pasteurized. Intimate exposure within the family or an epidemic population to measles, rubella, chickenpox, mumps or infectious mononucleosis warrants postponement beyond the incubation period. Too often inquiry is perfunctory and meaningless, especially of vagrant professional donors.

The source of donors is the important factor in safety; 90 per cent of hepatitis can be traced to commercially obtained blood (Allen).

Patient himself: Autologous blood is safest but is an almost wholly neglected source. One to four units can be drawn at intervals preoperatively without adversely affecting the hematocrit (Cuello et al.). Salvage of blood shed during surgery is feasible and safe. Equipment for autotransfusion is available (Klebanoff and Watkins).

Panels of donors: Sequential uncomplicated donations demonstrate safety.

Family and close friends: History is likely to be accurate and incidence of disease low.

Kindhearted neighbors: Depending upon motivation and education, this large source is safe.

The surgeon can determine the safety of his blood supply by anticipating needs and urging patients to recruit donors among their intimates. Collection of autologous blood should be urged. He should discourage the use of blood purchased for a pittance on skid row, because such blood is associated with a hepatitis attack rate ten times that of a family donor.

Hepatitis must be reported promptly to permit identification and quarantine of hazardous donors. According to a recent survey, only 4.2 per cent of hepatitis victims were reported to health authorities!

Tests for hepatitis: Complement fixation tests for hepatitis-associated antigen (Australian) and antibody persist in 35 per cent of those with serum hepatitis (MS-2). The test should be used to eliminate this proportion of dangerous donors. Currently there is no test for infectious hepatitis (MS-1) (Krugman and Giles).

COLLECTION OF BLOOD

Sterility and integrity of the coagulation mechanism are best preserved by collection in a restricted area by a skilled phlebotomist (Huestis et al.).

Asepsis requires continual supervision. Equipment design must encompass a closed system capable of hermetic sealing — such as a hemorepellent system based on a plastic bag and integral donor tube — and disinfection of the skin to prevent contamination of the bore of the needle. Scrub with soap to remove soil; flood off lather with 2 per cent aqueous iodine; rub the area to keep it moist with germicide for 2 minutes; and rinse with 60 per cent isopropanol.

Aseptic technique must be maintained by critical inspection.

1. Do not palpate the site of skin puncture.

2. Do not remove the protective sheath from the needle until ready for phlebotomy.

3. Do not finger the cannula. It is sharp, clean and sterile. It need not be tested.

4. Seal the container while the needle is still in the donor's vein.

Preservation of clotting factors is a critical aspect of phlebotomy. Avoid trauma to tissue, which initiates clotting. The laminar flow design of the needle protects the clotting mechanism. Platelets, trapped by aggregation on the rough bore of the needle, form a stringlike thrombus in the donor tube. A jelly-like clot results from slow flow or poor mixing with anticoagulant. Coagulant factors are consumed as plasma is converted to serum.

PRESERVATION AND STORAGE

Preservation. Blood is chilled immediately and rapidly following collection to retard metabolism and is processed for components promptly in a sequence illustrated in Figure 6–1.

Storage. Store blood under the control of a physician in a tamper-

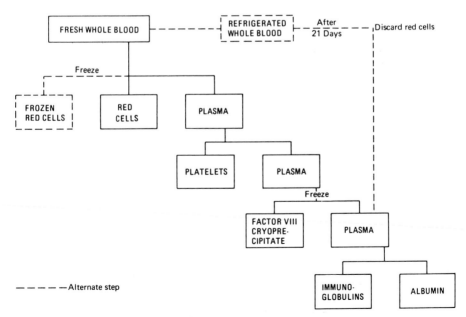

Figure 6–1. Common scheme of blood processing. (From An Evaluation of the Utilization of Human Blood Resources in the United States, Division of Medical Sciences, National Academy of Sciences–National Research Council, Washington, D.C., October 1970.)

proof refrigerator used exclusively for blood or its components. The temperature must be monitored continuously.

WHOLE BLOOD. Whole blood is stored at 39.2° F. (4° C. ± 1). The postinfusion survival of the formed elements varies with the anticoagulant-nutrient solution used, as can be seen in Table 6-1.

PACKED RED CELLS. Erythrocytes are separated promptly by centrifugation or by sedimentation during the first six days of storage. Two hundred ml. of plasma is expressed; the resulting hematocrit is 70 per cent. Infusion can be done without resuspension. Survival is comparable to whole blood stored at 39.2° F. (4° C.) (Szymanski and Valeri).

FROZEN RED CELLS. A widely used method exposes packed red cells to a solution of glycerol and invert sugar in a specially designed plastic bag. The glycerin stabilizes the intracellular solutes and permits freezing at −94° F. (−70° C.) and subsequent thawing without damage to the cell membrane (Haynes et al.). Storage has been accomplished for over five years. When cells are needed, the content of the bag is thawed and the cells are deglycerized by the addition of glucose. The red cells agglomerate (clump) and rapidly settle. The supernate is replaced with a series of sugar solutions to elute the glycerine; ultimately the agglomerated cells are resuspended in isotonic saline. In this form the erythrocytes can be stored at 39.2° F. (4° C.) for 24 hours (Huggins).

PLATELETS. These are easily harvested by differential centrifugation (Yankee et al.). Platelet concentrate can be stored at 72° F. (22° C.) for 48 hours (Murphy et al.).

Table 6–1. PRESERVATIVE-ANTICOAGULANT SOLUTION FOR THE COLLECTION OF 500 ML. OF WHOLE BLOOD

ANTICOAGULANT	STORAGE PERIOD (DAYS)	PRESERVATIVE-ANTICOAGULANT	VOLUME
4% sodium citrate	2	2 gm. trisodium citrate	50 ml.
Heparin	2	2250 units heparin	30 ml. buffered 0.85% NaCl
Ion exchange (resin decalcified)	2		$Ca^{++} \leftrightarrows 2Na^+$
ACD "A"	21	1.65 gm. trisodium citrate 0.6 gm. citric acid 1.84 gm. dextrose	75 ml.
ACD "B"	21	Same as ACD "A"	125 ml.
CPD	28	1.8 gm. trisodium citrate 0.22 gm. citrate acid 0.15 gm. sodium acid phosphate 1.75 gm. dextrose	70 ml.

Table 6–2. CHARACTERISTICS OF ACD "A" PLASMA DURING STORAGE AT $4 \pm 1°$C.*AS SUPERNATE OVER RED CELLS

	UNIT VALUE	DAYS STORED				
		0	7	14	21	28
Dextrose	mg. %	350	300	245	210	190
Lactic acid	mg. %	20	70	120	140	150
Inorganic phosphate	mg. %	1.8	4.5	6.6	9.0	9.5
pH		7.00	6.85	6.77	6.68	6.65
Hemoglobin	mg. %	0-10	25	50	100	150
Sodium	mEq./l.	150	148	145	142	140
Potassium	mEq./l.	3-4	12	24	32	40
Ammonia	μg. %	50	260	470	680	—

*From Strumia, M. M. (ed.): General principles of blood transfusion. Transfusion 3:303, 1963.

LEUKOCYTES. Unless garnered from donors with chronic granulocytic leukemia, the number of leukocytes that can be transfused is ineffective for the treatment of granulocytopenia. Such transfusions are limited to proliferative disease.

PLASMA. Single donor plasma is readily prepared in the blood bank. It should be administered to ABO-compatible recipients unless demonstrated to be free of antibodies. Fresh frozen plasma is harvested by centrifugation immediately after collection of the blood. When frozen promptly, labile clotting factors are preserved. It is stored at $-4°$ F. ($-20°$ C.). Plasma that is separated by sedimentation accumulates degradation products as listed in Table 6-2. Single donor plasma carries the same risk of hepatitis as single unit blood transfusion.

Plasmapheresis of stable donor populations is the source of commercial plasma and unpasteurized blood derivatives equivalent to one and one-half million units of blood annually.

Pooled plasma is too likely to be infected with hepatitis viruses to permit its use.

Cryoprecipitated human factor antihemophilia globulin (Factor VIII) can be concentrated by permitting freshly frozen plasma to thaw at 39° F. (4° C.) for 20 hours. The supernatant plasma is expressed, leaving a potent residue of cold precipitative Factor VIII (Pool and Shannon).

QUALITY OF STORED BLOOD

All blood in the refrigerator is not alike. Inspect the undisturbed container for leakage and color of plasma to cull that unfit for infusion. Leaks indicate potential contamination. The red stain of hemolysis, the brown hue of acid hematin, the purple of degradation by psychrophiles are unmistakable danger signals.

Criteria for Usefulness. Whole blood or packed cells separated in a closed system: "Stored whole blood is considered satisfactory for transfusion provided the method chosen for collection, storage, and transportation assures a minimum survival of 70 per cent of transfused erythrocytes 24 hours after transfusion" [United States Public Health Service; Dating period for citrated whole blood (human)].

However, the ability of erythrocytes to deliver oxygen to the tissues is not dependent merely upon cell survival. The oxygen dissociation curve of stored red cells gradually shifts to the left with age. A relatively tight bond develops between the hemoglobin molecule and oxygen which impedes oxygen delivery to the tissues. Twenty-four hours after transfusion, the dissociation curve of donor cells returns to normal. Blood over five days old in ACD or 10 days old in CPD should not be used in large quantities for patients requiring blood to promote tissue oxygenation or in patients whose cardiovascular systems are already working at capacity (Dawson and Ellis).

Plasma: Progressive degradation of plasma occurs as indicated in Table 14-2. After 10 days of storage in the form of supernate over red cells, the changes deleterious to patients with hepatic or renal insufficiency or to the extremely debilitated include increasing quantities of free potassium, hemoglobin and ammonia.

Categories of Whole Blood Beneficial to the Recipient. FRESH

Table 6–3. BLOOD CLOTTING FACTOR*

INTERNATIONAL NOMENCLATURE	SYNONYMS	TREATMENT OF DEFICIENCY
I	Fibrinogen	Fibrinogen concentrates
II	Prothrombin	Whole blood ⎫ Plasma ⎬ up to 3 wk. old
III	Thromboplastin	———
IV	Calcium	———
V	Proaccelerin Labile factor	Whole blood ⎫ Plasma ⎬ up to 7 days old Fresh-frozen plasma†
VII	Proconvertin Serum prothrombin conversion accelerator	Whole blood ⎫ Plasma ⎬ up to 7 days old Fresh-frozen plasma†
VIII	Antihemophilic factor Cryoprecipitated globulin	Whole blood ⎫ as fresh as possible, Plasma ⎬ <24 hr. old Fresh-frozen plasma†
IX	Christmas factor Plasma thrombo- plastin component	Whole blood ⎫ Plasma ⎬ up to 7 days old Fresh-frozen plasma†
X	Stuart–Power factor	Whole blood ⎫ Plasma ⎬ up to 7 days old Fresh-frozen plasma†

*From Grove-Rasmussen, M., Lesses, M. F., and Anstall, H. B.: Transfusion therapy. N. Eng. J. Med. *264*:1034, 1088, 1961.

†Fresh-frozen plasma may be used if whole blood or plasma < 7 days old not available.

BLOOD. Status limited to 3 hours post-collection. Platelets, leukocytes, accelerator globulin (Factor V) are still active.

36-HOUR BLOOD. Except in heparinized blood, oxygen dissociation by red cells dwindles after 24 hours. CO_2 transport and buffering capacity are progressively impaired. Leukocytes, platelets and accelerator globulin deteriorate. Remains of formed elements are scavenged upon transfusion.

12-DAY BLOOD. Red cell survival post-infusion is high (decrement is 0.83 per cent/day). Their ability to exchange oxygen is restored after 24 hours in recipient circulation. Plasma potassium, hemoglobin and ammonia remain at tolerable levels.

OLD BLOOD. The viable red cell mass dwindles to 80 per cent in ACD blood stored for 21 days in appropriate plastic; oncotic power persists. Plasma hemoglobin, potassium and ammonia increase. Coagulation factors are spent. Burden of particulates (red cell ghosts; protein aggregates) rises. Deleterious degradation products are listed in Table 6-2. Capacity for delivery of oxygen in the immediate postinfusion period is poor.

Status of Clotting Factors. See Table 6-3.

PRIORITY OF USE BASED ON NEEDS OF RECIPIENT

A demand for fresh blood must be justified by clinical or laboratory findings shown by the patient. In many, more adequate dosage of a vital component can be gleaned from several units of fresh blood (Medical Letter; Oberman).

Fresh Blood
1. Oozing hemorrhage without identifiable coagulation defect.
2. Anoxia in coronary or cerebrovascular disease, acute anemia, azotemia or liver disease.
3. Exchange transfusion.
4. Acute or invasive infection.
5. Preoperative preparation of a patient with idiopathic thrombocytopenic purpura with platelet count less than 50,000.

36-Hour Blood
1. Extracorporeal circulation.
2. Controlled hemorrhage.
3. Anemia with cardiorespiratory insufficiency (packed cells are indicated rather than whole blood).

12-Day Blood. The upper limit for marginal recipients, used in
1. Cardiac or pulmonary insufficiency.
2. Renal or hepatic disease.

Old Blood. Provides oncotic power and red cell mass, for
1. Uncontrolled hemorrhage.
2. Chronic anemia.
3. Emergency use when more appropriate blood is not available.

COMPLICATIONS OF TRANSFUSION

The reported frequency of complications varies widely among scattered authors around the world (Gruber). The incidence data in this chapter are taken from experience of the Cook County Hospital during 1961 to 1968, and are based on 131,614 units of blood and 47,909 recipients (Baker and Nyhus). During the four days following transfusion, 5.3 per cent of the recipients had reactions. Serious complications are largely iatrogenic and stem from panic, ineptness or disregard of proper technique.

Incompatible Blood.   A major proportion of incompatibility (ABO) reactions results from night raids on the blood bank by the distraught doctor. The common fault is failure to identify the recipient as party to the crossmatch by checking the label on the blood with the *number* of the patient and his recorded blood group and type. Laboratory error is minimal; physician error is great.

Transfusion is the homotransplantation of a tissue—blood. Donor erythrocytes senesce at the same rate as those of the host—the half-life being 34 days. Following infusion of serologically incompatible blood, a portion of both donor and host cells is destroyed. In about one third of transfusions, erythrocyte survival is shortened to 14 to 16 days. This is evidence of irregular antibody incompatibility found in 0.5 per cent of those without previous pregnancy or transfusion. After each transfusion and each pregnancy, antibodies increase and minor hemolytic reactions become more frequent. The risk of such isoimmunization is cumulative—about 1 per cent per transfusion. Immunization against thrombocyte and leukocyte agglutinins also plays an increasing role. Crossmatching before every nonsequential transfusion is good practice. Special assay of the compatibility of patients who have received multiple units of universal donor blood is essential prior to infusing blood of the patient's hereditary type (Barnes and Allen).

Isoimmunization underlies two thirds of hemolytic reactions. These are mild and delayed in contrast to ABO incompatibility reactions.

Hemolytic Reactions.   Some type of hemolytic reaction occurred in 0.53 per cent of recipients. Reports in the literature range from 0.2 to 1 per cent.

SIMULTANEOUS REACTIONS.   Serious immediate precipitous reactions occurred in 0.08 per cent of recipients with a 36 per cent mortality.

CLINICAL PICTURE.   Precipitous reactions begin after a small volume of blood (25 to 50 ml.) has been infused. There is stinging or burning along the course of the tributary vein; flushing of the face; headache; chills and fever; respiratory distress or oppressive feeling in the chest; pain in flanks or low back; tachycardia and perhaps shock. The wound may begin to ooze.

Anesthesia masks the symptoms. Intractable hypotension and bleeding direct attention to the reaction.

Look for hemolysis in the plasma and for hemoglobin or acid hematin crystals in the urine.

DELAYED HEMOLYTIC REACTIONS. These occur several days after transfusion in 0.45 per cent of recipients with a mortality of 1.8 per cent. Only occasionally severe, this type of reaction is a secondary antibody response to undetected incompatibility of donor cells. The transfused cells are usually destroyed.

TREATMENT

1. Stop transfusion.

2. Combat oligemic shock. Expand blood volume with plasma, albumin, dextran, and fresh compatible blood.

3. Establish diuresis with 25 per cent mannitol or 10 per cent dextran. Avoid vasoconstrictors and antidiuretics. Morphine acts as an antidiuretic.

4. Alkalinize the urine with sodium bicarbonate to prevent degradation of hemoglobin to acid hematin in the renal tubule.

5. Treat bleeding. Fibrinogenemia and fibrinolysis must be suspected.

6. Collect blood and urine samples, and impound and refrigerate equipment and residual blood for investigation.

Allergenic Reactions. An allergenic reaction occurs in 2 to 3 per cent of recipients. Itching, erythema and fever to 103° F. develop after the transfusion is nearly complete. Urticaria, myalgia and arthralgia are less common. Rarely dyspnea, wheezing or stridor is an alarming symptom. Previous allergenic reaction to blood predisposes the recipient to greater risk of another. Delayed reactions occur owing to sensitization to infused allergens.

PROPHYLAXIS. Avoid donors with allergy to prevent transfer of antibodies. For atopic recipients, give an antihistamine 20 minutes before starting transfusion.

TREATMENT. Use antihistamines for minor reactions and intravenous epinephrine for hypotension, bronchospasm or severe urticaria. Do not add medication to blood.

Pyrogenic Reactions. Pyrogenic reactions have become less frequent with the adoption of commercial transfusion equipment and improved clinical practices. Sporadic causes are:

1. Immunologic: arising from isosensitization against leukocytes following repeated transfusions.

2. Bacterial: bacteria are present in 2 per cent of banked blood (Walter et al., 1957). Cryophilic bacteria such as *Escherichia freundii* and *Aerobacter aerogenes* produce acid hematin, a nephrotoxin (Litwin, et al.). There may be shock resulting from endotoxin. Bacteria grow during protracted infusion or in residual liquid in reusable equipment.

The arresting symptom is fever higher than 103° F., usually following a chill. Hypotension or shock may ensue. Acute renal tubular necrosis may result.

Stop the infusion immediately.

Febrile Reactions. These occur in 2 to 3 per cent of recipients. This complication probably represents a mild degree of allergenic or pyrogenic reaction.

Oozing Hemorrhage. This results from either an overlooked history of coagulation disorder (an ultimately vital detail in the work-up of a patient); incompatible blood; large volume replacement (oozing occurs in 33 per cent of patients receiving 10 or more units); consumption or dilution of clotting factors by infusion of serum instead of plasma; and disseminated intravascular clotting in exanthematous viral or arborviral disease. The latter is treated, paradoxically, by heparinization and transfusion (McKay and Margarettsen).

A system for the detection of coagulation disorders is presented in Chapter 7.

Embolism. Air. Collapsible plastic containers have eliminated the major cause of air embolism — pumping air into a container to force more rapid flow. Air embolism also results from aspiration through an injection site in plastic tubing downstream from a flow regulator positioned adjacent to the drip chamber. *Regulators must be positioned lower than the heart.* Entrainment of air is prevented by the positive pressure of the liquid in the entire system (Reusch and Ballinger; Kerr).

Clinical Picture. Gasping respiration, venous distention, hypotension, apnea, and cyanosis, along with splashing, crunching noises in precordial area.

Treatment. Turn the patient on his left side; tilt his head down. Aspirate the heart through a No. 15 needle. If cardiac arrest occurs, open the chest and decompress both ventricles prior to manual systole.

Particulate. Clotted material in transfused blood forms microemboli that cause pulmonary congestion and loss of compliance, and occasionally hemorrhagic pulmonary edema (Mosley and Doty, 1970A).

Clinical Picture. The symptoms are tachypnea, increased expiratory effort and cyanosis unrelieved by oxygen. Inspiratory effort and hypotension develop as venous pressure increases.

Prevention. It is unwise to squeeze filter sets that are full of debris in the effort to acclerate flow (Mosley and Doty, 1970A).

Immunologic. Incompatible ghosts may cause renal tubular necrosis (Schmidt and Holland).

Circulatory Overload. Circulatory overload emerges as a major unrecognized factor in death during transfusion.

Anticipate hypervolemia caused by delayed dispersal of plasma in the elderly or debilitated or in those with chronic anemia, congestive failure, renal failure or pulmonary insufficiency. Packed cells are preferable to correct a red cell deficit. Monitor venous pressure to modulate transfusion. Infuse slowly: 1 ml./kg. body weight/hour.

CLINICAL PICTURE. Livid cyanosis, tachypnea, flushing of face and neck, hypertension, wide pulse pressure, distended jugular veins, loud heart sounds, cardiomegaly, pulmonary edema.

TREATMENT. Tourniquets on extremities, and phlebotomy.

Cardiac Arrest. ECG monitoring of a massive transfusion is desirable. In the absence of hypoxia, ventricular fibrillation and disturbances of rhythm and conduction may occur following rapid replacement of blood volume. These result from:

1. Hypothermia. Rapid infusion of cold blood may induce hypothermia. A crtical drop in temperature of the myocardium predisposes to fibrillation. Warming tubing through which blood is infused, 98.6° F. (37° C.), is desirable in energy-depleted patients.

2. Citrate toxicity. Two liters of citrated blood can be infused in 20 minutes without producing a deficit in ionized calcium in absence of liver damage, shock or hypothermia. When sequestration of calcium is suspected, 1 gm. of calcium gluconate is given per liter of blood infused. The hypothermic myocardium is dangerously sensitive to exogenous calcium.

3. Hyperkalemia. This stems from extracellular potassium that accumulates in aging blood (see Table 6–2).

Thrombophlebitis. Thrombophlebitis may follow venospasm after infusion of cold blood, venospasm after pressure infusion or venospasm after extravasation. Beware of infusing vasoconstrictors through a venous channel once used for pressure infusion. Gangrene may result as the drug extravasates. Thrombophlebitis results from vein injury from an indwelling needle or degradation of plastic tubing.

Delayed Transmission of Disease

HEPATITIS. Following transfusion there are 30,000 cases with jaundice; five times that number remain anicteric. There are 3300 deaths annually.

The incidence is 1 per cent for whole blood and 12 per cent for pooled plasma (Fig. 6–2). Pasteurized components such as albumin or plasmanate carry no hazard. Heat-labile fibrinogen and its products carry the risk of plasmapheresis in donor populations.

Recent progress on the study of hepatitis showed hepatitis-associated antigen consistently present in sera from 25,000 patients with the MS-2 strain of serum hepatitis (SH); it was not present in MS-1, infectious hepatitis (IH). Hepatitis-associated antigen was detected earlier after a parenteral exposure to SH than after an oral exposure. Antigen appeared two weeks to two months before onset of jaundice; it was transient in 65 per cent of patients, but persisted for four months to 13 years in 35 per cent of children. The average incubation period of IH (MS-1) was essentially the same following an oral or parenteral exposure (32 to 33 days); in SH (MS-2) it was 65 days after parenteral exposure and 98 days after oral exposure. Gamma globulin consistently neutralized the infectivity of IH (MS-1) serum; in most cases it did not neutralize the infectivity of SH (MS-2) serum (Krugman).

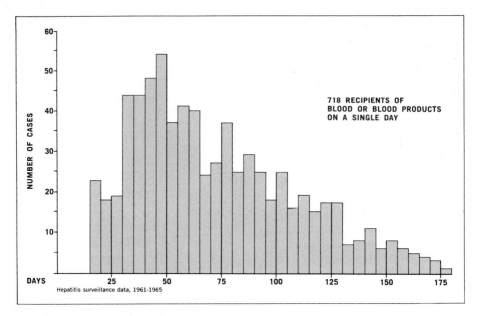

Figure 6–2. Distribution of incubation periods in post-transfusion hepatitis cases covered in Communicable Disease Center survey, showing unexpected clustering of cases in gap bridging traditional upper limit of infectious variety (50 days) and lower limit of serum hepatitis (60 days). A surprisingly high proportion (34.8 per cent) had an incubation period of less than 50 days. (From Antibiotic News, New York, October 27, 1965, p. 3, with permission of the publisher.)

POSTINFUSION SYNDROME.   Cytomegalic inclusion disease simulates infectious mononucleosis. Two to eight weeks after transfusion, fever, splenomegaly and atypical lymphocytes explain malaise and prostration. Absence of lymphadenopathy, hepatomegaly and heterophil differentiates from infectious mononucleosis. The cytomegalovirus (CMV) is demonstrable in urine, blood and saliva.

Infectious mononucleosis is also transmissible by transfusion. The Epstein-Barr virus (EBV) is found in urine, leukocytes and saliva. (Henle et al.).

Transmission of CMV and CBV during transfusion occurs more frequently than the viruses causing hepatitis.

SYPHILIS.   The incidence of syphilis varies with the source of the donors. The spirochete dies after 48 hours' refrigeration.

Other possible diseases are malaria, brucellosis and trypanosomiasis.

EQUIPMENT

Successful therapy depends upon selection of proper equipment and upon a realistic appraisal of the patient's need. Timeliness, rate and quantity are important factors. The complementary role of the transfusion in the total program of parenteral fluid therapy must be appraised. Simultaneous replacement of intravascular and extravascular deficits is optimal therapy.

Timely infusion depends upon selection of the recipient set. Three mechanical factors forestall predictable infusion. An occluded coupler, a partially immersed filter or an expediently inserted fine gauge intravenous needle becomes a barrier to lifesaving therapy.

Coupler. The piercing coupler that punctures the diaphragm and engages the outlet port of the container may provide but a slit, a cluster of small orifices or a narrow passage for the flow of blood. The intent is to retain clots in the container.

The channel through the coupler must be large enough to pass the stringlike clots of fibrin and platelets that often form in the donor tube during collection. These readily pass through a channel 4 mm. in diameter and are trapped in the filter. Bulky, jelly-like clots, sufficient to choke a 4 mm. bore, signal chemical degradation of blood and the need to discard the unit. When blood supply is scanty, such clots can be removed by filtration in the blood bank to provide a liquid suspension of red cells in serum suitable for emergent replacement of red cell mass and oncotic power.

Filter. Filters should be located between the container and the flow rate indicator; the sequence of the elements is significant. The specified drip spout breaks a milliter of blood into 16 drops under standard conditions of gravity flow. The drop from a spout partially occluded with a clot is smaller or may not be detectable. Indeed, a string clot may simulate a stream.

Filtration of blood during infusion is mandatory by the regulations governing transfusions [United States Public Health Service: Minimum requirements for citrated whole blood (human)]. It is essential to screen out particles that can embolize and obstruct significant arteriolar arborization patterns in the pulmonary arterial bed. Arterioles with a lumen 150 microns or smaller form a network of collaterals where the damage resulting from embolization is limited. The filter (USP Sieve Size No. 80) must trap hazardous particles.

Failure to fill the filter chamber diminishes the filtering capacity. This is little understood and results in unnecessarily slow flow and frustrated therapy. The ideal filter chamber is compressible so that it can be filled by squeezing the air into the container after timely occlusion of the tubing distal to the drip chamber (by folding it upon itself). Clots often can be dislodged from the piercing coupler by a similar maneuver. When used properly with good quality blood, a filter will process four or five units of blood. When the flow of blood is unaccountably slowed, it is prudent to replace the recipient set with a fresh one.

Cannula. A fine gauge needle is a barrier to effective therapy. At a pressure head of 30 inches, 35 ml. of blood will flow through a

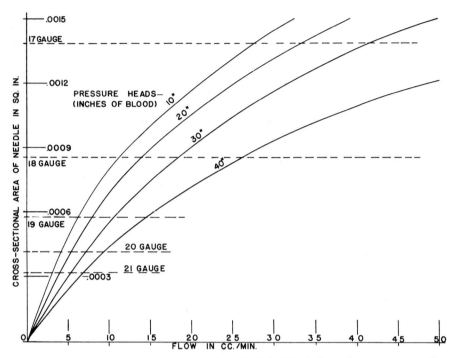

Figure 6–3. Flow in cc./min. of filtered whole blood through 1–1½ in. needles of various sizes at various pressure heads. (Net pressure.) (Modified from C. W. Walter et al.: Surg., Gynec. & Obst. *101*:115, 1955. By permission of Surgery, Gynecology & Obstetrics.)

standard 17 gauge needle in one minute. The flow rate increases as the square of the diameter of the bore (Fig. 6–3). It is imperative to insert a 17 gauge or larger needle when preparing a patient for major surgery or when treating hemorrhage.

RATE OF TRANSFUSION

Start each transfusion at 2 to 3 ml./minute. Symptoms of an untoward reaction are manifest during the infusion of the initial 50 to 100 ml. of *each* unit of blood; therefore, professional supervision is crucial prior to setting the rate of flow in accord with clinical requirements.

1. Elective transfusion into normal circulatory system: infuse 8 to 10 ml./minute; 60 to 80 minutes per transfusion permits dispersal of plasma.

2. Embarrassed cardiovascular system, particularly in the elderly: infuse 4 to 5 ml. per minute, 130 minutes per transfusion. Monitor with venous pressure.

3. Normovolemic requiring cellular components: infuse packed cells.

4. Acute hypovolemia: use maximal attainable infusion rates until systemic blood pressure of 100 mm. Hg is attained.

Emergency Transfusion for Active Hemorrhage. After checking for reaction, use a pressure infusion with extrinsic force. Avoid air pressure on blood. Warm blood to 95° F. (35° C.) to avoid hypothermia. *Accelerate replacement* by simultaneous infusion through multiple cannulas. Watch for extravasation. Venospasm owing to cold or to the stimulus of the jet of blood may impede flow.

Preoperative Transfusion. Chronic anemia with symptoms of anoxia involves an increased plasma volume. Therefore, anticipate an overload due to slow dispersal of plasma. In compensated chronic anemia, there is increased plasma volume, increased cardiac output, efficient gas exchange and satisfactory renal function. Hence transfusion is unnecessary. In cases of hemolytic anemia, multiple transfusions in the past result in isosensitization that may induce a hemolytic reaction.

CRITERIA FOR TRANSFUSION

The primary purpose of transfusion is to complement a deficient circulating blood volume to effect perfusion of the capillary bed. The microcirculation in turn maintains exchange with the reservoir of interstitial fluid that supports the metabolism of cells. During shock an inadequate blood volume is shunted through the obligatory circuit of heart, lungs and brain by arteriolar constriction at the periphery.

A secondary, often crucial purpose of transfusion is to overcome a specific deficit in the blood components, among either the formed elements or the protein constituents.

Each surgical patient presents a unique challenge in management of his extracellular fluid. Simple replacement in kind of overt losses fails to repair the more severe or complex defects. Recognition of the interplay between circulating blood and interstitial fluid is the key to the effective use of blood or its components as complements in a regimen of parenteral fluid therapy contrived to support the metabolism of tissue cells. This goal is achieved by bolstering the circulation to assure perfusion of the capillary bed and effecting venous return. Too many surgeons have neglected these vital parameters in their concern with treating the blood pressure with transfusions, plasma expanders and vasopressors. Depletion or sequestration of the extravascular fluid has resulted in disastrous hypotensive crises.

Extracellular fluid is a mobile, functional fluid comprising 20 per cent of body weight. But one quarter of it circulates intravascularly as blood or lymph; three quarters permeates the extravascular spaces as interstitial fluid and fluxes into the venous and lymph capillaries. An equilibrium of hydrostatic pressure and osmotic pressure maintains the relative volumes of the intravascular and extravascular fluid and determines the rate of exchange throughout the distribution, capillary and collection systems. It is clear that transfusion alone is inadequate therapy (see Chapters 3 and 10).

Transfusion is indicated:

1. To maintain blood volume and prevent or treat shock. Blood loss of less than 10 to 15 per cent of blood volume seldom causes symptoms or hemodynamic changes. Measured blood loss is replaced as it occurs. Blood loss measured at 500 ml. with hemodynamic changes requires 1000 ml. replacement. The degree of loss can be anticipated (Table 6–4). Measured blood volume is a feasible guide, and monitoring venous pressure is a practical aid. In hypovolemic shock, the degree of replacement depends upon clinical criteria—pulse, blood pressure, peripheral circulation, venous pressure and urine volume.

2. To improve or maintain oxygen carrying capacity. A low hemoglobin level is tolerated poorly by the injured, sick or aged. Acute anemia is more disabling than chronic anemia. Anoxia is threatening to patients with coronary or cerebrovascular insufficiency. Moderate hypovolemia results in dangerous hypoxia. Fresh blood is crucial when oxygen dissociation is expected (Reece and Beckett).

3. To promote or maintain coagulation. The recipient's deficiency must be defined (see Chapter 7). Storage lesions of blood and its components must be understood. The paradox of clot-induced bleeding must be appreciated.

4. For exchange of blood in neonates. Replace sensitized red cells before hemolysis results in hyperbilirubinemia. Cross-match with mother's serum. Consider heparinized blood.

5. As a prime for biomechanical apparatus (pump oxygenator). Inter-cross-match using pooled donors' serum or antibody screening.

Table 6–4.   AVERAGE BLOOD LOSS AT VARIOUS OPERATIONS*

Cholecystectomy	500 cc.
Thyroidectomy	500 cc.
Colon resection	1000 cc.
Hysterectomy	1000 cc.
Gastric resection	1500 cc.
Radical mastectomy	1500 cc.
Radical neck dissection and hemimandibulectomy	2000 cc.
Abdominoperineal resection	2500 cc.
Pulmonary lobectomy	2500 cc.
Resection of large aneurysm	3000–10,000 cc.

*From Artz, C. P., and Hardy, J. D.: Complications in Surgery and Their Management. 2nd Ed. Philadelphia, W. B. Saunders Co., 1967.

REFERENCES

Allen, J. G.: Commercially obtained blood and serum hepatitis. Surg. Gynec. & Obst. 131:276, 1970.

Artz, C. P., and Hardy, J. D.: Complications in Surgery and Their Management. 2nd Ed. Philadelphia, W. B. Saunders Co., 1967.

Baker, R. J., and Nyhus, L. M.: Diagnosis and treatment of immediate transfusion reaction. Surg. Gynec. & Obst. 130:665, 1970.

Barnes, A., and Allen, T. E.: Transfusions subsequent to administration of universal donor blood in Vietnam. J.A.M.A. 204:695, 1968.

Cuello, L., Vazquez, E., Perez, V., and Faffucci, F. L.: Autologous blood transfusion in cardiovascular surgery. Transfusion 7:309, 1967.

Dawson, R. B., Jr., and Ellis, T. J.: Hemoglobin function of blood stored at 4° C. in ACD and CPD with adenine and inosine. Transfusion 10:113, 1970.

Distinctions held blurred among forms of hepatitis. Antibiotic News, October 27, 1965, p. 3.

Grove-Rasmussen, M., Lesses, M. F., and Anstall, H. B.: Transfusion therapy. N. Eng. J. Med. 264:1034, 1088, 1961.

Gruber, U. F.: Blood Replacement. Translated by L. Oxtoby and R. F. Armstrong. Berlin, Heidelberg, New York, Springer-Verlag, 1969.

Haynes, L. L., Tullis, J. L., Pyle, H. M., Sproul, M. T., Wallach, S., and Turville, W. C.: Clinical use of glycerolized frozen blood. J.A.M.A. 173:1657, 1960.

Henle, W. H., et al.: Antibody responses to the Epstein-Barr virus and cytomegaloviruses after open-heart and other surgery. N. Eng. J. Med. 282:1068, 1970.

Huestis, D. W., Bove, J. R., and Busch, S.: Practical Blood Transfusion. Boston, Little, Brown and Company, 1969.

Huggins, C. E.: Frozen blood. J.A.M.A. 193:941, 1965.

Kerr, J. H.: Pneumatic hazards of intravenous therapy. Surg. Gynec. & Obst. 107:792, 1958.

Klebanoff, G., and Watkins, D.: A disposable autotransfusion unit. Amer. J. Surg. 116:475, 1968.

Krugman, A., and Giles, J. P.: Viral hepatitis: new light on old disease. J.A.M.A. 212:1019, 1970.

Litwin, M. S., Walter, C. W., and Jackson, N.: Experimental production of acute renal tubular necrosis. Ann. Surg. 152:1010, 1960.

McKay, D. G., and Margarettsen, W.: Disseminated intravascular coagulation in virus diseases. Arch. Int. Med. 120:129, 1967.

Moseley, R. V., and Doty, D. B.: Death associated with multiple pulmonary emboli soon after battle injury. Ann. Surg. 171:336, 1970A.

Moseley, R. V., and Doty, D. B.: Changes in the filtration characteristics of stored blood. Ann. Surg. 171:329, 1970B.

Murphy, S., Sayar, S. N., and Gardner, F. H.: Storage of platelet concentrates at 22° C. Blood 35:549, 1970.

Oberman, H. A.: The indications for transfusion of freshly drawn blood. J.A.M.A. 199:93, 1967.

Pool, J. G., and Shannon, A. E.: Production of high potency concentrates of antihemophilic globulin in a closed-bag system: Assay in vitro and in vivo. N. Eng. J. Med. 273:1443, 1965.

Reece, R. L., and Beckett, R. S.: Epidemiology of single-unit transfusion. J.A.M.A. 195:801, 1966.

Ruesch, H., and Ballinger, C. M.: Continuing hazard of air embolism during pressure transfusion. J.A.M.A. 172:1476, 1960.

Schmidt, P. J., and Holland, P. V.: Pathogenesis of the acute renal failure associated with incompatible transfusion. Lancet 2:1169, 1967.

Strumia, M. M., ed.: General principles of blood transfusion. Transfusion 3:303, 1963.

Szymanski, I. O., and Valeri, C. R.: Clinical evaluation of concentrated red cells. N. Eng. J. Med. 280:281, 1969.

Transfusion of blood components. Medical Letter, Vol. 9, No. 22, November 3, 1967.

United States Public Health Service: Dating period for citrated whole blood (human). Public Health Service Manual of Laws and Regulations, Section 73.306 of 42 CFR. Washington, D.C., United States Government Printing Office, 1961.

United States Public Health Service: Minimum requirements for citrated whole blood (human), paragraphs 4.50 and 4.52.

Walter, C. W.: Innovations in Transfusion Therapy (a motion picture, sponsored by the American College of Surgeons, 1962). Available from Fenwal Laboratories, Morton Grove, Ill.

Walter, C. W., Bellamy, D. J., and Murphy, W. P., Jr.: The mechanical factors responsible for rapid infusion of blood. Surg. Gynec. & Obst. 101:115, 1955.

Walter, C. W., Kundsin, R. B., and Button, L. N.: New technique for detection of bacterial contamination in a blood bank using plastic equipment. N. Eng. J. Med. 257:364, 1957.

Yankee, R. A., Grumet, F. C., and Rogentine, G. N.: Platelet transfusion therapy. New Eng. J. Med. 281:1208, 1969.

CHAPTER 7

HEMORRHAGIC DISORDERS

Edwin W. Salzman, M.D.

INTRODUCTION

Hemorrhagic complications are a frequent source of morbidity in surgical patients. In many cases, unexpected bleeding can be traced to a generalized defect in hemostasis. Recent years have seen an explosive growth in the understanding of hemostatic processes. Hemorrhagic problems can be approached with confidence based on detailed knowledge of the pathways to fibrin formation and insight into the function of blood platelets. Precise diagnosis of bleeding disorders is the rule. Specific therapy is effective and has become widely available.

MECHANISM OF HEMOSTASIS

When a blood vessel is divided, it constricts, and platelet aggregation and plasma coagulation combine to stanch flow from the constricted orifice. At the cut end of the vessel, exposure of subendothelial connective tissue provides a surface to which platelets adhere. Interaction with collagen fibers leads platelets to expel the contents of their secretory granules, including epinephrine, 5-hydroxytryptamine (serotonin), and adenine nucleotides, particularly ATP and ADP. The presence of these compounds in plasma as a product of the platelet "release reaction" leads to aggregation of further platelets and the eventual development of a platelet plug, which in small vessels is sufficient to stop the flow of blood and provide provisional ("primary") hemostasis. At the same time, exposure of plasma to connective tissue activates plasma enzymes ("clotting factors") and sets off a series of reactions that result in the generation of thrombin and ultimately in the conversion of fibrinogen to a fibrin clot. Tough fibrin strands reinforce the friable platelet aggregate ("secondary hemostasis"), and platelets and

157

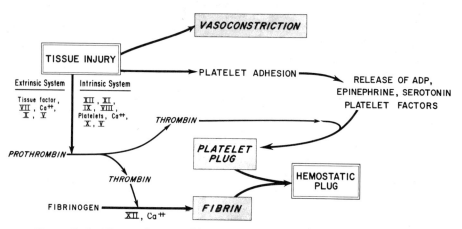

Figure 7–1. The mechanism of hemostasis. Vasoconstriction, platelet adhesion and aggregation, and the formation of fibrin cooperate to produce a hemostatic plug and arrest hemorrhage. Tissue injury causes the generation of thrombin and ultimately the formation of fibrin by provision of a clot promoting lipid tissue factor ("tissue thromboplastin") via the extrinsic clotting system, and by activation of plasma clotting factors through exposure of subendothelial connective tissue (intrinsic clotting system). Adhesion of platelets to connective tissue is followed by release of platelet constituents and aggregation of additional platelets. The release of biogenic amines from platelets is also induced by thrombin.

fibrin together produce a resilient composite hemostatic plug that can withstand the force of arteriolar pressure when the constricted vessel eventually relaxes.

In parallel with the course of hemostatic processes, initiation of coagulation leads also to the activation of plasminogen, a plasma globulin. In its active form, plasmin, the resultant proteolytic activity results in fibrinolysis, a natural defense against pathologic deposition of fibrin. Activation of plasminogen is also a feature of certain disease states (see below) and can be induced for therapeutic dissolution of intravascular thrombi.

The mechanism of hemostasis is summarized in Figure 7–1.

ROUTINE EVALUATION OF SURGICAL PATIENTS

The existence of a hemorrhagic diathesis should be regarded as a possibility in the initial consideration of every patient who is to undergo an operation, for, if present, a bleeding tendency may convert an otherwise straightforward surgical procedure into a catastrophe. No lengthy battery of laboratory examinations is required for routine evaluation. Most hemorrhagic disorders of significance can be suspected from a careful history and physical examination, if particular attention is directed to episodes of bleeding as a complication of previous surgery or trauma; hemorrhagic symptoms in other members of the family, especially if the pattern of inheritance follows the sex-linked recessive pattern characteristic of hemophilia; unusual swelling of joints or soft tissue not recognized as bleeding; and the ingestion of medications known to influence hemostasis adversely, such as aspirin, oral anticoagulants, phenylbutazone, and indomethacin.

Preoperative evaluation of every surgical patient should also include assessment of the number of circulating platelets. Thrombocytopenia may develop *de novo* as a result of drug ingestion or infection, or without known cause, and, if the patient has not been challenged by trauma or operation, may not be apparent to the examiner. Examination of a stained blood smear is sufficient for this assessment; six to ten platelets per high power field are usually visible. A platelet count is not necessary for this evaluation.

The use of tests of coagulation for indiscriminate screening is not recommended. Laboratory tests that are inexpensive and readily available, e.g., the whole blood clotting time and the bleeding time, are so insensitive that they offer no security. For example, the whole blood clotting time is normal in classic hemophilia if the level of Factor VIII (antihemophilic factor) exceeds 3 to 5 per cent of the average normal plasma concentration, but a plasma level at least 30 per cent of normal is required for safe surgical hemostasis. Tests of sensitivity and reproducibility sufficient for demonstration of a bleeding disorder (e.g., partial thromboplastin time, thromboplastin generation test, one-stage prothrombin time) are complicated and expensive. Their use for screening cannot be justified as a routine. A carefully taken history and physical examination will suggest the presence of an underlying bleeding disorder in patients whose hemorrhagic tendency is sufficiently severe to be of consequence, and this suggestion should lead to hematologic consultation and precise diagnosis.

HEMORRHAGIC DISORDERS

Congenital and acquired disorders affecting the various aspects of hemostasis have been described and can be identified by appropriate laboratory tests.

CONGENITAL BLEEDING DISORDERS

Defects in Blood Coagulation. Inherited deficiencies of plasma clotting factors exist. The most common of these is hemophilia, a deficiency of Factor VIII (antihemophilic factor). Hemophilia is inherited as a sex-linked recessive trait, transmitted by the female but manifest only in the male. The disease occurs once in approximately 10,000 male births. Factor IX deficiency (hemophilia B, Christmas disease) is clinically indistinguishable from hemophilia and has a similar pattern of inheritance but is due to the lack of a different clotting factor. The severity of the bleeding tendency in hemophilia and Factor IX deficiency is well correlated with the plasma concentration of the factor in question. Severely affected patients usually have less than 1 per cent of the normal value. Patients with more than 30 to 40 per cent of normal are in most cases asymptomatic. At intermediate levels, spontaneous hemorrhage is rare, but serious hemorrhage may follow surgery or trauma.

Inherited deficiencies of other plasma clotting factors have been described but are less common and, in most instances, less severe in their clinical effects than deficiencies of Factors VIII and IX.

Table 7-1 summarizes the important characteristics of the plasma coagulation factors.

Deficiencies of plasma clotting factors produce a defect in "secondary hemostasis." The initial arrest of bleeding by vasoconstriction and platelet aggregation is unimpaired, but the platelet plug that forms is not reinforced by fibrin and is unable to withstand the force of arteriolar pressure. When the protective effect of vasoconstriction abates, the flimsy platelet plug is apt to blow out and lead to delayed hemorrhage after hours or days. Tests of "primary hemostasis" such as the bleeding time and tourniquet test are normal in these conditions, unless there is also a defect in platelet function, as in von Willebrand's disease (see below). Diagnosis of inherited disorders of coagulation is summarized in Table 7-2.

Common clinical manifestations of congenital disorders of coagulation include bleeding into joints and soft tissues, occasionally into body cavities, and sometimes from the nose or the gastrointestinal or urinary tract. Affected patients rarely succumb to exsanguinating hemorrhage. The hypovolemic effects of blood loss are often overshadowed by the space-occupying nature of a hematoma, which predisposes to infection and ischemic necrosis of vital organs. Supportive measures such as immobilization of hemarthroses may be of value, but the mainstay of treatment is replacement of the deficient clotting factor by administration of blood, fresh or frozen plasma, or a relatively purified preparation concentrated from plasma by various fractionation procedures. The level of the several clotting factors required for hemostasis, their biologic half-life, their stability on storage, and the materials available for replacement therapy vary with different clotting factors (Table 7-1).

Surgery in a patient with a congenital coagulation disorder is a complicated undertaking. One must provide a safe blood level of the deficient clotting factor during the operation and the entire postoperative period until healing is complete. If the factor has a short half-life in the circulation (e.g., Factor VIII [antihemophilic factor] 4 to 5 hours) and is required in relatively high concentration for safe hemostasis (e.g., Factor VIII: 30 per cent of normal), infusions of 2 to 3 liters of plasma per day may be required. Circulatory overload is a hazard of such a program and can only be avoided through the use of concentrated preparations of the deficient factor with a low content of extraneous protein. Requirements for transfusion therapy increase with the magnitude of the surgical procedure and are also influenced by the size of the patient and his circulatory volume and by unusual metabolic demands, such as fever and infection.

The development of a natural anticoagulant inhibiting Factor VIII is a serious complication of transfusion therapy in a small fraction of patients with severe hemophilia. The plasma concentration of the inhibitor increases in response to infusion of the deficient clotting factor in such patients. The inhibitor neutralizes circulating Factor VIII and thus frustrates attempts at replacement therapy. Since transfusion raises the titer of the anticoagulant, administration of the deficient factor should be avoided except in an acute threat to life. In a desperate case, transient benefit may be obtained through the use of highly concentrated Factor VIII preparations of animal origin or by exchange transfusion. Because of the attendant requirement for several weeks of effective replacement therapy, elective operation is absolutely contraindicated in patients with an acquired inhibitor of antihemophilic factor. Acquired anticoagulants directed toward the other clotting factors have also been described but are less frequent than in hemophilia. An acquired inhibitor to Factor VIII has also been recognized in occasional elderly nonhemophilic male patients and less often in postpartum women, in whom it usually disappears with the passage of time. Other acquired anticoagulants are sometimes observed in leukemia and in disseminated lupus erythematosus.

Von Willebrand's disease is an inherited disorder of hemostasis transmitted as an autosomal dominant characteristic. It is the most common inherited coagulation disorder after hemophilia. The disease is characterized by a deficiency in Factor VIII and an associated decrease in platelet adhesiveness, resulting in a long bleeding time and simultaneous defects in primary and secondary hemostasis. Transfusion of fresh plasma leads to a transient correction of the abnormality in platelet function and a more sustained rise in Factor VIII level, apparently augmented by synthesis of new Factor VIII from precursor material contained in the transfused plasma. Spontaneous correction of the characteristic defects has been observed late in pregnancy.

Inherited Disorders of Platelet Function. Thrombasthenia (Glanzmann's disease) is a rare hereditary bleeding tendency in which the platelets do not aggregate with ADP, epinephrine, or other agents. Plasma coagulation is normal, but platelet clumping is completely absent. Transfusion of fresh viable platelets is effective.

In a more common qualitative disorder (Portsmouth syndrome, thrombocytopathia), the "release reaction" of platelets is impaired and platelet aggregation is therefore deficient, although the platelets re-

(Text continued on page 165.)

Table 7-1. Circulating Hemostatic Elements

Official Name	Common Synonyms	Life Span in Vivo (1/2 Life)	Fate During Coagulation	Stability in ACD Bank Blood (4°)	Ideal Agent for Replacing Deficit	Normal Level	Level Required for Safe Hemostasis
Factor I	Fibrinogen	72 hours	Consumed	Very stable	Bank blood; concentrated fibrinogen	200–400 mg./100 ml.	60–100 mg./100 ml.
Factor II	Prothrombin	72 hours	Consumed	Stable	Bank blood; concentrated preparation	20 mg./100 ml. (100%)	15–20%
Factor V	Proaccelerin, accelerator globulin, labile factor	36 hours	Consumed	Labile (40% at 1 week)	Fresh frozen plasma; blood under 7 days	100%	5–20%
Factor VII	Proconvertin, serum prothrombin conversion accelerator, SPCA, stable factor	5 hours	Survives	Stable	Bank blood; concentrated preparation	100%	5–30%
Factor VIII	Antihemophilic factor, AHF, antihemophilic globulin, AHG	6–12 hours	Consumed	Labile (20–40% at 1 week)	Fresh frozen plasma, concentrated AHF, cryoprecipitate	100% (50–150)	30%

Factor	Synonyms	Half-life	Survival in stored blood	Stability	Source for replacement	Normal level	Level for hemostasis
Factor IX	Christmas factor, plasma thromboplastin component, PTC, Hemophilia B factor	24 hours	Survives	Stable	Fresh frozen plasma, bank blood, concentrated preparation	100%	20–30%
Factor X	Stuart-Prower factor	40 hours	Survives	Stable	Bank blood, concentrated preparation	100%	15–20%
Factor XI	Plasma thromboplastin antecedent, PTA	Probably 40–80 hours	Survives	Probably stable	Bank blood	100%	<10%
Factor XII	Hageman factor	Unknown	Survives	Stable	Replacement not required	100%	Deficit produces no bleeding tendency
Factor XIII	Fibrinase, fibrin stabilizing factor, FSF	4–7 days	Survives	Stable	Bank blood	100%	Probably less than 1%
Platelets	—	8–11 days	Consumed	Very labile (40% at 24 hours; 0 at 48 hours)	Fresh blood or plasma, fresh platelet concentrates (not frozen plasma)	150,000–400,000/mm.³	60–100,000/mm.³

Table 7–2. Diagnosis of Inherited Disorders of Coagulation

Deficient Factor	Partial Thromboplastin Time	One-Stage Prothrombin Time	Thrombin Time	Bleeding Time	Fibrinogen Level	Platelet Adhesiveness	Remarks
I (fibrinogen)	Long	Long	Long	Long or normal	Low	Normal	Corrected by stored or adsorbed plasma but not by serum
II (prothrombin)	Long	Long	Normal	Normal	Normal	Normal	Corrected by stored plasma
V	Long	Long	Normal	Normal	Normal	Normal	Corrected by adsorbed plasma
VII	Normal	Long	Normal	Normal	Normal	Normal	Corrected by stored plasma or serum
VIII	Long	Normal	Normal	Normal	Normal	Normal	Corrected by adsorbed plasma
IX	Long	Normal	Normal	Normal	Normal	Normal	Corrected by stored plasma or serum
X	Long	Long	Normal	Normal	Normal	Normal	Corrected by stored plasma or serum
XI	Long	Normal	Normal	Normal	Normal	Normal	Corrected by stored plasma or serum
XII	Long	Normal	Normal	Normal	Normal	Normal	Corrected by stored plasma or serum
XIII	Normal	Normal	Normal	Normal	Normal	Normal	Clot is soluble in 6 M urea or 1% monoiodoacetic acid
Von Willebrand's disease	Long	Normal	Normal	Long	Normal	Low	Deficiency in Factor VIII

Defects may be correctable by mixture of abnormal plasma with shelf-stored plasma (deficient in V and VIII), plasma adsorbed with $BaSO_4$ or $Al(OH)_3$ (deficient in II, VII, IX, X), or serum (deficient in I, II, V, VIII). Suspected defects can be confirmed by special assays for specific factors.

spond in normal fashion to exogenous ADP. The bleeding tendency that results is, in many respects, analogous to that produced by aspirin (see below). In severe cases, the bleeding time is prolonged, but in its more mild form the disorder can be diagnosed only by specialized tests of platelet function. Only recently recognized, this disorder appears to be a frequent cause of hitherto unexplained mild bleeding tendencies. Transfusion of fresh viable platelets corrects the hemostatic defect.

ACQUIRED BLEEDING TENDENCIES

Many acquired disorders of hemostasis are complex and involve defects in several components of the hemostatic processes. An exception is the effect of administration of anticoagulant drugs, either heparin or derivatives of coumarin ("oral anticoagulants"). Heparin is a strongly anionic sulfated polysaccharide whose biological activity is due to its ability to form salt complexes with plasma proteins. Heparin inhibits coagulation by blocking interaction of thrombin with fibrinogen and by impairing the activation of Factor IX (Fig. 7-1). The aggregation of platelets by thrombin is inhibited by heparin, but in conventional clinical dosage the drug has no other effect on platelet function. Heparin is destroyed in the stomach and is not effective unless given parenterally. Its action is neutralized by protamine; 1 mg. of protamine will reverse the effect of 100 units of heparin, on the average.

Oral anticoagulants have no effect on coagulation *in vitro*. They competitively inhibit the synthesis of vitamin K dependent clotting factors (Factors VII, IX, X and prothrombin [Factor II]) by the liver. Their pharmacological effect is largely a function of their free blood level and is increased by a variety of other drugs, which may compete with coumarin derivatives for albumin binding sites and thus raise the free plasma level of the anticoagulant (e.g., phenylbutazone, sulfasoxazole), may reduce the rate of excretion by competition for degradative enzymes (e.g., tolbutamide, diphenylhydantoin), or may increase the affinity for the anticoagulant of enzyme receptor sites (e.g., quinidine, anabolic steroids) and thus reduce the dosage requirement for effective anticoagulation. The effect of coumarin derivatives is also subject to inhibition by drugs if they increase the activity of hepatic enzymes that degrade the coumarin (e.g., phenobarbital) and thereby reduce the effectiveness of the anticoagulant.

Administration of the oral anticoagulant blocks the synthesis of the four vulnerable clotting factors and is followed by a decline in their plasma concentration through natural processes of degradation. The initial effect is on Factor VII (half-life 5 hours). Factors IX and X disappear more slowly (half-life 24 hours and 40 hours, respectively), and prothrombin is even slower (half-life 72 hours). After discontinuation of the drug, restoration of plasma levels of these factors follows roughly the same course.

The bleeding tendency in anticoagulated patients is a direct function of their effect on hemostasis and increases in parallel with their antithrombotic effect. If a hemorrhagic complication is encountered when the level of anticoagulation is not excessive, an underlying lesion should be suspected. The propensity of unsuspected gastrointestinal neoplasms to bleed in anticoagulated patients is a frequent example.

Important acquired disorders of platelets include thrombocytopenia and abnormalities of platelet function. A decrease in platelet number without a defect in coagulation may develop as an allergic reaction to drug ingestion (e.g., quinidine, thiazide diuretics, chloramphenicol, anti-inflammatory agents), as a feature of leukemia, in association with marrow failure from metastases or other causes, or by autoimmunization (idiopathic thrombocytopenic purpura). The gravity of the hemorrhagic state is a direct function of the platelet count. Hemorrhagic complications at operation are uncommon if the platelet count exceeds 60,000 to 100,000/mm.^{3} Spontaneous bleeding is seen at platelet counts less than 20,000 to 30,000/mm.^{3} Intracranial hemorrhage is a major hazard if the platelet count is less than 10,000/mm.^{3} In idiopathic thrombocytopenic purpura, adrenal steroids often lead to a rise in platelet count. Splenectomy produces a remission in two thirds of cases, but relapse is not uncommon. Replacement therapy requires viable platelets in fresh whole blood, platelet-rich plasma, or concentrated preparations. In idiopathic thrombocytopenic purpura, platelet destruction is accelerated by immune mechanisms, and the response to infused platelets is often evanescent. Platelets withstand storage poorly, especially in the cold; few survive reinfusion after storage for 48 hours in ACD or CPD anticoagulant at refrigerator temperature, but if they are kept at room temperature, a useful rise in platelet count may be achieved with transfused materials 3 or 4 days old.

Acquired disorders of platelet function frequently result from ingestion of drugs that inhibit the "release reaction" of platelets and thus impair platelet aggregation. Aspirin is most commonly involved; it produces a profound effect after administration of only two or three tablets per day, the effect lasting 4 to 6 days. Many instances of faulty surgical hemostasis and diffuse wound bleeding, previously unexplained, appear to be the consequence of the use of aspirin by surgical patients. Other agents with a similar effect include phenylbutazone, sulfinpyrazone, antihistamines, indomethacin, chlorpromazine, and many tranquilizers.

A functional platelet defect is also seen after the infusion of dextran of average molecular weight 70,000 or, to a lesser extent, 40,000. In patients who receive more than 1.5 gm. dextran per kg. as a single infusion, a clinically significant bleeding tendency is common, and an increase in bleeding time and in operative blood loss is often seen.

The bleeding tendency of uremia is largely the result of abnormal platelet function. A qualitative platelet defect is a prominent feature of advanced renal failure. Defective platelet adhesiveness and impaired participation of platelet lipids in coagulation ("platelet factor 3") are characteristic. The gravity of the defect is roughly correlated with the degree of azotemia. Correction of the platelet abnormality has been described after dialysis and after renal transplantation.

Mixed hemostatic defects involving both clotting factors and platelets occur in patients with liver disease. All the clotting factors whose source is known appear to be made in the liver; the source of Factor VIII may be some liver cell other than the hepatocyte. Extrahepatic synthesis of Factor VIII, fibrinogen, and perhaps other clotting factors has also been claimed. Factors VII, IX, X, and II (prothrombin) require vitamin K for their synthesis; the others do not. Vitamin K is ingested in the diet and is produced by intestinal bacteria. A deficiency of this fat-soluble vitamin is seen in starvation and after the administration of broad-spectrum antibiotics with sterilization of the gut and is also observed from failure of absorption in cases of common bile duct obstruction or biliary fistula. In hepatic cirrhosis, a deficiency of these and other clotting factors synthesized in the liver occurs. If present, portal hypertension with secondary splenomegaly often leads to thrombocytopenia. Failure of the cirrhotic liver to remove activators of plasminogen accounts for the coexistence of fibrinolysis, aggravated by a pathologic plasminogen activator produced by the diseased liver. The circulating products of fibrinolysis ("fibrinogen digestion products") are potent anticoagulants and also impair platelet aggregation. Consumption coagulopathy (see below) is present in occasional patients with hepatic decompensation and may further embarrass hemostasis. Local causes of bleeding, such as esophageal varices, peptic ulcer, and gastritis, also play an important role.

Treatment of the hemorrhagic state accompanying hepatic failure is difficult because of the complicated nature of the hemostatic defect and in many instances because of inability to control the underlying disease process. Replacement therapy with fresh frozen plasma or concentrated preparations of the vitamin K dependent clotting factors may be transiently effective, and platelet concentrates are sometimes of value. Epsilon aminocaproic acid (EACA), an inhibitor of plasminogen activation, has been employed to reverse the fibrinolytic state in these patients, but the results have been less encouraging than with fibrinolysis in other clinical settings.

A hemostatic defect accompanies extracorporeal circulation for cardiopulmonary bypass. A complex abnormality results from the invariable development of thrombocytopenia, the activation of fibrinolysis, the administration of heparin for anticoagulation during the period of cardiopulmonary bypass, occasionally from the initiation of intravascular coagulation, and probably from nonspecific denaturation of blood proteins at air interfaces. The problem may be compounded by faulty replacement of depleted clotting factors, if cardiac cirrhosis has impaired hepatic synthetic mechanisms. Improvement in perfusion techniques and meticulous attention to surgical hemostasis have reduced the frequency of this problem in patients after open-heart surgery, but the solution awaits the development of nonthrombogenic surfaces for extracorporeal circuits.

Careful attention to neutralization of heparin with protamine will eliminate the most frequent source of a generalized bleeding tendency after open heart operations. Protamine has anticoagulant activity itself, but its effect is trivial compared to heparin, and a modest excess of the drug is well tolerated. If evidence of a generalized hemostatic defect persists after an adequate dose of protamine, diagnostic studies should be performed as for any case of an acute bleeding state (see below). The indiscriminate use of epsilon aminocaproic acid or other drugs is not recommended in the absence of specific diagnosis, but such agents may be useful if indicated by appropriate laboratory studies. This problem is also considered in Chapter 15.

ACUTE TRANSIENT BLEEDING DISORDERS

A transient hemorrhagic tendency may develop *de novo* in a surgical patient as a complication of many disorders in which bleeding is not a primary feature. Such a phenomenon can arise through dilution of hemostatic elements by massive transfusion with stored blood, by consumption of plasma factors and platelets secondary to intravascular coagulation, and by destruction of hemostatic plugs through fibrinolysis.

Massive Transfusion. Replacement of blood loss with bank blood induces thrombocytopenia and a defect in plasma factors V and VIII because of the lability of these hemostatic components during shelf storage (Table 7–1). Neosynthesis or mobilization of clotting factors from body stores prevents major coagulation deficiencies in most massively transfused patients, except in those with severe liver disease or hemophilia. However, since the storage pool of platelets is limited, thrombocytopenia is a frequent consequence of massive transfusion. If the volume of rapidly administered bank blood exceeds 8 to 10 pints, a platelet count less than $100,000/mm.^3$ may be expected, and if the transfused volume exceeds 7 or 8 liters, a long bleeding time and clinically significant hemorrhagic tendency are frequent. Treatment requires replacement of the deficient materials in the form of fresh blood or fresh platelet-rich plasma. Factors V and VIII may be supplied in frozen plasma, but this does not contain viable platelets. A practical preventive procedure is the administration of fresh blood during the course of rapid transfusion, one unit of fresh blood for each four or five banked units being sufficient to prevent the development of symptomatic dilutional thrombocytopenia.

Consumption Coagulopathy. At one time regarded as a curiosity, disseminated intravascular clotting has become recognized as a common mechanism of disease. A large number of disparate conditions are marked by entrance into the blood stream of materials that induce blood coagulation and platelet aggregation. In some instances, as in bacteremia, malaria, amniotic fluid embolism, or snakebite, the procoagulant substance is a specific chemically defined agent peculiar to the disease. In other cases, as in massive soft tissue crush injury or disseminated malignancy, the offending substance may be a less well characterized product of tissue destruction. Occasionally, as in hemolytic transfusion reactions or absorption of components of a retroplacental hematoma, the stimulus to intravascular clotting is a constituent of the blood itself. Sometimes, as in large hemangiomata or perhaps in the presence of gram-negative endotoxemia, a widespread vascular lesion may activate clotting and platelet alterations.

Disseminated coagulation within the circulation interferes with organ perfusion and may lead to a generalized hemorrhagic state, the consequence of a "consumption coagulopathy" resulting from consumption of labile hemostatic elements, including Factors V and VIII, prothrombin, fibrinogen, and platelets. Stable clotting factors, such as IX and X, may also be reduced since once activated they are filtered from the circulation by the liver.

Diagnosis of consumption coagulopathy depends on demonstration of a deficiency of the labile clotting factors and of platelets (Table 7–3). Alterations in erythrocyte morphology are often present, as a result of damage sustained by red cells in squeezing through fibrin clots. Products of fibrinolysis (see below) can usually be demonstrated, for activation of lytic mechanisms is a natural response to intravascular clotting. The common association of fibrinolysis with intravascular coagulation accounts for the failure to demonstrate occluding thrombi in autopsy material from patients who die following a clinical course typical of consumption coagulopathy.

Treatment of disseminated intravascular clotting is most likely to be effective if the source of the stimulus to clotting can be removed, e.g., evacuation of the uterus in "obstetrical defibrination," drainage of abscesses and administration of appropriate antibiotics for bacteremia, use of specific antivenins for snakebite. Replacement therapy is apt to be ineffective unless entrance of procoagulants into the blood stream can be controlled. Heparin may be of value to block consumption of hemostatic elements; sometimes, as in disseminated malignancy, it may be the only therapy available. The required dose is that needed to produce an improvement in fibrinogen levels and prothrombin time. Replacement of the consumed hemostatic elements can then be carried out with fresh blood or fresh platelet-rich plasma. The use of concentrated fibrinogen is not recommended, since it lacks the other clotting factors likely to be deficient and since it is a major source of serum hepatitis,

Table 7-3. ACUTE BLEEDING DISORDERS

	PLATELET COUNT	PROTHROMBIN TIME	THROMBIN TIME	FIBRINOGEN	FIBRINOLYSIS	REMARKS
Dilution (massive transfusion)	Low	Normal or long	Normal	Normal	Absent	—
Consumption coagulopathy	Low	Long	Long	Low	Absent or present	Clot lysis and euglobulin lysis time may or may not be abnormal; fibrinogen digestion products are usually demonstrable; abnormal erythrocyte morphology
Fibrinolysis	Normal	Normal or long	Normal or long	Normal or low	Present	Circulating plasmin demonstrable by clot lysis time, euglobulin lysis time, or fibrin plate
Circulating heparin	Normal	Normal or long	Long	Normal	Normal	Long thrombin time corrected by protamine
Underlying inherited coagulation disorder	Normal	Normal	Normal	Normal	Normal	Clinical evidence of generalized bleeding disorder but normal screening tests usually indicate pre-existing hemorrhagic state involving coagulation, most often hemophilia

Simple rapid screening tests for working diagnosis of acute hemorrhagic states sufficient to guide therapy. Confirmation requires detailed evaluation.

being prepared from pooled plasma. The role of inhibitors of platelet aggregation, such as aspirin and indomethacin, is at present under evaluation.

Fibrinolysis. Activation of plasminogen to plasmin is a regular accompaniment of hemostasis, but fibrinolysis can also exist as a pathologic process and can lead to a severe bleeding diathesis. In addition to dissolution of fibrin clots, plasmin digests fibrinogen and other clotting factors. The products of fibrinolysis and fibrinogenolysis are polypeptides with potent anticoagulant activity. They block the further polymerization of fibrin and also impede platelet aggregation.

Most often fibrinolysis arises as a consequence of disseminated intravascular coagulation. Although fibrinolysis has been described as an isolated finding after resuscitation from cardiac arrest and occasionally in other circumstances, many authorities believe that activation of plasminogen occurs only in response to intravascular clotting and that primary fibrinolysis does not exist. Under these circumstances the administration of epsilon aminocaproic acid, an effective antidote to plasminogen activation, is hazardous, for inhibition of lysis may remove the patient's only defense against widespread thrombosis. Unless one has laboratory evidence that fibrinolysis *does not* coexist with intravascular coagulation (in practice, this assurance requires a normal platelet count and fibrinogen level), EACA should probably not be used without the simultaneous administration of heparin.

Diagnosis of acute transient bleeding disorders is summarized in Table 7-3.

REFERENCES

Biggs, R., and Macfarlane, R. G.: Treatment of Haemophilia and Other Coagulation Disorders. Philadelphia, F. A. Davis Company, 1966.

Brinkhous, K. M.: Hemophilia and New Hemorrhagic States — International Symposium, New York, Chapel Hill, The University of North Carolina Press, 1970.

Britten, A., and Salzman, E. W.: Surgery in congenital disorders of blood coagulation. Surg. Gynec. & Obstet. *123*:1333, 1966.

McKay, D. G.: Disseminated Intravascular Coagulation — An Intermediary Mechanism of Disease. New York, Harper & Row, 1965.

Owen, C. A., Bowie, E. J. W., Didisheim, P., and Thompson, J. H., Jr.: *The Diagnosis of Bleeding Disorders.* Boston, Little, Brown and Company, 1969.

Poller, L.: Recent Advances in Blood Coagulation. Boston, Little, Brown and Company, 1969.

Ratnoff, O. D.: Treatment of Hemorrhagic Disorders. New York, Harper & Row, 1968.

Salzman, E. W., and Britten, A.: Hemorrhage and Thrombosis: A Practical Clinical Guide. Boston, Little, Brown and Company, 1965.

Tarnay, T. J.: *Surgery in the Hemophiliac.* Springfield, Charles C Thomas, 1968.

CHAPTER 8

VENTILATION AND VENTILATORY FAILURE

JOHN M. KINNEY, M.D., F.A.C.S.

The general surgeon has often regarded ventilatory problems as the concern of the anesthetist or of the thoracic surgeon, and only recently has attention been given to the ventilatory impairment associated with general surgical procedures or with problems of trauma or sepsis which may not arise from primary chest involvement. Every surgeon has a growing responsibility for the intelligent evaluation of ventilation because of the increasing number of operations on older people, the trend toward more extensive surgical operations and the increasing amount of surgical care required for trauma and other emergency surgical problems. The recognition of a decreased ventilatory reserve before operation, whether elective or emergency, may allow useful preoperative treatment and/or more intelligent postoperative management. Evidence indicates that ventilation is more compromised after abdominal operations than was formerly realized, and this may be particularly serious if unreplaced blood loss and other circulatory alterations also restrict tissue gas exchange.

Statistics regarding the exact incidence of pulmonary complications, following major abdominal or thoracic operations, are difficult to document accurately because of the variety of criteria used. A review of hospital records usually indicates an overall incidence of postoperative atelectasis and pneumonia of less than 10 per cent. Yet individual reports of patients undergoing upper abdominal surgery describe atelectasis in 25 to 50 per cent on the basis of detailed physical examination and chest x-ray. Despite such disparity of statistics, most authorities agree that between 10 and 20 per cent of patients undergoing abdominal or thoracic operations have atelectasis or pneumonitis of clinical significance.

The planning of surgical care for any patient should include the following questions:

1. Does the patient have decreased ventilatory reserve at the outset, either because of his surgical problem or because of underlying chronic lung disease?

2. How will my therapy, operative or otherwise, influence this patient's ventilatory reserve?

3. If initial loss of reserve is present, is it reversible? Does the plan of therapy include measures to treat pre-existing loss as well as minimize further loss of ventilatory reserve?

4. Will this patient require any special effort to monitor his ventilatory status and how will the information be obtained, organized and made available for optimal clinical care?

VENTILATORY SUPPLY AND DEMAND

It is common to expect an immediate decrease in ventilatory reserve in patients undergoing thoracic operations. However, the loss of ventilatory reserve associated with general surgical procedures, particularly those in the abdomen, as well as nonthoracic trauma and infection, has not received adequate attention. Ventilatory reserve is a general term which is used here to include various kinds of reserve capacity of the ventilatory apparatus, particularly in relation to three areas:

1. Volume and rate of air moved per unit of time. Dead space vs. alveolar ventilation (CO_2 excretion).

2. Stiffness of the lung, compliance, lung volumes and capacity. Work of breathing.

3. Oxygenation of blood, V/Q matching, "shunting."

Data on loss of reserve following various surgical conditions in each of these three areas of ventilation is incomplete, and undoubtedly the loss of reserve of one type is usually accompanied by loss of reserve to some degree in the other two. However, it is instructive to consider each type of functional loss separately, because the emphasis on both patient monitoring and steps in therapy will differ somewhat with each type.

It is a mistake to consider ventilation as a separate function from circulation, or ventilation and circulation as separate from the demands of tissue metabolism. Figure 8-1 is a diagram to indicate that appropriate tissue gas exchange is the primary consideration of monitoring and of therapy. This involves understanding the balance which must exist between the "supply" factors of the ventilation and circulation and the "demand" factors of tissue metabolism.

A part of the postoperative loss of ventilatory reserve was demonstrated by Anscombe, when he studied changes in vital capacity and maximal inspiratory and expiratory flow rate following twelve different

OVERALL GAS EXCHANGE

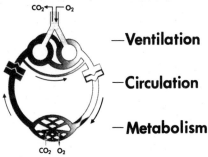

—Ventilation

—Circulation

—Metabolism

Figure 8–1. A diagrammatic representation of ventilation, circulation and tissue metabolism. This is to emphasize overall gas exchange as a primary objective in patient management.

types of abdominal operation. The influence of the surgical operation on each of these functions was quantitatively similar. A conventional uncomplicated gastrectomy caused reductions of 50 to 60 per cent of normal preoperative values for the first two days after operation, with a slow return toward normal during the following week. It is of particular interest that the loss of function following transthoracic gastrectomy was shown by Anscombe to be no greater than that seen with subtotal gastrectomy utilizing either of two upper abdominal incisions. Similar but less extensive decreases in ventilatory reserve were found after lower abdominal procedures.

The demands for resting gas exchange after major operation are seldom increased more than 10 per cent above the preoperative values, although complications and infection may cause increases of 10 to 30 per cent. Generalized peritonitis may cause sustained increases in resting metabolic demands of 20 to 50 per cent, whereas major burns may have prolonged increases of up to twice normal. Thus the supply and demand picture for ventilation in surgical patients may involve mild to moderate increases in demand, but the problems are more frequently related to factors which cripple the capacity for supply such as failure to oxygenate blood adequately, to clear CO_2 in sufficient amounts or to supply effective muscular work at a rising energy cost of breathing.

The balance between ventilatory supply and tissue demand is diagrammed in Figure 8-2. There is no single method for following the balance between ventilatory reserve and tissue demands. The ventilatory reserve is shown as decreased according to the data of Anscombe on vital capacity and air flow, but this is undoubtedly accompanied by some increases in retained secretions, dead space ventilation and shunting of blood past underventilated alveoli with a decrease in blood oxygenation. The tissue demands for gas exchange may be raised somewhat by fever, sepsis or extensive tissue trauma. This loss of ventilatory capacity and any increase in tissue demands result in a diminished reserve which slowly improves with normal convalescence. It takes

VENTILATORY "SUPPLY & DEMAND"

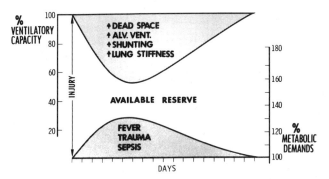

Figure 8–2. Ventilation following injury is a function of the balance between the ventilatory capacity for supply of gas exchange and tissue demand for metabolism. Therefore the available reserve can be restricted because of a decrease in capability for supply or an increase in tissue need.

little imagination to visualize the situation when the patient undergoes a major injury or extensive operation at a time when unsuspected lung disease has already reduced his ventilatory reserve to 75 per cent of normal. This level of loss is compatible with a moderately active life and a normal chest x-ray, yet causes unexpected ventilatory failure following operation or injury with little or no increase in tissue demands. A different pattern of onset is represented by the postoperative patient with progressive peritonitis. Here the initial loss of reserve does not improve, whereas the tissue demands increase until a lethal deficit develops after demands exceed the reserve capacity for supply (Fig. 8-3).

VENTILATORY FAILURE

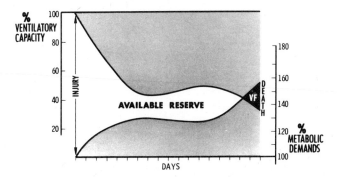

Figure 8–3. The available ventilatory reserve after injury may be progressively narrowed until the demand exceeds capacity and a period of ventilatory failure ensues. The onset of ventilatory failure must be recognized and treated promptly, because it is usually progressive and leads to a fatal outcome in a relatively short time.

MEASUREMENT OF BLOOD GASES AND pH

Many investigators feel that the most important advance in patient monitoring of the past decade has been the growth of blood gas and pH measurements on arterial blood. Part of the reason for the unique value of such measurements is the reflection they provide of the balance which exists between supply and demand for ventilation.

The introduction of electrodes and other new devices for the measurement of oxygen and carbon dioxide levels in blood has expanded the clinical usefulness of blood gas determinations. This advance is analogous to the introduction of the flame photometer which made serum sodium and potassium measurements a common part of surgical care during the 1950's. Several commercial instruments are currently available for the rapid analysis of small samples of blood and provide satisfactory accuracy for clinical purposes without requiring unusual technical skill. Arterial O_2 levels may be measured as per cent saturation or as partial pressure, the latter having certain advantages when considering the effectiveness of a given level of inspired oxygen to oxygenate the blood. The partial pressure of CO_2 in arterial blood has particular importance in reflecting the amount of effective alveolar ventilation. Neither the measurement of the carbon dioxide combining power nor the total carbon dioxide content of blood is useful in determining the adequacy of ventilation unless the total CO_2 content is combined with a pH measurement to allow the calculation of arterial P_{CO_2}.

The measurement of blood gases and pH on a sample of arterial blood requires more thought and care than does a routine chemical determination on venous blood. The arterial blood samples must be representative of the arterial blood prior to the needle puncture. Therefore, after introducing the needle into the artery, one should avoid withdrawing the blood sample until 30 seconds of normal ventilation have taken place in order to avoid nonrepresentative blood gas values as a result of breath holding or hyperventilation by an apprehensive patient. The blood sample must be absolutely free of bubbles in order to be anaerobic and must be sealed in a tightly fitting heparinized syringe. The laboratory technician should have been notified in advance so that the blood sample can be promptly analyzed following its withdrawal from the patient. It is not enough to record on the patient's chart the blood gas values with the date; the notation must also include the time of day when the blood was drawn and whether any oxygen, intermittent positive pressure breathing or other ventilatory therapy was in use at the time.

PREOPERATIVE EVALUATION OF VENTILATORY FAILURE

History. In order to detect the patient with previously unrecognized loss of ventilatory reserve, the surgeon must conduct his preoperative history with an increased index of suspicion and a special effort to notice certain red flags which may be clues to ventilatory trouble after operation:

1. Childhood respiratory infections.
2. Pneumonia or pleurisy before the discovery of antibiotics.
3. The bronchitis often associated with cigarette smoking.
4. Presence of morning sputum.
5. Old chest injuries, especially in epileptics or chronic alcoholics.
6. Current physical activity. Question a friend or relative. Limitation of activity for whatever reason may mask the insidious loss of ventilatory reserve (as in the furniture mover who changed to desk work because of a leg injury).

The common clinical signs indicating loss of ventilatory reserve (dyspnea, tachycardia, cyanosis and altered mental status) are often unreliable. Cyanosis is generally thought to be the most reliable indication of tissue hypoxia, but the blueness of the lips, nailbeds and mucosa depends upon the absolute amount of reduced hemoglobin in the surface capillary blood, rather than on the proportion of the reduced hemoglobin to the oxygenated hemoglobin. A minimum of 5 gm. of reduced hemoglobin per 100 cc. of blood must be present before cyanosis is clinically apparent. Furthermore, visual acuity affects the ability of the clinician to detect the color changes of cyanosis, so that it is often unrecognized until the arterial oxygen saturation is under 80 per cent.

The surgeon should also look for ventilatory red flags during the physical examination. Is there adequate excursion of the thoracic cage and diaphragm? Some patients who appear to have an increased anteroposterior diameter of the chest actually have moderately good thoracic excursion. Finding a maximal thoracic excursion of over 1 inch by a tape measure around the patient's chest suggests no serious restrictive disease in his thoracic cage.

Is there prolonged expiration or wheezing? These conditions increase the energy cost of breathing, seriously limit the ability to hyperventilate and predispose to the accumulation of pulmonary secretions. A rough idea of expiratory force and volume may be obtained by asking the patient to blow out a half-burned match held 6 inches from his mouth. To extinguish the flame is said to require a forced expiratory volume of approximately 1 liter, or a peak flow rate in excess of 100 liters/minute. Bringing the lips together while blowing must be avoided, because even a slight approximation could allow a patient with poor ventilation to extinguish the match.

Chest X-ray. An x-ray of the chest is commonly performed as part of the surgical work-up and is sometimes mistakenly regarded as a pulmonary function test. A chest film may be read as normal in a patient with significant loss of ventilatory reserve, and, conversely, lungs which are obviously diseased may have surprisingly good ventilatory capacity. Therefore a chest x-ray is of great importance to the evaluation and management of ventilation only when it is interpreted in the light of what it is—a static picture, not a test of pulmonary function. The combination of chest fluoroscopy with x-ray improves the correlation with pulmonary function. This enables the surgeon to observe which respiratory muscles are being used, to gain an impression of the uniformity of distribution of expired air and to better localize sites of pulmonary disease. Lag in motion of the diaphragm and air trapping may be observed on fluoroscopy after successive forced expirations.

Pulmonary Function Tests. The surgeon should divide the pulmonary function tests available in his hospital into those which are indicated by virtue of red flags in the history or physical examination and other studies which are indicated only to answer specific questions which may be raised if the preliminary tests are abnormal. Excellent discussions of pulmonary function tests are available (Comroe et al.).

The three tests of ventilatory function most readily available in hospitals are vital capacity (VC), maximum breathing capacity (MBC) and forced expiratory volume (FEV). The vital capacity is the total volume of gas that can be expelled from the lungs from a position of full inspiration with no time limit on duration of expiration. The vital capacity test used alone is an unsatisfactory method for evaluating preoperative pulmonary function. As a single screening procedure, it has been reported to detect only one third of the patients who had evidence of impairment by other pulmonary tests.

The MBC, sometimes referred to as the maximum voluntary ventilation (MVV), is the maximal volume of gas that can be breathed in 15 or 30 seconds by voluntary effort, usually reported as liters/minute. This test is a useful measure of the overall integration of the ventilatory apparatus and will detect up to two thirds of patients who have loss of pulmonary reserve if properly performed.

Patients with an MBC below 75 per cent of predicted normal can be assumed to have some degree of airway obstruction or emphysema and should receive extra attention when undergoing surgery. Values of 75 to 60 per cent of predicted normal indicate significant loss, whereas values of 60 to 40 per cent indicate patients with serious loss who carry a significantly higher postoperative mortality from ventilatory complications and justify maximum ventilatory care both before and after operation. The MBC has certain important limitations, particularly related to the requirement for considerable exertion on the part of the patient and being influenced by nonpulmonary factors such as patient understanding, motivation and endurance. For these reasons, the MBC has been replaced in many institutions by a single-breath method such as the FEV.

The forced expiratory volume is the volume of a maximally fast expiration starting from a full inspiration, timed for 0.5, 0.75 or 1.0 second. This is perhaps the most useful single procedure for preoperative evaluation of mechanical pulmonary function. An approximate correlation has been demonstrated between the $FEV_{0.75}$ multiplied by 40, or the $FEV_{1.0}$ multiplied by 30, and the MBC in liters/minute. Miller and coworkers have recommended the analysis of preoperative pulmonary function by comparing the ratio of observed to predicted values for vital capacity against the ratio of the half-second vital capacity to observed total vital capacity. When patients were studied in this manner and the findings plotted on a quadrant graph, the distribution of patients was reported to allow a ready separation between those with satisfactory, poor and prohibitive pulmonary function.

Tests for arterial blood gases and pH are not useful screening procedures but are important to perform if other evidence suggests ventilatory insufficiency and for the evaluation of therapy in improving abnormal blood gas levels.

PREOPERATIVE VENTILATORY THERAPY

Preoperative instruction has proved to be of great value, particularly in the elderly or chronically ill. Many patients are unfamiliar with techniques for achieving optimal ventilation and effective coughing. These techniques can be taught and practiced preoperatively with more beneficial effect than when they are imposed upon a frightened patient in postoperative pain. Professional physiotherapists are employed for this task on many hospital services, but a routine set of effective exercises can be taught by other trained personnel. Patients who are aware of the hazards of pulmonary complications will cooperate more actively in their prevention.

The potential danger of elective operation in a patient with an active upper respiratory infection has been emphasized. Individuals with colds, sinusitis, tonsillitis or acute bronchitis should not undergo surgery until completely well for one or two weeks. The most consistent source of postoperative pulmonary complications is chronic bronchitis of whatever source. One can classify bronchitis by the amount and character of the sputum—none, less than 1 ounce or more than 1 ounce, mucoid or purulent. Every effort should be made to decrease pulmonary secretions by postural drainage, inhalation of high humidity vapor and intelligent use of expectorants. A lung process seemingly may start as an infectious disease, but in its natural history asthmatic or bronchospastic elements begin to play a role and pulmonary emphysema may subsequently develop. If preoperative bronchoconstriction has been shown by the presence of a prolonged expiratory phase, wheezing or improvement in the FEV after administration of a bronchodilator drug, an important guide to preoperative therapy and postoperative management will have been obtained.

The most common cause of simple bronchitis is cigarette smoking.

Some patients seem to regard a chronic, persistent, productive cough as perfectly normal, dismissing it as a cigarette cough. Functional as well as morphologic abnormalities have been reported in the ventilatory apparatus of heavy smokers, leading to the conclusion that anyone who smokes in excess of 20 cigarettes per day can be assumed to have abnormal pulmonary function. Therefore, abstaining from cigarettes for two weeks before elective abdominal and thoracic operations is recommended.

The prophylactic use of intermittent positive pressure breathing to reduce the incidence of postoperative complications has been recommended, but the exact benefit has not been clearly established. In contrast, in patients with known preoperative pulmonary disease, the periodic employment of intermittent positive pressure breathing has been shown to be a useful part of the therapeutic program. Their postoperative care should be planned to allow the use of mechanical assistance in the most efficient manner.

In summary, a period of preoperative ventilatory therapy can be expected to correct excessive secretions and pulmonary infection and to improve bronchoconstriction, if present. Preoperative therapy cannot be expected to improve an absolute loss of alveolar diffusing surface, to increase alveolar perfusion, or to change a mechanical restriction of the thorax.

VENTILATION DURING OPERATION

Position during the operation should be planned with at least as much consideration for the patient's ventilatory function as for the surgeon's comfort. Visceral pressure against the diaphragm and lateral pressure against the chest wall are commonly employed to improve position. Surgeons would do well to test these positions on themselves to demonstrate their detrimental effects on breathing and their production of subsequent back pain and other discomfort. Vigorous retraction, heavy draping and careless leaning by members of the surgical team should be minimized.

Because of advances in anesthesiology and more careful attention to preoperative preparation of the patient, the chances of the patient's developing a serious problem in ventilation during the surgical operation are very small. It is not uncommon, however, to see a consultant's note in the record before operation which includes a statement such as: "This patient is probably a reasonable risk for surgery as long as anoxia and hypotension are avoided during the operation." Actually, the anesthetized patient who is completely relaxed and has an endotracheal tube in place, and whose ventilatory function is being watched continuously with regard to rate and depth of breathing and accumulation of bronchial secretions, could probably not be in a more advantageous position with regard to his ventilation. *Usually, the danger of ventilatory insufficiency is not during the operation, but thereafter.* The patient moves from the operating room to the recovery room in a sedated condition, still partially anesthetized, with the endotracheal tube removed and without the high concentration of inspired oxygen as well as the mechanical assistance of ventilation at the time when his need for gas exchange has been reduced and now begins to rise toward normal. At this time the margin between the tissue demand for ventilation and the ability to supply ventilation begins to narrow. It is now that the preoperative evaluation of the patient's ventilatory reserve begins to assume its real significance!

POSTOPERATIVE VENTILATION

A febrile response to general anesthesia and major surgery has been accepted by some clinicians as being inevitable and inconsequential. Still, an afebrile postoperative course is a reasonable objective after most operative procedures. Any rise in temperature should be interpreted as a physiologic disturbance beyond the normal process of wound healing and metabolic response to trauma. With diligent attention to preventive and therapeutic measures to maintain optimal pulmonary ventilation, most patients can undergo prolonged and complicated surgical procedures with postoperative temperatures never exceeding 100.4° F. (38° C.). The numerous factors logically predisposing to pulmonary complications suggest that a large proportion of the otherwise unexplained postoperative temperature elevations arise from a disturbance of pulmonary function.

Nearly every form of postoperative ventilatory failure is associated with some retention of *bronchopulmonary secretions.* Pre-existing bronchitis as well as shallow postoperative breathing and cough inhibition caused by pain or narcotics will accentuate the problem. *Beware of administering narcotics for restlessness; the problem may be cerebral hypoxia instead of pain.* If frequent coughing is not sufficient to control secretions, tracheal aspiration by nasal catheter may be needed. This will remove secretion not only directly, by suction, but also indirectly, by stimulating coughing and hyperventilation. Nasotracheal suction requires careful asepsis and should be used with specific indication, not as a routine. Its use will sometimes avoid the subsequent need for bronchoscopy to clear the major airways.

Dyspnea may be the most prominent clinical feature of postoperative ventilatory insufficiency. This increased ventilatory effort is due to the central stimulus of retained carbon dioxide and the lowered oxygen tension in blood, with whatever airway obstruction is present owing to secretions. Mental confusion can arise from either hypoxia or hypercarbia. In the early stages of failure the patient may be anxious, restless and irritable, whereas the skin of the extremities is warm, the pulse is full and the blood pressure is normal or slightly elevated. In the later stages of ventilatory failure, somnolence progresses to coma and then hypotension with progressive circulatory failure. In late peritonitis the mode of death is frequently sudden apnea at a time when there is still a satisfactory heartbeat.

Cyanosis in the immediate postoperative period may be due to drug-induced depression of the respiratory center, mechanical obstruction of the upper or lower respiratory tract, or interference with the muscles of respiration. Some of these are recognizable at a glance. Evidence of bronchiolar constriction, atelectasis or pneumothorax should be sought by inspection, percussion and auscultation of the chest. This examination should be performed at once on all patients who are cyanotic despite an open airway. Emergency x-ray examination of the chest, if quickly available, deserves consideration. In bronchospasm auscultation characteristically reveals rhonchi, wheezing and prolongation of expiration. In atelectasis expansion of the affected side of the chest is diminished and the heart and trachea are shifted to the affected side. There are dullness to percussion and absence of breath sounds over the involved area. Chest expansion is also decreased in pneumothorax, with diminished breath sounds on auscultation of the affected side, but the heart and trachea deviate to the opposite side, and there is hyperresonance on percussion.

The possibility of *tension pneumothorax* following intrathoracic operations is uppermost in the minds of all personnel involved, so that its occurrence is anticipated and treated. Even with nonthoracic operations, intermittent or sustained elevation of intrapulmonic pressure can produce rupture of the surface of a lung already damaged by preexisting disease. This results in one-way passage of air or gas into the pleural cavity where it accumulates under pressure. Respiratory embarrassment and cardiovascular collapse may shortly ensue. Both may be promptly relieved by the performance of simple thoracentesis with a large bore needle.

Oxygen should be administered at any time that the surgeon is in doubt of the adequacy of ventilation in the postoperative patient. Carbon dioxide narcosis in the patient with advanced respiratory insufficiency has been taught and discussed with such thoroughness that some surgeons are hesitant to give oxygen because of the possibility of removing the hypoxic stimulus to ventilation. The hypoxic stimulus to ventilation should never be preserved as part of surgical therapy! If there is any question of cyanosis or inadequate ventilation, oxygen should be administered promptly, recognizing that the patient's minute ventilation must be carefully followed thereafter. The use of oxygen may actually increase the need for ventilatory assistance, because the oxygen may convert the signs of cyanosis and dyspnea in the patient with alveolar hypoventilation to a satisfactory pink color, as well as relieve restlessness and sometimes disorientation. Unfortunately, the alveolar hypoventilation may become more severe with progressive respiratory acidosis. One must be alert to factors which may decrease the percentage of alveolar ventilation without reducing minute ventilation — such as progressively shallower ventilation, atelectasis or pneumonia.

The six common methods of O_2 administration were compared by Kory and co-workers for efficiency, comfort and economy. The adult O_2 tent was found to be a costly and inefficient means of providing O_2 therapy and constituted a serious fire hazard. The environmental cooling of a tent can be provided by other means such as a cooling blanket, which does not interfere with professional care. This study also indicated that with appropriate flow rates the administration of O_2 by nasal catheter or cannula was effective regardless of the extent of mouth breathing.

The inability to clear pulmonary secretions is accepted to be part of the problem of postoperative atelectasis, but the influence of *humidity* on the character of the secretions is seldom examined. It is appropriate to note the importance of temperature in controlling the amount of water vapor which the inspired gas mixture can hold (Fig. 8-4), because this holds a key to understanding the clinical problem and providing effective therapy. The water content of the average indoor air is seen to contain approximately one quarter of the water which is required when this air reaches the alvcoli. The obligatory addition of water (and heat) to inspired air is performed readily by the mucous membranes of the normal upper airway. The presence of hyperventilation, fever or reduced oral intake of water will contribute to drying of the upper airway and hence aggravate any tendency toward drying of the mucous blanket which normally coats the lower airway. This problem is accentuated if the water contribution of the upper airway is bypassed by a tracheostomy or if oxygen is given without adequate humidification.

It is common knowledge that oxygen from any commercial source is supplied in a completely dry form, and therefore therapeutic oxygen is passed through a humidifier jar before reaching the patient. The effectiveness of this humidifier is limited by temperature, and a moment spent at the bedside will confirm that such jars are cool when in use. The vaporizational cooling will have lowered the water temperature in the humidifier from 10 to 20° F. below room temperature, depending on the flow rate of oxygen. The maximum amount of water vapor which can be added to the dry oxygen (point A in Figure 8-4) will amount to essentially the same small proportion (point B) of alveolar requirements as is provided in normal indoor air. It is possible to increase the water content of oxygen passing through an unheated humidifier by suspending water particles in the gas; however, much of this suspended water collects on the walls of the tubing or in the oropharynx and does not reach the lower airway where it is most needed. The most effective way

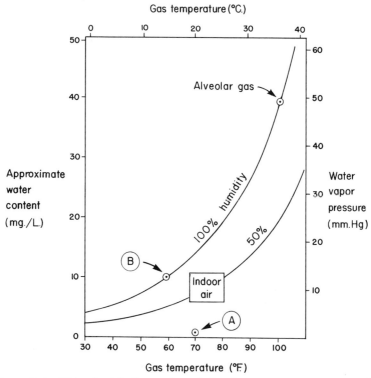

Figure 8–4. This chart indicates the relation between vapor tension and water volume per unit gas volume at various temperatures. The unit weight of water per unit volume of gas is only approximate, because values for these units have been extrapolated to correct for changes in gas volume as a function of changes in temperature. (Modified from Wells, R. E., Perera, R. D., and Kinney, J. M.: Humidification of oxygen during inhalational therapy. New Eng. J. Med. 268:644, 1963.

to improve a problem of bronchopulmonary secretions is to provide a high humidity gas mixture (100 per cent relative humidity between 90 and 100° F.) by using one of the commercially available heated humidifiers. The efficiency of the heated humidifier requires extra attention to maintain the proper water level. Such a humidifier should be located on a level below the patient so that most of the extra condensate in the oxygen tubing will run back to the humidifier and not down onto the patient.

Postoperative patients with no known pulmonary disease may demonstrate stridor, wheezing or labored ventilation suggesting *bronchospasm* whenever marked hyperventilation occurs or secretions accumulate. The administration of bronchodilator medications into the upper airway may be particularly valuable under these conditions. Medications such as isopropylarterenol (Isuprel) are commonly used, but it should be remembered that warm moist air is also an important bronchodilating agent. In those patients with pulmonary insufficiency prior to operation, aminophylline by vein or rectal solution should supplement the short-acting effect of intra-airway medication.

It is important to suspect the presence of *bronchitis* or *bronchopneumonia* in any postoperative patient with ventilatory difficulty. Routine systemic antibiotic therapy is usually not justified on a prophylactic basis after operation, although it has been recommended by some as a means of reducing postoperative pulmonary complications in the aged. The presence of high diaphragms, excessive secretions or long periods of hypoventilation should make the surgeon recognize the increased likelihood of sepsis. Any patient who has had difficulty with the removal of pulmonary secretions for a period of 48 hours should have the pulmonary secretions cultured and antibiotic therapy begun.

VENTILATORY FAILURE IN SHOCK, TRAUMA AND SEPSIS

Pulmonary insufficiency has come to be recognized as one of the leading causes of death in fatal cases of shock, trauma and serious infection. Because abnormal blood gas levels have been found in both civilian and military patients after injury and shock which appeared not to have involved the thorax or lungs, the term "shock lung" has been used to refer to the functional abnormalities and to the pathologic changes seen at autopsy. Many investigators object to this term, because it may not represent a discrete entity but rather the end result of various forms of pulmonary damage. The lungs of such patients, at the time of autopsy, are characteristically congested and heavy, although the pathologic changes may not be homogeneous. The most frequent finding is pulmonary vascular congestion with some interstitial edema, associated with widened alveolocapillary septa, scattered areas of pericapillary hemorrhage and a proteinaceous exudate within the alveoli. If the process has been developing over a number of days, there may be hyaline membrane formation in some alveoli, early fibrosis in interstitial areas and variable numbers of small pulmonary emboli. The extent of alveolar collapse may vary from scattered atelectasis to massive consolidation. Fat particles may be seen with appropriate stains of lung sections after death from acute pulmonary insufficiency, regardless of whether major skeletal injury was present.

Certain factors have been suggested as contributing to the etiology of acute ventilatory failure in surgical patients:

Fluid Overload. Buffered sodium solutions have become widely accepted as appropriate therapy for acute surgical conditions. However, the net balance of forces which keeps fluid from seeping from the pulmonary capillaries is approximately 1 cm. of water. Anything that alters this narrow balance, such as acutely reducing colloid osmotic pressure, will tend to cause interstitial fluid accumulation. Thus, overenthusiastic use of such colloid-free solutions may have contributed to pulmonary insufficiency in some cases.

The hazard of interstitial accumulation of fluid in the lung has been emphasized by many workers. The central venous pressure may not rise to dangerous levels during prolonged infusion, but the interstitial space of the lung will tend to accumulate fluid faster than elsewhere in the body. Interstitial pulmonary edema develops insidiously over many hours or days, often without the production of pulmonary rales or distended neck veins. This lesion is rarely emphasized in postmortem findings, even in patients who died with a lethal alveolar-arterial oxygen gradient, because of being overshadowed by atelectasis, congestion, hemorrhage or pneumonia.

Intravascular Coagulation.   The problem of pulmonary macroemboli arising from thrombosis in peripheral veins is well established and is discussed elsewhere. However, other related conditions deserve mention. The central role of intravascular coagulation in various forms of shock and trauma has been studied extensively by Hardaway, who suggests that various vital organs, including the lung, may be damaged after shock as a result of disseminated intravascular coagulation. The similarity of pathologic changes in the lungs, after many types of shock, led Blaisdell and coworkers to conclude that pulmonary changes were more common when shock was associated with severe tissue damage from shock or trauma than following hemorrhage alone. The lungs are a site for trapping or sequestration of fibrin and platelets from the peripheral capillary bed. Such microemboli can produce pulmonary vascular obstruction as well as local pharmacologic effects, owing to the release of vasoactive material such as serotonin or histamine.

The studies of several investigators have confirmed the presence of considerable debris in ACD banked blood. This debris is filtered primarily by the pulmonary capillary bed and secondarily by the peripheral capillary bed. This offered a reason for the partial correlation between the degree of postoperative hypoxemia in trauma cases and the volume of transfused blood which the patients had received. Various filters are under development to allow blood flow without high resistance or red cell damage and to remove platelet aggregates and other debris which appears to accumulate in banked blood.

Fat Embolism.   Fat embolism is a condition in which fat appears in the circulating blood in droplets which are large enough to obstruct arterioles and capillaries. These droplets of fat are larger than the triglyceride particles which circulate with a lipoprotein coating in metabolic lipemia. At the time that this fat gains entrance to the vascular system, it is not emulsified or stabilized with a lipoprotein coating. Such neutral fat droplets, when intravenously injected into animals, are almost completely sequestered in the pulmonary circulation. The examination of patients dying of fat embolism reveals that only about 25 per cent of such patients have evidence of fat embolism in the systemic circulation. This small amount of fat which does pass through the pulmonary filter accounts for the fat which appears in the urine and becomes of diagnostic significance. Fat embolism is a frequent complication of fractures, particularly of multiple fractures of the long bones, pelvis and ribs. Pulmonary embolism with droplets of neutral fat results not only in the mechanical blockage of the pulmonary vascular bed, but also in the chemical effects on the endothelial and lung parenchyma. The pulmonary emboli of neutral fat are removed from the lung over a period of days by the action of a lipase produced by the lung parenchyma. Extracellular lipase may appear in the systemic circulation with fat embolism and the level of lipase becomes of diagnostic value. The products of hydrolysis of this neutral fat are the fatty acids, and they are much more toxic than the neutral fat itself, therefore causing serious damage to the pulmonary capillary endothelium and diminishing lung surfactant activity.

Aspiration of Gastric Contents.   Massive aspiration of gastric contents results in prompt and dramatic pulmonary impairment. Less spectacular but of disturbing frequency is the aspiration of small amounts of gastric fluid in association with general anesthesia, especially in emergency cases.

Experimental studies have shown that the dilute hydrochloric acid produces alveolar collapse with consolidation, loss of compliance and a markedly increased pulmonary vascular resistance. Such changes are consistent with damage to the alveolar cells, loss of surfactant and the development of hyaline membranes.

Mechanical Ventilation.   During the past decade, an increasing number of surgical patients have received mechanical ventilation for periods of days to weeks; thus it seemed possible that the mechanical ventilation in itself might be a primary etiologic agent. Some clinicians and pathologists have spoken of the findings of "respirator lung" cases. A detailed animal study by Nash et al. demonstrated that animals exposed for prolonged periods to room air had normal lungs whether or not a mechanical ventilator was used. Examination of these lungs, by both light and electron microscopy, revealed that abnormalities were correlated with breathing increased concentrations of inspired oxygen and appeared within three or four days regardless of whether the animal was breathing with or without a mechanical ventilator.

Oxygen Toxicity.   The recent interest in the use of hyperbaric oxygen has increased the general awareness of the toxic effects of oxygen when administered for prolonged periods at pressures exceeding 1 atmosphere. A by-product of this interest in hyperbaric therapy has been the recognition of potential damage to pulmonary alveoli by oxygen therapy at pressures of less than 1 atmosphere. A conventional means of providing oxygen therapy in the past has involved the use of a tent or nasal catheter. The concentration of inspired oxygen provided by these methods seldom exceeded 35 per cent. These apparently inefficient methods of oxygen administration may have provided a built-in protection for the patient. However, critically ill patients who are maintained with mechanical ventilation may receive inspired oxygen levels of from 60 to 100 per cent for days at a time, which thus may contribute to alevolar collapse and progressive atelectasis. Pulmonary oxygen intoxication begins insidiously with physiologic changes occurring several hours before the onset of clinical symptoms. The latent interval appears to be inversely proportional to the partial pressure of the inspired oxygen, and a minimum of 300 mm. Hg of oxygen is usually required to produce damage. Hyaline membranes are the most conspicuous features of pulmonary intoxication with oxygen but are not pathognomonic. Recovery after the development of hyaline membranes is uncommon, but if life can be maintained the membranes will be removed by phagocytosis. Oxygen toxicity is only partially understood. At the molecular level excessive oxygen activates certain enzymes and interferes with the formation of high energy phosphate bonds as well as inhibiting proteolysis, thus stimulating histamine release and decreasing pulmonary surfactant. Once the alveolar-capillary block is initiated, the process appears to be self-perpetuating, because increased concentrations of inspired oxygen are then required to maintain the pulmonary alveolar oxygen tension. This in turn produces further lung damage, hypoxemia and eventually death.

Surfactant. It has become evident that normal ventilation would be difficult without the action of an agent to help keep the millions of tiny alveoli expanded in their normal configuration. Such an agent has been described and great importance has been attributed to it. It has been characterized as a lipoprotein, the active part of which is the phospholipid component of the molecule. The substance has been termed surfactant, and it appears to line the alveolar surface as a continuous acellular layer. The development of congestive atelectasis following shock or trauma has been attributed to the loss of integrity of this membrane. It has been suggested that the pneumatocyte II cells in the lung are responsible for the production of this surface active material and that when they are damaged by a period of low flow the subsequent decreased production of surfactant results in atelectasis.

Clowes and others have emphasized the hemodynamic changes which are associated with the pathologic changes in the lung and have suggested that there is a common response in the lungs of patients or animals who have been subjected to shock, extensive tissue damage or sepsis. This concept holds that the pulmonary lesion which may be fatal is the result of a nonspecific inflammatory response of the lung to insult anywhere in the body which involves tissue injury or infection. The relationship between a decrease in pulmonary blood flow, the presence of circulating toxic materials or microthrombi is not known. An increase in pulmonary vascular resistance appears to follow each type of insult, and inadequate perfusion or toxic materials result in the loss of alveolar surfactant production. The concept of a final common pathway in acute pulmonary insufficiency is appealing and may help to resolve some of the dilemmas in this difficult field.

MANAGEMENT OF ACUTE VENTILATORY FAILURE

When faced with a comatose, apneic patient, the ability to act independently of equipment may decide between life and death. The supply of oxygen is the most delicate link between man and his environment. The almost total lack of oxygen storage in the body makes acute ventilatory failure the most urgent of emergencies. In the acute postoperative ventilatory emergency, all other ventilatory therapy is secondary to the maintenance of adequate minute ventilation. It is clear that positive pressure inflation with expired air, using mouth-to-mouth breathing, provides more effective gas exchange than the older manual methods which manipulated the thorax. The upper airway from the lips to the glottis is often a keystone to successful emergency ventilation. Obstruction from secretions, foreign bodies, local trauma or swelling must be eliminated immediately or bypassed by a tracheostomy. More subtle but equally serious obstruction to the upper airway may occur in the unconscious patient as a result of the position of his head and neck which may kink the airway and produce ventilatory insufficiency. Accordingly, to be effective, artificial respiration or intermittent positive pressure breathing must be conducted with the head and neck extended. A semiconscious or stuporous patient in a semi-sitting position may have the same difficulty when his head falls forward on his chest.

When a ventilatory emergency occurs in the emergency ward, it is common practice to insert an endotracheal tube for further ventilation. Unless an experienced person is available to insert the tube promptly, initial efforts at ventilation should be tried by inserting an oropharyngeal airway and manually ventilating the patient with one of the portable bellows ventilators, attached to a face mask. The insertion of the endotracheal tube can usually be postponed until ventilation has been stabilized by such means. However, the use of an endotracheal tube will probably be required if the patient remains comatose and is expected to require ventilatory assistance beyond the acute episode.

The advantages of tracheal intubation, whether with an endotracheal tube or a tracheostomy tube, include the following: the tracheobronchial tree can be isolated, the removal of pharyngeal secretions is facilitated, the respiratory dead space is reduced by approximately one third, the resistance to respiratory effort is lessened if the tube size is adequate, and mechanical ventilation is simplified. The disadvantages of tracheal intubation are largely related to the introduction of airway infection and mechanical damage to tissues from the presence of the tube or the balloon cuff. Strict asepsis is essential in the care of any patient with tracheal intubation. This is particularly true in the manner of handling the suction catheter, which is a common path of entry for pathogenic organisms. The catheter should always be sterile and used only by individuals wearing sterile gloves. Every effort should be made to avoid trauma to the mucous membrane during aspiration of secretions. Cultures with antibiotic sensitivity tests of the tracheal aspirate should be performed at least twice weekly. When the nose and pharynx are bypassed, their air conditioning role is lost, as is the protective function of arresting the entry of bacteria and dust into the lungs. Therefore it is necessary to warm and humidify the inspired air mixture (preferably achieving 100 per cent relative humidity at close to body temperature) by means of a small plastic canopy overlying the end of the tracheostomy tube.

The early diagnosis of ventilatory impairment depends upon proper evaluation of vital signs and blood gases. Pontoppidan and coworkers have utilized additional information from the bedside measurement of vital capacity, inspiratory force, the alveolo-arterial O_2 gradient $(A-aDO_2)$ and the ratio of dead space to tidal volume (VD/VT) to monitor ventilation. These investigators have summarized extensive clinical experience in Table 8-1.

Details of performing these measurements and their interpretation are available in the general references at the end of this chapter. The trend in any of these values is of the utmost importance. The values given are for adults and do not apply to infants and small children.

The management of a patient requiring mechanical ventilation must include constant attention to airway humidification, removal of secretions, the lowest concentration of inspired O_2 which will achieve a satisfactory blood O_2 level and periodic hyperinflation of the lungs. The majority of patients who die of acute ventilatory failure are found to have some degree of pulmonary infection. The air path through a mechanical ventilator may become contaminated, especially in the

Table 8-1.*

		ACCEPTABLE RANGE	CHEST PHYSICAL THERAPY, OXYGEN, CLOSE MONITORING	INTUBATION TRACHEOTOMY VENTILATION
Mechanics	Respiratory rate	12–25	25–35	>35
	Vital capacity, ml./kg.	70–30	30–15	<15
	Inspiratory force, cm. H_2O	100–50	50–25	<25
Oxygenation	$A-aDO_2$, mm. Hg†	50–200	200–350	>350
	p_aO_2, mm. Hg	100–75 (air)	200–70 (on mask O_2)	<70 (on mask O_2)
Ventilation	V_D/V_T	0.3–0.4	0.4–0.6	>0.6
	p_aCO_2, mm. Hg	35–45	45–60	>60‡

*From Pontoppidan, H., Laver, M. B., and Geffin, B.: Acute respiratory failure in the surgical patient; *in* Welch, C. E. (ed.): Advances in Surgery, Volume 4. Chicago, Year Book Medical Publishers, 1970, p. 163.
†After 15 minutes of 100% O_2.
‡Except in chronic hypercapnia.

moist areas of the humidifier, nebulizer and distal tubing. The patient attached to such contaminated equipment is caught between an obligatory, continuous exposure to bacteria and his crippled lungs, which can neither provide adequate gas exchange nor clear bacteria in normal fashion. The humidifier and tubing should be sterile when starting mechanical ventilation and should be replaced as frequently as serial cultures indicate that this is appropriate.

The proper mechanical use of a ventilator requires attention to (1) the tidal volume, (2) inspiratory and expiratory flow rates and pressures, and (3) the duration of inspiration and expiration. The optimal pattern of ventilation is not known and varies from patient to patient, depending upon the underlying problem and the response of the patient. Equipment must therefore be capable of providing ventilation over a wide range of patterns, as is true of modern, volume-limited ventilators.

Sladen and others have described a clinical syndrome in patients receiving prolonged mechanical ventilation characterized by a positive water balance with a gain in weight and radiologic changes suggesting pulmonary edema, poor pulmonary mechanics and deteriorating blood-gas exchange. Average weight gain in the patients that were studied was 2.6 kg., a value easily overlooked unless patients are weighed accurately. Water retention and pulmonary edema were noted in the absence of clinically evident cardiac failure and in the presence of a normal central venous pressure. It must be remembered that patients receiving artificial ventilation lose little or no water from the airway if inspired gas is properly saturated with water vapor near body temperature. The reasons for the reduced ability to handle free water during prolonged mechanical ventilation are not known. Diuretic therapy and some fluid restriction will usually lead to an improvement of pulmonary congestion and associated respiratory function.

Mechanical ventilation may involve conflicting considerations when circulation and blood-gas exchange are marginal. Safe management requires a knowledge of how different patterns of ventilation influence pulmonary mechanics, alveolocapillary gas exchange and the systemic circulation. This is particularly true in regard to the recent revival of interest in continuous positive pressure ventilation (CPPV) as a means of treating the refractory hypoxemia of late ventilatory failure. This technique prevents the pressure from dropping to atmospheric levels during each expiratory phase. Kumar has presented clinical data on the hemodynamics and lung function with CPPV. It appears that this technique is often effective in providing a high blood O_2 level with a lower inspired O_2 concentration. However, the resulting increase in mean intrathoracic pressure will decrease venous return. The systemic transport of O_2 (cardiac output times arterial O_2 content) must be considered. One must be careful not to reduce cardiac output more than the improvement achieved in arterial O_2 content. The major complications of CPPV are alveolar rupture and pneumothorax. This risk is apparently increased by the method used to establish the CVVP. An uncooperative patient may develop dangerous levels of inspiratory pressure if a static flow resistance is inserted in the expired air tubing. The pressure threshold approach appears to be of less danger.

Concepts in the use of artificial airways and the management of acute ventilatory failure have undergone major changes over the last decade. Prolonged tracheal intubation (4 to 7 days) has received widespread acceptance, and the need for tracheostomy has in many cases been obviated. For most cases of acute respiratory obstruction, the speed and ease with which intubation can be accomplished has made it the technique of choice. Emergency tracheostomy has thus become justifiable only when tracheal intubation is not possible. There is little to choose between prolonged oral and nasal tracheal intubation. The nasal tubes are better tolerated in conscious patients, permit closure of the mouth and are more easily anchored. However, tube size is limited by the nostrils and nasal structures. With prolonged intubation, sudden occlusion by plugging or kinking is a major hazard, especially in the presence of lower airway bleeding. Obstruction by secretions is uncommon with good humidification; however, this is not always preventable. Therefore facilities for prompt replacement of tracheal tubes must be available at the bedside. Endotracheal tubes can produce discomfort in the conscious patient and may be an irritant to the upper airway with the production of increased pharyngeal secretions. Ulceration of the larynx is the main lesion that follows endotracheal intubation. However, this may be aggravated by motion of the head, chemical irritation from toxic materials within the tube substance or tissue reaction to residual ethyline oxide used for sterilization. The many complications mentioned make it impossible to precisely define a "safe period" for prolonged endotracheal intubation. In some centers endotracheal tubes are used for up to a week in adult patients and up to 3 weeks in infants and children.

A growing number of reports have appeared over the past three years concerning tracheal deformity following tracheostomy for artificial ventilation. Trauma to the trachea from tracheostomy tubes may occur at the tip of the tube, at the level of the stoma or opposite the inflatable cuff. The maximal damage and deformity typically develop at the level of the inflatable cuff. Impaired circulation aggravates the damage caused by pressure from the cuff. The technique of prestretching the balloon cuff in warm water can produce a large-volume cuff which can provide an airtight seal at reduced balloon cuff pressures and thus reduce the extent of tracheal damage with prolonged intubation.

Weaning from Mechanical to Spontaneous Ventilation. Every step during management of the patient in acute ventilatory failure should be directed toward relieving the patient of his dependency on the ventilator. The transition from artificial to spontaneous ventilation can be attempted only when objective evidence indicates that lung function is adequate to permit this change. The weaning process must proceed gradually, particularly if the patient has required prolonged mechanical ventilation or has residual evidence of chest wall instability as seen following thoracic trauma. According to Pontoppidan et al., sustained spontaneous respiration in patients recovering from respiratory failure requires the ability to produce the minimal vital capacity of 10 ml./kg. or a volume essentially twice as large as the predicted normal resting tidal volume. Independence of ventilatory support for a minimum of 24 hours and removal of the endotracheal or tracheostomy tube are generally possible when the vital capacity exceeds 15 to 20 ml./kg. Weaning from the ventilator when the alveolar-arterial oxygen gradient is greater than 350 mm. Hg. or the dead space to tidal volume ratio is above 0.6, is rarely successful. Difficulty in weaning from the ventilator may be due to abnormal pulmonary mechanics and blood gas exchange, a low cardiac output, a hypermetabolic state or muscle weakness. Patients who have required prolonged ventilation show marked variation in their response to the discomfort or dyspnea associated with weaning. Most are apprehensive and display wide fluctuation of vital signs when first faced with the need to breathe spontaneously. Hypotension and bradycardia are indicative of hypoxemia and occur infrequently, whereas hypertension, tachycardia and tachypnea are common. The need for careful monitoring of blood gases during the initial phase of the weaning cannot be overemphasized. Initial trials with spontaneous ventilation must be made under close supervision while supplying added concentrations of oxygen to compensate for an anticipated increase in right-to-left shunting.

REFERENCES

General References

Bendixen, H. H., et al.: Respiratory Care. St. Louis, C. V. Mosby Company, 1965.

Comroe, J. H., Jr., Forster, R. E., II, Dubois, A. B., Briscoe, W. A., and Carlsen, E.: The Lung: Clinical Physiology and Pulmonary Function Tests. 2nd Ed., Chicago, Year Book Medical Publishers. 1962.

Moore, F. D., et al.: Post-Traumatic Pulmonary Insufficiency. Philadelphia, W. B. Saunders Company, 1969.

Peters, R. M.: The Mechanical Basis of Respiration. Boston, Little, Brown and Company, 1969.

Pontoppidan, H., Laver, M. B., and Geffin, B.: Acute respiratory failure in the surgical patient; in Welch, C. E. (ed.): Advances in Surgery, Volume 4. Chicago, Year Book Medical Publishers, 1970, p. 163.

Proceedings of Conference of Pulmonary Effects of Non-thoracic Trauma. Edited by Eisenan, B., and Ashbaugh, D. C. National Academy of Sciences-National Research Council. J. Trauma, 8:623, 1968.

Safar, P.: *Respiratory Therapy.* Philadelphia, F. A. Davis Company, 1965.

Selected Articles

Anscombe, A. R.: Pulmonary Complications of Abdominal Surgery. Chicago, Year Book Medical Publishers, 1957.

Blaisdell, F. W., Lim, R. C., Jr., and Stallone, R. J.: The mechanism of pulmonary damage following traumatic shock. Surgery, *130*:15, 1970.

Clowes, G. H. A., et al.: Circulating factors in the etiology of pulmonary insufficiency and right heart failure accompanying severe sepsis (peritonitis). Ann. Surg., *171*:663, 1970.

Hardaway, R. M.: The role of intravascular clotting in the etiology of shock. Ann. Surg., *155*:325, 1962.

Hedley-Whyte, J.: Causes of pulmonary oxygen toxicity. N. Eng. J. Med., *283*:1518, 1970.

Kory, R. C., Bergmann, J. C., Sweet, R. D., and Smith, J. R.: Comparative evaluation of oxygen therapy techniques. J.A.M.A., *179*:767, 1962.

Kumar, A.: Continuous positive-pressure ventilation in acute respiratory failure. Effects on hemodynamics and lung function. N. Eng. J. Med., *283*:1430, 1970.

Miller, W. F., Johnson, R. L., Jr., and Wu, N.: Half-second expiratory capacity test: Convenient means of evaluating nature and extent of pulmonary ventilatory insufficiency. Dis. Chest, *30*:33, 1965.

Nash, G., Bowen, J. A., and Langlinais, P. C.: "Respirator lung": A misnomer. Arch. Path., *21*:234, 1971.

Sladen, A., Laver, M. B., and Pontoppidan, H.: Pulmonary complications and water retention in prolonged mechanical ventilation. N. Eng. J. Med., *279*:468, 1968.

Wells, R. E., Perera, R. D., and Kinney, J. M.: Humidification of oxygen during inhalational therapy. N. Eng. J. Med., *268*:644, 1963.

CHAPTER 9

CIRCULATION AND CARDIAC FAILURE

John W. Kirklin, M.D., F.A.C.S.

The cardiovascular subsystem (the patient as a whole being a complex system composed of numerous interrelated subsystems) has as its business the circulation of blood. The *analysis* of the subsystem in a given patient requires knowledge of its *performance*, the *adequacy* of the performance, and the used and unused *reserves* of the subsystem. Its performance is assessed primarily in terms of cardiac output. Regional arterial blood flow, or the distribution of cardiac output, is usually appropriate to the level of cardiac output in surgical patients, and in the absence of specific arterial occlusive lesions usually does not require special attention. Arterial blood pressure is determined by systemic arteriolar resistance as well as cardiac output, necessitating consideration of the large and small arteries. The systemic venous component of the cardiovascular subsystem is importantly related to cardiac output, because central venous pressure, mean right atrial pressure and the pressure in the right ventricle at end diastole are determined by both systemic venous blood volume (a function of total blood volume) and the distensibility or tone of the venous system. The veins also may develop acute thromboses.

EVALUATION (ANALYSIS) OF THE CARDIOVASCULAR SUBSYSTEM

Performance. The performance of the cardiovascular subsystem is traditionally analyzed by noting the pulse rate and blood pressure. The chief merit of this practice is that these variables are easily measured. In fact, particularly in surgical patients, the performance of the subsystem should be evaluated primarily in terms of *cardiac output*. The cardiac output in normal persons at rest averages 3.5 liters/minute/-square meter of body surface area, with the range being between 2.5 and 4.4. Although the cardiac output in normal individuals convalescing normally from major surgery or major trauma is elevated appropriate to the elevated oxygen consumption, in most postoperative situations a cardiac index above 3.0 liters/minute/square meter can be considered usual or normal. An exception is septic shock. Unfortunately, only in special intensive care units is cardiac output measured as a routine. Therefore it is necessary to estimate it from available data at each visit to the patient early after major surgery or trauma. Our own data indicate that reasonable success can be had in doing this, using the character of peripheral pulses (dorsalis pedis, posterior tibial, and radial), extremity skin temperature, capillary refilling time of fingers and toes, color of lips and nail beds and arterial blood pressure. The cardiac index is usually low (less than 2.2), and thus the patient is seriously ill when he appears anxious, the peripheral pulses are absent or weak, the skin of the feet cool, fingernails and toenails blue, and the skin moist. The arterial blood pressure may be low, but *it and pulse rate may be normal or elevated* in a patient with low cardiac output. When cardiac output is greater than 3.0, the patient usually has full peripheral pulses, warm skin, pink fingernails and toenails, and normal or elevated arterial blood pressure. He is obviously well as regards the cardiovascular subsystem. His cardiac index is estimated to be between 2.2 and 3.0 when his clinical condition is intermediate to the aforementioned extremes, and as regards his cardiovascular subsystem his condition is regarded as suboptimal.

Adequacy. Adequacy refers to the relation of cardiac output to the function of other organs and subsystems (including that of the heart itself related to the coronary blood flow) and to the general metabolic activity. The latter relation is described by mixed venous oxygen levels, and when they are normal the relation between cardiac output and metabolic rate is normal, unless there are nonperfused areas of the microcirculation in which an oxygen debt is developing. There is not a necessary relation between the adequacy of cardiac performance and the level of cardiac output.

Observations of urine flow, cerebration, and the cardiac rhythm, particularly as regards premature ventricular contractions, are useful in analyzing the cardiovascular subsystem of the surgical patient for the adequacy of its function. If a catheter is in the pulmonary artery, measurement of the oxygen saturation of mixed venous blood is helpful. If a central venous catheter has been advanced to the right atrium, a sample of right atrial blood may be analyzed instead, since it is similar to, though not identical with, pulmonary artery blood as regards oxygen levels. Although mixed venous oxygen saturation is normally about 75 per cent, a level of 65 per cent is adequate if most of the microcirculation is being perfused. A urine flow of 20 ml./hour is adequate unless there is an unusual solute load or impaired renal function.

Reserves. Identification of the used and unused reserves of the cardiovascular subsystem in the surgical patient is needed in order to know its capability for increasing its performance when sudden new demands develop because of fever, atelectasis, increased work of breathing, restlessness, arrhythmias, and the like. The reserves of the heart are in the determinates of cardiac output, namely heart rate, the end-diastolic stretch of ventricular sarcomeres (preload or the Starling effect), the load resisting shortening of the sarcomeres (afterload), and myocardial contractility. Systemic venous tone is a reserve mechanism of the subsystem, and increase in it results in increased preload, other things being equal. Systemic arteriolar resistance is a reserve mechanism of the cardiovascular subsystem, and increase in it can maintain an arterial blood pressure adequate for perfusion of the brain, kidneys, and heart when cardiac output is low. The peculiar properties of the hemoglobin molecule, as reflected in its oxygen dissociation curve, are an important reserve of the organism as a whole for oxygen transport when cardiac performance is poor.

When the cardiac rhythm is sinus and heart rate is increased, this reserve mechanism for increasing cardiac output is being employed. When heart rate reaches about 180 beats/minute it is being maximally employed and is not available as a further reserve. When pulmonary arterial or systemic arterial systolic blood pressure is high, the heart is being stressed, because there is an inverse relation between afterload and the energy of ventricular contraction and thus stroke volume, other things being equal. The reserve of the heart is therefore diminished in this situation. The contractile state of the myocardium is a continuously active reserve mechanism when it is normal, being responsible for heterometric and homeometric autoregulation and some of the responses of the heart to sympathetic and humoral stimulation. When contractility is depressed by severe coronary heart disease, advanced valvular heart disease, long-standing hypertensive heart disease, sepsis, or other factors, the reserve of the cardiovascular subsystem is impaired. When central venous or right atrial pressure is high, and the tricuspid valve is not stenotic and thus right ventricular end-diastolic pressure is about the same, the reserve of the Starling effect is being utilized maximally and is not available for further augmentation of cardiac output. The same analysis and reasoning can be used on the left side of the heart.

When systemic arteriolar resistance is high, as suggested by cool and pale extremities, this reserve mechanism is being used and further stresses to the subsystem will probably not be well tolerated. Systemic venous tone is moderately elevated for about 48 hours after operations, and thus most surgical patients are using this reserve mechanism.

PREOPERATIVE EVALUATION

Preoperative evaluation is concerned with the performance and adequacy of performance of the cardiovascular subsystem in the patient about to undergo surgery, but most importantly with the used and unused reserves of the subsystem. It is these which enable the patient to withstand the stress of the surgical procedure under consideration.

History.   Good exercise tolerance denotes a good cardiovascular reserve. Dyspnea on mild exertion, paroxysmal nocturnal dyspnea, or orthopnea suggests the presence of pulmonary venous hypertension owing to mitral valve disease or impairment of left ventricular performance. These suggest serious heart disease, and operation should be advised only when urgently necessary and when preoperative, operative, and postoperative care can be precise. Dyspnea only on severe exertion, episodic ankle edema, and mild abdominal swelling suggest heart disease of considerably less severity, and in these patients operation is usually well tolerated, providing that care is precise and proper.

Angina on effort or a history of myocardial infarction can be considered presumptive evidence of coronary heart disease. If exercise tolerance is good and angina occurs only on strenuous exercise, cardiac reserve is good. When angina or significant dyspnea develops on mild effort, left ventricular end-diastolic pressure and thus pulmonary venous pressure can be considered elevated during exercise. This indicates a limitation of cardiac reserve and under these circumstances the risk of operation is higher than usual. In any case, the tendency for arrhythmia, myocardial infarction, or pulmonary edema to develop in such patients indicates the need for scrupulous attention to the details of operative and postoperative management.

Physical Examination.   The patient is examined for dyspnea, increased venous pressure and evidence of fluid retention. Chronic marked fluid retention and hepatomegaly indicate long-standing and far advanced heart disease, and in these patients cardiac reserve is low and the risk of operation is high. Operation should be advised only for life-threatening emergencies. When the heart beats rapidly and seems to be overactive on auscultation, further investigation of its reserve is warranted. Fine rales heard over both lungs suggest pulmonary venous hypertension, and the patient should be questioned closely as to dyspnea and orthopnea.

The *thoracic roentgenogram* is of some indirect value in assessing cardiac reserve because it allows an estimate of cardiac size. The *electrocardiogram* gives additional indirect data. Evidence of left ventricular hypertrophy and strain indicates that the reserve of the left ventricle may be limited, and patterns suggestive of a previous myocardial infarction indicate significant coronary artery disease.

Certain cardiac lesions increase the risk of operation even though cardiac reserve seems to be good. Patients with severe aortic stenosis or incompetence are particularly susceptible to the development of ventricular fibrillation; general surgical procedures should be performed only when urgently indicated. Patients with mitral stenosis but few symptoms tolerate such operations well, but particular care must be taken to avoid undue increase of left atrial pressure and consequent pulmonary edema. Patients with coronary artery disease and good cardiac reserve tolerate general surgical procedures well but require particular attention to the details of management.

POSTOPERATIVE EVALUATION AND TREATMENT

The evaluation or analysis of the cardiovascular subsystem in the patient early after surgery or other forms of trauma proceeds concomitantly with analysis of the other subsystems. Decisions concerning intervention are based on analysis of all subsystems and thus of the integrated complex system that is the patient as a whole.

The analysis of the cardiovascular subsystem proceeds as described earlier. The *present performance* is defined by the values for *cardiac output*, *arterial blood pressure* (reflecting the systemic arteriolar resistance), and, when available, *central venous or right atrial pressure* and *pulmonary venous or left atrial pressure* (these reflecting respectively tone and blood volume in the systemic venous system including the right atrium and during diastole the right ventricle, and in the pulmonary venous system and left atrium and during diastole the left ventricle). The adequacy of the present performance is judged by methods previously described, as are the used and unused reserves of the subsystems.

Decision-making with regard to interventions directed at the cardiovascular subsystem depends on the previous analyses. When cardiac output is low (<2.2 L./min./m.^{2}), or when it is suboptimal (2.2 to 3.0 L./min./m.^{2}) and less than adequate, attempts to increase it are indicated. When cardiac output is suboptimal but adequate and the reserves are being used maximally, efforts to increase output and relieve some of the reserve mechanisms are indicated.

The possibilities for increasing cardiac output are to increase heart rate and/or stroke volume. When heart rate is less than 60 beats/minute under these circumstances, it should be increased. Under some special circumstances (after intracardiac surgery and after myocardial infarction, for examples), when heart rate is less than 85 beats/minute cardiac output is increased by increasing heart rate to about 100 beats/minute. When the heart is in sinus rhythm the rate is most controllably increased by atrial pacing, and when there is atrial fibrillation or atrioventricular dissociation, by ventricular pacing. Stroke volume is, generally, directly related to the stretch of the ventricular fibers at the end of diastole (preload) and to myocardial contractility, and inversely to the load resisting shortening of ventricular fibers. Unless the ventricular end-diastolic pressure (similar to mean atrial pressure and thus to central venous pressure in the case of the right side and pulmonary venous pressure in the case of the left) is already high, that is, over about 15 to 18 mm. Hg, and unless ventricular compliance is severely decreased or intrapericardial pressure severely increased, stroke volume and cardiac output can usually be increased by increasing blood volume and thus ventricular end-diastolic pressure and volume. This is probably the most commonly used therapeutic maneuver in surgical patients having low cardiac output. When cardiac output is low, systemic arteriolar resistance high, and thus arterial systolic blood pressure and left ventricular afterload high, stroke volume can often be increased and left atrial pressure decreased by decreasing left ventricular afterload with Arfonad, Thorazine, or morphine. The response of cardiac output to these interventions is variable, and therefore they generally should not be used unless cardiac output is being measured. Since morphine is also a venodilator, and decreases venous tone and pressure also, care must be taken in using it in this situation. When cardiac output is low, atrial and venous pressure high, pericardial tamponade absent, and systemic arterial blood pressure not high, efforts are made to increase myocardial contractility with digitalis or, if the situation is acute and severe, with epinephrine or isoproterenol (see below).

Postoperative Cardiac Arrhythmias

The optimal cardiac mechanism is sinus and the optimal rate is one that is proportional to the physiologic needs of the patient; deviations can affect cardiac output adversely. The management of various arrhythmias is guided by their effect on cardiac output or by their lethal potentiality. Since each arrhythmia differs in these respects, they must be considered individually.

Premature Ventricular Contractions. In general surgical patients, these are generally benign if infrequent and of the same configuration. If frequent, they can cause reduced cardiac output. In patients who have undergone open intracardiac operations, premature ventricular contractions are particularly important, since they may indicate inadequate myocardial perfusion and may signal the possibility of ventricular fibrillation. Particularly if premature ventricular contractions are of varying configurations, they may be the harbingers of ventricular tachycardia or fibrillation. Arterial desaturation (or an abnormally low arterial P_{O_2} and electrolyte abnormalities, particularly hypokalemia and acidosis, should be searched for. Excess digitalis can be the cause. Ventricular ischemia or infarction may have occurred without other obvious signs or symptoms.

The first step in treatment is an attempt at correction of these factors. Administration of oxygen by mask should be tried, because increasing the arterial P_{O_2} to abnormally high levels is sometimes helpful. Without very much delay, however, lidocaine (Xylocaine) should be employed. The initial effort should be with 50 mg. administered in a bolus intravenously. If this does not abolish the premature ventricular contractions or if they return, then an intravenous infusion of lidocaine should be begun. After control has been obtained with the intravenous medications, it will probably be wise to switch to an oral drug. For this purpose procaine amide (Pronestyl) is used. Diphenylhydantoin (Dilantin) is occasionally helpful and carries almost no risk.

When premature ventricular contractions are frequent and particularly if they are of differing configurations, monitoring of the electrocardiogram must be done because of the increased possibility of ventricular fibrillation.

Atrial Tachycardia. This is a common postoperative arrhythmia which often occurs in persons without evidence of heart disease. The ventricular rate is usually 160/minute or more and should be slowed. In some persons the tachycardia can be terminated by carotid sinus massage or induced vomiting. Morphine given subcutaneously may cause conversion in a few minutes. Phenylephrine (Neo-Synephrine) intravenously in hypotensive patients is often particularly useful; 0.3 ml. of a 1 per cent solution is diluted to 1 ml. and given slowly until the blood pressure increases, at which time the tachycardia often ceases. Digoxin given intravenously may abolish the arrhythmia, but care is needed since digitalis toxicity may actually cause atrial tachycardia.

Atrial Fibrillation. This is a frequently encountered arrhythmia which can occur in the absence of recognizable heart disease, particularly postoperatively. In addition, disease of the mitral valve or ischemic heart disease predisposes to it.

Although it renders the heart somewhat less efficient, atrial fibrillation is usually not a problem unless the ventricular rate exceeds 100/minute. In the aged, the rate may be normal and no treatment is required. When the rate is excessive, the treatment of choice is digitalis. In most instances, the rate serves as an excellent guide to the adequacy of digitalization.

Often, the arrhythmia will revert spontaneously to a sinus mechanism, particularly if it is a postoperative occurrence. If not, a decision regarding reversion must be made. Either quinidine or electronic cardioversion can be employed; the latter is more effective but rarely necessary as an emergency procedure, and it is probably best used after the early postoperative period.

Atrial Flutter. This is less common than atrial fibrillation but is more difficult to manage. It occurs under the same circumstances as atrial fibrillation and the approach to treatment is similar. However, the ventricular rate may not be so easily controlled, and early elective electronic cardioversion is more appropriate. Often, a small amount of direct electrical current (50 watt seconds) will immediately correct the arrhythmia. It is better to carry out early cardioversion than to use toxic doses of digitalis in an effort to control the rate.

Ventricular Tachycardia.   This is generally a grave arrhythmia, for several reasons. Its presence is usually indicative of organic heart disease. It results in a reduced cardiac output because of the rapid rate and abnormal contraction. This arrhythmia can be a prelude to ventricular fibrillation and sudden death.

The analysis and general management of the patient are similar to those for the premature ventricular contractions described above. An additional specific treatment is generally required, consisting of either electronic cardioversion or lidocaine administered parenterally. The former is indicated if the patient is hypotensive or otherwise in critical condition. The latter can be tried, cautiously at first, if the patient is tolerating the arrhythmia well.

Even after restoration of normal sinus rhythm, it is best to monitor the electrocardiogram of the patient. Lidocaine or procaine amide can be used if very frequent premature ventricular contractions persist. Diphenylhydantoin is also useful, for its sedative as well as its direct myocardial effect (doses are similar to those for premature ventricular contractions).

Complete Heart Block.   This may be present preoperatively with no symptoms. In all patients with this arrhythmia there is the possibility of fatal asystole developing during or after operation. Therefore, prior to operation, temporary electronic pacemaking should be established, preferably by the insertion of an intravenous catheter-pacemaker into the right ventricle. The heart should be paced during and after operation until the patient is up and walking.

Ventricular Fibrillation.   This requires immediate recognition for successful resuscitation. Patients who have had very frequent premature ventricular contractions, ventricular tachycardia or recent myocardial infarction are susceptible to this catastrophe and should be monitored electronically or observed closely postoperatively.

The patient should have immediate and continuous external cardiac massage and pulmonary ventilation by the quickest means available while the defibrillator is being set up. In a patient who suddenly becomes pulseless and cyanotic, time should not be wasted on prolonged electrocardiographic interpretation prior to the first countershock. If the first countershock is unsuccessful, cardiac massage and ventilation should be continued while the electrocardiogram or monitor screen is studied. Repeated countershock may be required, but it is essential to maintain circulation (coronary and cerebral) and ventilation during treatment (see below). Reliance on countershock alone is an error which may prevent resuscitation.

Cardiac Arrest.   This term is applied in situations in which the heart rather suddenly stops. By implication, ventricular end-diastolic

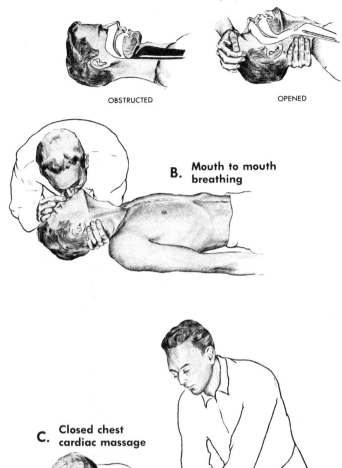

A. Airway opened

OBSTRUCTED   OPENED

B. Mouth to mouth breathing

C. Closed chest cardiac massage

Figure 9–1. Heart-lung resuscitation. The patient is placed in a supine position on a rigid support. Firm pressure is applied downward about 80 to 100 times a minute. At the end of each pressure stroke the hands are relaxed to permit full expansion of the chest. The position of the operator should be such that he can use his body weight while applying the pressure. Sufficient pressure should be exerted to move the sternum 3 or 4 cm. toward the vertebral column. The effectiveness of the presternal compression should always be monitored by having another person palpate the femoral pulse. No more force should be exerted than is necessary to produce a peripheral pulse of good volume. Rapid ventilation of the lungs using positive pressure should be permitted after each series of three compressions. (Reproduced with permission from National Academy of Sciences–National Research Council. J.A.M.A. *198*:372, 1966.)

203

pressure is adequate and the cessation of effective heart action is unexpected. The causes are numerous, but include hypoxia, hypercarbia, certain forms of electrolyte disturbance, stimulation of the pharynx, and electrical shock. Because of the development of irreversible brain damage within 3 minutes of cessation of cerebral blood flow, cardiac arrest demands immediate and effective intervention.

The initial interventions are cardiac massage (by closed-chest massage or, if the thorax is already open, by direct cardiac massage) to provide some blood flow, and ventilation (by mouth-to-mouth breathing, or with a simple device such as the Ambu bag with a face mask) to provide air flow (Fig. 9–1). Only then is an electrocardiogram obtained. Endotracheal intubation is done only after arrival of an individual competent to perform it skillfully and quickly.

If the heart is in asystole, cardiac massage may quickly provoke cardiac action and the crisis subsides. If no cardiac action develops after about 1 minute of massage, about 5 ml. of 1:10,000 epinephrine is injected into the heart (preferably the right ventricle) and massage continued. This may be repeated four times if no or feeble cardiac action continues. If no effective response is obtained, 5 or 10 ml. of 10 per cent calcium chloride is injected into a cardiac chamber. Because the low systemic blood flow quickly produces metabolic acidosis, sodium bicarbonate (44 mEq.) is given intravenously.

If the heart is in ventricular fibrillation, electric defibrillation by direct-current countershock is required. The instrument available in one's own institution should be studied and understood. If several attempts are unsuccessful, between which, of course, cardiac massage and pulmonary ventilation are continued, the drug therapy presented above is tried as attempts at successful conversion are continued.

Resuscitation continues to be attempted until effective cardiac action has been restored, or a calm collaborative appraisal indicates the probable irreversibility of the situation. Usually the efforts continue for at least 1 hour.

ACUTE ARTERIAL OCCLUSION

Acute arterial occlusion can occur postoperatively as a result of embolization or in situ thrombosis.

Preoperative Evaluation. This should include measures to determine whether the patient has a propensity for development of acute arterial occlusion, as indicated by evidence of polycythemia, occlusive arterial disease, popliteal aneurysm or generalized arteriosclerosis (predisposing to in situ thrombosis); or by evidence of arterial aneurysm, atrial fibrillation, mitral stenosis or myocardial infarction (which may give rise to an arterial embolus).

Postoperative Care. This should include measures to minimize the possibility of occurrence of an arterial embolus, consisting of (1) attention to the general hemodynamic state and hydration of the patient and (2) prophylactic anticoagulant therapy (see below) in patients with associated conditions predisposing to formation of arterial emboli and without contraindications to anticoagulant therapy.

Treatment. Details of treatment of arterial emboli are beyond the scope of this manual. In general, when the occlusion is embolic and involves a major artery, embolectomy is indicated unless within 2 hours of onset there is clear evidence of regression of symptoms and signs (suggesting that the embolus is small and has perhaps moved to a distal minor artery). When the embolus appears to be located in an easily accessible artery (femoral, popliteal or brachial), its direct removal is usually advisable. When it is located more centrally, insertion centrally of a Fogarty embolectomy catheter through an easily accessible artery (femoral or brachial) is usually effective at an extremely low operative risk. Anticoagulant therapy is indicated postoperatively to prevent another episode of embolization.

It may be difficult to know when acute arterial occlusion is due to in situ thrombosis rather than embolization. If operative exposure of the area indicates the former to be the case, complete removal of the thrombus (which may be extensive) and attention to any local obstructing arterial lesion are indicated. Anticoagulants are advisable postoperatively.

Venous Thrombosis and Thromboembolism

Venous thrombosis in pelvic veins and lower extremities is of significance because of the tendency of the thrombi to embolize and move to the lungs and because of the late sequelae in the legs. Less than 1 per cent of pulmonary emboli in postoperative patients originate in the heart or in veins of the upper extremities. Certain conditions, identifiable preoperatively, increase the risk of venous thrombosis, as do certain operations. In the presence of these, particular effort must be made postoperatively to prevent and treat thrombosis, thrombophlebitis and pulmonary embolism.

Preoperative Evaluation. Evaluation of all patients being considered for operation should include search for situations which impose an unduly high risk of postoperative thrombosis, thrombophlebitis or thromboembolism. These include heart disease, previous thrombophlebitis or pulmonary embolism or both, obesity and polycythemia. When any of these is present, anticoagulant drugs should be administered postoperatively on a prophylactic basis unless there is a specific contraindication to their use.

Postoperative Care. The goal is the prevention of venous thrombosis and thromboembolism or the treatment of these conditions if they occur. Although practices differ widely with regard to use of drugs or venous ligation for this purpose, choice of management can be based on the following facts:

The incidence of fatal pulmonary embolism after major surgery is low (approximately 0.2 per cent) even if no special measures are taken (Barker et al.). This makes it difficult to insist on a special regimen of prophylaxis postoperatively or to evaluate one.

Of all the pulmonary emboli that occur postoperatively, three fourths are not initially fatal (Priestley and Barker).

A patient who has sustained a nonfatal pulmonary embolism has a significant possibility (18 per cent) of sustaining a subsequent fatal pulmonary embolism (Priestley and Barker).

Certain operations are followed by a somewhat higher incidence (1.5 to 2.5 per cent) of postoperative pulmonary embolism than occurs generally. Included are abdominal hysterectomy, splenectomy, repair of bilateral inguinal hernias and resection of terminal portions of the colon.

The institution of anticoagulant therapy in a patient who has sustained a nonfatal pulmonary embolism postoperatively significantly reduces the probability of a subsequent fatal pulmonary embolism (Hermann et al.).

The prophylactic use of anticoagulant therapy significantly reduces the incidence of pulmonary embolism (Sevitt; Bottomley et al.).

Anticoagulant therapy in the postoperative patient has small but real hazards and problems. Accomplishment of a steady, adequate reduction of prothrombin values (to approximately 20 per cent of control values) is not always achieved and thromboembolism may occur in the periods of inadequate deficiency. Fatal bleeding is rare and, under proper circumstances, its risk is probably about 0.2 per cent. Troublesome bleeding may occur in about 2 per cent of cases. The risk of bleeding as a result of anticoagulant therapy is greater than average following certain operations (exploration of the common bile duct, partial gastrectomy, vaginal hysterectomy and insertion of arterial grafts or prostheses).

Partial interruption of the vena cava (plication, insertion of a filter or application of a nonocclusive clip) appears to be as effective as vena caval ligation in the prevention of postoperative pulmonary embolism and has a significantly lower incidence (about 5 per cent) of undesirable serious sequelae in the legs (Spencer et al.). There is a risk to this operation (15 to 30 per cent). When there is septic thrombophlebitis, vena caval ligation is indicated.

About 30 per cent of patients who have iliofemoral thrombophlebitis have late sequelae (edema, varicose veins or chronic ulcers) (McCallister et al.). It is not clear whether thrombectomy significantly reduces this.

A rational and recommended regimen is the following (assuming there are facilities for daily determination of prothrombin time):

1. Anticoagulant therapy is routinely begun 48 hours postoperative-

ly following abdominal hysterectomy, combined abdominoperineal resection or segmental resection of sigmoid colon, and in patients over 40 years of age undergoing repair of bilateral inguinal hernias.

2. Anticoagulant therapy is begun similarly in all patients with conditions imposing an undue risk of thromboembolism (see above).

3. When a patient who is not receiving anticoagulant therapy has a nonfatal pulmonary embolism, anticoagulant therapy is instituted immediately. Therapy is begun by the administration of heparin, usually in intermittent doses given intravenously every 4 hours with testing to assure an adequate prolongation of clotting time. Heparin therapy is continued for 3 to 7 days, during which time any evidence of active thrombophlebitis usually subsides. Then the administration of warfarin (Coumadin) is begun and after an adequate prothrombin deficiency has developed, heparin is discontinued. Warfarin should be continued for about 6 weeks after the patient has been dismissed from the hospital.

4. Patients who are not receiving anticoagulant therapy and who manifest clinical evidences of thrombophlebitis (calf tenderness, pain in calf on dorsiflexion of foot or swelling of lower extremity) should be started on an anticoagulant regimen. They should remain in bed with application of hot packs and elevation of legs for at least three days after institution of therapy with heparin is begun. Coumadin is gradually substituted for heparin as described above.

5. Partial vena caval interruption should be reserved for the rare instances in which the patient has sustained a nonfatal pulmonary embolism, but anticoagulant therapy is contraindicated or has been ineffective in preventing further pulmonary emboli.

6. Venous thrombectomy is controversial at present. Its clearest indications are phlegmasia cerulea dolens and early massive edema from acute iliofemoral thrombophlebitis.

Pulmonary Embolectomy. Indications for this procedure are few since most patients with large pulmonary emboli either survive or die immediately; however, in a few patients the operation is life-saving. When a patient suddenly becomes critically ill but is surviving, and it is likely that a pulmonary embolus is the cause, an emergency pulmonary arteriogram should be done. If the diagnosis is confirmed, emergency embolectomy with cardiopulmonary bypass is indicated.

DRUGS

Heparin. This drug is employed when an immediate anticoagulant effect is desired. The injection of 5000 units intravenously every 4 hours is satisfactory. This may be discontinued when an adequate prothrombin deficiency has been effected by administration of warfarin.

Warfarin. This is the anticoagulant agent of choice because an adequate prothrombin deficiency (10 to 20 per cent of control value) can be obtained in about 36 hours. In adults the initial dose, orally, is about 25 mg., with about 15 mg. being given 24 hours later. The maintenance dose varies between 2.5 and 12.5 mg./day. Initial and maintenance doses should be reduced in patients with liver disease or inanition because these patients usually have a greater sensitivity to the effect of the drug. This drug must *not* be used unless there are facilities for daily determination of prothrombin time. When prompt reversal of the effect of the drug is desired, phytonadione (vitamin K_1, Aquamephyton) is administered intravenously in a dose of 5 to 25 mg. When only some diminution in effect is desired, menadione (Hykinone) in doses of 36 to 72 mg. is given intravenously.

Digitalis. Surgeons should select one digitalis preparation for use. Digoxin is recommended. It can be given intravenously, orally, or intramuscularly. An effect can be seen within 30 minutes when it is given intravenously. If toxicity develops, its relatively rapid excretion is useful.

The dose required for full action without toxicity in most people is 0.9 mg./square meter of body surface area when given intravenously, or 1.6 mg./square meter of body surface area when given orally. *Any individual may require more or less than this estimated digitalizing dose,* and the patient must be carefully observed for digitalis toxicity during each step of the digitalizing process. When the situation is urgent and the patient has received no digitalis previously, one half or two thirds of his estimated digitalizing dose is given as a bolus intravenously. After 2 hours, if no signs of toxicity have developed and the desired effect is not achieved, one sixth of the estimated dose is given. This process may be continued until the total estimated digitalizing dose has been administered. For maintenance of digitalization one quarter of the estimated digitalizing dose is administered daily, usually by administering one eighth of the estimated digitalizing dose twice daily.

The oral route of administration is chosen when digitalization is not urgently needed. Ordinarily the initial dose in an adult is 0.5 mg., given three times in the first 24 hours. The following day 0.25 mg. is usually given two or three times, and the day after that the remainder of the estimated digitalizing dose is given. Thereafter maintenance is attained by giving one quarter of the estimated digitalizing dose each day, again usually in divided doses.

Patients in atrial fibrillation with a rapid ventricular response present a special situation in which accurate monitoring of the amount of digitalis needed is available by use of the ventricular rate. Therefore the initial dose is usually somewhat smaller and the estimated digitalizing dose is used only as a precaution against giving too much of the drug. Thus in an adult with atrial fibrillation and a rapid ventricular response, usually about 0.25 to 0.5 mg. is given intravenously, depending upon the ventricular rate. If after 2 hours there is no significant slowing of the rate, an additional 0.25 mg. is given. The patient is "titrated" subsequently by giving about 0.15 to 0.25 mg. intravenously every 2 to 6 hours until the ventricular rate reaches about 105 beats/minute. Usually an interval of 12 hours is allowed to pass and then a maintenance dose is started.

Epinephrine. Epinephrine is a potent drug for use in proper circumstances in patients with low cardiac output. Its infusion should be through a line preferably in a central vein or if in a peripheral vein through a needle that is extremely securely in position. A relatively strong solution, containing 4 mg. of epinephrine and 250 ml. of 5 per cent glucose in water, is used and infused through a microdrip apparatus. It is carefully regulated so as to give the minimal amount of drug that will produce a proper effect. If it is found that the drug is needed in very small amounts, the solution can be made more dilute.

Isoproterenol. Isoproterenol stimulates myocardial contractility, increases heart rate, and has a tendency to decrease systemic arteriolar resistance. Although it is a very useful drug, in patients in severe shock needing catecholamines epinephrine is apt to be more effective. Isoproterenol should, however, be tried first. Its method of administration is as indicated above. The solution is made by placing 0.5 mg. of isoproterenol in 250 ml. of 5 per cent glucose in water.

Lidocaine (Xylocaine). As indicated above, the drug may be given intravenously in a single injection of 50 mg. If there is need for further lidocaine, a solution containing 1 mg./ml. of fluid can be made, using 5 per cent glucose in water as the diluent. This may be infused intravenously at a rate which will control the ventricular premature contractions. Rather large amounts of lidocaine may be safely given. When lidocaine is given in excessive amounts, central nervous system irritability and depression of myocardial contractility may result.

Procaine Amide (Pronestyl). Procaine amide is best used orally for the more chronic control of the tendency toward premature ventricular contractions. Ideally for maximal benefit the drug should be given every 3 hours, and if this dosage schedule is utilized, 250 mg./dose is indicated. It may be given at 4 to 6 hour intervals, in which case 250 or 500 mg./dose is used.

Diphenylhydantoin (Dilantin). This drug is not commonly used but can be effective in patients whose premature ventricular contractions result from an overdosage of digitalis. One hundred mg. every 8 hours is a usual dosage schedule.

REFERENCES

Barker, N. W., Nygaard, K. K., Walters, W., and Priestley, J. T.: A statistical study of postoperative venous thrombosis and pulmonary embolism. I. Incidence in various types of operations. Proc. Staff Meet. Mayo Clin. 15:769, 1940.

Bottomley, J. E., Lloyd, O., and Chalmers, D. G.: Postoperative prophylactic anticoagulants in gynaecology: A ten year study. Lancet 2:835, 1964.

Harrison, D. C., Kerber, R. E., and Alderman, E. L.: Pharmacodynamics and clinical use of cardiovascular drugs after cardiac surgery. Amer. J. Cardiol. 26:385, 1970.

Hermann, R. E., Davis, J. N., and Holden, W. D.: Pulmonary embolism: Clinical and pathologic study with emphasis on the effect of prophylactic therapy with anticoagulants. Amer. J. Surg. 102:19, 1961.

Kirklin, J. W., and Theye, R. A.: Cardiac performance after open intracardiac surgery. Circulation 28:1061, 1963.

Litwak, R. S., Kuhn, L. A., Gadboys, H. L., Lukvan, S. B., and Dakurai, H.: Support of myocardial performance after open cardiac operations by rate augmentation. J. Thorac. Cardiovasc. Surg. 56:484, 1968.

McCallister, B. G., Shick, R. M., and Kvale, W. F.: Iliofemoral thrombophlebitis: A ten year study of conservative treatment. Circulation 28:766, 1963 (abstract).

Mueller, H., Giannelli, S., Ayres, S. M., Conklin, E. F., and Gregory, J. J.: Effect of isoproterenol on ventricular work and myocardial metabolism in the postoperative heart. Circulation 37:(suppl. 2) 146, 1968.

Priestley, J. T., and Barker, N. W.: Postoperative thrombosis and embolism: Their treatment with heparin. Surg. Gynec. & Obstet. 75:193, 1942.

Ross, J., and Braunwald, E.: Study of left ventricular function in man by increasing resistance to ventricular ejection with angiotensin. Circulation 29:739, 1964.

Rushmer, R. F.: Cardiovascular Dynamics. 3rd Ed. Philadelphia, W. B. Saunders Company, 1961.

Sevitt, S.: Venous thrombosis and pulmonary embolism: Their prevention by oral anticoagulants. Amer. J. Med. 33:703, 1962.

Sheppard, L. C., Kouchoukos, N. T., Kurtts, M. A., and Kirklin, J. W.: Automated treatment of critically ill patients following operation. Ann. Surg. 168:596, 1968.

Sonnenblick, E. H., and Downing, S. E.: Afterload as a primary determinant of ventricular performance. Amer. J. Physiol. 204:604, 1963.

Spencer, F. C., Jude, J., Rienhoff, W. F., III, and Stonesifer, G.: Plication of the inferior vena cava for pulmonary embolism: Long-term results in 39 cases. Ann. Surg. 161:788, 1965.

CHAPTER 10

THE PATIENT IN SHOCK

Lloyd D. MacLean, M.D., F.A.C.S.

INTRODUCTION AND DEFINITION OF THE PROBLEM

Shock is best treated when the cause is known and the response to therapy is quantitated in a meaningful way. The greatest single contribution to our knowledge of the subject in this century was the recognition by Blalock[1] and by Parsons and Phemister[2] that traumatic shock is due to hypovolemia. The continuous measurement of central venous pressure has provided a simple method to quantitate response to treatment, particularly valuable in patients with hypovolemia or cardiogenic shock.

Clinical descriptions of patients in shock usually list the signs of hypovolemia and are misleading in that other causes of shock can be overlooked. In seeking a suitable definition for shock, we have passed through several phases. Early in this century, a patient would be considered in shock only if he had a thready pulse and a low blood pressure. A suitable definition at that time might have been "hypotension associated with pallor and sweating following injury or bleeding." More recently, the importance of blood flow to vital organs was recognized and many patients were seen who had a low cardiac output and a normal blood pressure who eventually died of this as a result of vital organ failure. In similar patients with low cardiac output and low blood pressure, the augmentation of blood pressure alone by vasoconstrictors without increase in cardiac output was rarely successful.[3] A suitable definition of shock at that stage of our understanding was "inadequate blood flow to vital organs."

Today we recognize patients in shock who have a higher than normal cardiac output but abundant evidence of organ failure and lacticacidosis. A suitable current definition of shock is "inadequate blood flow to vital organs or failure of the cells of vital organs to utilize oxygen." A classification based on this definition appears in Table

Table 10-1. Classification of Shock

I. Hypovolemic
   1. Blood loss
   2. Plasma loss
   3. Water loss

II. Cardiogenic
   1. Infarct
   2. Arrhythmia
   3. Tamponade
   4. Late hypovolemia
   5. Epidural and general anesthesia

III. Peripheral pooling
   1. Loss of tone in resistance vessels
      Spinal anesthesia
   2. Trapping in capacitance vessels
      Endotoxin shock in the dog

IV. Cellular defect
   Decreased oxygen utilization despite high flow and normal oxygen content of blood
   as in septic shock in man.

10-1. The purpose of any classification is to facilitate recognition and to promote correct and specific therapy as quickly as possible. This classification suggests that a hemodynamic diagnosis should be made as soon as possible and treatment based on this started before a clinical diagnosis is established. The ultimate welfare of the patient will depend also on excellent medical and surgical care directed to the clinical diagnosis. For example, it would be of importance to repair surgically a perforated duodenal ulcer in a patient in shock, but the recognition that hypovolemia is the cause of the shock and the correction of it are equally as important.

ASSESSMENT OF PATIENTS IN SHOCK

Eight measurements are extremely useful in the initial assessment and follow-up on all patients in shock (Table 10-2). Seven of the eight are readily measured in most hospitals. Only cardiac output is difficult to measure accurately. Fortunately in most instances, the information provided by the other measurements alone establishes a hemodynamic diagnosis.

THE IMPORTANT RELATIONSHIP OF OXYGEN SATURATION, HEMOGLOBIN CONCENTRATION AND CARDIAC OUTPUT IN SHOCK

The central problem in shock is the impairment and eventual failure of cellular oxygenation. As will be emphasized later, my col-

Table 10–2. THE EIGHT CRITICAL MEASUREMENTS FOR
PATIENTS IN SHOCK

	NORMAL VALUES IN ADULT MAN
1. Arterial blood pressure	120/80
2. Pulse rate	80/min.
3. Central venous pressure	5 cm. H_2O
4. Urine flow	50 ml./hour
5. Cardiac index	3.2 L./min./m.²
6. Arterial blood PO_2	100 mm. Hg
$\quad$ pCO$_2$	40 mm. Hg
$\quad$ pH	7.4
7. Arterial blood lactate	12 mg. %
8. Hematocrit	35–45%

leagues and I believe that in hypovolemic and cardiogenic shock, cellular damage follows the development of a tissue oxygen debt caused by low tissue perfusion. In contrast, in shock caused by a cellular defect, as seen in many patients with sepsis, a primary cellular defect occurs characterized by low oxygen utilization. The hyperdynamic circulation seen in many patients with septic shock is then a compensatory mechanism.

Nunn and Freeman[4] have quantitated the available oxygen in hypovolemic shock in the following way:

Available oxygen = Cardiac output × Arterial O_2 saturation × Hemoglobin concentration × 1.34

which becomes

$$\frac{1000}{ml./min.} = \frac{5250}{ml./min.} \times \frac{95}{100} \times \frac{15}{100} \underset{gm./ml.}{\times} \frac{1.34}{ml./gm.}$$

We utilize approximately 250 ml./min. in the resting state, which might at first glance suggest a large reserve. More specifically, this formula suggests that, if normally 5 volumes per cent of oxygen is extracted from arterial blood containing 20 volumes per cent, a reserve of 15 volumes per cent remains. This supposition must be modified in two ways:

1. A certain partial pressure gradient is needed for transfer of oxygen from capillary to tissue, and below a critical partial pressure of oxygen in capillary blood, tissue hypoxia will result. The critical value may vary from tissue to tissue and, of course, with pH and temperature,

but a reasonable range is approximately 20 to 30 mm. Hg. This corresponds to an oxygen saturation of 35 to 55 per cent. This in turn means that of the 20 volumes per cent of oxygen normally carried in arterial blood, approximately 7 to 11 volumes per cent are unavailable to the tissues.

Of the original 1000 ml./min. of oxygen potentially available, only about 600 to 700 ml./min. is actually available to the tissues when circumstances are ideal.

2. There is also a variation in oxygen uptake and requirements by different tissues of the body. While the overall oxygen uptake per 100 ml. of blood is approximately 5 volumes per cent, the chemoreceptors of the body have no measurable oxygen uptake, the kidney 1.5 volumes per cent, and the heart approximately 11.5 volumes per cent with little or no oxygen reserve.[4] Only a selective increase in coronary blood flow can prevent the heart from being the first organ to suffer in general hypoxia. This offers an explanation as to why cardiac failure (inadequate cardiac output with high filling pressure) may supervene in certain patients with hypovolemia who have, at first, inadequate volume replacement followed later by large volumes because of persistent or recurrent hypotension. Vigorous and quick volume replacement in the beginning would likely avoid the secondary form of shock which is, from the hemodynamic viewpoint, cardiogenic.

Having established that available oxygen has a limited reserve and is dependent upon cardiac output, arterial O_2 saturation and hemoglobin concentration let us follow the calculations of Nunn and Freeman[4] for specific deficits. If any one of the three variables is reduced, the available oxygen is reduced proportionally. Therefore, if saturation and hemoglobin remain constant, a halving of cardiac output will halve the available oxygen, and a small margin of safety still exists.

If two of the variables are lowered at the same time, the effect on available oxygen will equal the product of the individual changes. Thus, if cardiac output and hemoglobin are both half of normal, the available oxygen will be reduced to one quarter or 250 ml./min. This is a most dangerous level in critically ill patients and is compatible with life for only short periods.

If all three factors are moderately reduced, the effect on available oxygen will be great, because this will reduce available oxygen by a factor equal to the product of the three individual changes. Thus, if cardiac output, hemoglobin and saturation are each reduced by one third, the available oxygen will be only 300 ml., a level which is rapidly fatal. For example,[4] available oxygen = cardiac output × O_2 saturation × hemoglobin concentration × 1.34.

$$300 \text{ ml.} = \frac{3500}{\text{ml./min.}} \times \frac{64}{100} \times \frac{10}{100} \times 1.34$$

In this circumstance, none of the values are particularly alarming and all are seen individually with great frequency during shock and anesthesia. All three should be looked at carefully and corrected in seriously ill patients before irreversible damage has occurred.

HYPOVOLEMIC SHOCK

"J. J., a college student aged 21 years, was run over one morning by a truck, and both legs were severely crushed. He became temporarily unconscious but was able to talk on the the way to the hospital. Three broken bones were easily set; there was no visible bleeding, and after taking a sedative he felt well enough to smile and appeared to be on the road to recovery. In the afternoon, however, he became restless; his face showed an anxious expression, with pallor; his pulse became weak and rapid, his skin cold and clammy and his breathing labored and shallow; he sank into coma despite a 500 ml. blood transfusion and, toward evening, died."[5]

This boy, seen over 25 years ago and reported by Rhoads and Harkins, died of hypovolemic shock.[5] There is no form of shock in which our ability to save life has shown greater progress than in the treatment of hypovolemic or post-traumatic shock.

To Archibald and McLean[6] in World War I, the clinical picture of shock was equally sharp—"a low-tension pulse, usually rapid, shallow breathing, pallor, sometimes going on into a light cyanosis, lack of apparent suffering, carelessness as to one's surroundings, preservation of a clear though lethargic mind up to the very last." Of 17 patients admitted to a casualty clearing station in France with systolic blood pressures below 75 mm. Hg, none survived. Saline, gelatin with saline and, in three patients, 16 to 20 ounces of blood were given by Archibald and McLean for volume replacement at that time.

In contrast, in Korea and in Vietnam, Howard and Brown[17] report that "pre-operative irreversible shock is not recognized, for, without exception, the blood pressure can be returned to normal in the preoperative period if bleeding can be controlled." "Continued hypotension means continued bleeding or inadequate transfusion."

One recalls the course of a 77-year old patient seen in civilian practice in 1956 with a crushing injury of both legs, with fractures of both femora and both tibae and fibulae. The patient required 8000 cc. of blood over a seven-hour period to stabilize his vital signs. There was no external blood loss. The frequent use of chest auscultation was the only means available to avoid overtransfusion in this elderly, vulnerable patient. The need for a quick, easy method to guide one in blood volume replacement was obvious at that time. Measurements of central venous pressure now make replacement of blood volume in hypovolemic shock rapid, simple and safe.

Central venous pressure (CVP), according to Jacobson,[8] is the function of four measurable and independent forces: the volume of blood in the central veins; the distensibility and contractability of the right heart chambers; venomotor activity in the central veins; and intrathoracic pressure. If one can rule out abnormal causes of elevated intrathoracic pressure, e.g., hemothorax, the CVP reflects principally the volume of blood returning to the heart and the ability of both the right and left ventricles to propel it. One is impressed with the great value of serial measurements of the CVP and the advantages of this over individual or serial measurements of blood volume. Figure 10-1 summarizes a comparison in 16 patients of the normal blood volume and the effective blood volume after treatment for hypovolemic shock at a time when blood pressure, urine flow and tissue perfusion has returned to normal. The effective blood volume exceeded the normal blood volume in all of these patients soon after the correction of hypovolemic shock. The CVP at that time was between 10 and 20 cm. of water in all patients and

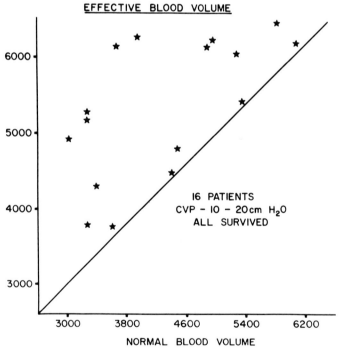

Figure 10-1. Effective blood volume, or that volume which restored arterial blood pressure, urine output, and tissue perfusion, exceeds the normal blood volume for each of these patients in hypovolemic shock. The central venous pressure is an excellent guide for replacement of effective blood volume, whereas the measurement of the blood volume can be quite misleading. With normal blood volume many patients will remain in shock with a low central venous pressure. (By permission of Surgery, Gynecology & Obstetrics.)

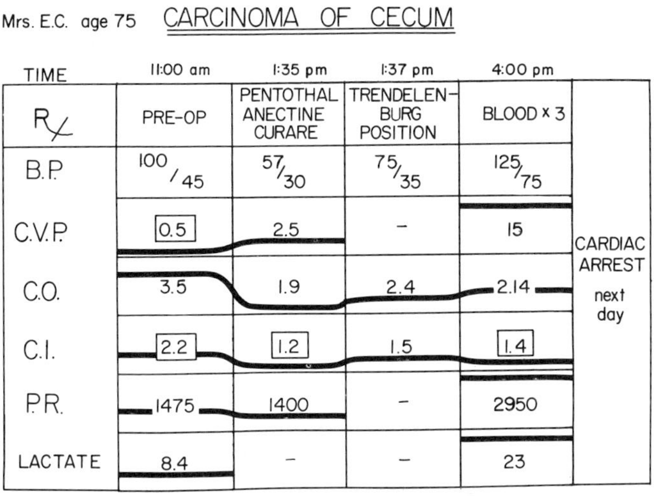

Mrs. E.C. age 75   CARCINOMA OF CECUM

TIME	11:00 am	1:35 pm	1:37 pm	4:00 pm	
Rx	PRE-OP	PENTOTHAL ANECTINE CURARE	TRENDELEN-BURG POSITION	BLOOD x 3	
B.P.	100/45	57/30	75/35	125/75	
C.V.P.	0.5	2.5	-	15	CARDIAC ARREST next day
C.O.	3.5	1.9	2.4	2.14	
C.I.	2.2	1.2	1.5	1.4	
P.R.	1475	1400	-	2950	
LACTATE	8.4	-	-	23	

Figure 10-2.   Patient E. C. presented for surgery with a low CVP, low cardiac index, high peripheral resistance and normal blood pressure, suggesting hypovolemia. With induction of anesthesia there was a marked drop in blood pressure and flow. Following the operation and after 3 units of blood, the patient had a normal blood pressure but an elevated CVP with a very low cardiac index (CI) and an elevated arterial blood lactate, all suggestive of cardiogenic shock. The patient had a cardiac arrest the following day but recovered. There was no evidence of myocardial infarction. Improperly treated hypovolemia became cardiogenic shock in this patient.

between 10 and 15 cm. of water in 15 of the 16 patients. In some the data suggest that the measurement of blood volume would persuade one not to transfuse and would thereby be misleading rather than helpful.

The late recognition of hypovolemic shock or inadequate volume replacement can lead to another syndrome even in young adults without a history of cardiac disease. Hypovolemic shock, seen early, is characterized by a low CVP, low blood pressure, low cardiac output and high peripheral resistance, all of which respond favorably to adequate and rapid volume replacement. In contrast, the patient with hypovolemic shock not adequately replaced, can present, when vigorous attempts are made to elevate blood pressure and promote urine output, with a high CVP, low blood pressure and persistently low cardiac output. At this point, the patient has cardiogenic shock (Fig. 10-2).

Arterial Blood Lactate.   Cannon in 1918[9] recorded a rough correlation between the severity or duration of hypotension and the decrease in carbon dioxide combining power of the blood. Peretz et al.[10] in 1964 were the first to show, in man, in shock, a close correlation between arterial blood lactate levels and survival. Their observations suggested that inadequate perfusion of tissues results in partial arrest of glycolysis at the anaerobic phase, with accumulation of lactate and other ions as a consequence of decreased tissue pO_2. Crowell and Guyton[11] showed that inevitable death occurs in dogs subjected to hemorrhagic shock when an oxygen debt of 150 ml. of oxygen per kg. occurred regardless of what measures were taken.

There is no advantage in shock studies to measure "excess lactate," i.e., the disproportionate elevation of the level of lactate in relation to that of pyruvate. There is no correlation between blood pressure and lactate elevation, but Figure 10-3 shows a close correlation between the lactate level when the patient is first seen and prognosis. Serial measurements of arterial blood lactate are of great prognostic importance (Fig. 10-4), and are a valuable measurement with which to follow the adequacy of treatment.

Some investigators have questioned the cause-and-effect relationship between lactate rise and tissue hypoxia or oxygen debt, and it is known that nonhypoxic hyperventilation will cause a marked elevation of blood lactate.[12] In the latter experiments on dogs, the pCO_2 was markedly decreased to 10 to 15 mm. Hg. The experiments of Cain[13] have resolved this controversy in a convincing manner which substantiates the value of the clinical measurement of lactate clinically. Cain showed a correlation between lactate elevation and oxygen debt. Furthermore, the lactate elevation was greatest with hypocapnic hypoxia, less with eucapnic hypoxia and least with hypercapnic hypoxia. However, lactate increase at any carbon dioxide tension correlated positively with oxygen debt.

In summary (Table 10-3), most patients with hypovolemic shock present with a low blood pressure (under 90 systolic); rapid pulse (over 100); low CVP (under 2 cm. water); low cardiac index (under 2.5

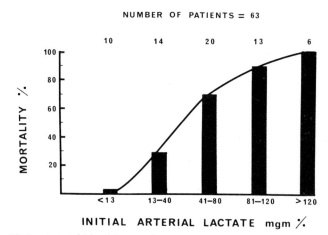

Figure 10-3. Arterial blood lactate determinations in 63 patients in shock, measured when the patients were initially seen and before treatment was begun. This value was of prognostic significance, whereas a similar plot of initial blood pressure vs. mortality was not.

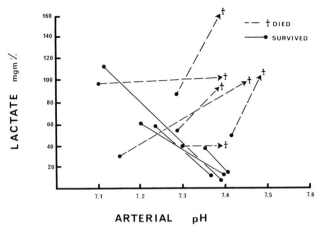

Figure 10-4. A summary of 32 patients in whom serial measurements of arterial blood lactate reflect prognosis. In ten patients (represented by the broken lines) the lactate rose and all patients died. In 22 patients (represented by the solid lines) the lactate dropped quickly to normal and all survived.

L./min./m.^{2}); low urine flow (under 20 ml./hour); near-normal arterial pO$_2$; increased arteriovenous oxygen difference; and a moderately elevated arterial blood lactate (20 to 30 mg. per cent). There is a dramatic response to rapid volume replacement first with normal saline, Ringer's lactate or buffered saline (44 mg. of sodium bicarbonate in each liter of saline), followed by the fluid lost, which is usually blood or plasma. If bleeding can be arrested and the replacement is prompt (the patient has normal vital signs within one to two hours of onset), the prognosis is excellent even in the elderly.

The hematocrit is useful as a guide of what to give for replacement rather than when to give it. Therefore one would give plasma and

Table 10-3. HEMODYNAMIC AND METABOLIC DIFFERENCES IN VARIOUS TYPES OF SHOCK

	BLOOD PRESSURE	PULSE RATE	CVP	CARDIAC INDEX	URINE FLOW	RESPONSE TO VOLUME LOAD	ARTERIAL pO$_2$	ARTERIO-VENOUS O$_2$ DIFFERENCE	ARTERIAL BLOOD LACTATE
Hypovolemic shock	↓	↑	↓	↓	↓	↑	→	↑	↑
Cardiogenic shock	↓	or ↑↓	↑	↓	↓	↓	↓	↑	↑
Peripheral pooling	↓	↑	↓	↓	↓	↓	↑↓	↑	↑
Cellular defect	↓	↑	↑	↑	↓	↓	↓	↓	→↑

saline for a patient with hypovolemic shock caused by pancreatitis who might have a hematocrit of 60. This patient will improve as evidenced by an increased cardiac output, urine flow, blood pressure and decreased pulse rate if the hematocrit is promptly lowered from 60 to 35 by saline alone. Conversely, the patient in shock with a bleeding duodenal ulcer who has a hematocrit of 20 will require blood. Maximum oxygen carrying capacity is achieved with a hematocrit between 35 and 45.

In experimental animals, resistance to hypovolemic shock, produced by bleeding to a mean blood pressure of 30 mm. Hg, was greatest if the animal started with a hematocrit of 42 per cent.[14] It was found that available oxygen reached its highest values at the same hematocrit. Resistance to hemorrhage and available oxygen both fell with higher or lower values.[14]

A decrease in peripheral resistance is achieved by volume replacement alone in hypovolemic shock. The use of vasodilators for this purpose does not seem justified. The lowering of blood pressure induced by phenoxybenzamine in a hypovolemic patient will promote rapid volume replacement but does not seem necessary. Increased peripheral resistance is the result, not the cause, of shock.

CARDIOGENIC SHOCK

Cardiogenic shock may be defined as "inadequate blood flow to vital organs due to inadequate cardiac output despite a normal cardiac filling pressure." Although it is classically associated with myocardial infarction, many patients with problems, primarily surgical, appear with this form of shock. Mr. J. F., aged 53, was admitted to the Royal Victoria Hospital with a perforated and mildly bleeding duodenal ulcer. He was believed to have hypovolemic shock caused by hemorrhage, when in fact the cause was peritonitis. Before this was recognized, the patient had received several units of blood and had a markedly elevated hematocrit. At this time he had a low cardiac output, low blood pressure, low urine volume and high CVP, i.e., cardiogenic shock. Correction of the hematocrit only, by administration of saline, caused return of all values toward normal. Recovery thereafter was uneventful.

A second dramatic example of cardiogenic shock, one which occurred in the operating room during lung transplantation, was recently encountered. The operation commenced with a patient with normal blood pressure and CVP despite abnormal blood gases. Severe shock supervened, characterized by a falling blood pressure and a rising CVP. It was important to know, promptly, if hypovolemia or cardiogenic shock was the cause. The latter was likely because of the falling blood pressure and rising CVP, and an excellent response to intravenous isoproterenol was achieved despite markedly abnormal blood gases and pH which existed at that time. Prompt recognition of the hemodynamic diagnosis permitted one to correct the fundamental clinical problem (pulmonary failure) by lung transplantation.

Isoproterenol when used for the therapy of shock should be diluted 1 to 2 mg. in 500 cc. of dextrose 5 per cent in water, and should be given at a rate that does not elevate pulse rate over 120 to 130. Larger doses are not useful and may be dangerous.

Arrhythmias. Arrhythmias are frequently encountered in poor risk patients and patients in shock. The continuous monitoring of EKG and blood pressure in these patients is extremely important. Some common problems and their therapy follow:

1. In bradycardia, if manifested by sinus or a slow nodal rhythm, atropine, 1 to 1.2 mg. intravenously with elevation of the legs, is usually effective; isoproterenol is also effective in treating complete heart block with slow idioventricular or nodal rhythms. A continuous infusion of 1 to 4 micrograms/min. is recommended. Percutaneous transvenous endocardial pacing should be immediately resorted to if response to this therapy is not prompt.

2. In ventricular extrasystoles, lidocaine is the preferred agent. It is given initially as a 1 to 2 mg./kg. bolus, followed by a continuous infusion of 1 to 4 mg./min. If a patient shows fewer than one in ten ventricular extrasystoles, one is inclined to observe but treat as above for more frequent occurrences on the monitor. Intravenous procainamide or quinidine can be used, but hypotension and myocardial depression may occur. Serum potassium must be watched carefully, especially in digitalized patients. Specifically, digitalis toxicity may have initially caused the arrhythmia, which will persist or recur if a low potassium persists.

Output after Recovery of Rate and Rhythm. Agents with positive inotropy can restore circulation in those circumstances that frequently follow cardiac arrest. Calcium chloride, isoproterenol, dopamine and glucagon all increase myocardial contractility. In normotensive man dopamine, 2 to 6 micrograms/kg./min., has been reported to produce fewer arrhythmias and chronotropic effects than isoproterenol, 0.01 to 0.16 per kg./min. Further studies of dopamine during shock are needed, particularly with larger doses (10 to 20 micrograms/kg./min.) Glucagon may also be a useful agent. The mode of action in producing increased contractibility is unknown, but it is independent from that of digitalis. The dose used is 5 mg./kg. repeated every 30 minutes, or 100 mg./min. as a continuous infusion.

The Poor Risk Patient. Age, obesity, specific organ failure, chronic illness and infection are all well-known causes of increased operative risk. Many of these factors cannot be corrected, but optimal hemodynamic status can be evaluated conveniently preoperatively by measuring the eight factors used to assess patients in shock (Table 10-2).

An example of the possible use of this technique to evaluate the "risk status" of a patient has already been described (Fig. 10-2). This patient probably would not have developed shock and subsequently a cardiac arrest if she had been prepared so that at the time of operation her CVP was between 5 and 10 cm. of water and her cardiac index (CI) over 3.2 L./min./m.^{2}

Cardiopulmonary resuscitation for cardiac arrest has been most useful. Presently, 30 per cent of patients in hospital are resuscitated and 15 per cent leave the hospital. It is also clear that most patients who survive have myocardial infarction or reversible pulmonary failure as the cause. Complicated surgical problems as illustrated in Figure 10-3 are best treated by prevention. Many cardiac arrests on surgical wards could be avoided by correction or even partial correction of the eight measurements outlined above in Table 10-2.

Epidural and General Anesthesia. Most general anesthetics decrease cardiac output without changing or actually causing a rise in CVP, indicating a compromise of cardiac function. Profound and prolonged declines in blood pressure and cardiac output with induction of anesthesia are best treated by correction of venous return as assessed by CVP, blood gases and pH, hematocrit, and urine flow before the operation rather than by emergency measures after the fall in blood pressure.

It is not as generally realized that epidural anesthesia or high spinal blockade can result in cardiac sympathetic block which causes decreased cardiac index with an elevated central venous pressure. The cardiac deficit occurs mainly through loss of rate control, resulting in bradycardia as well as further loss of performance through decreased myocardial contractibility despite adequate filling.

Epidural anesthesia or analgesia offers excellent relaxation for abdominal surgery and has been very successful in relieving pain associated with thoracic trauma and pancreatitis. However, several instances of hepatorenal failure after epidural and spinal blockade not prevented by the use of vasoconstrictors suggest that cardiogenic shock was the cause. Restoration of cardiac output to normal is easily accomplished with isoproterenol. Norepinephrine on the other hand failed to restore cardiac performance to control.[15] It is likely that cardiac sympathectomy occurs even in those instances in which the analgesic is administered in the lumbar region. Total epidural block adds peripheral dilatation and pooling to the cardiac effect and further decreases output by decreasing venous return. A vasoconstrictor is useful for this abnormality.

In summary, cardiogenic shock is seen in a wide variety of surgical patients and may be due to (1) myocardial infarction, (2) arrhythmias, (3) cardiac tamponade, (4) delayed and inadequate volume replacement in hypovolemia, (5) inappropriate volume replacement in hypovolemia with the creation of a high hematocrit, (6) epidural anesthesia with resultant cardiac sympathectomy, and (7) adrenal insufficiency.

The patient usually presents with a lowered blood pressure, a slow or rapid pulse, an elevated CVP, decreased urine flow, decreased cardiac index, lowered arterial pO_2, moderately elevated lactate (15 to 30 mg. per cent) and increased arterio-mixed venous difference (Table 10-3).

PERIPHERAL POOLING

This hemodynamic abnormality is classically seen in experimental hemorrhagic or endotoxin shock in the dog. The syndrome is characterized by a low blood pressure, rapid pulse, low CVP despite massive volume replacement, low CI caused by failure of venous return, low arterial pO_2 but increased arteriovenous oxygen difference caused by increased oxygen extraction.[16] Many studies have revealed that in the dog the area of trapping is principally in the liver and splanchnic bed. This syndrome is not characteristic of hypovolemic or septic shock in man, but is observed in patients with untreated hypotension caused by spinal anesthesia.

CELLULAR DEFECT

Septic shock in man is the principal cause of a primary cellular defect in shock. Evidence will be presented in this section that sepsis causes a cellular defect which inhibits oxygen utilization, and that this occurs before the hemodynamic changes. All patients with septic shock do not present with a cellular defect, but hypovolemia and even cardiogenic shock are occasionally seen as a consequence of sepsis. Hence, the fourth and final section in the classification of shock is called "cellular defect" rather than septic shock.

Septic shock has emerged as the main unsolved problem in shock, both in understanding the mechanisms involved and in successful therapy. It is now common practice to successfully resuscitate soldiers in Vietnam or civilians with devastating injuries and associated hypovolemic shock. Many of these patients, however, succumb days or weeks later from septic shock.

There are several factors that predispose to sepsis in medical and surgical patients. These include underlying neoplastic disease, diabetes mellitus, old age, hypovolemia, steroid therapy, immunosuppressive therapy, indwelling urinary or intravenous catheters, indiscriminate use of prophylactic antibiotics, overconfidence in the effectiveness of antibiotic agents, cancer chemotherapy, cirrhosis of the liver, tracheostomy and radiation therapy. These patients are especially prevalent on surgical services in which larger operations are being performed with increasing frequency on patients with many of the aforementioned predisposing factors.

PATTERNS OF SEPTIC SHOCK

Hyperdynamic or Warm Shock. These patients present with the syndrome summarized in Table 10-4 and are now recognized commonly.[17] Hyperventilation is especially valuable as an early sign of septic shock. The true cause of hyperventilation may be overlooked, especially after operation when atelectasis, pneumonia, pulmonary embolism or even myocardial infarction is likely to be thought of first. The typical patient with this hyperdynamic type of septic shock presents with hypotension, rapid pulse rate, high cardiac index, elevated arterial blood lactate, hypoxia, respiratory alkalosis, a high normal CVP and elevated plasma volume.

A summary of the hemodynamic findings before and after therapy, including the survival rate of 28 patients with hyperdynamic septic shock, appears in Figure 10-5. Salvage is related to maintaining a higher than normal flow rate, and to prompt and complete drainage or excision of the source of infection (Table 10-3).

Hypodynamic Septic Shock. In contrast to the hyperdynamic state, this form of septic shock is seen in patients with evidence of a "third space" loss prior to the septic process. Most have gangrenous intestinal obstruction, mesenteric thrombosis or peritonitis. The clinical presentation suggests hypovolemic shock with a low CVP, hypotension, low cardiac output, increased peripheral resistance, elevated lactate, low urine output and cold cyanotic extremities. A summary of the hemodynamic findings and mortality rate in ten patients appears in Figure 10-6.

In both the hyperdynamic and hypodynamic types of septic shock, patients present early with respiratory alkalosis and the mortality rate is lower than if seen late when they are overwhelmed with severe metabolic acidosis and an elevated arterial blood lactate. An early case of hypodynamic septic shock caused by gangrenous small bowel obstruction occurred in a 52-year-old female who several years previously had received radiotherapy for carcinoma of the cervix and presented at this time with abdominal distention, rigidity and a blood pressure of 80/40, pulse of 140, and CVP of 0. Her extremities were cold, moist and

Table 10–4. HYPERDYNAMIC SEPTIC SHOCK IN MAN

Hyperventilation
Respiratory alkalosis
High central venous pressure
High cardiac index
Low peripheral resistance
Hypotension
Oliguria
Lacticacidemia
Warm, dry, pink or suffused extremities

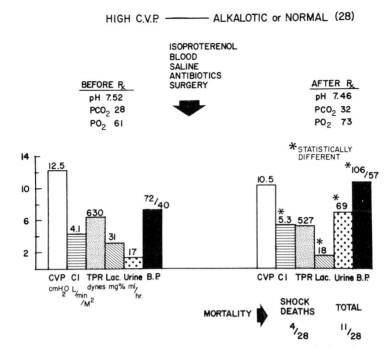

Figure 10-5. Summary of hemodynamic findings before and after therapy in 28 patients with hyperdynamic septic shock. (By permission of Annals of Surgery.)

slightly cyanosed, and there was no urine output. Arterial blood gas studies showed a pO_2 of 86 mm. Hg; pH of 7.42; pCO_2 of 25 mm. Hg; and base deficit of 6.5 mEq./L. Hemoglobin concentration was 10 gm./100 ml. hematocrit 34 per cent and white blood count 16,000/cm. Prior to resuscitation, the cardiac index was 2.8 L./min./m.^{2}

Preparation for surgery over a four-hour period included blood, saline, mannitol and sodium bicarbonate which brought the CVP to 6 cm. of water and the cardiac index to 3.2 L./min./m.^{2}

At operation, massive small bowel infarction caused by volvulus was found and extensive resection was carried out with a successful outcome. During operation, the CVP was maintained at 7 to 14 cm. of water by administering blood, and the patient remained normotensive.

Postoperatively, blood pressure was 130/80 mm. Hg and the CVP was 6.5 cm. of water, yet disturbingly the cardiac index had declined to 2.7 L./min./m.^{2} Repeat hematocrit was 51 per cent, indicating a marked hemoconcentration. With correction of this disorder, the cardiac index promptly rose to 5.4 L./min./m.^{2} and there was a marked improvement in urine flow. Twelve hours later, blood lactic acid had declined from the inital value of 61 mg. per cent to 15 mg. per cent. The patient was discharged well 10 days later.

Summary. Preoperative preparation based on the eight key measurements can be quickly and easily accomplished in hypodynamic

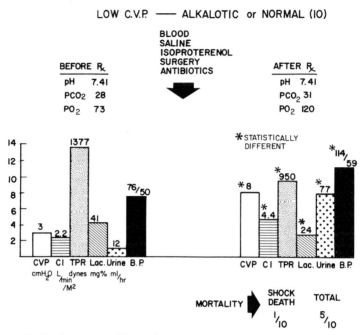

Figure 10-6. Summary of hemodynamic and metabolic findings in hypodynamic septic shock before and after treatment. There is an excellent response to volume replacement. (By permission of Annals of Surgery.)

septic shock. There is a tendency to treat hypotension occurring during surgery especially for gangrenous small bowel obstruction, with blood and this is good. In the illustrative patient, this was overdone and a larger quantity of Ringer's lactate or saline could have been used. It is here suggested that a hematocrit between 30 and 40 per cent should be maintained. Massive quantities of Ringer's lactate that lower the hematocrit below 30 to 35 per cent would be equally bad.

GRAM-NEGATIVE VERSUS GRAM-POSITIVE INFECTIONS

A summary of the organisms found in 56 patients with septic shock and the presenting syndrome, either hyperdynamic or hypodynamic, appears in Table 10-5. Gram-negative organisms were by far the most common cause, and were associated with both types of shock. Gram-positive organisms and fungi, with only one exception, produced a hyperdynamic syndrome. The offending fungus was Candida in all cases. These data do not indicate that there is a different hemodynamic response to the products of gram-negative and gram-positive organisms but rather that the causes of "third-space" losses differ and hence a hypodynamic response is more frequently associated with intestinal or

Table 10–5. MICROORGANISMS CULTURED AND TYPE
OF SHOCK ENCOUNTERED

	HYPERDYNAMIC	HYPODYNAMIC
Gram-negative	27	15
Gram-positive	9	1
Fungus	3	1

genitourinary infections and therefore with gram-negative organisms. Either response is seen with a wide variety of organisms and should not be used as a guide to antibiotic therapy. The question might be asked at this point if there is any difference between hypodynamic septic shock and any other form of hypovolemia. Although not as yet proved, there is a strong possibility that this form of shock produces direct cellular damage not seen until much later in hypovolemic shock.

DEFECTIVE OXYGEN CONSUMPTION IN SEPTIC SHOCK

Using accurate methods of collection and analysis of inspired and expired air, oxygen uptake has been shown to be decreased in patients with septic shock who have a normal or increased cardiac output. Furthermore, these same patients have an elevated arterial blood lactate and an inappropriately low arterio-mixed venous oxygen difference.

In exercise, in which the need for oxygen increases, there is an increased cardiac output and at the same time an increased oxygen extraction and increased arteriovenous difference. In hypovolemic shock, cardiogenic shock and endotoxin shock in the dog there is a decreased cardiac output but an increased oxygen extraction and therefore a wide A-V difference, which is an appropriate response. Patients with septic shock have a need for a larger than normal oxygen uptake (fever, rapid pulse and infection) but have a normal or low uptake. This might be due to a failure of oxygen transport in the lungs; failure of flow to the tissues of utilization; failure of oxygen release from hemoglobin in the tissues; arteriovenous shunting in the periphery or failure of oxygen utilization by the cells of vital organs. Although the arterial oxygen content of arterial blood is decreased in most patients with sepsis, correction of arterial pO_2 does not improve oxygen uptake, (Fig. 10-7), and large increases of arterial blood pO_2 as accomplished by hyperbaric oxygen therapy have been of no value.[17] The second possibility is a failure of flow; but we have already established that increased cardiac output is a characteristic of this form of shock. Failure of oxygen release from hemoglobin owing to a decrease in 2,3-diphosphoglycerate (2,3-DPG) is a possibility. As 2,3-DPG falls, the HbO_2

PATIENTS WITH SEPTIC SHOCK

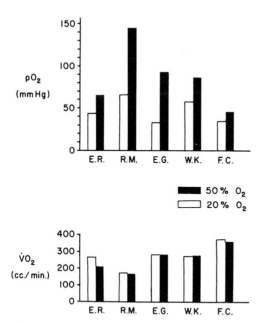

Figure 10-7. Comparison of oxygen uptake ($\dot{V}O_2$) and pO_2 in five patients on either 50 or 100 per cent oxygen. Raising the arterial pO_2 does not increase oxygen uptake.

dissociation curve swings to the left; that is, for a given pO_2, the hemoglobin per cent oxygen saturation is higher. Miller and his associates[18] reported that the 2,3-DPG level was decreased in clinical septic shock, and they postulated that this contributed to poor tissue oxygenation, which in turn was the cause of the low oxygen uptake. No measurements of tissue pO_2 were made, however, and the overall effect in vivo of the many factors known to influence HbO_2 dissociation remains speculative. It is known that in septic shock and experimental endotoxemia, the synthesis of adenosine triphosphate (ATP) is improved and the fall in 2,3-DPG level may merely reflect the accumulation of AMP and ADP in the red cell as part of a widespread metabolic upset.

The final two possibilities to account for the decreased oxygen uptake in septic shock are arteriovenous shunting and a primary cellular defect caused by a direct effect of sepsis. Using the model of Clowes et al.[19] to produce hyperdynamic septic shock in dogs, Wright et al.[20] measured cardiac output, blood flow in skeletal muscle, oxygen uptake and femoral and total arteriovenous oxygen differences. Muscle blood flow was determined by Xenon-133 clearance which measures only tissue capillary flow. There was a highly significant correlation between the rise in cardiac index and the increased muscle blood flow in animals with hyperdynamic sepsis, demonstrating that no capillary arteriovenous shunting was taking place but that the decreased oxygen uptake was likely due to a primary cellular defect. The hyperdynamic circulation is probably a compensatory mechanism to increase flow and oxygen supply to those deficient cells.

In summary, the patient with hyperdynamic septic shock presents with hyperventilation, a low blood pressure, rapid pulse, high CVP, low urine flow, high cardiac index, low peripheral resistance, normal hematocrit, narrow arteriovenous oxygen difference, low oxygen uptake, mild lacticacidosis and, if seen early, respiratory alkalosis, but later when the prognosis is poor uncompensated metabolic acidosis (Table 10-3).

Hypodynamic septic shock presents as hypovolemic shock, with the addition of narrow arteriovenous oxygen difference and subnormal oxygen uptake, indicating a cellular defect in addition to the consequences of hypovolemia.

THE LUNG LESION IN SHOCK

Interstitial or diffuse air space pulmonary edema can be the result of sepsis, fat embolism, cardiac failure, lung contusion or oxygen toxicity. The resulting pulmonary insufficiency is a major cause of death in injured patients and patients receiving intensive care.[21] A single cause for "shock lung" has not been described, and any or all of the above may be implicated. The lung lesion which occurs with septic shock is usually sudden in onset and for that reason easier to study.

McLean et al.[22] described 24 patients with septic shock who presented with pulmonary insufficiency within hours of the onset of shock. All patients were treated in an intensive care unit, and determinations were made serially of the eight key measurements. In one patient, measurements were made of pulmonary artery pressure and pulmonary capillary wedge pressure during a period of shock associated with pulmonary edema. In 17 of the 24 patients, pulmonary edema was present. This varied from early interstitial edema to massive, diffuse edema involving air spaces. In only three could this be accounted for on the basis of congestive heart failure. The CVP was elevated to 23, 22 and 21 cm. of water in these three patients. In the remaining 14 patients, the CVP was 12 cm. of water or less. In one patient, with a low CVP and massive pulmonary edema, the pulmonary capillary wedge pressure was also low. In 16 of the 17 patients who presented with pulmonary edema and septic shock, the serum albumin was normal.

The pulmonary edema seen on radiologic examination was associated with a severe decline in arterial blood oxygen tension. This did not rise to normal on breathing 50 to 100 per cent oxygen. In all, severe shunting in the lung resulting from ventilation-perfusion admixture was thought the best explanation for the persistent hypoxia. The pulmonary edema in septic shock on the basis of these observations, i.e., a normal CVP and normal serum albumin, must be attributed to increased pulmonary capillary permeability. One might expect the pulmonary lesion to account for a failure of oxygen uptake by these patients. In fact, this appears to be a minifestation of impaired peripheral utilization. Raising the arterial blood oxygen tension does not increase oxygen uptake nor does it lower the arterial blood lactate concentration in these patients.

Lowery et al.[23] have produced a model in the pig to study the lung lesion in hemorrhagic shock and have shown the onset of pathologic lesions in the lung and hypoxemia only after the return of shed blood. This suggests that blood products might be of importance in the etiology of the shock lung.

Treatment of Septic Shock

The treatment of septic shock is much more difficult than treatment of either hypovolemia or cardiogenic shock and must appear to us now as traumatic shock did to Archibald and McLean[6] in World War I.

Prophylaxis. Antibiotics. This therapy has not reduced the incidence of infection with complicating septicemia. Furthermore, intensive or prolonged antibiotic therapy permits the emergence of antibiotic resistant strains of gram-negative bacteria and their invasion of the blood stream.[24] Most studies of the use of prophylactic antibiotics in surgery are not definitive. One excellent, prospective, double-blind decisive study by Polk and Lopez-Mayor on patients undergoing elective surgery on the gastrointestinal tract strongly supports the use of prophylactic antibiotics.[25] They advise the prophylactic use of cephaloridine, 1 gm. intramuscularly on call to surgery, and at five hours and 12 hours postoperatively. This short course avoided toxicity, provided a high blood level at the time of risk, did not result in emergence of resistant strains and greatly lowered the infection rate in clean contaminated cases. Prophylactic antibiotics are not bad; it is the regimens of use that have been faulty.

Hemodynamic Stability. Although not proved, one has the strong conviction that regulation to normal of the eight key measurements before surgery decreases the incidence of postoperative sepsis and shock.

Avoidance of Tracheostomy. It is not established that positive pressure ventilation will elevate arterial pO_2 over that accomplished by mask delivery except when hypoventilation as evidenced by a elevated arterial pCO_2 exists or when exhaustion is imminent. The incidence of pneumonia and septicemia is high after tracheostomy.

In-line bacterial filters for intravenous feedings. This safety measure is now being evaluated in patients who require centrally placed catheters for hyperalimentation or the measurement of pressure and may be of prophylactic value.

Urinary bladder irrigation. The urinary tract is still a frequent source of gram-negative septicemia. Continuous irrigation via a "three-way" catheter using 1 L. of saline containing 40 mg. of neomycin and 200,000 units of polymyxin B each 24 hours provides good antibacterial coverage.

AN INFECTION CONTROL COMMITTEE. This committee in the hospital can control a large number of procedures to lower the infection rate.

Treatment. EARLY RECOGNITION. Table 10-4 illustrates the early signs of septic shock. Hyperventilation is a particularly valuable warning sign. Mortality of sepsis is decreased when recognized before the onset of shock.[24]

APPROPRIATE ANTIBIOTICS. Altemeier et al.[24] have showed in a large series of patients a mortality rate of 54 per cent for sepsis when the patient was placed on an inappropriate antibiotic and 28 per cent when an appropriate antibiotic guided by culture sensitivities was used.

RESTORATION OF NORMAL HEMODYNAMICS. A higher than normal cardiac output with normal filling pressure and normal hematocrit should be sought. This may require blood, saline, isoproterenol or all three. Unfortunately, many patients die of a cellular defect despite this treatment. However, the survival rate is better in patients who are capable of elevating their cardiac index 1 L./min./m.[2] than in those who are incapable of this with treatment.[17]

DRAINAGE OF ABSCESSES. Patients who have a septic source amenable to surgical treatment and who are treated surgically have a better prognosis than patients who do not satisfy this criterion. Adequate and continuous drainage of abscesses and fistulae of the gastrointestinal tract is best accomplished using continuous suction with air-vent catheters.

Decompression of the small intestine via a long tube without enterostomy is important in small bowel obstruction to lower the incidence of peritonitis and sepsis.

CORTICOSTEROIDS. This therapy, although not of proved value, is widely used. The basis for the large doses used (50–150 mg./kg. of hydrocortisone in a single bolus) is threefold. First, clinical observation suggests benefit, particularly in pulmonary and renal function. Second, steroids stabilize cellular and subcellular membranes. The most important of the organelles are the lysosomes, which may release hydrolytic enzymes that adversely affect the mitochondria which in inactivity prevent oxygen utilization. Third, corticosteroids stabilize the membranous portion of the microcirculation. A summary of the large literature on this subject, which generally supports the use of steroids, especially in septic shock, appears in a recent monograph.[26]

REFERENCES

1. Blalock, A.: Experimental shock; the cause of the low blood pressure produced by muscle injury. Arch. Surg. 20:959, 1930.

2. Parsons, E., and Phemister, D. B.: Haemorrhage and "shock" in traumatized limbs: An experimental study. Surg. Gynec. & Obst. 51:196, 1930.
3. MacLean, L. D., Duff, J. H., Scott, H. M., and Peretz, D. I.: Treatment of shock in man based on hemodynamic diagnosis. Surg. Gynec. & Obst. 120:1, 1965.
4. Nunn, J. F., and Freeman, J.: Problems of oxygenation and oxygen transport during haemorrhage. Anaesthesia 19:206, 1964.
5. Harkins, H. N., and Rhoads, J. E.: Shock; in Rhoads, J. E., Allen, J. G., Harkins, H. N., and Moyer, C. A. (eds.): Surgery, Principles and Practice. 4th Ed. Philadelphia, J. B. Lippincott Co., 1970, pp. 121–148.
6. Archibald, E. W., and McLean, W. S.: Observations upon shock, with particular reference to the condition as seen in war surgery. Ann. Surg. 66:280, 1917.
7. Howard, J. M., and Brown, R. B.: Military Surgery; in Rhoads, J. E., Allen, J. G., Harkins, H. N., and Moyer, C. A. (eds.): Surgery, Principles and Practice. 4th Ed. Philadelphia, J. B. Lippincott Co., 1970, pp. 599–648.
8. Jacobson, E. D.: A physiologic approach to shock. N. Eng. J. Med. 278:834, 1968.
9. Cannon, W. B.: Acidosis in cases of shock, haemorrhage and gas infection. J.A.M.A. 70:531, 1918.
10. Peretz, D. I., McGregor, M., and Dossetor, J. B.: Lacticacidosis: a clinically significant aspect of shock. Canad. M. A. J. 90:673, 1964.
11. Crowell, J. W., and Guyton, A. C.: Further evidence favoring a cardiac mechanism in irreversible hemorrhagic shock. Amer. J. Physiol. 203:248, 1962.
12. Zborowska-Sluis, D. T., and Dossetor, J. B.: Hyperlactatemia of hyperventilation. J. Appl. Physiol. 22:746, 1967.
13. Cain, S. M.: Effect of pCO$_2$ on the relation of lactate and excess lactate to O$_2$ deficit. Amer. J. Physiol. 214:1322, 1968.
14. Baue, A. E., Tragus, E. T., Wolfson, S. K., Cary, A. L., and Parkins, W. M.: Hemodynamic and metabolic effects of Ringer's lactate solution in hemorrhagic shock. Ann. Surg. 166:29, 1967.
15. McLean, A. P. H., Mulligan, G. W., Otton, P., and MacLean, L. D.: Hemodynamic alterations associated with epidural anesthesia. Surgery 62:79, 1967.
16. Duff, J. H., Malave, G., Peretz, D. I., Scott, H. M., and MacLean, L. D.: The hemodynamics of septic shock in man and in the dog. Surgery 58:174, 1965.
17. MacLean, L. D., Mulligan, W. G., McLean, A. P. H., and Duff, J. H.: Patterns of septic shock in man—a detailed study of 56 patients. Ann. Surg. 166:543, 1967.
18. Miller, L. D., Oski, F. A., Diaco, J. F., Sugerman, H. J., Gottlieb, A. J., and Delivoria, P. M.: The affinity of hemoglobin for oxygen: its control and in vivo significance. Surgery 68:187, 1970.
19. Clowes, G. H., Zuschneid, W., Turner, M., Blackburn, G., Rubin, J., Toala, P., and Green, G.: Observations on the pathogenesis of the pneumonitis associated with severe infections in other parts of the body. Ann. Surg. 167:630, 1968.
20. Wright, C. J., Duff, J. H., and MacLean, L. D.: Regional capillary blood flow in severe sepsis. Surg. Gynec. & Obst. 132:637, 1971.
21. Moore, F. D., Lyons, J. H., Pierce, E. C., Morgan, A. P., Drinker, P. A., MacArthur, J. D., and Dammin, G. J.: Post-traumatic pulmonary insufficiency. Philadelphia, W. B. Saunders Co., 1969.
22. McLean, A. P. H., Duff, J. H., and MacLean, L. D.: Lung lesions associated with septic shock. J. Trauma 8:891, 1968.
23. Lowery, B. D., Mulder, D. S., Jayal, E. M., and Palmer, W. H.: The effect of hemorrhagic shock on the lung of the pig. Surg. Forum 21:21, 1970.
24. Altemeier, W. A., Todd, J. C., and Inge, W. W.: Gram-negative septicemia: a growing threat. Ann. Surg. 166:530, 1967.
25. Polk, H. C., and Lopez-Mayor, J. F.: Post-operative wound infection: a prospective study of determinant factors and prevention. Surgery 66:97, 1969.
26. Schumer, W., and Nyhus, L. M.: Corticosteroids in the treatment of shock. Urbana, Ill., University of Illinois Press, 1970.

CHAPTER 11

RENAL FUNCTION AND RENAL FAILURE

SAMUEL R. POWERS, JR., M.D.

Renal function is said to be normal when the internal environment is maintained within sharply defined limits. Maintenance of a normal internal environment requires that various metabolic products be selectively cast out of the body while normal constituents are carefully preserved. The kidney accomplishes the removal of these metabolic products in a remarkably inefficient manner. First the glomeruli of the kidney permit the escape of a quantity of water equal to the entire body water stores every eight hours of each day and, with this, the entire body supply of sodium and other essential dissolved substances. This enormous quantity of water and dissolved materials, amounting to approximately 200 liters per 24 hours, must then be actively resorbed back into the circulation, at considerable energy cost, by the tubular mechanism. Normal renal function will only be present, therefore, when the kidney is first capable of discarding the entire internal environment and then selectively resorbing the 99 per cent which is necessary for survival, leaving for excretion the tiny fraction of metabolic waste. In a sense, the kidney operates on the presumption that it is best to throw out the baby with the bath water and then go outside to pick up the baby and bring him back into the house.

There are, therefore, two control systems required to regulate the kidney; one determines the quantity discarded and the other the exact proportion of this which will be resorbed.

The first mechanism acts by control of glomerular filtration rate, and the second by governing the resorption of sodium, water or both. If a insufficient quantity of extracellular fluid fails to pass through the glomeruli into the tubular lumen, then no amount of tubular function can maintain the levels of urea, creatinine and other metabolic end products at a normal level in the blood. Likewise, if tubular function is

impaired, then the enormously complex job of putting the lost extracellular fluid back into the body may not be carried out. Evaluation of
these two systems, glomerular filtration and tubular resorption, constitutes the methods of assessing renal function. Disorders of renal
function will be considered as representing (1) the normal functioning
of these systems operating to preserve the organism in the face of a
disordered internal environment, or (2) a breakdown of the systems
owing to specific organ failure.

The quantity of glomerular filtrate depends upon the hydrostatic
pressure gradient between the glomerular capillary lumen and the
space of Bowman's capsule. If this gradient is less than approximately
40 mm. of mercury, then all filtration ceases and no fluid enters the
tubular lumen. It is apparent that, since this is a simple mechanical
process governed by hydrostatic laws, there would tend to be a wide
variation in the quantity of glomerular filtrate, with alterations in systemic blood pressure. These alterations may occur as a result of hemorrhage, surgical stress, dehydration, or other factors. In order to minimize the wide fluctuations that would take place in an uncontrolled
system, the kidney has developed a highly specialized control mechanism which keeps the quantity of glomerular filtrate remarkably constant over wide ranges of systemic blood pressure. This control mechanism, known as autoregulation, acts by controlling the vasomotor tone
in the afferent and efferent arterioles. Whatever the exact mechanism
may be, this, like any other control system, requires a comparator to
monitor the product being operated upon, and a control mechanism to
adjust the product to a predetermined set point. Increasing evidence
suggests that the product being tested is the concentration of sodium at
the end of the tubule and that this is measured by the cells of the
macula densa. The rate of glomerular filtration is then adjusted so as to
bring the sodium concentration back to an optimal value for that particular situation.

Estimations of the quantity of glomerular filtrate can be obtained
by measuring the quantity in the urine of a dissolved substance which
is not resorbed by the tubular mechanism. Creatinine is such a substance, and therefore every milliliter of glomerular filtrate contains precisely the same quantity of creatinine as 1 ml. of plasma. Thus, if the
concentration of creatinine in plasma is 1 mg. per 100 ml., and the total
quantity of creatinine excreted in the urine in a 24 hour period is 1 gm.,
then it is clear that 100 liters of plasma must have passed through the
tubular mechanism to provide this quantity. This value, spoken of as
creatinine clearance, is an excellent and simple measure of the quantity
of glomerular filtration in a given period of time.

Normal tubular function accomplishes the resorbing of the vast
quantities of water and dissolved electrolytes which have been lost
through the glomeruli. Resorption of water will clearly result in a
change in concentration of dissolved materials in the tubular lumen and

will be reflected by the urine-plasma concentration ratio of substances such as creatinine or urea. Since sodium is also absorbed from the urine, it is entirely possible for the concentration of dissolved materials in the urine to actually be less than that of plasma, and indeed, under certain circumstances a hypotonic urine may result. The important point here is that tubular function alters both the amount of water and the concentration of dissolved materials and makes them different from plasma. Measurement of tubular function is therefore best carried out by determining the urine-plasma ratio of some substance or substances and finding that it is different from unity. Because of the variability of individual dissolved materials, the most useful measurement appears to be the urine–plasma osmolar ratio, because this method measures the ratio of the concentration of all dissolved materials.

In certain circumstances such as a decreased sodium intake to the body, it is desirable that adjustments be made to allow a greater conservation of sodium stores. On the other hand, following a period of dietary sodium excess it is equally desirable that some control mechanism permit the excretion of the increased filtered sodium load. The control of sodium resorption in addition to fluctuations in glomerular filtration, as mentioned above, is also influenced by the hormone aldosterone. It is now generally agreed that the quantity of circulating aldosterone is determined by the level of angiotensin in the blood, which in turn is determined by the secretion of renin by the kidney. It is interesting that renin granules are found in the juxtaglomerular apparatus adjacent to the sodium-sensing cells of the macula densa available for release into the circulation in response to changes in sodium concentration. Nature thus provides two mechanisms for controlling the excretion of sodium; first, the total quantity of sodium delivered to the tubules is influenced by glomerular filtration rate, and, second, the quantity of sodium resorbed back into the circulation is determined by the circulating level of aldosterone and its effect upon the tubular cell.

The final renal control mechanism that appears to be of clinical importance in the surgical patient is associated with the excretion of water. The antidiuretic hormone of the posterior pituitary gland (ADH) appears to act on the collecting tubules by governing the amount of water which can pass through these cells back into the blood stream. It will be recalled that as a result of tubular activity the fluid in the bottom of the loop of Henle as well as the interstitial fluid surrounding it in the depths of the renal medulla is markedly hypertonic. Therefore when urine passes down the collecting tubule through the renal medulla, there is an osmotic force of considerable magnitude acting to pull water from the collecting tubules. ADH acts by governing the rate at which this absorption takes place. Release of antidiuretic hormone and its consequent facilitation of water resorption may occur from a number of causes but is seen most frequently in the clinical setting of acute volume depletion. It is important to realize that antidiuretic hormone

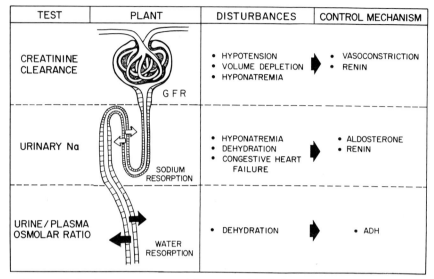

TEST	PLANT	DISTURBANCES	CONTROL MECHANISM
CREATININE CLEARANCE	GFR	• HYPOTENSION • VOLUME DEPLETION • HYPONATREMIA	• VASOCONSTRICTION • RENIN
URINARY Na	SODIUM RESORPTION	• HYPONATREMIA • DEHYDRATION • CONGESTIVE HEART FAILURE	• ALDOSTERONE • RENIN
URINE/PLASMA OSMOLAR RATIO	WATER RESORPTION	• DEHYDRATION	• ADH

Figure 11-1. The three principal functions of the kidney. Filtration, sodium absorption and water absorption are considered as "plants" that react to disturbances of the internal environment. The control systems are separate but interrelated.

can act only when there is a large osmotic gradient between urine and plasma, that is, in association with normal tubular function. Failure of the tubules to establish an increased concentration of solutes, or alternatively, the administration of an increased solute load, such as an osmotic diuretic, can eliminate the concentration gradient across the collecting tubule and limit or negate the effect of antidiuretic hormone.

Normal renal function can, therefore, be described as the interaction of glomerular filtration, tubular activity and water resorption; both of these processes fall under the command of interrelated feedback control systems (Fig. 11-1).

THE ASSESSMENT OF RENAL FUNCTION

The response of the kidney to various therapeutic maneuvers provides a reliable guide to the state of renal function. Alteration of the input to any system, biological or physical, will produce a change in output that can provide useful information concerning the system under study. Renal function under one set of conditions and at any one instant in time provides little reliable information concerning the status of the kidneys. The urine volume may be abnormally high in conditions in which glomerular filtration rate is reduced to the point of renal failure and the increased urine volume represents a supplemental failure of tubular function. Likewise, an abnormally low urine volume may occur in the presence of perfectly normal kidneys. In the same manner, a low blood pressure in the range of 90 mm. Hg may be associated with perfectly normal renal perfusion, whereas under circumstances such as the crush syndrome a normal blood pressure may be associated with severe renal vasoconstriction and almost complete cessation of glomerular filtration. In each of these situations, however, the response to an administered fluid load is characteristic of the state of the organism at the time the fluid is administered and is frequently diagnostic of the underlying condition.

It is important to emphasize that no single response can be considered as a reliable guide, but rather that the response of the entire organism should be considered. In the face of severe volume depletion, the patient will generally be oliguric with a rapid heart rate and a low central venous pressure. The administration of isotonic saline solution at a rate of 400 to 500 ml. per hour will immediately provide information concerning the overall status of the patient. If dehydration is in fact present, the central venous pressure will remain low in spite of the rapid rate of infusion, but the pulse rate will likely come down and urine output will at least transiently improve. On the other hand, an increase in central venous pressure with the first 300 to 500 ml. of infused fluid, especially if this is accompanied by a failure to increase urine output, suggests that fluid volume is normal or slightly expanded and that the difficulty lies elsewhere. Frequent determinations of the serum sodium concentration are likewise of great importance, because failure of the serum sodium concentration to increase following an infusion of isotonic saline suggests overall volume depletion. Such a load in a normally hydrated individual will result in either a marked increase in sodium excretion in the urine or an increase in the serum sodium level. In either case, the test infusion provides valuable information concerning the state of the patient.

A word should be said concerning the measurement of central venous pressure. Although this technique is frequently carried out, it is not always appreciated that the details are so important that, if they are not rigidly adhered to, the measurement can be misleading and even dangerous. The term central venous pressure means that the tip of the catheter must be in either the vena cava or the right atrium. Certain knowledge of this position can be obtained only by means of a chest x-ray. Measurements of the distance that a catheter is inserted are totally unreliable, because catheters introduced through the arm may pass up the jugular vein into the jugular bulb or downward into the abdomen, lodging in the hepatic veins or in certain cases even in the renal veins. It is a part of the technique of central venous pressure monitoring to include a chest x-ray to ascertain the position of the catheter. The bed must be completely flat, because changes in position of the patient exert a variable gravitational effect on the manometer and may provide totally erroneous results. In addition, the bottom of the manometer must be placed at the level of the midaxillary line and, of more importance, should be repositioned to the same point each time the central venous pressure is measured. If the measurement is carried out in this way, the response of central venous pressure to fluid therapy can be a useful clinical guide.

The accurate and continuous measurement of urine volume is essential in the management of any patient with suspected renal failure. The risk of an indwelling urethral catheter must be accepted in order to obtain the moment-to-moment information concerning urine output which is essential for the successful management of these cases. Modern collecting devices provide a closed system between the catheter and a graduated measuring flask, which can be emptied from the bottom without disconnecting the catheter. In this way, the danger of gross contamination is minimized while still providing the necessary monitoring facility.

Persistent oliguria below 25 ml. per hour for more than two hours constitutes a true medical emergency requiring the most urgent and aggressive corrective therapy. Oliguria produces the clinical setting in which renal cell necrosis may develop. Failure of the urine volume to increase with a fluid load, especially if associated with an increase in central venous pressure, indicates that the normal renal control systems may no longer be operative. Determination of the urine–plasma osmolar ratio will provide an answer to this question. This determination can be carried out in most laboratories, but if the equipment is not available, the urine-plasma-urea ratio may also be used.

The finding of identical concentrations of dissolved materials in both plasma and urine is proof that acute renal failure has taken place. It needs to be emphasized that renal failure may occur in the presence of a diminished urine volume, in the face of complete anuria, or with a normal or excessive urine output.

It is the quality rather than quantity of the urine that provides the diagnostic information. The ratio of creatinine in the urine to that of the plasma provides a rough index to the state of tubular function. If the creatinine concentration in the urine is only twice that in plasma, one may assume that approximately half the glomerular filtrate has been resorbed. To put this in a slightly different manner, the glomerular filtration rate was twice the urine volume. Under these circumstances, measures designed to increase glomerular filtration rate will improve the ability of the kidney to clear nitrogenous wastes, although in the face of severely disturbed tubular function this cannot approach a normal state.

There is a transition phase between depression of renal function by a normally acting control mechanism and the beginning breakdown of renal function that is spoken of as functional renal failure. An opportunity to reverse the chain of events leading to renal cell death exists during this period. The rationale for pharmacologic manipulation of the renal control mechanisms in the prevention of acute renal failure is predicated on a knowledge of the sequence of events which leads through the period of functional renal failure to renal shutdown.

Much of the recent information concerning the development of acute renal failure has come from studies of regional renal blood flow carried out using the radioactive gas washout technique. The principle of this technique consists in delivering a quantity of highly diffusible material into the kidney by means of an injection in the renal artery and then following the rate at which the material is removed from the renal parenchyma. If the solubility of the diffusible gas in blood is known, then the rate at which the substance is removed depends only on the quantity of blood flowing through the tissue. When the diffusible gas is radioactive, then the measurements of rate of removal can be carried out with an external scintillation detector. An example of a normal washout is shown in Figure 11–2, along with the technique of analysis. The most important feature of the analysis is the three different slopes or three different washout rates. This implies that there are three different rates of blood flow through different portions of the kidney, and indeed, it is the variations among these regions that appear to be of paramount importance in the pathogenesis of renal failure. Redistribution of blood flow between the outer cortex, the juxtamedullary area and the medulla is a constant finding during the development of experimental renal failure. Studies have been carried out which suggest that hypotension and dehydration can result in selective ischemia of the outer portions of the cortex of the kidney. This portion is the site not only of many of the glomeruli, but also of the peritubular capillaries which surround the distal tubule, the site of the maximal damage in acute renal failure. The occurrence of selective vasoconstriction in the outer cortex suggests that this portion of the kidney has a blood supply different from that of the bulk of the cortex. It seems likely that the autoregulatory mechanism in the kidney preserves blood flow through portions of the juxtamedullary cortex while allowing other portions of the cortex to become selectively ischemic. If this condition is allowed to persist, acute renal failure may well develop. The key to reversal of functional renal failure toward normal lies in restoring blood flow to the superficial portions of the cortex along with the blood supply to the distal tubule. This is carried out by deliberately manipulating the feedback control system that appears to govern glomerular filtration rate in this portion of the kidney.

It will be recalled that the sodium concentration in the distal tubule appears to be a determinant factor in the control of glomerular filtration rate, especially following a period of hypotension. The decrease in blood pressure results in a decreased filtration into the tubule, and hence a fall in the sodium load. Tubular urine which has passed through the loop of Henle arrives with a very low sodium concentration, and in some manner this signals to the control system that volume must be conserved so that a further reduction in glomerular filtration occurs in these nephrons. If the sodium concentration in the distal tubule could be artificially increased, a false signal would be provided to the control mechanism suggesting that conditions were actually satis-

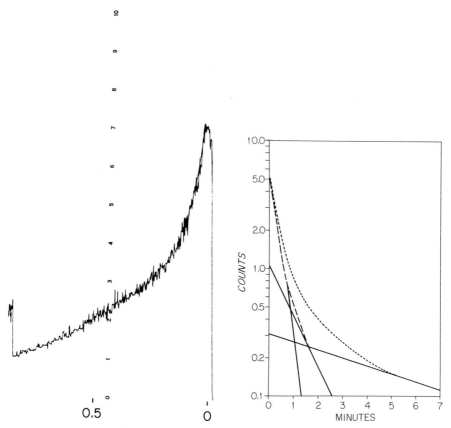

Figure 11–2. Technique of exponential stripping to determine the separate blood flow rates in three different areas of the kidney. The dotted line represents the original tracings as transferred from the count rate meter. The compartments with the most rapid blood flow have been completely cleared of the radioactive xenon by five minutes. Therefore, a straight line can be drawn from five minutes to the end of the washout period representing the rate of blood flow through only the compartment with lowest blood flow. Extrapolating the straight line to zero time allows the number of counts at any time which are due to the slowest compartment to be accurately known and subtracted from the initial curve. The dashed line represents the second curve, and it will be seen that after about two minutes the fastest compartment is completely washed out and a new straight line can be drawn which represents the rate of washout of the intermediate compartment. Extrapolation of this line by a second solid line back to zero time permits subtraction of the intermediate compartment, leaving only the most rapid compartment indicated by the solid line with a washout between zero and one and a half minutes. The three solid lines, therefore, represent the rate of blood flow through the three compartments within the kidney.

factory and that glomerular filtration rate could be maintained. Modern pharmacologic therapy, using either the osmotic diuretic mannitol or one of the loop diuretics such as ethacrynic acid or furosemide, appears to protect the kidney from tubular necrosis by artificially increasing sodium concentration in the distal tubule.

Variations in renal function seen in the surgical patient can be divided into two large groups. The first consists of variations that represent an appropriate response of the renal control mechanisms to an abnormal physiologic stress; the second consists of failure of the renal control systems resulting from damage or inappropriate action. The distinction between these two conditions may be clinically obscure, because in each case there may result a low or a high urine volume, and the urine may consist of dilute or concentrated fluid. The distinction is clearly important, because on the one hand a superbly functioning system is carrying out its appointed task, and on the other a pathologic state which can lead to the death of the patient is taking place. The distinction hinges on the ratio of concentrations of dissolved material between plasma and urine being different from unity. Normal responses are invariably associated with some processing of the glomerular filtrate during its passage through the tubular system. This processing may result in a urine that is more or less concentrated than plasma, but can never result in a urine whose composition is identical with that of plasma.

Evidence of tubular activity is given by the result of the transport of sodium ions out of the tubular lumen back into the interstitial fluid of the kidney and into the blood stream. Disorders of renal function that represent normally functioning control mechanisms can, therefore, be considered under the general headings of those mechanisms which control sodium excretion. The quantity of sodium excreted in the urine depends, first, on the rate of glomerular filtration, that is, on the quantity of sodium deposited in the tubules, and, second, on the presence of the hormone aldosterone, which governs the rate of sodium resorption. The concentration of sodium in the urine depends also on the amount of water excreted with the sodium, and this in turn is controlled by the antidiuretic hormone.

DISORDERED RENAL FUNCTION DUE TO DECREASES IN GLOMERULAR FILTRATION RATE

Glomerular filtration rate is measured in milliliters per minute and is a quantitative statement of the amount of fluid that must have passed through the glomeruli to account for the quantity of a nonresorbable substance such as creatinine, which appears in the urine. It will be recalled that if 100 mg. of creatinine appears in the urine in one minute and the plasma concentration is 1 mg. per milliliter, then 100 ml. of plasma per minute must have been filtered through the glomeruli. It is clear that the quantity of plasma which is filtered will depend on the total quantity of blood perfusing the kidney, but it is not so obvious that the quantity which passes across the glomerular capillary membrane depends on the difference in resistance of the afferent and efferent arterioles. It is this latter variation in resistance that enables the kidney to maintain glomerular filtration rate at a nearly constant level in spite of wide fluctuations in systemic arterial blood pressure. Studies in experimental animals and man suggest that a fall in blood pressure down to a level of around 80 mm. Hg is not associated with a significant change in glomerular filtration rate, whereas a fall in blood pressure below this produces a precipitous decline. When glomerular filtration rate falls, there is a marked fall in the sodium concentration of the urine. Under extreme circumstances as little as 2 mEq. of sodium per liter of urine may be lost, indicating a maximal tubular effort. If the quantity of a metabolic end product such as urea is produced faster than it is cleared into the glomerulus, the blood level of this substance will rise. This rise may occur in the presence of normal tubular function.

Decreases in glomerular filtration rate occur not only in the shock state when the blood pressure is below 80 mm. of mercury, but occur also if there is a marked decrease in the state of hydration of the individual. This decrease occurs even though blood pressure is normal and represents further evidence of normal function of the control system for conserving water and electrolytes. The location and mode of action of these volume receptors is unknown at the present time, but it is clear that the total body water can be maintained within narrow limits through this mechanism.

The aforementioned considerations suggest that severe oliguria and even increased concentration of waste materials in the blood stream may be a normal response of the kidney in the face of markedly decreased blood pressure, total body water depletion and severe hyponatremia. In all such circumstances the urine-plasma-urea ratio will be high and markedly different from unity.

The therapy for an acute decrease in glomerular filtration rate is to correct the disordered internal environment. This frequently entails correction of the quality as well as the quantity of the extracellular space. Replacement of a diminished ECF must be carried out by an electrolyte solution. The administration of dextrose in water or of half normal saline is a practice to be deprecated. ECF depletion requires ECF replacement.

DYSFUNCTION DUE TO SODIUM RESORPTION

Sodium restriction, especially when accompanied by water restriction for even a few hours, may result in activation of the aldosterone mechanism. This is another example of a normal control system that acts to enhance sodium resorption under circumstances in which further loss of sodium from the body would represent a threat to survival. This is considered a disorder of renal function, because a normally functioning kidney will excrete almost any administered sodium load. Inability to excrete excess administered sodium poses a potential threat in the postoperative period.

The mechanism for activation of aldosterone appears to depend on the release of renin from the kidney with its subsequent action on a plasma globulin to produce angiotensin. The control mechanism is again the cells of the macula densa in the distal tubule which appear to detect alterations in sodium concentration and to govern the release of renin granules from the juxtaglomerular apparatus. This mechanism is of considerable clinical importance because of its relatively long time of action. The release of aldosterone from the adrenal cortex requires several hours from the time of sodium depletion. Once this substance has been released, it will continue to circulate for a period of many hours or even days, and during this time the ability of the kidney to excrete sodium is markedly reduced. The clinical implications of this are apparent when one considers that the release of aldosterone is initiated by a sodium lack, but when sodium is replaced intravenously the kidney is unable to excrete quantities which may result in serious sodium overloading. Patients with congestive heart failure and expanded extracellular volumes may well suffer from such aldosterone effects, especially if they are prepared for surgery by a period of fasting and dehydration. Attempts to restore sodium balance by the intravenous administration of sodium chloride solutions can easily result in further overexpansion of the extracellular space owing to the kidney's inability to excrete the administered sodium load. This control mechanism has undoubted survival value in situations in which sodium cannot be readily replaced. Unfortunately the ability of the physician to administer sodium chloride by vein is an unanticipated bit of human meddling which removes the necessity and even the survival value of this control system. Sodium retention as a result of activation of aldosterone might be considered as a failure by the physician to understand and correctly manipulate internal environment to the advantage of his patient. The preoperative intravenous administration of salt and water will assure that the patient enters the stress of surgery with the sodium control mechanism set for free excretion of sodium ion. Continued administration of electrolyte solution during the course of surgery will prevent the activation of the renin-angiotension-aldosterone axis with its consequent restrictions for intravenous fluid therapy and undesirable sodium retention.

DYSFUNCTION DUE TO APPROPRIATE RELEASE OF ADH

This control mechanism is designed to preserve water in the face of water depletion and acts independently of the excretion of dissolved

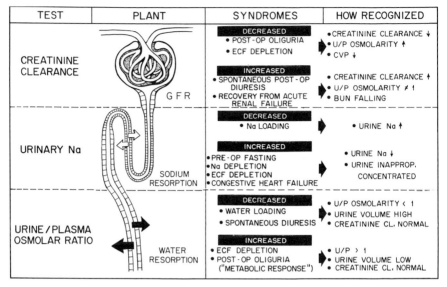

TEST	PLANT	SYNDROMES	HOW RECOGNIZED
CREATININE CLEARANCE	G F R	**DECREASED** • POST-OP OLIGURIA • ECF DEPLETION	• CREATININE CLEARANCE ↓ • U/P OSMOLARITY ↑ • CVP ↓
		INCREASED • SPONTANEOUS POST-OP DIURESIS • RECOVERY FROM ACUTE RENAL FAILURE	• CREATININE CLEARANCE ↑ • U/P OSMOLARITY ≠ ↑ • BUN FALLING
URINARY Na	SODIUM RESORPTION	**DECREASED** • Na LOADING	• URINE Na ↑
		INCREASED • PRE-OP FASTING • Na DEPLETION • ECF DEPLETION • CONGESTIVE HEART FAILURE	• URINE Na ↓ • URINE INAPPROP. CONCENTRATED
URINE / PLASMA OSMOLAR RATIO	WATER RESORPTION	**DECREASED** • WATER LOADING • SPONTANEOUS DIURESIS	• U/P OSMOLARITY < 1 • URINE VOLUME HIGH • CREATININE CL. NORMAL
		INCREASED • ECF DEPLETION • POST-OP OLIGURIA ("METABOLIC RESPONSE")	• U/P > 1 • URINE VOLUME LOW • CREATININE CL. NORMAL

Figure 11-3. Alterations in renal function which result from a normal kidney acting to correct or preserve an abnormal internal environment. The quantity and quality of urine are appropriate for preserving the entire organism but may if uncorrected result in renal damage.

material. ADH can be effective only when the countercurrent mechanism of tubular urine concentration is functioning normally and a high osmotic gradient exists across the collecting duct. ADH acts by facilitating the transfer of water across this duct and can markedly reduce the urine volume. It is important to realize that since the transfer of water is passive and under the influence of an osmotic difference, there is a limit beyond which further water cannot be resorbed, namely, when the concentration of dissolved materials in the collecting ductule becomes equal to the concentration in the interstitial fluid. For this reason the oliguria seen in the presence of ADH does not fall to a level that simulates acute renal failure.

A normal-functioning renal parenchyma can, therefore, produce urine of high or low specific gravity and in high or low quantities. The normal kidney, however, will rarely if ever produce a urine volume of less than 15 ml. per hour, and under no circumstances will it produce a urine whose concentration of dissolved material is identical with that of plasma (Fig. 11-3).

ALTERATIONS OF FUNCTION DUE TO FAILURE OR INAPPROPRIATE ACTION OF RENAL CONTROL SYSTEMS (Fig. 11-4)

The control systems mentioned above are designed to preserve the integrity of the internal environment under conditions of stress and are predicated on a normally functioning renal cell mass. Under conditions in which profound hypotension, severe renal vasoconstriction, the presence of abnormal protein pigments, and perhaps other unknown factors are present, acute renal failure may develop. During the period of renal functional deterioration these control mechanisms may have a severely deleterious effect on the kidney in an attempt to preserve the integrity of the internal environment. The distinction here is important, namely, that the control mechanisms are designed to preserve the organism as a whole even at the expense of renal damage. Under these circumstances, it is to the advantage of the physician to deliberately alter the control mechanism response because the organism can be preserved by resuscitative methods and the prime requirement is the maintenance of renal function. We have indicated in earlier sections that alterations in the internal environment which produce a decrease in the sodium concentration of the distal tubule may result in further reductions in glomerular filtration rate, and that, in addition, this may be accompanied by regional shifts in renal blood flow which produce progressive ischemia of the outer cortex and medullary portions. Figure 11-5 depicts the Xe washout curve from a dog in profound hypovolemic shock. When compared with Figure 11-2 it is apparent that Xe removal is markedly slowed. In addition a "compartment analysis" indicates the principal reduction in flow to be in the outer cortex. If a false signal, namely, an increase in sodium concentration in the distal tubule, can be artificially produced, then those controls that tend to reduce glomeru-

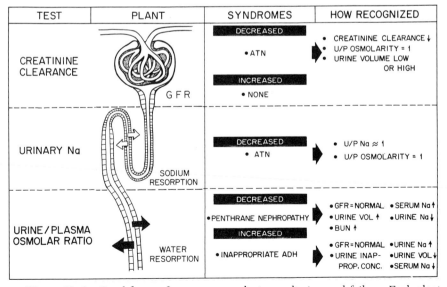

Figure 11-4. Breakdown of one or more plants results in renal failure. Each plant requires adequate function of the previous plant for its own activity, i.e., water resorption cannot occur unless the tubular mechanism is operative.

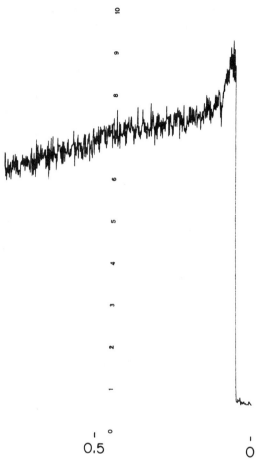

Figure 11–5. Xe washout curve from dog in hypovolemic shock. The disappearance rate is markedly slowed and conforms to a single compartment. The rapid component from the outer cortex has disappeared.

lar filtration rate and decrease the excretion of water and sodium can be circumvented with a restoration toward normal renal hemodynamics. This aim can be accomplished with either an osmotic diuretic or, in selected cases, the use of one of the loop diuretics such as furosemide.

The clinical setting in which renal failure develops is precisely that in which sodium and water conservation by the organism is maximal. Hypotension, volume depletion and hyponatremia, especially in the presence of abnormal circulating hemoglobin pigments, may lead to renal failure, especially if these conditions are allowed to persist for a matter of many hours. As suggested previously, these control mechanisms are designed to preserve body water and sodium, and therefore they can initially be reversed by the simple expedient of restoring blood pressure to normal by means of adequate volume replacement and adequate control of electrolyte composition. When such correction is not carried out for many hours, urine volume may not be restored merely by correcting the internal environment. Under these circumstances mannitol or furosemide may still reverse impending renal tubular necrosis. An example of the effectiveness of this form of therapy is indicated in Figure 11-6, which depicts the course of a patient who had sustained severe trauma with prolonged hypotension without adequate therapy for approximately 48 hours. Urine volume had fallen to less than 10 ml. per hour, and such urine as was obtained had an osmolar concentration almost identical to that of plasma. Creatinine concentrations in the urine were approximately twice that of serum, suggesting that only half of the filtered load had been resorbed. It will be recalled that under normal circumstances approximately 99 per cent of the filtered load is resorbed. The calculated glomerular filtration rate was between 10 and 20 per cent of the predicted normal. The patient was initially treated with the osmotic diuretic mannitol without response. Following this, sequentially increasing doses of furosemide were administered, starting with 40 mg. and doubling it until a total dose of 1.3 gm. was administered. Following this there was a diuresis with urine volume approaching 100 ml. per hour, and these values were main-

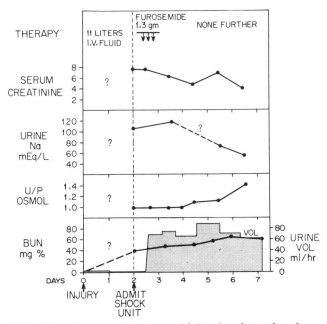

Figure 11-6. Clinical course of 28-year-old female admitted with apparent established acute renal failure. Response to loop diuretic therapy suggests that there was a recruitment of the remaining functioning nephrons which were then adequate to correct the disordered internal environment.

tained throughout the patient's course. It is apparent from the rising serum creatinine that true renal failure was present, but the presence of a large urine volume and the prompt recovery of tubular function as indicated by falling serum creatinine in the ensuing days suggests a marked amelioration of the picture of renal failure.

The suggested treatment for severe oliguria not responsive to adequate fluid and electrolyte replacement is, therefore, the administration of increasing doses of furosemide up to and including doses as high as 1 gm. It has been found that there is a threshold dosage below which one attains no response whatever and above which a maximal diuresis will occur. We have observed no toxic effects from the drug, even at this high dose, and therefore recommend its use. It should also be emphasized that in some patients a relatively small dose, such as 20 mg. of this drug, may be adequate to induce adequate urine flow. The mechanism of action is believed to be a result of the interference with sodium resorption in the loop of Henle, resulting in an increased distal tubular sodium concentration. This high level of sodium provides the false signal to the control mechanisms, tending to increase glomerular filtration rate to a maximum.

This technique may result in the reversal of functional renal failure and restoration of normal tubular function as evidenced by an increase in the urine–plasma osmolar ratio. If tubular damage is already severe before therapy is begun, the loop diuretics are still useful, because they appear to provide a maximal glomerular filtration rate through the still functioning portions of the kidney. In the absence of tubular function there will still be chemical evidence of renal failure as evidenced by an increasing creatinine and blood urea nitrogen, but the continued urine volume will make problems of water and electrolyte balance considerably easier to manage than they have been in the anuric state.

Acute renal failure is a generally preventable complication of severe injury. Prophylaxis can almost invariably be accomplished if aggressive therapy is carried out within a short time of the acute process. A high index of suspicion for the clinical setting in which acute renal failure may occur, combined with frequent measurements of the quantity and composition of the urine, provides an early clue to impending difficulty. Measurements of the urine–plasma osmolar ratio are most helpful, but additional useful information is obtained from urinary Na and creatinine determinations. A urine volume that is inappropriately low (less than 40 ml./m.) or high (greater than 80 ml./m.) deserves further investigation and immediate corrective action. Prevention of acute renal failure is usually accomplished when a series of steps designed to restore the sodium concentration in the distal tubule is carried out. This can be accomplished in many cases by the simple administration of adequate quantities of isotonic sodium chloride, but may, under special circumstances, require the addition of an osmotic or loop diuretic. Each of these maneuvers should be carried out rapidly, one after the other, until urine volume is restored to a level of approximately 60 ml. per hour. Because of the ever present danger of fluid overload, it is essential that this type of aggressive therapy be carried out with a central venous pressure cannula in place and that the urine volume be monitored at least every 15 minutes. Under these circumstances this form of prevention is highly successful and can be accomplished with a minimum of risk.

ALTERATIONS IN FUNCTION DUE TO UNDESIRED ACTIVATION OF THE ALDOSTERONE MECHANISM

The secretion of aldosterone by the adrenal cortex occurs in response to a decrease in sodium concentration secondary to either a fall in glomerular filtration rate or a decrease in the serum sodium composition. In either case, this activates a sodium-conserving mechanism which acts by facilitating sodium resorption across the renal tubule. Once this mechanism has been set in motion by the body, it will persist even though volume is restored and sodium concentration returned toward normal. It is therefore important that this mechanism be recognized and that appropriate modifications in intravenous therapy be carried out. Evidence for increased aldosterone secretion consists mainly of a markedly lowered sodium concentration in the urine, reaching levels as low as 2 to 3 mEq. per liter. When this has occurred, the physician must use extreme caution in the administration of sodium-containing solutions, because the kidney will be unable to excrete the increased sodium load. Patients who are treated early and aggressively with adequate volume restoration and sodium-containing solutions will rarely develop the clinical picture of increased aldosterone excretion. The common routines of preoperative preparation of patients result all too frequently in this difficulty. The usual preoperative orders of "nothing by mouth after the early evening" results in a period of 12 to 18 hours without water or sodium intake. This may be sufficient to produce an activation of the aldosterone mechanism so that sodium chloride administration in the postoperative period easily results in fluid overload. If the patient is adequately prepared with intravenous sodium chloride prior to surgery, then activation of the aldosterone mechanism need not occur. Measurements of urinary sodium concentration are diagnostic in this situation and, if the level is extremely low, are indicative of a normally functioning control mechanism which need not be disturbed, in most patients. It is clear that the situation cannot occur unless the tubular system is functioning normally, and therefore oliguria in the face of a very low sodium should not be confused with impending tubular damage. It is only when tubular necrosis has developed that the aldosterone mechanism will become nonoperative.

The principal undesirable side effects of activation of the aldosterone control mechanism are, therefore, the restrictions that must be placed on intravenous fluid administration. The normal kidney can excrete large quantities of sodium and provide a safety margin for the patient who is receiving intravenous fluids. This safety margin is desirable, and therefore every effort should be made to prevent the activation of the aldosterone mechanism. Adequate preparation of the patient and early administration of adequate volume and sodium concentration will usually allow this control mechanism to remain in the "off" position.

DISORDERS DUE TO AN INAPPROPRIATE OR FAULTY WATER RESORPTION CONTROL SYSTEM

Conservation of water under circumstances of volume depletion represents a normal functioning of this control system. It is important to realize that the control system also operates in the other direction by suppressing release of ADH under circumstances in which excretion of excess water from the body is desirable. These circumstances would apply with overexpansion of the extracellular fluid compartment, particularly if this is in association with a low serum osmolality, such as would occur secondary to hyponatremia. Serious abnormalities of the internal environment would clearly occur if the ADH control system was inoperative or ineffective under conditions of water depletion or, conversely, if the system was activated by the secretion of ADH under circumstances in which an excess of water was present in association with hyponatremia.

INAPPROPRIATE ADH SECRETION

This recently described syndrome consists of a clinical entity in which water retention occurs in the face of an expanded extracellular space in conjunction with hyponatremia. The syndrome is characterized by an inability to raise the serum sodium by exogenous administration, because such administered sodium will be quantitatively excreted in the urine. At a time when the internal environment calls for excretion of urine that is maximally dilute, a urine is processed which is more concentrated than one would anticipate. It is important to realize that the urine may be relatively dilute under these circumstances but is still more concentrated than the serum which has been further diluted by expansion of the extracellular space. Recognition of this disorder is important, because treatment by the usual program of sodium administration is doomed to failure; indeed, if the sodium is administered as an isotonic solution, it may actually worsen the situation because water will be retained in preference to sodium. Once the diagnosis has been established, the only effective therapy is rigid water restriction with the aim of increasing the serum osmolarity. Fortunately this disorder is self-limited, and, if further overloading of the extracellular space can be avoided, no serious consequence will ensue. The differential diagnosis from other causes of hyponatremia is easily made if urinary sodium concentrations are obtained. Other causes of hyponatremia will present with low urine sodium, whereas patients with inappropriate release of ADH will excrete almost any sodium load administered with resultant high urinary sodium values.

PENTHRANE NEPHROPATHY

Complete failure of the ADH control system may occur under special circumstances clinically typified by the syndrome of Penthrane nephropathy. It has been known for many years that complete absence of ADH such as that seen in patients with diabetes insipidus produces a clinical picture of massive water loss in the urine and severe dehydration. The urine under these circumstances is characteristically maximally dilute, being much more dilute than plasma. The tubular mechanism is functioning normally as is glomerular filtration rate. Sodium resorption is maximal, as one would expect from adequate functioning of the aldosterone mechanism. The characteristic feature of Penthrane nephropathy, therefore, consists of the clinical picture of the total absence of ADH activity. Patients will become severely dehydrated owing to the excessive water loss, and since sodium is not excreted along with the water, severe hypernatremia may ensue. This syndrome is differentiated from true diabetes insipidus in that administration of ADH fails to correct the abnormality. Because of the findings of ADH resistance, the condition is often referred to as nephrogenic diabetes insipidus. The marked dehydration that may occur in this condition if uncorrected will result in elevations of the blood urea nitrogen simulating the picture of high output acute renal failure. The distinction, however, is of great importance when one remembers that the glomerular filtration rate and tubular function in this disorder are within normal limits. In acute renal failure tubular function is reduced, and therefore the urine emerges with the same osmolarity as plasma. Once the basic underlying abnormality is appreciated, the therapy is a logical consequence. The loss of volumes of water in the urine requires that these volumes be replaced quantitatively. Several patients in our own series have required as much as 9 liters of water per day to maintain resonably normal hydration. Under these circumstances the blood urea nitrogen will return to normal; since this disorder is self-limited, restoration of a normal urine volume and normal urine-plasma osmolar ratio will soon spontaneously occur. Penthrane nephropathy can, therefore, be considered as an example of failure of the control mechanism of water resorption owing to inability of the collecting tubule to respond to ADH.

SEQUENTIAL DECISIONS FOR ANALYSIS OF POSTOPERATIVE VARIATIONS IN RENAL FUNCTION

The preceding analysis suggests that postoperative disturbances of renal function may be considered as either the normal functioning of a control mechanism in order to correct an abnormal internal environment or the abnormal or inappropriate activity of these control systems working in renal functional deterioration. In the former case, rational therapy consists in correcting the internal environment so that the control systems are turned back to normal operations. In the latter situation, it may be necessary to manipulate the control systems to function in a way other than that intended by nature so that preservation of organ function can occur. In order to distinguish these two main classes of renal functional alteration, the accompanying decision charts (Tables 11-1 and 11-2) are recommended. It is suggested that in each case the decision be based on standard clinical measurements of renal function and that each disturbance of renal function be clearly identified. Application of these principles, along with the appropriate therapeutic modality, should result in a significant decrease in the incidence of renal failure as a complication of major surgical procedures.

MANAGEMENT OF ESTABLISHED RENAL FAILURE

Failure to obtain a urine flow of 40 ml. per hour or better is tantamount to the diagnosis of acute renal failure. Complete absence of urinary output is most unusual, however, in the early stages of tubular necrosis. Indeed, the appearance of immediate anuria suggests that the difficulty lies in obstruction of the outflow of urine rather than in its production. Obstruction of the lower urinary tract at the bladder neck is a common postoperative experience, although unfortunately not always immediately diagnosed. A less common form of immediate anuria will occur following intra-abdominal operations in which the ureters may have been inadvertently damaged. It is most unusual for a surgeon to feel that his operative procedure could conceivably have resulted in damage to the upper urinary tract, but the facts speak loudly that even in the hands of the most experienced surgeon, occasional obstruction to the ureters may be an unwanted complication of intra-abdominal surgery. The appearance of immediate postoperative anuria is diagnostic of urinary tract obstruction until appropriate x-ray contrast studies have been obtained which eliminate this diagnostic possibility.

MANAGEMENT OF ESTABLISHED ACUTE TUBULAR NECROSIS

Acute tubular necrosis is established when the kidneys are no longer able to maintain the composition of the internal environment

Table 11–1.

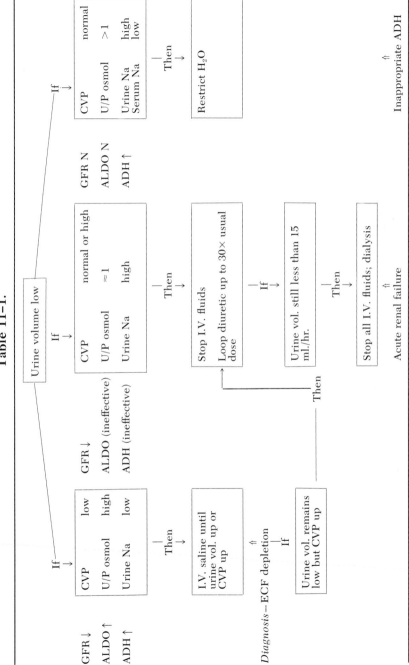

Table 11-2.

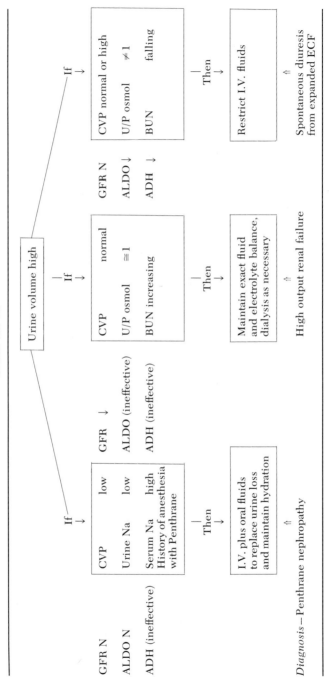

within normal limits. The exact point in time at which this diagnosis becomes manifest is impossible to identify, because a large fraction of the renal parenchyma can be destroyed before evidence of renal insufficiency can be demonstrated. It is likely that many patients with the clinical syndrome of functional renal failure who respond to the use of loop diuretics do indeed have a significant number and perhaps even a majority of the nephrons severely damaged. Acute tubular necrosis is, therefore, a quantitative estimate of the proportion of the kidney which is damaged rather than a simple statement that damage is present. The patient described in Figure 11-6 undoubtedly suffered from acute tubular necrosis, and yet a sufficient number of functioning nephrons were available so that with appropriate therapy the internal environment was rapidly returned toward normal. This clinical observation is borne out by pathologic studies which indicate that tubular necrosis has a patchy character with microscopic areas of apparently normal renal tissue interspersed between areas of severe tubular damage. The cardinal principle of the management of acute tubular necrosis is the maintenance of a normal internal environment; when the kidneys are unable to do this, supplemental measures must be utilized.

Acute renal failure may occur in either an oliguric or a polyuric form, and the management of each of these is somewhat different. In either case, the management is best divided into considerations of the metabolic consequences of inadequacy of renal function and later of the complications that arise from the background of disordered metabolism. The clinical syndrome of oliguric renal failure is associated with retention of potassium, water and sodium, and nitrogen and anion accumulation. The most serious of these disorders is the retention of potassium. Hyperkalemia can cause sudden death from cardiac arrest with little or no warning, whereas the other aspects of renal insufficiency proceed slowly with ample time for leisurely considered selection of the best method for correction. Potassium intoxication may be associated with a patient who is symptom-free one hour and dead from cardiac arrest the next. For this reason, the diagnosis of acute tubular necrosis demands that an immediate serum potassium level be obtained and, further, that an electrocardiogram tracing be recorded. Cardiac arrhythmias can develop more rapidly than the clinical laboratory can determine the electrolyte concentration. For this reason electrocardiographic monitoring assumes a place of prime importance in the management of this disorder. The typical electrocardiographic changes of hyperkalemia, as shown in Figure 11-7, should be brought to the attention of the entire staff, including those nurses who are engaged in the immediate care of the patient. The changes seen in Stage III indicate an urgent emergency requiring the most energetic measures for rapid restoration of the potassium level toward normal. Early stages are indicative of impending disaster but can generally be managed by more conservative means. Management of hyperkalemia includes first and foremost cessa-

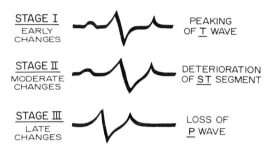

Figure 11-7.   Stages of electrocardiographic evidence of hyperkalemia.

tion of potassium intake. It is surprising how often one finds patients in renal failure receiving oral food or intravenous solutions containing potassium. Fruit juice, coffee, tea and broth are all sources of considerable potassium and should be rigidly eliminated from the diet of anyone with acute renal failure. An oral diet consisting of water and special dishes composed only of fat and carbohydrates should be used.

Hyperkalemia in oliguric renal failure can usually be controlled by a combination of cessation of potassium intake and removal of potassium from the body by sodium polystyrene sulfonate. This material (Kayexalate) is administered in 30 ml. of sorbitol to which has been added sufficient water to make the mixture ingestible. This combination is best given by mouth, but if the gastrointestinal tract is not functioning it can also be administered by rectum. Repeated instillations of Kayexalate will result in control of the level of serum potassium in the vast majority of patients, and indeed hyperkalemia as an indication for dialysis should rarely arise.

The next most serious compound retained in oliguric renal failure is water. Most patients will enter the phase of oliguric renal failure with an expanded ECF because vigorous attempts will usually have been made to institute urine flow. Careful avoidance of overhydration and the liberal use of loop diuretics in the early phase will help to minimize the likelihood of overhydration, although its presence must be assumed in the majority of instances. The day-to-day water requirement of a patient in oliguric renal failure is much less than is generally appreciated. If there are no extrarenal losses of water, then the total loss consists of the basal insensible water loss from the skin and lungs and amounts to 12 ml. per kilogram per day. This loss is partially offset by the metabolic production of water which results from the metabolism of glucose. In the postoperative period this may yield 300 to 400 ml. of water per day so that the patient's deficit is as little as 500 to 600 ml. A useful guide to the state of hydration is the level of serum sodium. If there are no extrarenal sodium losses, then accurate water replacement will result in a constant concentration of sodium in the extracellular fluid. When extrarenal sodium and water losses are present, such as will occur from gastric drainage, enterotomies, and fistulae, then this loss must be accurately measured as regards both volume and electrolyte composition, and should be quantitatively replaced. A second useful guide to the degree of hydration is careful daily weighing of the patient. If the patient is fasting, then a weight loss of approximately 1 pound per day should occur. Maintenance of a steady weight indicates a continuing degree of overhydration.

Modern dialytic therapy is aimed at maintaining the internal environment within normal limits. There is considerable recent evidence that the maintenance of the blood urea nitrogen in the normal range by appropriate dialytic therapy will markedly lessen the incidence of infection and wound disruption which are so frequently the terminal complications of the patient with acute renal failure. It is now our practice to prepare patients for dialysis with a Scribner arteriovenous shunt as soon as the diagnosis of tubular necrosis has been made. The frequency of dialysis will be determined by the metabolic state of the patient, the degree of tissue damage, and the presence of infection. Clinical evidence of uremia should never be allowed to develop in these patients, and indeed with frequent and adequate dialysis a near normal metabolic state can be maintained.

Peritoneal dialysis can be used in situations in which the necessary equipment for hemodialysis is not available. Unfortunately, this latter technique is frequently inapplicable in the surgical patient because of the presence of intraperitoneal drains and open retroperitoneal areas or other factors that destroy the fluid-containing properties of the parietal peritoneum. Peritoneal dialysis may have a place in the treatment of acute renal failure in association with open heart or thoracic surgical procedures when the peritoneal cavity has not been violated. This is particularly true when the presence of suture lines in the heart or major blood vessels makes the use of heparin dangerous. Several recent studies have indicated that early aggressive peritoneal dialytic therapy is of help in the management of postperfusion renal tubular necrosis.

Once the patient has been successfully managed through the period of oliguric renal failure, a period of polyuric renal failure will generally occur before complete recovery has taken place. This period of polyuric renal failure is identical with the high output form of acute renal failure which is frequently seen in patients who have been well hydrated prior to the development of the renal insult. It is most imperative that an appreciation of the nature of the diuresis and the overall state of hydration of the patient be continually assessed. In certain patients the magnitude of the diuresis represents a restoration toward normal hydration in a patient who was previously suffering from fluid overload. In these circumstances it is a serious therapeutic error to attempt to keep up with the diuresis. The replacement of the lost fluid will result in the development of further fluid overload and possible congestive heart failure. On the other hand, the excessive urine volume may result from failure of the tubular mechanism to produce a concentrated urine and, therefore, is a representation that glomerular filtrate is being quantitatively lost from the body. Measurements of urine-plasma osmolar ratio and the level of central venous pressure are helpful. Certain patients in the recovery phase of oliguric acute tubular necrosis will demonstrate a continuing rise of the blood urea nitrogen in the diuretic recovery phase. If the plasma-osmolar ratio remains at unity, further dialysis may be required, just as in the cases of high output renal failure. Therapy should not be terminated until the internal environment has returned to normal.

REFERENCES

Auger, R. G., Dayton, D. A., Harrison, C. E., et al.: Use of ethacrynic acid in mannitol-resistant oliguric renal failure. J.A.M.A. 206:891, 1968.

Bartter, F. C., and Schwartz, W. B.: The syndrome of inappropriate secretion of ADH. Amer. J. Med. 42:790, 1967.

Carrico, C. J., Coln, C. D., Lightfoot, S. A., et al.: Extracellular fluid volume replacement in hemorrhagic shock. Surg. Forum 14:10, 1963.

Hollenberg, N. K., et al.: Acute renal failure due to nephrotoxins. N. Eng. J. Med. 282:1130, 1970.

Porter, G. A., and Starr, A.: Management of postoperative renal failure. Surgery 65:390, 1969.

Powers, S. R., Jr.: The maintenance of renal function following massive trauma. J. Trauma 10:554, 1970.

Powers, S. R., Jr., Kiley, J. E., and Boba, A.: Current Problems in Surgery, November, 1964.

Thurau, K.: Influence of sodium concentration at macula densa cells on tubular sodium load. Ann. N.Y. Acad. Sci. 139:388, 1966.

CHAPTER 12

TRANSPLANTATION

Paul S. Russell, M.D.

The demands upon the team caring for transplant patients can be as great as in any branch of medicine. Enlightened decisions require not only the close involvement of a varied group of clinicians (in the case of kidney transplantation, the central group must surely comprise at least a general surgeon, urologist, nephrologist, psychiatrist, pediatrician, and an infectious disease expert), but also the close support of an able serologist and a geneticist. Results are improving steadily, but there is no immediate prospect of moving to a greatly expanded application of transplantation treatment to the point that it will be readily applicable in most hospitals, although it is likely that this will take place in time. For the present the evaluation and safe control of transplant rejection remains the most formidable obstacle. Methods of donor selection according to compatibility also continue in a state of flux. The severe limitation of insufficient numbers of donor organs is yielding only gradually to a variety of approaches aimed at different aspects of this difficult problem. All these factors add greatly to the fascination of this growing field in which the success of an operation, achieved by the most careful planning and by constant vigilance, can be a supremely rewarding event for doctor and patient alike.

This chapter will be directed toward the clinical principles of transplantation as they are currently understood. An effort will be made to pay special attention to selected developments in the clinical arena, but it would be shortsighted to neglect altogether the newer discoveries emerging from many laboratories upon which the promising future of this arm of medicine must depend. Many of these have been reviewed recently in greater detail than can be devoted to them here.[1]

This work was supported in part by grants AM07055 and AI06320 of the United States Public Health Service.

Since kidney transplantation has been so much more widely practiced than the transplantation of any other organ, it will be treated in particular detail as a kind of specimen piece for all organs.

KIDNEY TRANSPLANTATION

Since the early 1950's something over 5000 kidney transplants have been performed throughout the world. For a number of reasons the kidney is a particularly suitable organ for transplantation. These reasons include the simple anatomy of the renal pedicle (although multiple arterial vessels are found in some 20 to 30 per cent of kidneys); the fact that complete lack of kidney function is compatible with life for at least a few days, and that artificial external support in the form of hemodialysis is a well-developed mode of therapy; that lethal diseases largely or completely confined to the kidney are quite common; and finally that uncontrollable infection is not a usual accompaniment of such renal disease. Since a single well-functioning kidney is sufficient to maintain normal life, a recipient need have only one new kidney, and a normal living donor can, under carefully controlled circumstances, donate one of two kidneys without undue risk. Roughly half of the kidneys transplanted so far have come from living donors, usually closely related members of the patient's family.

Although the use of normal living donors must be a matter of deep concern for transplant groups which employ them, it is believed by many that this risk can be made acceptable, at present, for three reasons: (1) The donor organ can be procured in an optimal physiological state. (2) The transplantation operation can be scheduled and performed at a time selected for the benefit of the patients concerned. (3) Considerably greater compatibility between donor and recipient can be assured by present typing methods than with unrelated donors because of the special circumstances involved in the inheritance of histocompatibility factors (see below).

Selection of Patients and Preoperative Preparation. Transplantation is designed, of course, to make good the deficiency of a given organ or structure. If the disease responsible for the condition to be treated is a generalized one involving other organs in such a way that the replacement of, say, a kidney will still leave the patient with severe disease elsewhere, then kidney replacement is contraindicated. Accordingly, renal failure associated with such conditions as diabetes or systemic lupus erythematosus is usually not treated by transplantation at the present time, although it is interesting that certain metabolic defects involving renal failure, such as cystinosis, have been successfully treated by transplantation. Infection, wherever located, must be controlled prior to transplantation.

Hemodialysis is often instituted preoperatively in order to convert the patient's uremic state as much as possible toward normal. This will improve nutrition and blood-clotting potential, and restore fluid spaces and electrolytes toward normal. Usually much can be accomplished in a period of about two weeks of intensive dialysis so that transplantation from a living donor can be planned as soon as this. Since the availability of a donor in the nonliving category is unpredictable, the preoperative period of hemodialysis may be much more prolonged. Frequently it is advisable to construct an arteriovenous fistula between the radial or ulnar artery and a superficial vein. In a few weeks the venous network will become greatly dilated in response to the arterial pressure and a thrill is palpable throughout the forearm. Large bore needles can be placed temporarily into these vessels for intermittent hemodialysis, thus avoiding inlying percutaneous cannulae.

A point for special emphasis is the dual danger of ordinary blood transfusions for these patients. In the past, because of the anemia which is so characteristic of uremia, most patients undergoing prolonged hemodialysis treatment have received frequent blood transfusions. This resulted in a high incidence of serum hepatitis which has not infrequently been transmitted from one patient to another and even to nurses and physicians in dialysis units. Also, of great importance is the frequency of sensitization to histocompatibility antigens by the leukocytes present in the transfused blood. Repeated transfusions have often left patients sensitized to these antigens, which are also present in kidneys, so that it may be difficult or impossible to identify a donor whose tissues will not bear at least some of the antigens to which the patient has been previously exposed. Transplantation in the face of known presensitization regularly results in very acute rejection of the transplant, with circulatory stasis occurring within minutes or hours because of the presence of humoral antibodies. Suitable tests should be done in an effort to avoid this catastrophe. The simplest of these is to perform a "cross match" test in which donor leukocytes are mixed with the serum of an intended recipient in the presence of complement. Evidence of specific cytotoxicity is a strong contraindication to the use of the donor in question.

We have been particularly satisfied with blood which has been stored in the frozen state with glycerol for transfusions to these patients. The extensive washing, along with freezing and thawing, which is employed in the processing of the erythrocytes, eliminates virtually all the leukocytes and leukocyte fragments, thus greatly reducing the likelihood of sensitization to transplantation antigens. The incidence of serum hepatitis has also been very much less with transfusions prepared in this way,[2] and our results with transplant patients support this.

In preparing a patient for renal transplantation, several special problems are often encountered. For example, the hypercalcemia so frequently accompanying uremia should be evaluated. This condition, which calls forth secondary hyperparathyroidism, may be associated with evidence of calcification of tissues throughout the body, especially arterial vessels. Management of electrolytes, and particularly the conduct of hemodialysis treatments, must take this condition into account. The parathyroid hyperplasia which occurs may go on to relatively autonomous hypersecretion, sometimes with adenoma formation, a state which has been called "tertiary hyperparathyroidism." Although the hypercalcemia usually returns to normal in time after a successful transplant, parathyroidectomy has been recommended by some when control of calcium levels becomes difficult.

The peripheral neuropathy of uremia is usually most marked in the lower extremities with sensory symptoms of burning pain being most common. Motor deficiencies, particularly involving the peroneal nerve, are sometimes severe and may be only partially reversible. Incomplete emptying of the urinary bladder can sometimes occur with neuropathy as well. This is usually fully reversible.

Accordingly, the complete preoperative management of these patients must be designed not only to correct as well as possible the complex metabolic problems concerned, but also to attend to muscular conditioning by general physical therapy, and by pulmonary physiotherapy to give training in deep breathing and the evacuation of secretions.

The Operation. Usually the operative procedure consists of bilateral nephrectomy as well as kidney transplantation, although there are circumstances in which prior nephrectomy may be advisable, as mentioned above. The transplant is commonly placed in the iliac fossa on the side opposite its location in the donor, since this provides better alignment with the iliac vessels for anastomosis with the renal vessels. The left kidney of the donor is preferred because of its slightly longer vessels, but also because the iliac vessels on the right side of the recipient are slightly more accessible than those on the left. The nephrectomies are performed in a transabdominal fashion through a single incision by some groups. We have preferred to remove the ipsilateral kidney through the transplantation incision. This is a lower oblique abdominal incision used to provide wide exposure of the retroperitoneal structures on that side. The contralateral kidney is removed through a standard flank incision thereafter. Continuous spinal anesthesia has proved to be quite satisfactory for the recipient. When the time of availability of the donor kidney is not certain, as in some cases in which the donor is nonliving, the catheter can be placed but administration of the narcotizing agent delayed until the operation is to proceed when it can be given promptly.

A Foley catheter is placed, with careful skin preparation, after anesthesia induction. This is valuable as a guide if the bladder is to be opened in order to place the donor ureter to the trigone by the submucosal tunneling technique. When the donor renal pelvis is anastomosed to the recipient ureter, as we normally prefer, prompt bladder drainage is also important since early diuresis is so common. Wherever performed, reconstruction of the urinary drainage system must be done with extreme care, since leakage, usually an avoidable complication, can be very serious.

Operation on the Donor. The donor nephrectomy must be performed with especial gentleness to avoid trauma to the kidney. Tugging or twisting the pedicle can result in severe vascular spasm with added ischemic damage even when the vessels are still in continuity. All vessels must be carefully ligated on the specimen side to avoid bleeding after restoration of blood flow. This is most difficult when a kidney is removed from a nonliving donor after circulatory arrest. Simple, low pressure perfusion with a balanced electrolyte solution at 4° C. is performed immediately. Other, more elaborate preservation schemes are also being used.

Early Postoperative Care. Function of the transplanted kidney is almost invariably prompt, ranging from a few minutes to a few hours after restoration of blood flow to the organ, when a living donor has been employed. With nonliving donors, the course is less predictable, although the level of early function will correlate roughly in an inverse manner with the apparent degree of ischemic damage to the kidney. A diuresis of well over 1 liter of urine per hour is common. Thus, replacement with appropriate electrolytes is a demanding assignment. Frequent checks of serum and urine constituents are necessary. Many patients are extremely hypertensive as a consequence of their renal disease. Edema fluid is often present throughout the body, in spite of hemodialysis, preoperatively. Thus, the central venous pressure is of especial value in the early hours and days as a guide to circulatory dynamics.

Immunosuppression usually consists of several agents given simultaneously; azathioprine (Imuran) remains the most commonly used drug. As a purine analogue it interferes with cell replication, which is a central aspect of immunological responses. Initially it is given in a dose of 10 mg. per kg. by mouth on the evening before operation. A sodium salt of this drug is also available, and this can be given intravenously until oral medication can again be accepted. The dose is reduced over the first three to five days to between 100 and 150 mg. per day, with daily adjustments according to changes in peripheral leukocyte counts in such a way as to preserve counts of at least 5000/mm.[3] Individual susceptibility to leukopenia varies widely, and changes in peripheral counts can be precipitous. Cortisone is also used in almost all cases, although with closely matched family donor combinations we do not employ cortisone at all unless rejection activity is uncontrolled by azathioprine. In other donor-recipient combinations, prednisone or prednisolone therapy is begun on the day of operation. We begin at a dose of 60 mg. per day and hope to diminish this dose over the first two to three weeks to about 15 mg. daily. Early rejection reactions may appear as soon as three to four days postoperatively, even in unsensitized recipients. At present the management of such early rejection, which is characterized morphologically by heavy mononuclear cell infiltration and edema, is best accomplished with short periods of greatly increased steroid dosage. Only three or four days of treatment at 300 mg. per day may be required to produce a marked diuresis with improvement in creatinine clearance and serum electrolytes (Fig. 12–1). Interestingly enough, rapid reduction of steroid dosage is usually not met by a recrudescence of rejection. A number of other chemical agents have been employed for immunosuppression, including actinomycin C or D, azaserine, and cyclophosphamide. These can be useful adjuncts under some circumstances.

Other approaches to nonspecific immunosuppression, such as thoracic duct drainage of lymph to reduce the body's pool of small recirculating lymphocytes or extracorporeal irradiation of the blood or lymph, have also received considerable attention. The list of known chemical agents with immunosuppressive properties is also a long one, and it remains likely that useful new drugs will continue to emerge, particularly as more is learned about antibody synthesis and the intimate

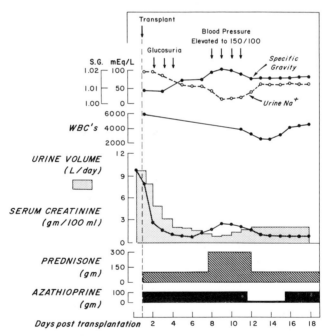

Figure 12–1. Typical early postoperative course of a kidney transplant recipient. This is a composite diagram assembled from experience with many patients and represents observations to be expected when the patient has received a kidney which is moderately incompatible with the recipient but in which the early rejection reaction (from days 6 to 13) can be overcome by increased immunosuppression. It will be noted that the rejection reaction is associated with decreased urine volume, a rising serum creatinine, a lowered urine sodium excretion, and a transient elevation of blood pressure. Leukopenia, depicted as beginning on the eleventh day, usually responds to decreasing azathioprine dosage.

events involved in the production of sensitized, immunologically competent cells.

One class of agents of particular biological importance, which has been much studied in very recent years, consists of antibodies produced in one species against the lymphocytes of another, so-called *"antilymphocyte serum."* The subject has been reviewed thoroughly elsewhere[3, 4] but will be summarized here because of its interest.

In brief, it has been found that sera resulting from repeated immunization of one species with lymphoid cells from another may have very powerful immunosuppressive effects in any member of the donor species, particularly for cell-mediated reactions such as transplant rejection. Sera with the best immunosuppressive properties result from mixing the immunizing cells with Freund's adjuvant, and the sera should be collected after only a few immunizing injections.[5] Since virtually all the immunosuppressive activity of a given serum resides in the gamma globulin fraction, indeed in its 7S or IgG portion, it is possible to remove a great deal of extraneous foreign protein from the whole serum by fractionation.

Confusion easily arises here. Methods of preparing and fractionating serum have varied in different laboratories, and reports of the use of serum or serum fractions have rarely been in terms which can be evaluated elsewhere. Furthermore, different batches of serum may vary considerably in potency even though they have been prepared according to the same plan. Unfortunately, no *in vitro* test of antibody activity which correlates reliably with *in vivo* immunosuppressive activity has yet been widely accepted, so that final comparison of sera prepared by different methods, or even at different times by the same method, must be in an *in vivo* test system. The fact that antilymphocyte sera prepared against cells of one species in another may have rather strong immunosuppressive effects in a third species has proved to be a most interesting biological fact which is also probably of value as an assay. Thus, sera prepared in horses against human lymphocytes or thymocytes can be compared in regard to toxicity and immunosuppressive capacity in monkeys which have received test skin allografts.

Further difficulties are raised by the fact that these sera obviously contain mixtures of many antibodies. Some of these will attach widely to tissues throughout the body when injected into individuals of the donor species. Other antibodies will bind solely to lymphoid cells. The former class of antibodies can be very undesirable if such sera are to be used in patients, although it now appears that they can be removed by absorption. Another problem stems from the fact that even the most highly purified foreign protein is likely to be immunogenic on its own when injected into another species. Thus, any of these serum fractions can provoke antibody against themselves in treated recipients, and this can lead to serum sickness and other undesirable effects. Various approaches to combating this possible drawback are now being taken.

Even with the considerable complexity of this approach to immunosuppression, however, its importance and possible value are impressive. ALS (here used to refer to the whole class of anti-lymphocyte sera) is clearly the most powerful immunosuppressive agent available. Even a brief period of treatment of a mouse, for example, with rabbit anti-mouse lymphocyte serum can allow survival of a strongly incompatible mouse skin allograft for several weeks. A rat skin xenograft to such a mouse may survive almost a month. Dog kidney transplants can survive for many months with horse anti-dog serum treatment alone. Treatment results in a profound peripheral lymphopenia within hours of the first injection, and most of the evidence now favors the interpretation that it is through the elimination of some lymphoid cells that the immunosuppressive effect is achieved. Suppression of humoral antibody responses also occurs but probably to a lesser degree.

The use of sera, or serum fractions, prepared in various ways in human organ transplantation is now being evaluated. From the aforementioned brief description of some of the complexities involved, it will be apparent why progress has been slow in collecting reliable information concerning a single uniform serum product in a standard clinical setting. From the substantial information of animal experiments, however, it seems virtually certain that it will be possible to produce powerful immunosuppressive agents in this manner and that they can be remarkably well tolerated.

Complications. Complications related directly to various aspects of the treatment program are common. The greatest menace is infection. Although a constant threat in any surgical patient, the increased likelihood of infection in these patients is associated with immunosuppression. It can be in an incision or elsewhere. Pulmonary infection is common and is very frequently an important contributor to death. Although common organisms, such as staphylococci, Klebsiella, *E. coli,* and *Pseudomonas aeruginosa,* are regularly seen, it is now widely recognized that various bacteria and viruses not usually considered to be systemic pathogens may also be dangerous in immunosuppressed patients. *Pneumocystis carinii,* monilia, and others are in this category. Policies differ widely in regard to isolation of patients. In many institutions minimal precautions are taken and these are maintained for only a few days. Satisfactory factual information is unfortunately not available concerning the general incidence of infection or the efficacy of isolation procedures of one kind or another. For the present it has been our practice to employ gown, glove, and mask precautions throughout the entire period of high dose immunosuppressive treatment.

Other complications attributable to immunosuppressive treatment, perhaps especially its steroid component, include peptic ulceration, sometimes with its further complications of perforation or bleeding, pancreatitis, emotional disturbances, and aseptic necrosis of bones, especially the femoral head.

The wives of transplant patients have conceived offspring which have developed normally, and female patients have even been able, in a few instances, to carry normal babies through to delivery even though they are receiving immunosuppressive treatment. Nevertheless, children may exhibit considerable impairment of normal growth and development, even though the function of the transplanted kidney remains satisfactory.

Late Results. The most recent results in two major groups of kidney transplant patients, reflecting the worldwide experience collated from reports received by the Kidney Transplant Registry (now maintained by the American College of Surgeons with the sponsorship of the National Institutes of Health),[6] can be found in Figure 12-2. This figure depicts the percentage of transplants reported as surviving from among the number which were performed long enough ago to permit their inclusion at any given time interval. The reports of individual centers naturally differ from this overall mean, but the striking difference between the *likelihood* of survival of a transplant from a related, as against an unrelated, donor is now generally acknowledged. The function of surviving kidneys, and consequently the degree of rehabilitation of the patients, varies considerably. In this respect, too, related donors have, in general, been distinctly superior. They have experienced fewer complications, require less immunosuppression, and have a smaller rate of late functional failure as the postoperative years go on. This difference appears to be heavily dependent upon the immunogenetic differences involved between donors and recipients (see below).

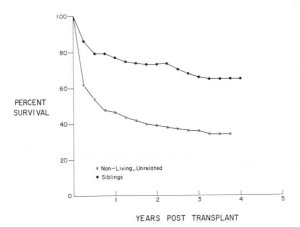

Figure 12-2. Survival of kidneys from sibling and unrelated (nonliving) donors compared. These are the aggregate data from the world experience as compiled by the Kidney Transplant Registry. The difference in survival of kidneys from these two sources is impressive. Transplanted kidneys from parents result in an intermediate level of survival. Patient survival is generally 15 to 20 per cent higher than transplant survival since hemodialysis support is available. (Data courtesy of Dr. Benjamin A. Barnes.)

Late failure of transplant function is usually a gradual process. Slowly declining renal clearance is frequently associated with rising hypertension and often with increasing proteinuria. Kidney biopsies at this stage characteristically show pronounced narrowing of the arteriolar lumina (Fig. 12-3), interstitial fibrosis, and moderate mixed inflammatory cell infiltration.[7]

In some cases, the pathological changes associated with gradual late decline of kidney function may be indistinguishable from glomerulonephritis.[8] Since these changes may occur in kidneys transplanted even to patients who did not suffer from glomerulonephritis before transplantation, it is difficult to be certain how frequently "return of the original disease" actually takes place. This aspect of transplantation immunologically is a particularly interesting one at the present time.

In optimal circumstances the patient is completely rehabilitated in that he works a full day, eats a normal diet, and regains his normal sense of well being. At this stage, when he received a stable dose of azathioprine and perhaps some prednisone, his susceptibility to infection and the other complications of immunosuppressive therapy does not seem to be very high, although care should be taken to treat promptly and thoroughly any infections which do occur. Urinary tract infection is a special problem in these patients. If looked for carefully,

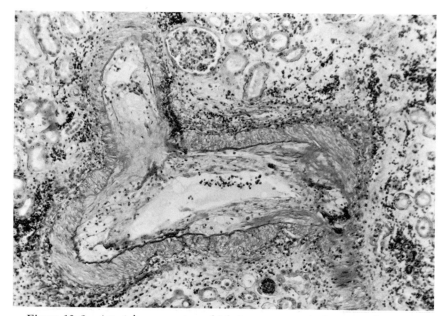

Figure 12–3. Arteriolar narrowing which is so common in late transplant rejection. This vessel, sectioned at a point of branching, was found in a biopsy of a transplant at six months. The evidence favors the interpretation that this change is mediated by humoral antibodies directed against the foreign antigens in the donor endothelium. Similar arteriolar changes are also seen in transplants of other organs.

it is found to be frequent in the early weeks after operation, especially in patients who have suffered leaks at the ureteral anastomosis or who have had urinary tract infection preoperatively. The longest survivor with an allotransplant (from an older brother) in the author's series is entirely well with normal renal function over eight years after transplantation.

OTHER ORGANS

Transplantation of a number of other vital organs besides the kidney, such as the heart, lung, pancreas, and liver, is quite feasible technically. It is important to note that, in general, the rejection reaction to different organs and tissues is the same. Indeed, it has long been believed that nucleated cells throughout the body of any individual display the same group of histocompatibility antigens in a combination which is specific for the individual concerned. It is these antigens which are determined by "typing" techniques which make use of leukocytes. According to this principle, a graft of one tissue from a donor to a given recipient would be expected to immunize or sensitize that recipient to a later graft of *any* tissue, and all tissues would be rejected in a basically similar manner and at about the same time. Although these propositions are still held to be fundamentally correct, advancing knowledge has shown that considerable variation in survival of different organs can occur in animal experiments in which the immunogenetic differences between donor and recipients can be standardized. Thus, there is some suggestion that the heart may survive better as a transplant between rats than the kidney or a skin graft.[9] The experience from transplantation in patients is much too scanty to afford evidence as to differences of this sort in the human being, but it is important to be aware that such differences may exist. Another major set of considerations of consequence, when the success of transplantation of additional organs beyond the kidney is being considered, concerns the urgency with which function of the transplant is needed by a recipient, along with the availability of assist devices to assume the functions of the needed organ on a temporary basis. Thus, the need for early function of a heart transplant at a high level of efficiency is great, since the availability of long-term assist devices is still limited. As assist devices improve, they will provide greater opportunity for the treatment of temporary derangements of transplant function from any cause, including rejection. Similar considerations apply for the liver and the lung.

The urgency of the need for a new organ from a nonliving donor, which is generated by these clinical circumstances, has meant that it is often impossible to maintain needy recipients in a sufficiently good physiological state to allow a suitable donor to be found, so that the number of transplants of such organs which have been performed under optimal circumstances has been relatively limited.

The scope of this presentation cannot include full consideration of the extensive information available pertinent to transplantation of each organ. The reader will accordingly be referred elsewhere for more extensive study and only the briefest summary will be presented here for each important organ or tissue.

Liver. Transplantation of the liver, like other organs, can be done with placement of the donor in its normal location and with its normal vascular connections in *orthotopic* style or in an unnatural position as a *heterotopic* transplant. The latter may be preferable in certain situations in which the patient's condition is precarious and removal of the liver would be particularly hazardous, as in some examples of advanced portal hypertension. Removal of the liver must, of course, be planned when this organ is involved with malignant neoplastic disease.

The indications for liver transplantation have been several.[10] Congenital biliary atresia is probably the best of them, although advanced cirrhosis and certain toxic destructive states can offer circumstances in which liver replacement is the only hope at present. Malignant disease may be an appropriate indication, especially when the tumor is primary in the liver.

Since liver decomposition is rapid when the blood supply is compromised, every precaution must be taken to afford an organ which is in optimal condition for transplantation. The best set of circumstances is afforded when the liver can be removed from a patient who has undergone "brain death" (see below) without cessation of circulation and when cooling by perfusion with a chilled balanced salt solution is instituted at the time of its removal.

Immunosuppression for liver transplantation has followed closely that established for the kidney. The use of anti-lymphocyte globulin in liver transplantation has coincided with a distinct improvement in survival of transplants.[10]

Although early and vigorous rejection of human liver allotransplants is unquestionably seen, it is not yet entirely clear whether or not the liver behaves as the kidney in man. Much interest has been aroused by the fact that liver transplants in certain pigs have been shown to survive longer than transplants of other tissue among the same stock of animals. Furthermore, it appears that in these animals a surviving liver transplant will also promote the survival of other tissues transplanted from the same donor.[11] The mechanism underlying these phenomena remains to be established.

So far about 130 human liver transplants have been performed throughout the world. Of these, the longest survivor was for 29 months, and 11 are reported as surviving at present.[6]

Lung. Transplantation of the lung has been performed relatively little. This is true even though death from pulmonary failure is a common occurrence, so that many patients could be considered for transplantation. Unfortunately, pulmonary insufficiency is usually associated with active infection, even when a chronic underlying process exists. Thus, the likelihood of devastating pulmonary sepsis is high as efforts are pressed to overcome the rejection of the transplanted tissue which is derived from an unrelated donor. A further problem, especially relevant to the lung, is that of restricted function of a lung, the lymphatic and nervous connections of which have been recently severed. Thus, the immediate function of such a lung, whether it is merely removed and replaced or is transplanted between individuals, is considerably reduced. This functional impairment has been associated with high vascular resistance and the development of edema and hemorrhage in the pulmonary parenchyma. Since pulmonary transplantation would only be performed in situations in which the contralateral lung, if still present, is very severely impaired, the early maintenance of pulmonary function could be difficult. Problems of the partition of flow and ventilation to the two sides are also involved.[1]

So far 25 pulmonary transplants have been recorded. The longest survivor was a patient who received a left lung transplant for terminal pulmonary insufficiency from silicosis; he survived for about 10 months before succumbing, probably to the consequences of slow rejection. At present no recorded pulmonary recipients are living.[6]

Heart. In the period of over three years to this writing since the first human heart transplant, about 165 of these procedures have been performed. All have been placed by modifications of the technique of Shumway and Lower,[12] and in all cases, even where both donor and recipient sino-auricular nodes have coexisted in the recipient, the heart rhythm has been governed by the donor node. A transplanted heart can assume the circulatory load with remarkable early success and great initial benefit to the patient. By humoral mechanisms, such as catecholamine stimulation, and by stretch receptors in the transplanted muscle, a transplant can respond quite well with increased output to exercise demands.

The problem of detecting transplant rejection early, and of distinguishing it with assurance from other conditions is a difficult one in the case of the heart as it can be for other organs. Since no direct immunological test for rejection, as such, exists, only indirect evidence of its presence is available. For the heart a decline in electrocardiographic voltage, especially in lead 2, the development of conduction disturbances, ST-segment changes, and supraventricular arrhythmias all suggest rejection. Elevation of certain serum enzyme levels, such as lactic dehydrogenase (LDH-1) may also be helpful. As in the case of other organs, rejection reactions can often be managed successfully. The pathology of transplant rejection, including the early edematous phase associated with cellular infiltration and the later period of parenchymal fibrosis often associated with pronounced arteriolar stenosis, is seen in the heart as in other organs.

Once again, as with other organs, it is the process of rejection which has been the central problem in managing patients with heart transplants, since, from a technical and physiological standpoint, they have shown remarkable potential. It is encouraging to note, however, that 27 heart recipients have lived for more than one year and seven for more than two years.[6]

Pancreas.   Transplantation of the pancreas as a means of supplying the endocrine secretions of this organ has definite attraction. Particularly in diabetes recognized early in life, metabolic control may be very difficult, in part because of varying demands for insulin. A living pancreas may thus have considerable superiority over treatment with exogenous hormones in some patients. As renal failure may accompany diabetes, the dual transplantation of both a pancreas and a kidney can be tested, and a few such procedures have been done.[13] The most successful technique for pancreatic transplantation has been the placement of the pancreas, with or without its attached duodenal loop, into a lower abdominal quadrant with appropriate vascular anastomoses to the iliac vessels and drainage of an end of the duodenal loop either as an external fistula or into the recipient's ileum.

Current information has it that about 19 pancreatic transplants have been performed and that one of these recipients has survived for at least a year.[6]

Bone Marrow and Thymus.   Considerable interest and effort have been directed toward the possibility of transplanting lymphoreticular cells in order to restore these cell populations selectively in certain circumstances. For example, accidental whole body exposure to single doses of irradiation at about 500 to 700 r is a condition particularly appropriate for bone marrow infusion. Although such accidents have been rare, encouraging results with bone marrow infusions in a few instances, and much evidence from animal experimentation, have led to expanded trials of marrow transplantation in other conditions in recent years. Bone marrow infusion following large dose chemotherapeutic or irradiation treatment of leukemia is now being attempted, for example. Most successful have been a few well-studied cases in which congenital lymphoid cell deficiencies, which are sometimes related to thymic aplasia, have been treated by thymic implants or bone marrow infusion.[14]

Technically both the harvesting and the administration of bone marrow is simple. After careful and full preliminary evaluation, living donors are normally placed under light general anesthesia and marrow is withdrawn into a heparinized medium from multiple needle aspiration sites along the sternum, both iliac crests, and the sacrum. Administration of marrow cells is best accomplished by the intravenous route and can be done, in our experience, with safety by direct infusion without filtration.

A consideration of special importance to the success of transplantation of cells of this type depends upon the fact that they represent a population which is itself "immunologically competent." In other words, the grafted cells are quite capable of mounting a destructive immunological reaction against those antigens which they recognize as foreign in the recipient, a phenomenon which has been called a "graft-versus-host reaction." Thus, severe anemia, diarrhea, and an impressive skin eruption have been described in patients receiving infusions of immunologically competent cells. These changes may be ameliorated with immunosuppressive therapy and may abate with survival of the progeny of the grafted cells in the recipient or with the rejection of the grafted cells by the recipient. The most effective measure for avoiding severe, or even fatal, graft-versus-host disease lies in careful selection of donors for close histocompatibility, but this must be compatibility in *both directions* so that neither donor nor recipient presents a large number of new antigens to the other. In practical terms, this is most likely if highly compatible siblings are employed (see below).

Endocrine Glands. The transplantation of endocrine glands has been an ancient subject of interest. With the advent of modern endocrinology and knowledge of the composition of many hormones, synthetic or biologically derived hormone supplements can be administered to correct most hormone deficiencies, including those which would otherwise be incompatible with life. The advantage of restoration of secretions by a transplant would, therefore, lie mainly in the greater responsiveness to physiological requirements of which a transplant would be capable. When an endocrine gland supplies several hormones, the relative balance of these secretions and their full restoration might be much better achieved by a transplant. Nevertheless, the clear dangers of immunosuppressive treatment have discouraged efforts to transplant most endocrine glands in recent years. Should improved methods of managing rejection be discovered this situation could change.

Other Organs and Tissues. Many other intriguing possibilities for utilizing living tissue transplants in "constructive surgery" exist. One of particular importance at present is the potential for use of living skin grafts for prompt coverage of extensively burned patients. Here it is already clear that such burned individuals are in a state of relative immunological incapacity in that skin grafts survive somewhat longer on them than on normal recipients. Still, the greater the compatibility of the donor skin to the recipient, the longer it will live in a healthy state.[15] The best timing and technique for performing extensive burn excisions and the optimal management of grafted burn wounds of this kind, along with the problem of patient selection, will be much considered in the immediate future.

Transplantation of the stomach and intestines is feasible technically. Especially in the case of the latter, there may be occasional patients who could benefit greatly by receiving tissue from another individual. With improved methods of intravenous alimentation such patients may survive their original illnesses more commonly so that their numbers will increase.

This section should not close without at least a mention of the great success which has been achieved with corneal transplantation. The immunological isolation of this structure, which also extends to the anterior chamber of the eye, permits prolonged survival of transplanted cells in the absence of a direct blood circulation. Thus, no immunosuppression is usually used. Presensitization to antigens of the donor is to be avoided in this situation, however, as this can result in rejection even in "immunologically privileged" sites.

HISTOCOMPATIBILITY TESTING

The immunological rejection reaction is generated by antigens which are apparently structural components of cell membranes. It is known that these antigens are closely determined by the genetic constitution of the individual concerned and that transplants of all tissues are accepted without rejection by genetically identical individuals. The extensive knowledge gained from several decades of research with mice has been of great importance in understanding the fundamentals of histocompatibility genetics, as these principles seem to apply to all other mammalian species analyzed. In both mouse and man, the genetic system governing the major histocompatibility antigens, particularly those which appear to be most important to rejection, seems to involve either a single locus with very many alleles or several closely linked loci, giving rise to many pseudoalleles. In man this whole genetic system has been termed the Human Leukocyte A (HL-A) locus, since the leukocyte has been used almost entirely as the test cell.

Graft rejection, multiple transfusions containing leukocytes, or several pregnancies may provoke the formation of humoral antibodies, each one of which will react against leukocytes, or other cells, of some individuals but not of others. Since the great majority of sera from individuals sensitized in these ways contain antibodies against multiple specificities, and different sera may contain overlapping activities against partially shared specificities, the analysis of the immunogenetics of this complex system presents a demanding task. Nevertheless, a number of individual antigens have been recognized and characterized well enough by several investigators so that they have been included in the list of approved antigens accepted by an international committee sponsored by the World Health Organization. Although more antigens will still be discovered and little is yet known of the comparative strength of individual antigens, several important facts of great value in transplantation surgery have emerged already.

As in other species, the major genes of histocompatibility (HL-A) of man are situated on a single pair of chromosomes. This has been determined from studies of the distribution of antigens as they are detected by serological tests of the leukocytes of members of the same family using a large number of suitable antibody reagents. The identity of the chromosome involved is not yet established, but when the tests are technically satisfactory the family pattern always falls into some variation of that depicted in Figure 12–4. Thus, the chances are that 25 per cent of siblings will have received the *same* two chromosomes of histocompatibility from their common parents and will accordingly be "HL-A identical." We are now convinced, from our own observations and those of others, that HL-A identical combinations will generally provide a far more favorable clinical outlook than any other except for identical twins. Even though identical with respect to these multiple important antigens, however, a pair of individuals will not necessarily be identical in their complements of certain other, and usually less important, antigens not sponsored by genes on this one chromosome so that rejection can still occur. Nevertheless, rejection between HL-A

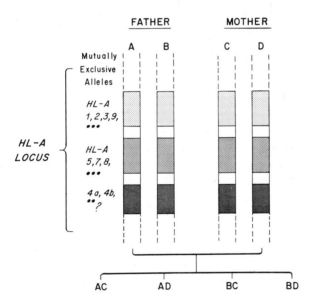

25 % chance that 2 siblings are identical
50 % chance that 2 siblings share one chromosome
25 % chance that 2 siblings share no chromosome

Figure 12–4. Diagram of histocompatibility chromosome distribution in families. The strong HL-A antigens are determined by multiple genes situated on a single pair of chromosomes in each individual. These are apparently grouped into two or three subloci, as diagrammed. On each chromosome a sublocus is represented by only one allele, although an individual may have an identical gene on the other of his two chromosomes and thus be homozygous for a given antigen. Some of the possible antigenic specificities which occur at each sublocus are listed in this figure, but others, as yet undetermined, will surely be added. The fact that the entire block of chromatin responsible for all these factors is transmitted to the offspring of common parents in a limited number of ways makes it possible to select highly similar siblings by genotypic family analysis even though all the antigens concerned are not identified. It is further shown that some siblings are quite incompatible and must be considered undesirable donor candidates.

identical siblings is much easier to control with immunosuppression, and smaller doses of medication are required. Another system of antigens which is clearly of importance to graft acceptance in man is the A, B, O blood group system. Here, as with other antigens, compatibility, but not identity, must be assured. Other red cell antigens, such as the Rh antigens, are not known to be involved in rejection, although there is some suggestion that mismatches for the P antigen are undesirable.

The fact that leukocyte antigen phenotyping in families provides such a strong indication of the success of an intrafamilial transplant, combined with the wealth of information from other species, makes it virtually certain that the class of specificities which are detected by methods now available are indeed central to the rejection process. The data available from some sources, however, have not shown a clear correlation between the clinical result following transplantation and the degree of compatibility as currently assessed by tissue typing. Others report a distinctly positive correlation between compatibility, as judged by leukocyte typing, and transplant survival. From what has been stated previously, it would seem that in those studies in which no correlation was found, this result must be explainable on the basis of the incompleteness of the test sera used, and on multiple technical factors such as the strength and polyspecificity of available antisera. The well-recognized variability of the immunological response would also be expected to produce occasional situations in which defined incompatibilities fail to produce vigorous rejection, especially in the presence of immunosuppressive treatment.

Other tests for compatibility also exist and can still be helpful.[1] Most significant of these is the measurement of compatibility which can be gained by quantifying the metabolic reaction that occurs between the peripheral leukocytes of two individuals maintained for several days in tissue culture.

In summary, it must be emphasized that histocompatibility testing is still in the developmental stage but that its present and future utility is, in the opinion of this author, assured.

ORGAN PROCUREMENT AND PRESERVATION

There is a severe shortage of suitable organs for transplantation. This applies even to the kidney, although the patient in need of a kidney transplant has a distinct advantage over those needing a heart, liver, or lung simply because he can be maintained by artificial means so much better during the waiting period. Because of problems of presensitization or relative difficulty in histocompatibility matching, some recipients must wait much longer than others. This is illustrated by the relative ease of finding a blood group compatible donor for a patient who is group AB as against group O. In the former case *any* organ donor would be acceptable, so far as blood groups are concerned, since in no instance would a new specificity be presented to the recipient. In the latter instance only blood group O donors can be considered.

A kidney deprived of circulation at room temperature will undergo rapid deterioration so that after an hour or so its future, after restoration of circulation, will be uncertain and even then function will usually be restored only after a period of severe limitation manifested as "acute tubular necrosis" or ischemic injury. Much effort is now being exerted to increase public awareness of the need for suitable donor organs. Considerable progress has been made in restructuring the laws of the various states to permit an individual to donate his own tissues at the time of his death and to make family donation of a relative's tissues simpler.[16]

A particular category of donor, but by no means the only potential group to be considered, is composed of patients who have undergone irreversible, generalized brain damage. It has been accepted by many experts that certain patients of this sort can be reliably declared to be dead, and continuing efforts are being made to identify absolutely sound criteria for "brain death." Thus, in many institutions when "brain death" has been declared by the individual patient's physician, and the informed consent of relatives and, when necessary, of legal authorities, has been obtained, organs are removed from a dead body before cessation of circulation.

At present the working criteria for brain death are the following, not all of which are felt to be required simultaneously in certain patients for the diagnosis to be made:[17]

1. Complete unresponsiveness.
2. No spontaneous movements or breathing.
3. No reflexes.
4. Isoelectric electroencephalogram (on two occasions separated by 24 hours).

The current technology for preservation of organs in a state of reliable viability is limited.[18] Although small tissue fragments or suspensions of living cells, such as blood, can be frozen and thawed with excellent retention of viability in the presence of certain solutes such as glycerol or dimethylsulfoxide, this is not yet possible in the case of any organ. Cooling to near freezing temperatures by brief perfusion with balanced salt solutions will provide several hours of satisfactory preservation, at least 8 to 10. This will allow transportation of the organ outside the body of the donor and will afford some time to identify and prepare a potential recipient. The use of constant perfusion with oxygenated fluid probably extends this period of preservation to some degree, perhaps to 20 to 24 hours, but one of its main advantages is in affording a means of testing kidney function by clearance studies before a patient is committed to receiving it.[19] This field will receive much attention in the future, and progress on presently available methods will be important in transplantation.

THE FUTURE OF TRANSPLANTATION SURGERY

The practical accomplishments of transplantation have already been appreciable, but there are several obstacles to a much wider and more successful application of transplantation in the solution of clinical problems. These include the need for a major innovation in immuno-suppression which will permit the *specific* alteration of recipient respon-siveness exclusively to those new antigens that will be presented in the transplant, leaving general immunological responses intact. There are several approaches to this goal, and there is now evidence at hand which suggests that it is attainable.[20] Should this be achieved, the risk associated with transplantation would be decreased substantially so that the transplantation of non-life-sustaining organs and tissues could be an acceptable practice. Thus, the restoration of lost extremities or the renovation of endocrine secretions by transplantation could be-come a reality.

The critical shortage of donor organs which can be appreciated even now would be much more acute if the dangers of transplantation were substantially reduced through improvements in immunosuppres-sion. Although some estimates of the number of suitable kidneys which might be available are encouraging in that they suggest that there could be enough to go around to potential recipients, this does not appear to be true for hearts. Thus, if heart replacement with living tissue, rather than an implantable machine, is to be generally available for all patients who could benefit from a new heart with current pat-terns of heart disease, at least some of these new organs must come from animals. As more information is gained regarding the immunologi-cal response of one species to another, the control of xenograft rejection looks somewhat less formidable, especially for organs such as the heart which apparently would not synthesize and release potentially immu-nogenic donor-specific proteins into the recipient as would the liver.

As the field of transplantation develops, it is clearly remaining as a healthy link between surgery and many other branches of medicine and biology, a link which may lead to new understanding of reactions to malignant cells, to the genesis and control of autoimmune conditions, and perhaps also to hints concerning the mechanism of aging.

REFERENCES

1. Russell, P. S., and Winn, H. J.: Transplantation. Medical progress. N. Eng. J. Med. 282:786, 896, 1970.
2. Huggins, C. E.: Frozen blood. Europ. Surg. Res. 1:3, 1969.
3. Proceedings of the Conference on Antilymphocyte Serum. Eds., D. B. Amos, R. E. Billingham, H. S. Lawrence, and P. S. Russell. Federation Proceedings, January-February, 1970.
4. Antilymphocyte Serum. A Ciba Foundation Study Group No. 29. Eds., G. E. W. Wolstenholme and M. O'Connor, J. and A. Churchill, Ltd., 1967.

5. Cosimi, A. B., Skamene, E., Bonney, W. W., and Russell, P. S.: Experience with large-dose intravenous use of antithymocyte globulin in primates and man. Surgery 68:54, 1970.
6. ACS/NIH Organ Transplant Registry, 55 East Erie Street, Chicago, Illinois. John J. Bergan, M.D., Director. Report as of October 23, 1970.
7. Porter, K. A.: Rejection in treated renal allografts (symposium on tissue and organ transplantation). J. Clin. Path. (Suppl.) 20:518, 1967.
8. Dixon, F. J., McPhaul, J. J., and Lerner, R.: Recurrence of glomerulonephritis in the transplanted kidney. Arch. Int. Med. (Chicago) 123:554, 1969.
9. Bildsoc, P., Sorensen, S. F., Pettirossi, O., and Simonsen, M.: Heart and kidney transplantation from segregating hybrid to parental rats. Trans. Rev. 3:36, 1970.
10. Starzl, T. E.: Experience in Hepatic Transplantation. Philadelphia, W. B. Saunders Company, 1969.
11. Calne, R. Y., Sells, R. A., Pena, J. R., et al.: Induction of immunological tolerance by porcine liver allografts. Nature (London) 223:472, 1969.
12. Lower, R. R., and Shumway, N. E.: Studies on orthotopic homotransplantation of the canine heart. Surg. Forum 11:18, 1960.
13. Kelly, W. D., Lillehei, R. C., and Merkel, F. K.: Allotransplantation of the pancreas and duodenum along with the kidney in diabetic nephropathy. Surgery 61:827, 1967.
14. Ammann, A. J., Meuwissen, H. J., Good, R. A., and Hong, R.: Successful bone marrow transplantation in a patient with humoral and cellular immunity deficiency. Clin. & Exp. Immunol. 7:343, 1970.
15. Batchelor, J. R., and Hackett, M.: HL-A matching in treatment of burned patients with skin allografts. Lancet 2:581, 1970.
16. Sadler, A. M., Jr., Sadler, B. L., and Stason, E. B.: The uniform anatomical gift act: a model for reform. J.A.M.A., 206:1949, 1968.
17. A definition of irreversible coma: report of the Ad Hoc Committee of the Harvard Medical School to examine the definition of brain death. J.A.M.A. 205:337, 1968.
18. Robertson, R. D., and Jacob, S. W.: The preservation of intact organs. Adv. Surg. 3:75, 1968.
19. Belzer, F. O., and Kountz, S. L.: Preservation and transplantation of human cadaver kidneys. Ann. Surg. 172:394, 1970.
20. Russell, P. S.: Immunological enhancement. Transplant. Proc. 3:960, 1971.

CHAPTER 13

PROBLEMS OF INFANTS AND CHILDREN

William B. Kiesewetter, M.D., F.A.C.S.

Much of the improvement in surgical results in adults in the last two decades has been rightly attributed to the attention given to pre- and postoperative care. Pure technical prowess has played its part, particularly in the cardiovascular field; but even here the definition of the physiological perimeters and the staying within them or the restoration of them have played a major role in success. If all of this be true in the adult, with his large reserves and ability to make homeostatic ajustments, it is even more important in the pediatric surgical patient. It has been well said that the infant or child undergoing surgery has "more bounce but less reserve" than his adult counterpart. This chapter will deal, therefore, with those considerations which will best put the child in the best condition for his operation, keep him there during the procedure, and maintain his postoperative ability to cope with the healing processes. It will be dealt with under the two main headings: (1) those general considerations that have to do with any condition requiring surgery, and (2) those specific considerations that bear particular reference to surgery in a certain area of the body or organ system.

GENERAL CONSIDERATIONS

Preoperative Diagnosis. Fundamental to all preoperative care is an accurate diagnosis of the condition with which one is faced. Without this, a rational approach to understanding what imbalances may exist, or come to exist, is quite impossible.

A careful *history* will often suggest both the diagnosis and the preparation necessary for surgery. A polyhydramnic mother with a vomiting or distended newborn suggests the strong possibility that he has intestinal obstruction; the emeses portend an alkalosis and dehydration that go along with it. An obstructed newborn, whose family has lost a sibling from "bowel stoppage" or who has a sibling with cystic fibrosis, may himself be a patient with mucoviscidosis manifesting itself as meconium ileus; such a child may tolerate general anesthesia poorly, or it may cause respiratory complications postoperatively. To have the mother of a four year old with hematemesis and melena tell of prolonged neonatal jaundice or an infected umbilical stump is frequently the historical key to recognizing portal hypertension.

Adequate physical examination is the sine qua non to diagnosis and preoperative preparation of any surgical child. If the vomiting is progressive after the onset at a few weeks of age and an epigastric mass is felt at the end point of gastric peristaltic waves, pyloric stenosis is the most likely cause. Attention must be directed toward possible dehydration and alkalosis resulting from the emeses. Bile-stained vomitus at any age is almost pathognomonic of true intestinal obstruction as opposed to the clear, functional vomitus of "nerves," reflex pain, gastroenteritis or the like. Bubbling, frothy mucous from the nose or mouth of a newborn in respiratory distress should alert one to the possible presence of esophageal atresia in the infant.

Finally, the ancillary use of *roentgen study* is mandatory for diagnosis in a reasonably high proportion of surgical problems. Simple plain films of a vomiting infant will often clinch a diagnosis by the presence of excessive gas in the stomach when a tracheosophageal fistula without atresia is present; or such a condition may result from pyloric or duodenal obstruction. A distended colon with a narrow anorectal area suggests megacolon as the cause. Pneumoperitoneum, when revealed, is of ominous import, and suitable antibacterial preparation is indicated preoperatively. Gas-filled loops shown on the simple chest film of a dyspneic child are of paramount interest in suggesting diaphragmatic hernia as the causative factor. Although many specialized examinations can be very helpful, three seem of singular importance: (1) an intravenous pyelogram in a child with an abdominal mass may suggest tumor or obstructive disease with lowered renal reserve; (2) a barium enema which reveals microcolon in a newborn means obstruction above this unused narrow bowel, as in meconium ileus; (3) a barium study of the distal colon will suggest Hirschsprung's disease when a narrow segment becomes large in the rectosigmoid area of a lifelong constipated child.

Optimal Condition. To put an infant or a child in optimal preoperative condition, many things must be considered and done when indicated. Foremost, of course, is to determine the *fluid and electrolyte balance* and to adjust it to as near normal as possible. At best, dehydration is an estimation and may be classified as mild (5 per cent), moderate (10 per cent) and severe (15 per cent). To make such an estimation, one may judge:

1. Skin turgor—pinching the skin and counting 1 per cent dehydration for each second it takes to flatten out.

2. Eyes—degree of recession.
3. Fontanelle—flatness or concavity.
4. Urine output.

Electrolyte status may be determined by either the micro or conventional intravenous techniques and should include the basic four studies: Na, Cl, K and CO_2. With the state of electrolyte and fluid balance compositely determined and evaluated, the regimen to be utilized is plotted out.

An infant or child suffering from pure dehydration from poor intake and a proportional electrolyte loss in all components needs *reconstitution* by the administration of water and physiological amounts of electrolytes with it. Table 13-1 suggests a method of estimating the correct fluids and electrolytes needed in each of the mild, moderate and severe dehydration states. The rate of administration is individually calculated and usually takes from 3 to 12 hours to accomplish, depending on the severity of the dehydration.

Correction of dehydration of any degree may be accomplished by the administration of appropriate combinations of 5 per cent dextrose in water, 5 per cent dextrose in normal saline and 5 per cent dextrose in lactated Ringer's solution. Dextrose in water is useful in "pure" dehydration without electrolyte shift; dextrose in saline is applicable to dehydration from vomiting, and dextrose in lactated Ringer's is most useful in diarrheal dehydration.

In moderate (10 per cent) dehydration, it may take 15 to 20 hours to obtain correction; fluids given at the rate of 10 cc./kg./hr. will accomplish this without danger of overloading.

Severe dehydration is best corrected by non-glucose-containing solutions to start with to prevent a hyperosmolar diuresis with its loss of fluid and electrolytes that defeats the repletion scheme. About one fourth of the calculated fluid and electrolyte is given in the first four hours at a rate of 20 cc./kg./kr. The remainder of the need is then spread out over the next 18 to 24 hours.

Potassium is given only after urination has been initiated by the fluid replacement so as not to run the risk of hyperkalemia from poor urinary output. At no time does one exceed the concentration of 40 mEq./liter of this ion, even though the deficits might seem to dictate it; again, the risks of hyperkalemia are thus avoided.

Of course, *maintenance* amounts of fluid and electrolytes must be

Table 13-1

WT. LOSS	WATER	Na	Cl	K
5% (mild)	50 cc./kg.	5 mEq./L.	5 mEq./L.	3 mEq./L.
10% (moderate)	100 cc./kg.	10 mEq./L.	10 mEq./L.	6 mEq./L.
15% (severe)	150 cc./kg.	15 mEq./L.	15 mEq./L.	9 mEq./L.

Table 13–2

WATER	Na	Cl	K
100 cc./kg./day (up to 10 kg.) 50 cc./kg./day (10–20 kg.) 25 cc./kg./day (over 20 kg.)	3 mEq./kg./day " "	2 mEq./kg./day " "	2 mEq./kg./day " "

given coincidentally, as Table 13–1 applies only to correction of deficits present. Such maintenance is given on the basis shown in Table 13–2. These maintenance amounts can be given in proper proportions by simply estimating the total fluid requirements and making them up one fifth as 5 per cent dextrose in saline and four fifths as 5 per cent dextrose in water; the potassium is added as KCl in the number of milliequivalents needed.

When specific deficits occur because of a differential loss of a single or two ions, correction must be made on the calculated deficit of that ion or ions. It should always be done so as to undercorrect rather than overcorrect the deficit. It can be done as follows on the basis of the serum Na determination, as the Cl will be corrected by the same means, allowing renal function to make any finer adjustments:

$$Na^+ \text{ needed} = mEq./L. \text{ deficit} \times wt. \text{ (kg.)} \times 70\% \text{ (infants)}$$
$$\times 60\% \text{ (children)}$$

Usable, or extracellular fluid, is estimated as 70 per cent of body weight in infants under 3 years and 60 per cent in children over 3 years. These deficits are added to the estimated dehydration and maintenance amounts and given to reconstitute the child.

Although admittedly serum electrolytes do not reflect fully the cellular condition, repeat determinations will be a rough guide to the effectiveness of therapy. They should be done with this purpose in mind.

In addition to fluid and electrolyte adjustments, the determination of a pediatric patient's *acid-base status* must be undertaken. This is often referred to as knowing what a patient's "blood gases" are. They are calculated from a whole blood sample and include pH, pCO_2, pO_2, standard bicarbonate and base excess. They suggest the total body reaction to a given state of hydration and acid production or loss at the tissue level. They also give a reasonable assessment of the state of tissue perfusion when combined with the clinical observation of respiration, heart action and peripheral circulation.

Basically, any of the four classic deviations from normal that have been so helpful in adults can occur in children. We refer to metabolic acidosis and alkalosis, as well as respiratory acidosis and alkalosis. They may also occur in combinations. For all intents and purposes, respiratory acidosis seldom occurs; it may be dismissed because pathologic conditions that lead to this aberration are not very often found in children. We are left with metabolic acidosis, metabolic alkalosis and respiratory alkalosis, which are met in this order of descending frequency.

Metabolic acidosis is the abnormality that most frequently confronts the pediatric surgeon. It is the result of dehydration, volume reduction and tissue hypoperfusion. A typical set of blood gases would show a pH of 7.24, a pCO_2 of 40, and a pO_2 of 60, with a standard bicarbonate of 18 and a base excess of -10. An estimate of the degree of dehydration is made and fluids and colloids are administered to restore volume and combat dehydration. Base is given in the form of bicarbonate. It is calculated by the following two formulas:

If the pH is between 7.20 and 7.30:
(Weight in kg. $\times$ 0.3) $\times$ base excess = mEq. bicarbonate
If the pH is below 7.20:
(Weight in kg. $\times$ 0.6) $\times$ base excess = mEq. bicarbonate

Redetermination of acid base is carried out in 2 to 3 hours and further adjustment made by bicarbonate administration only if no clinical and chemical improvement has occurred or the pH remains severely depressed. "Clinical improvement" means restitution of circulation and renal function.

In metabolic alkalosis, a lesion causing vomiting usually underlies the problem. Loss of hydrogen ions through the vomitus leaves an excess of serum bicarbonate, with eventual shift of the potassium ions from the cells into serum. This shift shows sodium and hydrogen ions transferring into the cells. This increased serum potassium is excreted by the kidneys, and the "blood gases" will reflect the whole picture as a pH of 7.50, a pCO_2 of 50, a pO_2 of 70, a standard bicarbonate of 40 and a base excess of $+11$. The correction involves restoration of circulating volume and the provision of potassium and chloride. This involves dehydration correction as detailed above, and chlorides are provided by 5 per cent dextrose in normal saline in the severely dehydrated or by one half 5 per cent dextrose in water and one half 5 per cent dextrose in saline in the modestly depleted child. Potassium is added as soon as urinary output is established and should be pushed at that point at a rapid rate.

Respiratory alkalosis is known to occur most often while a child is on artificial ventilation. The washing out of CO_2 results in less oxygen carrying capacity of the blood and a decrease of serum CO_2. Paradoxically, the poorer O_2 perfusion results in some tissue metabolic acidosis along with the respiratory alkalosis. Sudden cessation of the artificial ventilation makes for a rapid rise of pCO_2. This can be obviated by gradually weaning the child from a ventilator while blood gas monitoring assures that the acid-base equilibrium is being maintained.

Although fluid and electrolyte management is essential, *vitamin* requirements are important, especially in the newborn infant. Vitamin K_1 oxide in a dose of 2.4 mg. is sufficient for the infant, and higher doses are dangerous; in older children, larger doses may be given over several days parenterally when absorption from the intestine is in doubt in a jaundiced patient. Vitamin C in doses of 300 to 500 mg. is a safety factor that should be employed in all newborns preoperatively and will do no harm in any other depleted child.

To provide an *intravenous route for administration* of fluids, electrolytes, vitamins or blood, a large bore plastic cannula or needle is required. If parenteral administrations are planned for some days before and/or after surgery, a plastic tube inserted into a large venous channel should be employed. These can be placed through a needle in older children or can be threaded over a metal stylet in young children, so as to get maximum size into the vein. A cut-down insertion is the surest method, but uses up veins quite quickly, as they are tied in and thrombose more rapidly than in a free-flow vein. The medial malleolar saphenous is most commonly employed, or, in abdominal cases near the vena cava, an antecubital vein is preferable. As a last resort, when long-term intravenous work or frequent blood sampling is anticipated, a Silastic catheter can be placed through the saphenofemoral junction into the iliac or inferior vena cava, or a Silastic tube introduced via the jugular into the superior vena cava.

When identification of the urethra or bladder is important and decompression at and after surgery becomes necessary, a Foley self-retaining *catheter* is introduced immediately before surgery.

A child with a *temperature* above 101° needs the following done before surgery:

1. Rehydration to eliminate this as a cause of fever.

2. Administration of antibiotics of the broad-spectrum type or penicillin and kanamycin to combat sepsis as a fever cause.

3. Application of ice bags immediately before anesthesia to bring temperature into normal range and reduce the chance of hyperthermic convulsions.

The final step in putting the infant or child in optimal condition for his surgery is the adequate use of *preoperative medication*. It is employed for the following purposes:

1. To allay fear and apprehension.

2. To minimize respiratory secretions.

3. To control an exhausting and excessively rapid respiratory rate.

4. To facilitate anesthesia.

5. To obtund harmful reflexes.

It should be remembered that the medication (usually some combination of an opiate, barbiturate and scopolamine) as shown in Table 13-3 must have 30 to 45 minutes to achieve maximal effect before anesthesia is started.

Operative Handling. It is beyond the scope of a manual like this

Table 13–3. PREOPERATIVE MEDICATION TABLE

AGE	WEIGHT (lbs.)	MORPHINE-IN-ATROPINE OR (mg.)	SCOPOLAMINE (mg.)	SECONAL (INTRAMUSCULAR) (mg.)
Premature	Under 5½	–	Atr. 0.075	–
0–1 month	5½–7	–	Atr. 0.1	–
2–3 months	8–12	–	Atr. 0.15	–
4–5 months	13–14	–	Atr. 0.2	–
6–7 months	15–16	0.5	Scop. 0.1	15 (0.3 cc.)
8–11 months	17–20	0.6	Scop. 0.1	20 (0.4 cc.)
12–18 months	21–25	0.8	Scop. 0.15	25 (0.5 cc.)
19–24 months	26–30	1.0	Scop. 0.15	30 (0.6 cc.)
2–3 years	31–35	1.5	Scop. 0.15	40 (0.8 cc.)
4–5 years	36–45	2.0	Scop. 0.15	50 (1.0 cc.)
6–8 years	46–65	3.0	Scop. 0.2	75 (1.5 cc.)
9–10 years	66–80	4.0	Scop. 0.2	75 (1.5 cc.)
11–12 years	81–90	5.0	Scop. 0.3	100 (2.0 cc.)
13–14 years	91–120	8.0	Scop. 0.3	100 (2.0 cc.)
Over 14 years	Over 120	10.0	Scop. 0.3	100 (2.0 cc.)

1. The doses of opiate and barbiturate are very conservative and are calculated to complement each other. Each alone will be inadequate. No codeine is to be substituted. Demerol may be substituted for morphine, and must be in asthmatics.

2. Atropine and scopolamine doses are large; do not order more than the suggested dose. Do not use scopolamine for outpatients.

3. Barbiturates are most effective intramuscularly. Absorption by the oral or (especially) the rectal route is slower and less predictable.

to deal at length with *anesthesia* in children. It is a specialized branch of anesthesiology, and to acquire skill, safety and versatility in it requires training and care. The occasional pediatric anesthetist is not the one to give anesthesia to a child under one year or for a cardiovascular operation. Almost all the modalities and techniques of anesthesia used in adults are employed in children, but with much more specific indications. The margin of safety is much narrower and must be constantly borne in mind. To assist in determining basic body reactions during surgery, a number of *monitoring devices* are employed. A precordial stethoscope is a "must" in all cases, as is a readily available peripheral pulse-taking spot and a good light to see color and pupillary reflex. Any long or serious case demands a rectal thermometer and electrocardiogram to correlate electrical activity with observable peripheral vascular signs. Some people consider an electroencephalogram the most sensitive indicator of hypoxia and impending peripheral collapse, but it is not widely used.

Temperature control is very important when combined with the indwelling thermometric monitor. Normothermia is the ideal to be aimed at, and placing the child on a refrigeration-heating mattress can usually make it possible of attainment. Small infants seldom elevate their temperatures, but only drop them, so a controllable heating pad may suffice for them. Older children should have the benefit of a heat-cold device if at all possible.

Fluid and electrolyte administration during the course of surgery must provide adequate solute and volume without overwhelming the child's ability to excrete it through a kidney that has the ability to do so but which is somewhat altered by the stress of surgery. A scheme that has proved useful in our hands in the intraoperative management of fluids in all but the premature is outlined in Table 13-4. Prematures are physiologically incapable of managing these full fluid loads, and adjustments downward must be made. Something between one half to three quarters of the suggested amount can be safely used.

Operative *blood loss* must be constantly borne in mind and estimated by the surgical team, and replaced in a volume-for-volume manner. This is of paramount importance in children under two years because their blood volumes are small and the losses incurred are much greater relative to the margin of safety. Methods for determining this loss may be so simple as the combined estimate of the operating team or so sophisticated as by radioactive substances and as expensive a machine as the Volumetron. In between lies the weighing of sponges. Such losses must be matched against an estimated blood volume of 65 to 75 cc./lb. of body weight. It goes without saying that appropriate cross-matching procedures in sufficient quantity should be carried out preoperatively. It then becomes a matter of administering the blood through any one of a number of measuring devices calibrated for children so that accurate, small quantitation can be carried out. Most people feel that, when using the ordinary ACD bank blood, 1 to 2 cc. of 10 per cent calcium gluconate should be administered with each 100 cc. of blood given to help combat any lowering of calcium by the blood given.

The control of fluid and blood administration is the surgeon's responsibility, but he may (and usually does) delegate it to the anesthetist to supervise.

Table 13-4.   INTRAOPERATIVE FLUIDS IN MODERATE TO
SEVERE TRAUMA

	OPERATIVE	
2.5–5 kg.	½ D5W – ½ D5RL 10 ml./kg./hr.	+potassium
6–20 kg.	½ D5W – ½ D5RL 10 ml./kg./hr. × 2 hrs. 5 ml./kg./hr. thereafter	+potassium
20 + kg.	D5RL 5 ml./kg./hr.	+potassium

D5W = 5% dextrose in water.
D5/0.2% NaCl = 5% dextrose in 0.2% saline.
D5RL = 5% dextrose in lactated Ringer's.

Postoperative Care. Careful management of the *recovery period* from anesthesia is most important to the well-being of all patients after surgery. It is best managed by specially trained personnel in a recovery room where facilities for emergencies (tracheotomy, broncoscopy, pharyngeal intubation and cardiac massage) are readily available. There should be a nurse or nurses in constant attendance until consciousness is regained. The vital signs should be checked and recorded every 15 minutes or less until they have stabilized. In infants, vital signs are best recognized by color, the character of respiration and the rapidity of the heart rate. The child should be put in a position to favor normal, unobstructed breathing, and oxygen and suction must be available.

The moderately to severely ill pediatric surgical patient needs the benefit of an intensive care unit where *monitoring* of his vital functions can be the responsibility of a specially trained staff. A central venous pressure line via the superior vena cava provides much information as to the functional intravascular volume. It also allows for fluid, electrolyte and caloric intake. Pulse rate and electrocardiographic monitoring can be done in electronic fashion as in the adult, using smaller electrodes. If arterial pressure is a necessity, an arterial line into the aorta by way of the umbilical artery or, in extreme cases, via the femoral is sufficient; these lines also provide a ready way for blood gas sampling. Electronic breathing sensors are simple and helpful in managing a child's respiratory needs. The temperature regulation of a very small infant can be implemented by electronic thermocouples attached to the skin and the heating devices. Urine output and specific gravity of the urine give a reliable index of volume expansion and state of kidney function. When all these monitoring determinations are combined with serum electrolytes and acid-base balance, more precise guidelines for postoperative care can be outlined.

Attention to the *airway* is of utmost importance in the careful postoperative management of the child. Atelectasis is not nearly so frequent as in adults, but it still presents problems. It can best be dealt with by change of position and by adequate suctioning when there are secretions in the oropharynx. Such suctioning should not be so frequent as to irritate, but not so infrequent as to allow material to accumulate. There is adequate reason for using a humidified atmosphere in which to loosen the secretions and enable them to be brought up spontaneously by the coughing or crying of the child. If the child's secretions are particularly thick, it has been helpful to use some acetylcystine in the humidifying solution. If a child is badly played out after surgery, it may be of benefit to leave the endotracheal tube in and give him assisted ventilator respiration for 12 to 24 hours after surgery.

From a practical standpoint, the only real indication for use of a respirator is in a patient who is breathing inadequately, whatever may be the cause. It has been our experience that a volume-regulated (as opposed to pressure-regulated) respirator, with proper humidification and nebulization, offers the best assistance in the pediatric age group. $PO_2 < 40$, $pCO_2 > 65$ and pH under 7.25 are generally accepted, absolute indications for respiratory assistance. Relative indications are not as easily outlined but should be made by the full-time staff who attend on an intensive care unit; this staff of doctors and nurses are essential to any type of postoperative care of the very ill patient, but they are indispensable when artifical or assisted ventilation is used. In general, adjustments, weaning and withdrawal of respirators are judged by clinical and blood gas determinations.

Early and complete *ambulation* is generally the sign of a child who is recovering and is certainly the desirable goal to aim for as quickly as possible. A sick child or a child in pain will not move, and this may indicate a surgical complication or continuing illness. Although restraint of the extremities and the use of a "crib-top" are necessary in infants and children, particularly when intravenous infusions are maintained, it is desirable not to maintain this type of restraint except under specific indications and for as short a period of time as possible.

The use of *antibiotics* is a field in which there is considerable controversy and difference of opinion. There are specific situations in which antibiotics should be used. These include prematures, infection in the mother or amnionitis, children with known congenital heart disease, and situations in which gross infection is already present at the time of surgery. Under such circumstances, by culture and sensitivity testing, one can give a specific antibiotic for the bacteria present. In general, antibiotics should be reserved for these situations and should not be given routinely as prophylaxis after clean surgery. The change of flora caused by such antibiotic administration may produce complications more severe than those from the original bacteria themselves.

Specific attention to bowels and bladder is seldom necessary postoperatively in children because bowel movements are usually unaltered by surgery. Dehydration and inactivity may induce constipation and fecal impactions. Preoperative cleansing enemas and an awareness of this postoperative possibility will usually suffice to keep it under control. Catheterization is seldom necessary, except in neurologic and anorectal problems when a catheter is usually left in place at surgery to overcome this possibility.

One of the distressing abnormalities of the postoperative period, when it occurs, is *convulsions*. There are many possible causes for this, but those which are of most common occurrence in childhood are hyperthermia, anoxia, hypocalcemic tetany and toxemia resulting from infection or drug sensitivity. All these considerations and others must be investigated and specific therapy directed toward their correction.

Probably the most important postoperative consideration in pediatric surgery embraces *fluids, electrolytes* and *feedings*. Assuming that a child has been brought to a reasonable state of fluid and electrolyte balance prior to surgery, that which must be done after surgery is the maintenance of the state of hydration and the replacement of any abnormal losses of electrolytes. The aforementioned scheme for maintenance fluids and electrolytes should be carried out postoperatively, and any abnormal suction from the gastrointestinal tract, or from fistulas, should be replaced cubic centimeter for cubic centimeter. Upper gastrointestinal losses should be replaced in the child under six months by half normal saline, and in the child of over six months with two thirds normal saline. In addition to the above, the potassium replacement should be based on a 10 to 15 mEq./liter replacement. Lower gastrointestinal tract losses of abnormal degree should be calculated by an assay of the fluid lost, which will probably be higher in sodium and potassium than the upper intestinal tract losses. Mouth feedings should be restored as promptly as possible as the only adequate way to make up calories. In certain types of surgery, the use of a gastrostomy tube and in others a nasogastric tube can be employed to give alimentation when the child will himself be unwilling to take food in the conventional fashion. In recent years, schemes for providing adequate parenteral alimentation both for caloric intake and to attain positive nitrogen balance and weight gain have been devised. These are dealt with in another section of this manual.

Intestinal decompression must be employed in most cases of gastrointestinal surgery. The smaller the child, the more imperative it is to undertake this through an intermittent nasogastric tube insertion, rather than the continuance of a tube which may very well interfere with the child's breathing and cause upper respiratory complications. Of late, it has been desirable in upper gastrointestinal surgery to use a gastrostomy as a means of decompression prior to its use as a means for feeding. Finally, one should not fail to remember the usefulness of the oxygen tent in keeping the accumulation of gases to a minimum.

Attention to *pain* relief is of utmost importance in the adult. It seldom plays the same role in the child. Pain should be relieved by sedation, rather than by narcosis, and it has been our experience that infants rarely require narcotics. Pain relievers should not be ordered on a schedule, but should be given as needed for comfort after the child has been evaluated by a member of the house staff.

Finally, *temperature control* must be adequately managed in the postoperative period, with the aim of keeping the child as near normothermia as possible. A few of the frequent causes of an increased temperature are found in an elevated Isolette temperature, unsuspected infection in the patient, and simple dehydration by allowing the child to get behind in his fluid intake. Correction of these is easy and obvious.

It goes without saying that the best postoperative care is rendered to children in a special unit manned by nurses who are particularly competent in the postoperative management of surgical patients. The older children can be best handled in a small (five to six bed) ward, particularly if any amount of cardiac surgery is done in the institution.

Neonates receive the best chance for recovery by being put in a small unit managed by specialized pediatric surgical nurses who are trained in the management of such infants in Isolettes and who know how to handle particular problems.

SPECIAL CONSIDERATIONS

THORACIC SURGERY

Preoperative. A number of factors demand the attention of a surgeon preoperatively when there is a thoracic surgical condition present, but *dyspnea* and *cyanosis* are among two of the most important. Both of these indicate a lack of adequate oxygenation of the blood, and every effort should be made to correct this, in order to put the patient in the best possible condition for his surgery. The inherent basic problem may be such that this is impossible, but the employment of judicious suctioning, bronchoscopy and liberal administration of oxygen and oxygen carriers (blood) are certainly indicated. *Atelectasis* may be one of the causes for the dyspnea and cyanosis owing to infection or to simple mechanical blockage of a pulmonary segment or lobe. Stimulation of the cough reflex by voluntary coughing or endotracheal suctioning, together with the administration of appropriate antibiotics in the presence of a rich oxygen atmosphere, is an obvious step to be undertaken. Another contributing cause to the dyspnea and cyanosis may be the presence of an unsuspected *pneumothorax.* Physical examination may suggest the presence of this, but a chest x-ray should be undertaken to be sure that it is present. If it is found, aspiration of the pneumothorax should be undertaken promptly, and if it is due to a bronchopleural fistula, the insertion of an intercostal tube is mandatory.

Postoperative. Many things are required in the management of the postoperative thoracic patient. Adequate attention to the intercostal drainage set-up is most important, so as not to allow any pneumothorax to occur that would collapse portions of the lung and make adequate ventilation less certain. Children have a great tendency to lie inertly in bed and to avoid the necessary deep breathing and voluntary coughing which will keep their airways free, thus preventing atelectasis. On the other hand, the very small child will cry as an indication that he is unhappy or in some pain, and this involuntarily helps in the maintenance of a clear airway. It has been our custom through the years to insist upon as little in the way of dressings on the chest as possible, since all of these limit the child's ability to breathe; whenever possible, no dressings whatsoever are employed.

Any form of anoxia, temporary or prolonged is apt to exceed the lowered threshold for convulsive seizures in the central nervous system of a child, and every effort should be made to assure adequate oxygenation in order to prevent these detrimental convulsions.

Several infectious problems arise in the postoperative period in the child, as well as in the adult. Tracheobronchitis is not an infrequent problem, and is usually due to anesthesia and operation having been undertaken when incipient coryza was present. It is also possible that endotracheal intubation itself may be a contributing factor. A cold steam vaporizer, together with antibiotics, may be necessary to help correct this situation, but in spite of it the child may go on to a frank pneumonic situation which will demand symptomatic treatment with higher dosages of antibiotics and an oxygen tent. The final infectious problem which one sees with some frequency in thoracic surgery is the accumulation of fluid in the pleural cavity after the intercostal catheter has been removed. Simple tapping may take care of this problem satisfactorily, but all too often the pleural sera becomes infected and a frank empyema results. An intercostal catheter will have to be reinserted and, after appropriate culture, the specific antibiotics instituted which will combat his infection.

Finally, two aids to the management of the thoracic cavities after surgery may have to be undertaken—tracheostomy and ventilators. In many cardiovascular situations, a tracheostomy is done electively after surgery in order to maintain an adequate thoracic toilet. In other thoracic surgery, or following traumatic endotracheal intubation, it may be necessary to institute tracheostomy in order to overcome the effects of subglottic and laryngeal edema. A child who has undergone extensive surgery with depletion of his ability to respire may have to have a ventilator instituted in order to carry out his respiratory functions for him for a shorter or longer period of time. With the institution and understanding of these artificial respirators, many children have been helped over the difficult phase of their respiratory exhaustion and have gone on to recovery.

GASTROINTESTINAL SURGERY

Preoperative. In addition to the many general considerations alluded to previously, a few specific matters demand attention in the preoperative phase of pediatric intestinal surgery. Distention caused by intraluminal or extraluminal gas can be a very real problem as far as the child is concerned, because it elevates his diaphragms and makes respiration very difficult. This adds to the already vicious cycle that is present in the sense of debilitating the patient and making him less able to withstand his subsequent surgery. Intraluminal gas is difficult to manage, but it should be attempted through the usual means of intestinal decompression (tube, nothing by mouth, oxygen, etc.). Pneumoperitoneum can be dealt with much more efficaciously in the form of simply inserting a needle into the abdominal cavity and drawing off the necessary air to relieve the respiratory problem.

Shock is not nearly so often met in the preoperative pediatric patient as in the adult, but, when present, it should be dealt with by the usual measure of placing the patient in the Trendelenburg position, combined with intravenous fluids and antibiotics as indicated. Blood, or other plasma expanders, should be utilized when necessary. Hemorrhage, as a contributing factor to the shock or as an entity in itself, requires the administration of blood and an obvious early attempt to correct the cause of the loss of circulating blood volume.

Postoperative. Ordinary postoperative distention and paralytic ileus can be met by the usual measures for intestinal decompression referred to above. However, if prolonged (beyond 72 hours), one should think in terms of the possibility of an unrelieved intestinal obstruction being present, a localized abscess forming, or a pneumoperitoneum having occurred; all of these require prompt corrective action. Ambulation and enemas may be helpful in adynamic ileus, but parasympathomimetic drugs are usually no more effective in a child than they are in an adult.

Dressings of the abdominal wall should be minimal in extent and, whenever possible, should not be placed transversely so as to further limit the ability of the abdomen to distend, causing elevation of the diaphragm. Hiccups are usually transient, but, when protracted, may indicate a serious gastrointestinal complication such as peritonitis. Their main danger, if prolonged, is exhaustion, and they should be treated by simple rebreathing, or by use of a carbon dioxide-oxygen mixture.

Gastrointestinal fistulas do occur but may be of such minor degree as to make it difficult to be certain of their presence; the feeding of a carmine red or a charcoal solution will establish this. Their management should be toward the prevention of local tissue destruction by the use of protective ointments, or the removal of the fistulous matter by suction devices. The definitive closure of the fistula is of first importance.

Fecal impaction has been referred to above, and should be prevented by appropriate preoperative enemas. Should it occur postoperatively, a saline enema with or without the previous digital breaking up of the impaction will usually take care of the problem.

GENITOURINARY SURGERY

Preoperative. Three things may characterize the preoperative urologic patient—urinary retention, infection, and azotemia. Urinary retention may be due to blockage of the urinary tract at any point from the renal pelvis to the distal urethra. Appropriate steps must be taken to establish proximal diversion of the urine before corrective surgery. This may necessitate nephrostomy, ureterostomy or cystostomy. Infection is a constant factor in urologic problems, because it always superimposes itself upon obstruction, neoplasm or calculus. This should be dealt with by low grade antibiotic therapy until such time as the cause for the infection can be corrected surgically; it seems unwise to use one's strongest weapon before corrective surgery has been accomplished. The most serious complication preoperatively is that of azotemia, in which there may be such massive destruction of renal function that the blood cannot be adequately cleared of its waste products. Dietary measures and relief of any obstruction should be used to relieve the azotemia, and as a last resort dialysis should be employed. Transplantation of kidneys may also be considered.

Postoperative. Urinary retention postoperatively is most frequently encountered in specific urologic operations. Decompression by an indwelling Foley catheter or by a suprapubic cystostomy is definitive for this condition. Should urinary retention occur in the renal pelvis because of ureteropelvic surgery, appropriate decompression measures must be undertaken in the area above the obstruction. When other catheters are used, it is imperative that they be placed under aseptic conditions and that low-grade antibiotic therapy be given during the course of their presence to reduce the incidence and amount of infection if it occurs. The catheter must not be so large as to distend the urethra or other area where it is placed and thereby create a condition in which infection can easily ensue.

Stricture of an anastomotic site in the urologic tract can be dealt with by appropriate dilatation methods if it occurs in the urethra; above the bladder such dilatation is usually ineffective and the stricture must be corrected by further definitive surgery.

A fistula may occur at a site of anastomosis or above a point of obstruction when drainage procedures have been carried out; many fistulas will resolve spontaneously, given time for the edema to subside. Failure to do so indicates the continued presence of obstruction and must be dealt with definitively.

Finally, true anuria, or lack of formation of urine can occur, and may be due to a lower nephron nephrosis resulting from prolonged surgery with shock or from an incompatible blood transfusion. Another cause for anuria may be an error in surgical technique whereby ureters or urethra may have been ligated. The cause should be ascertained and appropriate action taken to correct this. If it is a surgical error, the treatment is obvious. The handling of shock and the limiting of fluids in the case of lower nephron nephrosis will be great helps in this situation. One may have to resort to temporary use of an artificial kidney to overcome the anuria.

EXTREMITIES

Preoperative. Every infant undergoing surgery should have his extremities wrapped in cotton wadding so as to preserve the body temperature by preventing undue radiation at this point. It also protects the extremities as one institutes immobilization procedures to keep them from movement during the course of surgery.

Postoperative. Phlebitis and its sequelae are the only extremity problems that seem to ensue postoperatively. Phlebitis seldom occurs spontaneously and is usually the result of continued intravenous fluid administration by a cut-down or needle. It carries with it the danger of sloughing of the skin and sepsis along the course of the vein. The phlebitis should be managed by the removal of the offending intravenous needle or tubing and saline compresses; this usually makes the patient more comfortable and eliminates the inflammatory reaction.

Thromboembolism in the child is almost unheard of; its rarity is thought to be due to the fact that the child's circulatory system keeps the blood in adequate motion by constant movement in a bed or in an Isolette.

REFERENCES

Holliday, M., and Segar, C.: Parenteral Fluid Therapy. Indiana University Medical Center, 1956.

Mustard, W. T., Ravitch, M. M., Snyder,W. H., Jr., Welch, K. J., and Benson, C. D.: Pediatric Surgery. 2nd Ed. Chicago, Year Book Publishers, 1969.

Pediatric Clinics of North America, Pediatric Surgery. Philadelphia, W. B. Saunders Company, August 1969.

Surgical Clinics of North America, Pediatric Surgery. Philadelphia, W. B. Saunders Company, August 1970.

Wilkinson, A. W.: Recent Advances in Pediatric Surgery. London, J. & A. Churchill, Ltd., 1969.

Part II

SURGICAL CARE of ORGANS and SYSTEMS

CHAPTER 14

LUNG, ESOPHAGUS AND MEDIASTINUM

George L. Nardi, M. D., F.A.C.S.

PREOPERATIVE CARE

Techniques for preparation of the patient undergoing thoracic surgery—bronchopulmonary, mediastinal, esophageal—are becoming ever more precise. Because of these diagnostic developments, because the limits of surgical cure of neoplastic disease have been better defined, and partly because of advances in the medical treatment of inflammatory and granulomatous diseases of the chest, the extirpative role of thoracic surgery has been narrowed over the last decade.

A medical history is of the utmost importance, and details concerning previous pulmonary illnesses in the patient and members of his family should be carefully obtained. Geographic areas in which the patient has lived and traveled are of particular importance in relation to fungus diseases. Previous radiograms should be available for comparison with current x-rays.

Despite diminished emphasis on physical examination, simple inspection of respiratory excursions, symmetry and shape of the thoracic cage may be highly informative. Percussion and auscultation may be critical for the rapid recognition of emergency problems and the changing course of a disease during the postoperative period. Palpation of the neck and the supraclavicular regions for metastatic lymph nodes and of the liver and upper abdomen for metastatic masses is part of the examination of the thorax. Physical signs such as cyanosis, distention of cervical and anterior thoracic veins, clubbing of the fingers, Horner's sign, hoarseness and vocal cord palsy, and vascular or neurological abnormality of the upper extremities should be carefully noted.

299

Pulmonary function tests (see Appendix) are of value in assessing the nature and extent of the patient's pulmonary deficits and the extent of pulmonary resection that can be performed. Inspection and auscultation of the chest, fluoroscopy, and simple determination of the maximum breathing capacity (MBC) will usually give a good idea of the patient's ventilatory capacity. An exercise tolerance test by observation of the patient's pulse and respiratory rate before and after climbing stairs provides an indication of diffusion and ventilation. When these tests are borderline, more sophisticated tests in a pulmonary function laboratory are indicated.

Determination of preoperative arterial blood gases is becoming of increasing importance, not only in assessing the preoperative status of the patient, but also in evaluating the effectiveness of preoperative therapy and serving as a baseline for postoperative care. Such preoperative values may be of particular importance as baseline studies in the postoperative management of a patient who must be maintained on a ventilator (see Chapter 8).

Prior to surgery, the patient should be seen by a chest physiotherapist and taught to breathe deeply and cough effectively. If excessive secretions are present, percussion and postural drainage may be of value. Sputum should be cultured and appropriate antibiotics given. The patient should stop smoking, and the use of intermittent positive pressure breathing and bronchodilators should be considered.

Equally careful cardiovascular assessment is necessary. This will include electrocardiography and sometimes cardiac catheterization with measurement of pulmonary artery pressure. A systolic pressure of over 30 mm. of mercury suggests pulmonary vascular obstruction, and a resection of pulmonary tissue under these conditions is of considerable hazard. Consideration should be given to the use of digitalis, quinidine to reduce cardiac irritability, and the usual measures of diuretics and salt restriction.

Radiologic examination of the chest consists of posterior, anterior, and lateral views or stereoscopic chest films. Oblique views are often of great help. Overexposed grid films may outline pathologic lesions in greater detail. Fluoroscopy will define the relationship of abnormal masses to chest wall, mediastinum, and vascular structures. Barium swallow not only is important in the evaluation of esophageal lesions, but also helps to define the extent of pulmonary and mediastinal lesions in demonstrating displacement of the esophagus by mass lesions or enlarged lymph nodes. Apical lordotic views eliminate the shadows of the clavicles and upper ribs from apical lung tissues. Laminography is of special value in demonstrating calcification or cavitation and the exact plane in which a lesion may be located. A special application is in discovery of additional lesions in patients who appear to have a solitary metastasis from a distant primary neoplasm. Angiocardiography may be of value in the differential diagnosis of mediastinal shadows (elimination of aneurysms), the definition of involvement of major pulmonary vessels by neoplasms and the localization of pulmonary emboli.

With large hilar tumors or lesions in the posterior gutter, intracostal venous osseography (azygogram) performed by the direct injection of contrast medium into the marrow cavity of one of the lower ribs on the involved side will outline the azygos vein and provide information regarding curability since azygos vein obstruction is almost always associated with nonresectability or incurability of the primary tumor.

Pulmonary scanning with macromolecules labeled with a radioactive isotope (I-131) may be injected intravenously to delineate the distribution of pulmonary arterial blood flow. This technique has been of particular value as a screening test for pulmonary embolism.

Bronchography is a radiologic technique in which a radiopaque medium is instilled to outline the tracheobronchial tree. An oily, viscous iodine preparation is most commonly used to coat the tracheobronchial tree. Recently excellent results have been obtained with special dispersions of powdered tantalum. Thorough topical anesthesia of the pharynx, larynx, and tracheobronchial mucosa is essential to control coughing during examination. Coughing will result in "alveolar fill" or expectoration of the contrast substance with subsequent poor visualization. Filling is usually done under fluoroscopic control. The liquid contrast medium can be introduced through a catheter inserted at the tracheal bifurcation and positioning the patient to direct its flow. Another method consists of direct injection into a catheter placed through the cricothyroid membrane. Selective bronchography of a single segment may be performed with directable catheters. When extensive pulmonary disease is present, as in bronchiectasis, bronchography may better be performed in stages, filling first one side and then the other, because respiratory distress may follow simultaneous bilateral bronchograms. Bronchography should be avoided during the acute phase of inflammatory disease, because inaccurate interpretations may result from bronchi that are falsely obstructed or dilated. A full range of x-ray pictures, including posterior, anterior, lateral, and right and left oblique views, are needed to demonstrate all the segments properly. In children, general anesthesia is necessary.

Bronchoscopy is of value both diagnostically and therapeutically. It may provide a histologic diagnosis, identify the extent of lesions, recognize displacement of the tracheobronchial tree by extrinsic involvement, and clarify the origin of cough, hemoptysis, and obstruction even when the lesion has not been identified by x-rays. Therapeutically, bronchoscopy is employed to remove foreign bodies, to clear persistent bronchial obstruction caused by secretions which cannot be removed by physiotherapy or by aspiration with a directed catheter and to assist in the bronchial drainage of lung abscesses.

A variety of bronchoscopes are available, but all consist of a hollow tube through which examination of the tracheobronchial tree is made by direct vision. The larynx and vocal cords should be seen in the course of the procedure. Examination can be done under either topical or general anesthesia, utilizing a "ventilating" bronchoscope which has a side arm permitting continuous ventilation during the examination. Angle telescopes permit examination of the upper lobe orifices and views into other bronchial orifices. Biopsy, aspirates, and washings are obtained selectively for histologic, bacteriologic and cytologic study. New small-diameter, flexible fiberoptic bronchoscopic systems may be passed through a ventilating tracheoscope and directed into segmental bronchi for direct visualization and procurement of material for study.

Esophagoscopy carries greater risk than bronchoscopy, because the thin-walled esophagus may be relatively easily perforated, particularly at the levels of the cricopharyngeus muscles and just above the diaphragm. Tracheal and hilar lesions require bronchoesophagoscopy for delineation of extent. Combined esophagogastroscopy is important in some cases of upper gastrointestinal bleeding in which no clear radiologic abnormality has been demonstrated. Diagnostic esophagoscopy most often follows an abnormal esophagogram performed because of dysphagia.

Scalene Node Biopsy. The highest lymph nodes in the thoracic drainage chain on both right and left sides lie at the junction of the axillary and internal jugular veins near the point of entrance of the lymphatic ducts. On the basis of Rouviere's classic studies of lymphatic anatomy, it has been accepted that the right thoracic duct drains the entire right lung and lower half of the left lung whereas the left upper lung field drains to the left thoracic duct. Recent studies, however, show that the entire left lung may drain to the left side and that in addition there are multiple crossings of lymphatics in the mediastinum. Too often lower cervical nodes have been excised mistakenly, in what has become known as a "scalene fat pad biopsy," instead of the upper thoracic nodes, thus vastly diminishing the diagnostic effectiveness of this procedure. When a palpable node is felt in the supraclavicular space, its excision alone is necessary for diagnosis. When nodes are not palpable, scalene biopsy may be diagnostic in about 80 per cent of cases of sarcoid and in 10 per cent of patients later shown to have carcinoma of the lung. Extension of such a scalene node biopsy to the deeper nodes of the thoracic chain by use of a laryngoscope increases the positive findings in carincoma of the lung. A safer and more informative method, however, is that of mediastinoscopy. This is performed by making a small incision in the supraclavicular notch. A tubular mediastinoscope is passed in the pretracheal plane to the subcarinal position. Lymph nodes may be visualized and biopsied in this location at the origin of the right and left main bronchi and paratracheally. Aspiration should always be performed before biopsy in order to avoid hemorrhage. By this technique accuracy in diagnosis of carcinoma of the lung without palpable supraclavicular nodes has been increased to 40 per cent.

POSTOPERATIVE CARE

The postoperative management of these patients requires first of all the application of the same basic principles applied to all postoperative patients in terms of fluid and electrolyte replacement, antibiotics, and chest physiotherapy and tracheal aspiration.

Until consciousness is regained, the primary consideration in management is maintenance of an adequate airway. While the patient is transported from the operating room, drainage bottles should be kept well below the level of the chest. Lowering the head below the feet (Trendelenburg position) should be avoided because elevation of the diaphragm may have a deleterious effect on ventilation. For similar reasons, slight elevation of the head may be desirable. In case of pulmonary resection, particular care must be taken not to overtransfuse or overhydrate the patient and cause pulmonary edema. In more complicated cases, frequent determination of arterial blood gases and support by means of ventilators with or without tracheostomy may be required (see Chapter 8).

Immediately postoperatively the patient should be turned frequently from lying upon his back to upon his operated side and back again. Turning him onto the nonoperated side should be avoided so as not to diminish ventilation.

Although numerous procedures on the chest and mediastinum can be performed without postoperative drainage, whenever fluid accumulation or air leaks are a possibility, chest drainage is advisable. When an air leak is not a problem, a single large posterior catheter placed through the posterior axillary line to the posterior gutter is utilized. Any serosanguineous collection is undesirable, because it interferes with re-expansion of the lung, provides a culture medium, and may result in a peel, interfering with pulmonary function. When an air leak is a possibility, a second, smaller catheter is placed anteriorly through the second interspace. These catheters should be attached to separate water seal bottles. If an air leak is present, controlled suction up to 15 cm. of negative pressure may be applied to facilitate re-expansion of the lung. The status of re-expansion of the lung and intrathoracic fluid accumulation is checked by daily x-rays. The lower tube may be removed when drainage is no longer obtained (usually 2 to 3 days). The upper tube is removed when the lung has remained expanded for 24 hours after discontinuance of negative suction, i.e., on water seal alone. The tubes may become easily occluded and may be irrigated with sterile saline or with a penicillin solution to restore their patency. Not infrequently tubes may be found to have been ineffectually placed at the time of operation, and additional drainage tubes for either air or fluid may have to be inserted by a trochar thoracotomy.

In the case of pneumonectomy it is customary to close the chest without drainage after operation to allow fluid to accumulate so that organization can occur. Such patients should be carefully followed with chest x-rays as well as needle taps to adjust the intrapleural pressure to minus 3 cm. of water as air and fluid are absorbed in the postoperative period. This is of utmost importance to prevent mediastinal shift capable of interfering with venous return, cardiac function, and ventilation.

The primary goal of treatment of acute empyema is restoration of respiratory function by prompt re-expansion of the lungs. An empyema is best localized by fluoroscopy. Once localized two dimensionally, thoracentesis should be performed. At the initial aspiration as much fluid as possible is removed, specimens are examined by bacteriologic smear and culture, and antibiotic sensitivities are determined. If the empyema is in its early stage, open drainage must be carefully avoided in order not to convert the infected effusion to a total empyema involving the whole pleural space. Repeated aspiration may be necessary. Closed intercostal catheter drainage may be useful if there is continued accumulation of fluid or if the patient's course does not show prompt response to aspiration and antibiotics. Such a catheter must be carefully placed, preferably with fluoroscopic identification of the most dependent point of the cavity. If the empyema is well localized and frank pus is obtained on aspiration, open drainage is achieved by rib resection. This is usually done under local anesthesia after careful localization of the most dependent portion of the cavity by both x-ray and aspiration at the time of drainage. Drainage must be maintained until the space is completely obliterated by cicatrization. The size of the cavity may be followed by x-rays using instilled radiopaque contrast injections or by measuring the amount of saline needed to fill the cavity. The length of the tube is gradually reduced and the diameter narrowed until the cavity closes.

Hemorrhage is a common complication of thoracic surgery. When the bleeding is massive the patient will demonstrate the signs and symptoms of hemorrhagic shock, inadequate aeration caused by pulmonary collapse, and mediastinal displacement. If a chest catheter is in place and functioning properly, the diagnosis is easily made by the volume and appearance of the drainage fluid. Postoperative bleeding may cease spontaneously, but continued bleeding demands re-exploration. Operation should be performed and the hemorrhage brought under control. Usually an intercostal vessel which had not been properly controlled or visualized at the time of the primary operation will be found to be the trouble-maker. Although respiratory motions usually defibrinate blood and prevent its extensive clotting, clotting may nevertheless occur and produce a constrictive peel. When a hemothorax or intrapleural peel persists postoperatively, serious consideration should be given to decortication within a few weeks to restore pulmonary expansion and function.

REFERENCES

Gibbon, J. H., Jr., Sabiston, D. C., Jr., and Spencer, F. C.: Surgery of the Chest. 2d Ed. Philadelphia, W. B. Saunders Co., 1969.

Hughes, R. K.: Thoracic trauma: A collective review. Ann. Thor. Surg. 1:778, 1965.

Johnson, J., and Kirby, C. E.: Surgery of the Chest. Chicago, Year Book Medical Publishers, 1970.

Palva, T.: Mediastinoscopy. Chicago, Year Book Medical Publishers, 1964.

Wilkins, E. W., Jr., and Head, J. M.: Pulmonary neoplasms: Surgical experience at Massachussetts General Hospital. Postgrad. Med. 37:584, 1965.

Wilkins, E. W., Jr., and Skinner, D. B.: Recent progress in surgery of the esophagus. J. Surg. Res. 8:41, 90, 1968; N. Eng. J. Med. 278:824, 887, 1968.

CHAPTER 15

CARDIAC SURGERY

W. Gerald Austen, M.D., F.A.C.S.

The field of cardiac surgery has undergone phenomenal progress and change during the past three decades. Cardiac operations, once a rarity, are now routinely performed in large numbers in many institutions. Although these patients are basically no different than other patients undergoing surgery, they are frequently very ill and therefore require particularly careful and precise management.

PREOPERATIVE CARE

No studies should be completely *routine*, but the following studies should usually be performed prior to cardiac surgery:

Chest x-rays and fluoroscopy
Electrocardiogram
White blood cell count and differential blood count
Hematocrit
Urinalysis
Serum electrolytes

Fasting blood sugar
Screening clotting and bleeding studies
Screening liver function tests
Screening renal function tests
Pulmonary function studies

These tests and other studies will be discussed in detail in the following pages of this chapter.

Naturally, the performance of the heart is crucial. The maintenance of adequate cardiac function and the avoidance of cardiac arrhythmias are of high priority. A preoperative electrocardiogram should be obtained to rule out any recent acute myocardial changes and to detect any cardiac arrhythmias or evidence of myocardial irritability. *Myocardial enzymes* (CPK, SGOT, and LDH), in conjunction with the electrocardiogram, are helpful to rule out recent acute myocardial necrosis. In patients with previous rheumatic fever and any suggestion of rheumatic activity, *serum antistreptolysin titers* should be obtained to rule out activity.

Patients with satisfactory cardiac reserve and in sinus rhythm are usually not taking a *digitalis preparation.* Some physicians would not recommend the institution of a digitalis preparation in this circumstance preoperatively because of the worry of digitalis toxicity intraoperatively and postoperatively. Others would suggest the use of a digitalis preparation because of the protective effect of this as regards both cardiac contraction and its limiting effects on the ventricular response to atrial tachycardias. The myocardial digoxin content has been studied in association with cardiopulmonary bypass. In some studies a decrease in content has been demonstrated, whereas in other studies the myocardial content has remained constant. In any event, clinical observations have suggested that the heart is more sensitive to a particular digitalis level following cardiopulmonary bypass. Because of these considerations, if a patient is taking a digitalis preparation, this drug should be stopped a number of days preoperatively so that its concentration will be less than what would normally be considered fully therapeutic at the time of surgery. With a long-acting agent such as digitalis, the medication should probably be discontinued five days before operation, whereas with a shorter-acting preparation such as digoxin, one or two days is satisfactory.

Cardiac arrhythmias should be brought under control prior to surgery. Patients in atrial fibrillation should be given sufficient amounts of a digitalis preparation to control their rate. As mentioned above, excessive amounts of digitalis should be avoided. Myocardial irritability must be carefully controlled. Ventricular ectopic beats are particularly worrisome and should be suppressed if they are frequent enough, i.e., greater than five or six per minute. Intravenous lidocaine in 50 mg. boluses* (maximum usually no more than 300 mg.) or intravenous drip (1 gm. in 250 cc. D/W) is usually effective, though it has a short duration of action. Alternatively, procaine amide may be given in 100 mg. increments intravenously, but because of its longer duration of action it is more difficult to titrate. Quinidine, 0.2 gm. every 4 to 6 hours or procaine amide, 250 mg. every 4 hours, may be given orally or intramuscularly for long-term suppression. Propranolol, 10 to 20 mg. every 6 hours, or Dilantin, 100 mg. every 6 hours, may also be effective. All these agents cause some suppression of myocardial contractility and should therefore only be employed when significant ventricular irritability is present. The subject of cardiac arrhythmias is discussed in detail on page 323.

Many patients undergoing cardiac surgery require *diuretics* preoperatively to control fluid volume. Naturally, these patients are also on a program of salt and fluid restriction. Although diuretics are, indeed, very helpful under these circumstances, they can cause serious prob-

---

*Dosages in this chapter in general refer to a normal sized adult.

lems with electrolyte imbalances and hypovolemia. In general, diuretics should be discontinued at least two days prior to surgery. Serum electrolytes should be carefully monitored and appropriate replacement undertaken, particularly potassium.

Impaired *renal function* preoperatively may be due to primary renal disease or may be secondary to inadequate cardiac output and/or the use of diuretic agents. An elevated blood urea nitrogen does not differentiate between these possibilities. The level of the serum creatinine is quite helpful, and a low serum creatinine (below 2 to 3 mg. per 100 ml.) would favor relatively normal kidney function with the cause of the elevated BUN being prerenal. Usually, there is no need to undertake extensive renal studies and, unless the renal abnormalities are very severe, cardiac surgery is not contraindicated. Occasionally, the BUN is sufficiently elevated and/or the fluid and electrolyte situation is sufficiently impaired that steps must be taken to improve the situation prior to surgery. Merely rearranging the medical cardiac program to improve the cardiac output, omitting diuretics, liberalizing fluid intake, and/or correcting the electrolyte imbalance by appropriate changes in intake will usually be sufficient. In an occasional instance, an elevated potassium requires treatment with ion exchange resin enemas and, in occasional instances, in addition intravenous glucose and insulin. The serum potassium must be carefully monitored. On rare occasions, peritoneal dialysis may be required to lower the BUN, correct electrolyte imbalances and/or rectify fluid volume overload. If the impaired renal function is due to inadequate cardiac performance, repair of the cardiac abnormality will frequently result in prompt improvement in renal function.

The state of the patient's *lungs* is one of the crucial determinants of the outcome following cardiac surgery. Many patients in the older age group suffer from unrelated chronic lung disease. Of course, the cardiac problem may have serious secondary effects on the lungs such as occurs in patients with pulmonary hypertension secondary to mitral valve disease or left-to-right shunts. Pulmonary function studies should usually be carried out prior to cardiac surgery. Whenever possible, cigarette smokers should give up smoking, preferably at least a month prior to surgery. All patients should have chest physiotherapy prior to surgery. The patient with severe pulmonary disease may benefit considerably from one to two weeks of intensive pulmonary physiotherapy, including in some instances bronchodilators. In patients with essentially normal lungs, a few days of chest physiotherapy is sufficient; here, the primary purpose is to teach the patient how to breathe and cough properly in the postoperative period. In all instances, it is extremely important to define any preoperative pulmonary infection, to isolate the offending organism, to treat the patient with appropriate antibiotics, and, if possible, to eradicate the infection prior to surgery.

The *liver* may be secondarily compromised in association with cardiac disease. Patients with congestive heart failure and elevated right-sided pressures may evidence an enlarged liver and impaired liver function. In addition, patients with low cardiac output may demonstrate parenchymal liver disease, probably secondary to inadequate liver perfusion. Measures to improve cardiac output and congestive heart failure will usually result in a decrease in the size of the liver and improved liver function. Surgical correction of the cardiac defect which results in improved cardiac performance will usually have a salutary effect on liver function. Occasionally, however, the liver damage is so severe that full recovery of liver function is not possible. In cases with severe liver disease special emphasis on bleeding and clotting studies should be made.

Hemostatic problems are not unusual in association with cardiac surgery. This is not surprising when one considers the extensive surgery required, the consumption and dilution of clotting factors associated with cardiopulmonary bypass and multiple transfusions, the need for heparinization during cardiopulmonary bypass, and the clotting defects particularly associated with cyanotic heart disease. All patients undergoing heart surgery should have certain simple screening studies, in addition to a careful inquiry into previous hemorrhagic difficulties. Laboratory tests should include a prothrombin time, a partial thromboplastin time and a platelet count. If any of these studies are abnormal, then appropriate further investigation and therapy should be undertaken prior to surgery (see Chapter 7).

Polycythemic patients rarely require a phlebotomy prior to surgery. The hemodynamic changes related to phlebotomy may be hazardous and result in a low output state. Reactive thrombocytosis is also an occasional consequence of phlebotomy and may lead to thrombotic complications. Hemodilution can be accomplished with ease during cardiopulmonary bypass. Platelet concentrations may be found to be decreased. If sufficiently low, the administration of platelets by transfusion with platelet concentrates or platelet-rich plasma may be helpful.

Anticoagulants are a special problem in the cardiac surgical patient, primarily because a sizable number of patients undergoing cardiac surgery will be on anticoagulant therapy (usually a vitamin K antagonist such as warfarin). The three main reasons that these patients are on anticoagulants include the presence of a prosthetic valve, coronary artery disease and previous embolization (usually in association with mitral valve disease). Because of the problem of intraoperative and postoperative bleeding, most surgeons reverse the anticoagulation. If possible, this should be done gradually over a number of days by omitting the anticoagulant drug. A prothrombin time of approximately 35 to 50 per cent of normal is satisfactory. Because of the risk of thrombosis or embolization, the prothrombin time should not be out of the therapeutic range for a longer time than absolutely necessary. Cardiac surgery should be undertaken as soon as the prothrobin level is appropriate and, when indicated, the prothrombin time should again be returned to the therapeutic range within a few days after surgery. If the risk of thrombosis and embolization is sufficiently great, it may be advisable to proceed with surgery with the prothrombin time in the therapeutic range. Under these circumstances, care should be taken that the prothrombin time does not exceed twice the control.

There are very few areas of surgery in which an *infection* has greater catastrophic implications than in cardiac surgery. Although it is difficult to prove that prophylactic antibiotics are helpful, most cardiac surgeons believe that this is the case. The usual routine includes an antibiotic that covers the gram-positive organisms (primarily staphylococcus) such as staphcillin or oxacillin. Many surgeons prefer to use, in addition, an antibiotic such as streptomycin to cover gram-negative organisms or a single agent that has a broad spectrum. Prophylactic antibiotics should be administered for a sufficient time preoperatively so that there is a satisfactory blood level at the time of surgery; thus, antibiotics should be started the night prior to operation or, at the latest, early on the morning of surgery. Antibiotics should be continued for a limited period of time following surgery. This subject is discussed in further detail on page 332.

On occasion, patients will require heart surgery in the face of *active intracardiac infection*. Certainly, eradication of sepsis is the ideal preoperative condition. Blood cultures should be taken and appropriate antibiotic therapy should be immediately undertaken based on the culture and sensitivities of the isolated organisms. Usually, high blood levels of antibiotics are best achieved by intravenous administration. Ideally, the patient should be treated for 6 weeks and then therapy should be discontinued and the patient should be carefully followed to be sure that the infection has been eradicated. After a reasonable interval (usually 4 to 6 weeks) following antibiotic therapy and no evidence of continued infection, the patient should be re-evaluated and cardiac surgery undertaken in appropriate cases. In some patients, rapid deterioration occurs because of the severe hemodynamic defect secondary to the cardiac infection. In such patients, there is insufficient time to follow the ideal preoperative antibiotic program, and early surgical intervention is required. This is particularly true in patients with bacterial endocarditis of the aortic valve and may also be true in patients with infection on previously inserted prosthetic valves.

Under rare circumstances, patients may require *assisted circulation* in preparation for cardiac surgery. This area is quite new and unexplored, and the value of assisted circulation is not well defined at present. It seems likely, however, that some patients with an extremely low cardiac output and/or severe cardiac failure may benefit from assisted circulation either to safely undergo necessary diagnostic studies in preparation for surgery, or to improve their general condition prior to surgery. There are a number of different approaches to circulatory assistance, and they are briefly discussed on page 323.

OPERATIVE CARE

Because cardiac surgical patients are frequently critically ill and cardiac procedures are usually quite extensive and frequently may involve major blood volume replacement, careful *monitoring* of the patient is required. Continuous monitoring of the arterial blood pressure is perhaps the most important physiologic parameter to follow. This is usually best accomplished by placing a cannula under local anesthesia in a peripheral artery (usually the radial artery) and connecting it to a strain gauge pressure transducer. The strain gauge output can be displayed on an oscilloscope screen, thus allowing observation of both the actual pressure and the pulse wave configuration. The data can, in addition, be recorded on a direct writing recorder for permanent preservation. In small infants, because of the small size of the radial artery, the brachial artery or umbilical artery may be chosen for cannulation. Monitoring of the central venous pressure is also crucial as an indicator of blood volume and cardiac performance. Cannulation is usually accomplished via a medial antecubital vein or via an external or internal jugular vein. An accurate central venous pressure requires that the catheter tip be within a vein in the thoracic cavity, and thus every effort should be made for the catheter to be located in the superior vena cava. An indication that the catheter is properly positioned is obtained by checking the pulse contour of the venous pressure; if the catheter is within the thoracic cavity, the venous pulse tracing demonstrates a small pulse wave in association with the respiratory excursion. This may also be checked by a preoperative chest film. The electrocardiogram should also be monitored during cardiac surgery. The patient should be prepared prior to surgery so that a full electrocardiogram, including limb leads, can be obtained if information regarding myocardial ischemia or a complicated arrhythmia is necessary. Usually during surgery, a simple torso lead electrocardiogram (such as lead II) is sufficient to give information regarding cardiac rate and rhythm. The patient's temperature should be monitored throughout the cardiac procedure. This can be done by a number of different routes, but the esophageal temperature appears to be most accurate. Arterial blood gases should be periodically obtained during cardiac surgery; if abnormalities arise, either metabolic or respiratory, they can be appropriately corrected. The measurement of urine output can also be helpful as an indication of adequacy of cardiac output and peripheral perfusion. The determination of serum electrolytes, especially potassium, is important, particularly in patients who have undergone cardiopulmonary bypass and/or are having a significant diuresis. Some surgeons feel that an electroencephalogram is helpful during cardiopulmonary bypass, but many surgeons have not found this particular parameter to be of great help.

Practically all *anesthetic agents* cause some myocardial depression. Therefore, in cardiac surgery, it is particularly important to use agents that cause the least amount of myocardial depression and to use these agents in the lowest amount consistent with satisfactory anesthesia. Many cardiac groups employ pentothal induction, muscle relaxation with intravenous d-tubocurarine or gallamine and supplemental anesthesia with nitrous oxide or halothane.

Narcotics and narcotic derivatives have little if any direct effect on the myocardium and have been found to be excellent agents for highly selected patients undergoing cardiac surgery. Doses of morphine up to 2 mg./kg. of body weight intravenously have been employed under these special circumstances. Advantages include no interaction with cardiotonic drugs (epinephrine or isoproterenol), no direct arrhythmogenic action, and a smooth and consistent level of anesthesia with the option of using 100 per cent oxygen to ventilate the patient. Induction of the patient with morphine or the narcotic derivative fentanyl may be associated with a considerable drop in blood pressure (secondary to a reduction in peripheral vascular resistance) preventable by the administration of intravascular colloid if the central venous pressure is less than 10 cm. of water. The additional use of a slow intravenous drip of epinephrine permits close adjustment of arterial blood pressure levels during induction of anesthesia. Narcotics or their derivatives, used alone, will not prevent the autonomic response to a surgical stimulus as expressed by an abrupt rise in blood pressure; occasionally, the arterial blood pressure may be high, and in such cases anesthesia is supplemented with 50 per cent nitrous oxide or small concentrations of halothane (0.25 to 0.5 per cent). Muscle relaxation is achieved with intravenous d-tubocurarine or gallamine.

It is essential that more than one large intravenous route be available for the administration of drugs, blood, and various fluids.

Once the chest cavity is opened, the *lungs* must be ventilated with large tidal volumes at low frequencies to keep arterial pCO_2 at normal levels and pO_2 optimally high. Whenever possible, the inspired concentration of oxygen should be maintained at a level adequate to insure an arterial pO_2 of 150 mm. Hg. This is not always feasible in the patient with a congenital defect and a right-to-left shunt. Use of an end-expiratory pressure will prevent collapse of terminal air spaces at the end-expiration. There is still considerable controversy regarding the optimal method of handling the lungs during cardiopulmonary bypass. Many feel that it really makes very little difference. One reasonable approach is to not ventilate the lungs during bypass, but to keep the lungs moderately expanded with a constant pressure of 10 cm. of water applied to the airway.

In cases in which *cardiopulmonary bypass* is required, pump flow must be carefully monitored. A reasonable blood flow in an adult is in the range of 55 to 70 cc./kg./min. With hypothermia, these flow rates can be reduced somewhat. Small children and infants require considerably greater flow per kilogram of body weight.

The increasing number of patients operated upon with extracorporeal bypass has placed a tremendous burden on the shoulders of blood banking facilities. For this reason, as well as the significant complications associated with multiple blood transfusions, many cardiac surgeons have chosen to eliminate blood from the pump prime, particularly when using a disposable bubble oxygenator. The clear prime consists principally of an electrolyte solution (saline or Ringer's lactate) or glucose solution or a combination of both. Some have added a protein solution (albumin, 3 to 4 gm. per 100 ml.). Some combine a clear prime solution with whole blood. The hematocrit of the patient on cardiopulmonary bypass will depend on the volume of priming solution, the presence or absence of whole blood in this priming solution, and the patient's initial blood volume. Loss of fluid from the patient-extracorporeal circuit is minimized by returning all suction from the operative field to the extracorporeal pump. Whenever an addition of fluid is necessary, whole blood or additional clear solution may be used, depending on the hematocrit. The oxygenator should provide a good equilibration with oxygen (pO_2 during bypass should normally range between 200 and 450 mm. Hg), depending on the magnitude of blood flow. Excessive loss of carbon dioxide from the blood can be prevented by adding CO_2 gas (3 to 5 per cent) to the inflow oxygen. pH corrections are unnecessary in the pump's priming solutions used for the adult patient. The lactate present is metabolized rapidly to bicarbonate, and the pH will be maintained within normal limits if blood flow is adequate. Urine flow can be promoted by adding 12.5 to 25 gm. of mannitol to the prime or intermittent addition of furosemide (5 to 10 mg.) during extracorporeal circulation. If hemolysis becomes excessive, as evidenced by hemoglobinuria, mannitol is best administered as a continuous drip (20 per cent solution) at a rate of 250 ml. (50 gm. of mannitol) per hour. Again, it should be pointed out that there is a significant potassium loss in this diuresis; the serum potassium should be monitored and, when necessary, potassium should be given intravenously.

Satisfactory *myocardial function* postoperatively is essential for recovery. Incision in the heart should be made in such a way as to minimize damage to the ventricles; interruption of coronary flow should also be kept to a minimum to preserve myocardial function. Care must be taken to avoid embolization from air or particulate matter. Damage to the conduction system (particularly the bundle of His or the SA node) should be carefully avoided. At the end of any cardiac procedure, and most particularly a procedure in which cardiopulmonary bypass has been employed, very careful hemostasis should be achieved. The surgeon should take sufficient time for the protamine to have counteracted the heparin and for all significant bleeding points to have been controlled. In patients who continue to exhibit excessive bleeding without an obvious anatomic source, bleeding studies should be performed in the operating room and appropriate therapy undertaken. A further discussion of bleeding problems in association with heart surgery can be found on page 319.

Patients who develop transient *heart block* during surgery should usually have temporary pacemaker wires inserted into the ventricular wall so that external cardiac pacing can be accomplished postoperatively, if heart block recurs. Even without difficulties with heart block, atrial and ventricular pacing wires may be very helpful in the postoperative period in the maintenance of the most effective cardiac rate and rhythm and also in the proper diagnosis of a complicated arrhythmia. Atrial pacing is helpful in patients with sinus bradycardia or a slow nodal rhythm or in suppression of ventricular irritability. Ventricular pacing, in addition to being invaluable in patients with heart block, may also help to suppress ventricular irritability. With both atrial and ventricular wires sequential atrioventricular pacing can be accomplished, and regulating the P-R interval may enhance cardiac performance. These temporary electrodes, therefore, should be frequently inserted at the end of the operative procedure.

It is sometimes helpful postoperatively to be able to monitor such *intracardiac pressures* as left atrial pressure and pulmonary artery or right ventricular pressure. In some circumstances, then, small catheters should be passed into these chambers at the end of the operative procedure; these catheters should be so inserted that they can be removed a few days postoperatively without intrathoracic bleeding. Additional discussion of these pressure recordings occurs on page 317.

Finally, some mention should be made regarding *the extremely sick patient* undergoing open heart surgery. Such a patient may not tolerate anesthesia and thoracotomy, and it may be very important to cannulate the femoral artery and vein for partial bypass under local anesthesia prior to initiation of general anesthesia. If the patient deteriorates hemodynamically, the partial bypass can be instituted and the patient should be sufficiently perfused while the thoracotomy is accomplished in preparation for total bypass. By the same token, the very sick patient may require a prolonged period of total or partial bypass following intracardiac surgery before his heart is able to handle the full hemodynamic burden. On occasion, an hour or even longer of circulatory support results in considerable improvement in myocardial function.

POSTOPERATIVE CARE

The cardiac surgical patient requires continued and careful observation in the immediate postoperative period. Ideally, there should be an intensive care unit, within reasonable proximity to the cardiac operating room, with proper facilities and trained nursing staff to continuously observe the patient's progress. Although the surgeon must be the individual responsible for the overall care of the cardiac surgical patient, he must also draw on the specialized knowledge of many expert consultants to assure his patient optimal care.

PATIENT MONITORING

A large number of parameters require monitoring in the postoperative cardiac surgical patient. The *arterial pressure* has already been mentioned in the section on operative care. Continuous monitoring of the arterial blood pressure is essential. In general, this pressure should be monitored, as it was in the operating room, via an arterial catheter connected to an oscilloscope. This method gives immediate visualization of the pressure trace. The level of the arterial pressure can give an indication of myocardial function and adequacy of intravascular volume.

A continuous *electrocardiogram* should also be employed. Usually, a torso lead electrocardiogram is sufficient for monitoring as far as cardiac rhythm and rate are concerned. Periodically, a full electrocardiogram should be done and certainly a full electrocardiogram should be undertaken if there is any question of myocardial ischemia or cardiac arrhythmia. As previously mentioned, epicardial electrodes, if present, can be helpful in the diagnosis and monitoring of cardiac arrhythmias. Care must be taken in using these electrodes to avoid dangerous electrical ground loops.

The *central venous pressure* is clearly of great value as an indication of both blood volume and cardiac performance. If the venous pressure is low and the blood pressure is low, a low blood volume is the most likely explanation. If the venous pressure is high and the blood pressure is low, then poor cardiac function or tamponade must be suspected.

Urinary output is particularly important as an indication of the adequacy of cardiac output and peripheral perfusion. Usually the measurement of output and the periodic determination of urine specific gravity is sufficient. In patients with renal difficulties, urine osmolarity and sediment, blood urea nitrogen, serum and urine creatinine and urine sodium and potassium concentrations are helpful in assessing renal function and distinguishing prerenal causes of impaired renal function from primary renal disease. This subject is discussed in further detail on page 326.

The respiratory status of the patient following cardiac surgery requires continuous and careful monitoring. The vital capacity, tidal volume and arterial blood gases are particularly pertinent. Usually, following cardiac surgery, patients receive ventilator support. When the patient's vital capacity, tidal volume, and arterial blood gases indicate adequate ventilation without assistance, removal of the endotracheal tube can be carried out.

Careful monitoring of *chest drainage* is of great importance following cardiac surgery. This is particularly crucial in the first 12 hours after surgery. Following open heart surgery, the chest drainage may be relatively large. A decision regarding re-exploration for continued bleeding should be made on the basis of the total amount of bleeding and the hourly rate of bleeding as assessed by chest drainage, the rate of transfusion, and the accumulation of blood in the chest on x-ray. It is essential that the chest tubes are patent to accurately judge intrathoracic bleeding; irrigation of the chest tubes with sterile saline may be indicated. If a patient continues to bleed at high rates for prolonged periods, re-exploration should be undertaken.

The *portable chest film* should be taken immediately after completion of surgery and at intervals postoperatively to evaluate lung expansion, pulmonary vascular congestion, and the presence and quantity of blood in the pleural spaces and mediastinum.

Careful monitoring of *fluid balance* and the weight of the patient is essential in the postoperative period.

Of the *electrolytes*, serum potassium concentration is unquestionably the most critical. Rapid shifts in extracellular concentration of potassium are not uncommon and may precipitate troublesome cardiac arrhythmias. Hyponatremia is common following cardiac surgery, particularly when dextrose and water hemodilution prime is used. Generally, the serum sodium corrects itself to normal or low normal range within 4 to 6 hours after perfusion. Extreme degrees of hyponatremia may contribute to lethargy and obtundation. Restriction of water intake and promotion of a diuresis will usually effectively correct the situation. Hypernatremia may occur, particularly if a large quantity of sodium bicarbonate has been required to treat a metabolic acidosis or if vigorous diuresis has been induced. There is probably little primary effect of sodium on myocardial contraction except through its inter-relationship with potassium and calcium transport across the myocardial cell membrane. It has been shown that with high extracellular calcium and low sodium concentrations, epinephrine is deprived of its positive inotropic action. The extracellular concentrations of calcium and magnesium have been shown to have a mutually antagonistic effect on myocardial contractility. An elevated magnesium concentration associated with a low calcium concentration decreases myocardial tonus, whereas the reverse improves contractility. Thus, in certain situations, particularly when large volumes of citrated blood have been transfused, measurement of the serum calcium and magnesium concentrations may be indicated.

Following cardiac surgery, the status of the *cardiac output* is usually assessed by the general clinical impression of the patient, including careful observation of the blood pressure, hourly urine output, appearance of peripheral perfusion and the metabolic status in terms of acid-base balance. With an inadequate cardiac output, a metabolic acidosis will supervene on the basis of inadequate tissue perfusion and oxygen transport at the cellular level. If there is a question regarding adequate tissue perfusion, a Siggaard-Anderson acid-base nomogram in the intensive care unit can be quite helpful in the assessment of the presence or absence of metabolic acidosis by allowing rapid calculation of the base deficit or excess in mEq./L. Occasionally, when there is a question of low cardiac output or when various forms of therapy to improve a low cardiac output are being compared, the determination of the cardiac output by the dye dilution technique or by the Fick principle may be very helpful.

Blood volume determinations are not often required. Generally, the blood pressure and pulse pressure, the central venous pressure, hourly urine output and appearance of peripheral perfusion are adequate indices of blood volume. Occasionally, however, there will exist a discrepancy in the observed central venous pressure and the clinical impression of blood volume. Usually, this occurs in the situation in which the central venous pressure is apparently normal or elevated at the time when the blood pressure is low, the urine output marginal, and the patient appears peripherally vasoconstricted. It has been shown that direct measurement of blood volume in the postoperative cardiac surgical patient may indicate hypovolemia in the presence of a normal or elevated central venous pressure. Although the accuracy of blood volume determinations is still questioned, in special circumstances it may be helpful to directly measure the blood volume with RISA (radio-iodine labeled albumin) or ^{51}Cr-labeled red cells.

Some cardiac surgeons feel that measurement of the *left atrial pressure and/or measurement of the pulmonary artery pressure and right ventricular pressure* is a better indication of adequate blood volume than central venous pressure. In addition, these direct intracardiac pressure measurements can be helpful to differentiate between right and left heart failure in the postoperative period.

A number of *routine laboratory studies,* including hematocrit, partial thromboplastin time, prothrombin time, bleeding time, platelet count, blood urea nitrogen, serum bilirubin, serum electrolytes and arterial blood gases should usually be monitored following cardiac surgery. In certain circumstances, the clinical situation may demand more detailed or special studies. These studies will be discussed in the section on the management of postoperative complications.

GENERAL MANAGEMENT

Fluids should be restricted during the first few days after heart surgery. Usually, intravenous fluids should be limited to 15 cc./24 hours for the average adult or approximately 750 cc./24 hrs./m.^{2} of body surface area. These fluids are normally given intravenously during the first 48 hours after surgery, and the usual preparation is 5 per cent glucose in water. The administration of sodium is usually avoided in the cardiac patient unless serum and urinary electrolyte studies indicate a need. Potassium also must be administered carefully and should be given only if the serum electrolyte studies indicate their requirement. Usually, the patient can begin to take fluids by mouth in approximately 24 to 48 hours after surgery. At this point, fluid restrictions are usually continued for a few additional days and then it is possible to gradually relax these restrictions. Sodium intake is usually restricted at about 200 mg./24 hours for 1 to 2 weeks postoperatively, depending on the patient's cardiac lesion and state of compensation.

The postoperative cardiac patient has considerable discomfort and certainly requires appropriate *sedation*. If sedation is not sufficient, the patient has excessive pain, and this may have a deleterious effect on the patient's blood pressure as well as on his respiratory function. Too much sedation may result in hypotension and respiratory depression as well. Initially, small doses of morphine (4 to 6 mg.) or Demerol (20 to 30 mg.) intravenously are advisable. Fentanyl, a synthetic morphine-like analgesic, may also be employed (0.012 to 0.025 mg. intravenously). Generally, if a narcotic has been relied upon as the anesthetic agent during surgery, little or no pain medication is required during the first 24 hours postoperatively. Once the patient is stabilized, moderate doses of this agent intramuscularly or subcutaneously should be given as needed. It is very important to differentiate between the discomfort of pain and the agitation of low cardiac output and/or anoxia; the latter requires immediate therapy for the basic problem and not the administration of pain medication or a sedative. When a sedative is required for agitation, diazepam (Valium) may be effective; it should be administered in single doses of not more than 5 mg. intravenously. The patient's discomfort can usually be controlled after 4 to 5 days with Percodan or Darvon by mouth.

The patient's *temperature* should be maintained at an approximate normal level: 37° C. Occasionally, if the patient has not been properly warmed in the operating room, he may be hypothermic and may require a heating blanket to achieve a normal temperature. Usually, the patient's temperature is elevated shortly after surgery, owing to the secondary effects of cellular destruction as well as atelectasis. A temperature up to 39° C. in the early postoperative period does not require treatment. Temperatures higher than this should be lowered with alcohol sponging of the skin and, in cases of severe hyperthermia, with the use of a cooling blanket.

Usually the postoperative cardiac patient is placed on *ventilatory assistance* for a variable period of time. In a patient with a straightforward, uncomplicated problem, such as an atrial septal defect, weaning and extubation may be accomplished early during the afternoon or evening of operation. More usually, it is best to keep the patient on respiratory support during the night following surgery and to consider weaning on the following day. Some patients with marginal cardiac function or significant pulmonary difficulty may require prolonged periods of respiratory support. When the patient's vital capacity, tidal volume, minute volume and arterial gases indicate adequate ventilation without assistance, weaning can then be accomplished by connecting the patient's endotracheal tube to a Briggs adapter with humidified oxygen of approximately 50 per cent concentration. If the above monitored parameters remain satisfactory, the patient may then be extubated.

Patients following cardiac surgery require considerable *rest*. Depending on the severity of their surgery and the function of their myocardium, they may begin to ambulate after one or more days following their operation. Thereafter, ambulation will be determined by the speed with which their strength returns. It is particularly important to emphasize to the patient that he will have good and bad days on the way to recovery. He should gradually increase his activity but should rest when he becomes tired. Patients who show evidence of low cardiac output or congestive heart failure should have a more restricted activity schedule.

Frequent *chest physiotherapy* should be afforded the patient in the postoperative period until he is fully active and has demonstrated that he can keep his lungs fully expanded without chest physiotherapy. The average patient requires 5 to 7 days of chest physiotherapy.

As mentioned on page 332, most surgeons feel that prophylactic *antibiotics* are helpful in avoiding postoperative infections in the cardiac surgical patient. In general, prophylactic antibiotics should be discontinued in four or five days following surgery. Antibiotics should be stopped at this point to avoid problems with overgrowth with resistant organisms. Specific infections should then be treated with appropriate antibiotics according to culture sensitivity tests.

Many patients following cardiac surgery require *anticoagulants*. Essentially all patients with presently available prosthetic valves should be treated with a prothrombin depressant drug such as Coumadin, unless there is a strong contraindication to anticoagulants. In addition, mitral patients with atrial clot, patients with large foreign surfaces in the heart (e.g., patch closure of atrial septal defect) should probably also be considered for anticoagulant therapy. Usually the prothrombin depressant drug is started at about 48 hours postoperatively with the plan to attain a therapeutic level in an additional 48 hours. A prothrombin time of approximately twice normal is considered a therapeutic level.

MANAGEMENT OF EARLY POSTOPERATIVE COMPLICATIONS

Hemorrhage. Following cardiopulmonary bypass, a number of alterations in the hemostatic mechanism may occur. The two most important of these are the presence of circulating heparin and the development of thrombocytopenia.

Usually, heparin reversal is accomplished by the administration of protamine. Protamine should be given slowly intravenously because of its hypotensive effect; some physicians have found the simultaneous administration of a vasopressor to be helpful. A reasonable dosage schedule is 1 to 3 mg. of protamine for 1 mg. of heparin used. Generally, a maximum of 3 mg. of protamine per 1 mg. of total heparin dose should not be exceeded; protamine in excessive amounts is an anticoagulant. The partial thromboplastin time may be used as an indication of adequate reversal of the heparin by the protamine; if the usual amount of protamine has been given and the partial thromboplastin time is still prolonged, it is helpful to obtain a protamine titration test as an indication of heparin reversal.

A significant platelet deficiency is usually present following cardiopulmonary bypass both from sequestration of platelets within the extracorporeal system and from dilution with non-blood prime and platelet-poor blood prime. Frequently, particularly in short perfusions, nothing specific need be done. Usually, if any blood volume deficit is replaced with platelet-rich fresh blood at the end of the procedure, the platelet count will be satisfactory (platelet count of approximately 100,000/cubic mm. or more). In rare circumstances, transfusion of platelet concentrates in addition to fresh whole blood is necessary to obtain adequate platelet levels.

Other less common aberrations in hemostasis after cardiac surgery, including intravascular coagulation, fibrinolysis, and problems of hemostasis related to liver disease, are discussed in Chapter 7.

Although a full understanding and careful documentation of possible coagulation problems are required in cardiac surgery, certainly the most important defense against postoperative hemorrhage is adequate mechanical hemostasis. The electrocautery can be very helpful, particularly in the handling of small bleeding points. Patience is essental; the chest should not be closed until hemostasis is very adequately controlled.

Careful monitoring of chest tube drainage postoperatively is essential. Care must be taken that the chest tubes are properly placed and functionally open. If there is any question regarding the patency of a chest tube, it should be irrigated with sterile saline. Periodic portable chest x-rays should be taken to determine the amount of fluid in the pleural spaces and the mediastinum. The clinical findings suggestive of cardiac tamponade should be carefully sought for. Patients who have no evidence of a coagulation defect and who continue to demonstrate excessive intrathoracic bleeding (in an adult, 150 to 200 cc. per hour for 6 hours without evidence of decreasing bleeding) should be re-explored. At the time of re-exploration, the blood in the mediastinum and pleura should be removed and mechanical hemostasis should be carefully accomplished. If re-exploration is performed at a time when the patient is still in satisfactory hemodynamic condition, the procedure is ordinarily extremely well tolerated and usually results in control of the bleeding problem.

Cardiac Tamponade. Cardiac tamponade is due to the pressure effects of clotted and unclotted blood in the confined mediastinal space. This situation usually occurs when excessive postoperative bleeding has continued for a number of hours and may be associated with malfunctioning of the chest tubes. To help avoid tamponade, most surgeons make it a practice to leave the pericardium widely open and to assure adequate drainage of the mediastinum into at least one pleural space. In spite of this, tamponade is a not infrequent occurrence following open heart surgery under the circumstances mentioned above. The compression of the heart causes limitation of diastolic filling and decreased cardiac output. The blood pressure is usually somewhat low and the pulse pressure is narrow. The venous pressure is elevated (unless the patient is hypovolemic, in which case the venous pressure may be normal or even low) and there may be a significant paradoxical pulse. The diagnosis, however, may be difficult to make because the systemic blood pressure and venous pressure findings are also consistent with cardiac failure; in addition, the paradoxical pulse may be difficult to identify, or it may be difficult to ascertain the significance of the paradoxical pulse in a patient on a respirator and/or with a cardiac arrhythmia. The presence of a large amount of mediastinal fluid on the portable chest x-ray may be helpful in the diagnosis. Certainly, a patient with significant cardiac tamponade should undergo re-exploration, removal of the offending blood and the accomplishment of hemostasis. Again, if such exploration is undertaken at a time when the patient is in a satisfactory hemodynamic state, the results are excellent.

Low Cardiac Output Syndrome and/or Cardiac Failure. Cardiac failure and/or the low cardiac output syndrome are common problems in the postoperative cardiac surgical patient. Cardiac failure and low cardiac output represent, in general, different manifestations of the same basic problem. The usual causes for both low cardiac output and cardiac failure include long-standing cardiac disease, myocardial depression associated with the operative procedure, inadequate surgical correction of hemodynamically significant anatomic defects, arrhythmias, metabolic aberrations, and special anatomic problems (such as left ventricular outflow obstruction resulting from too large a prosthetic mitral valve, etc.)

Cardiac failure may be isolated left ventricular, right ventricular, or biventricular failure. The cardiac output may be maintained until failure has progressed to the descending limb of the Starling curve, when cardiac output may be considerably decreased. The critical manifestations of cardiac failure in the postoperative cardiac surgical patient may be less clear cut than in the usual nonoperative situation. Positive pressure respiratory support may diminish or completely mask the physical findings of pulmonary rales and the x-ray appearance of pulmonary edema. The chest x-ray may show some pulmonary congestion; the arterial pO_2 will be decreased owing to the pulmonary arteriovenous shunt which occurs in association with pulmonary edema. In the presence of a normal blood volume, the central venous pressure is usually elevated. Of course, the central venous pressure may be elevated because of cardiac tamponade or secondary to certain arrhythmias (such as nodal rhythm); sometimes isolated left ventricular failure will occur and right-sided pressures will be normal.

Low cardiac output, like cardiac failure, is usually due to long-standing intrinsic myocardial disease, but may be associated with any of the entities mentioned above. A cardiac output determination is quite helpful whenever there is any question regarding adequacy of cardiac output. Effective management of the low cardiac output syndrome and/or cardiac failure is greatly assisted if its cause can be ascertained. When a relative hypovolemia is present, increased blood volume is very helpful. The central venous pressure may be misleading and some so-called low cardiac output states may be effectively treated by controlled left atrial hypertension. The arterial pO_2 must be closely monitored so as to detect the early signs of left ventricular failure in the form of increased pulmonary A-V shunting. Arrhythmias should be carefully looked for and properly treated. Myocardial depression should be minimized as much as possible during the operative procedure. The ventricular musculature should not be incised unless absolutely necessary, and as little as possible of the coronary circulation should be interrupted. Coronary perfusion should be maintained as closely to normal as possible. Every attempt should be made to completely correct hemodynamically significant anatomic defects at the time of surgery and to avoid anatomic problems such as prosthetic outflow obstruction. Metabolic aberrations may have a depressant effect on the myocardium and should be corrected. Acidosis is particularly important and, when present, should be immediately reversed. Hypocalcemia, hyperkalemia, hypokalemia and severe hyponatremia may have an adverse effect upon myocardial function and, if present, require therapy. Proper digitalization is an important aspect of treatment in a patient with congestive failure and/or low cardiac output. In congestive failure, the use of a diuretic such as ethacrynic acid or furosemide, or occasionally phlebotomy, may be valuable. With these latter maneuvers, left ventricular failure may improve and, with improvement in pulmonary congestion, the decrease in the pulmonary arteriovenous shunt results in a rise in the arterial pO_2. Of course, low cardiac output may be due to hypovolemia. If the central venous pressure is low, certainly the addition of blood volume should be the first order of business. The cardiac surgical patient may require a central venous pressure considerably higher than normal to achieve a satisfactory filling pressure and resultant cardiac output.

When all these maneuvers are insufficient to maintain an adequate cardiac output and/or to avoid cardiac failure, most physicians turn to positive inotropic agents such as isoproterenol and/or epinephrine. Isoproterenol combines the advantages of an inotropic agent with peripheral vasodilatation but may have a considerable cardiac chronotropic effect. Epinephrine has a strong inotropic effect but may also have a significant peripheral vasoconstrictor effect. Both agents may cause cardiac irritability, particularly epinephrine.

In recent years, there has been considerable enthusiasm for peripheral vasodilatation as the primary objective in the treatment of these patients with low cardiac output. In so doing, there is a decrease in the degree and duration of left ventricular isometric contraction and subsequently a decrease in left ventricular oxygen consumption. The commonly used agents include phenoxybenzamine (20 to 200 mg. daily) and corticosteroids (30 mg./kg. of methylprednisolone). Thorazine and, to some extent, isoproterenol have similar benefits. When significant vasodilatation is accomplished, volume replacement must also be simultaneously accomplished to maintain adequate systemic pressure and cardiac output.

In recent years, there have been some encouraging reports regarding the use of assisted circulation in the treatment of low cardiac output. Total cardiac replacement and partial (left ventricular bypass) devices have been developed, but there are still problems with thrombosis and blood-formed element destruction. Various temporary assist systems have been developed, including counterpulsation, veno-arterial pumping (cardiopulmonary bypass), left atrial-to-femoral arterial bypass, left ventricular-to-femoral artery bypass, external synchronous assist, implantable cardiac compression device (Anstadt cup), and body acceleration. Temporary cardiopulmonary bypass has been employed clinically for short periods with some success. Various forms of counterpulsation have also had considerable clinical trial. The intra-aortic balloon assist device has been used in a limited number of patients suffering from low cardiac output secondary to a myocardial infarction or following intracardiac surgery; clearly, this counterpulsation system is reasonably safe and has a significantly beneficial affect on cardiovascular hemodynamics.

Cardiac Arrhythmias. Virtually any cardiac arrhythmia may occur following cardiac surgery, just as arrhythmias may occur following other types of surgery. Certainly, the incidence of cardiac arrhythmias is far more common following cardiac surgery because of many factors to be discussed below. In addition, these arrhythmias may have more serious consequences because of the fact that they are occurring in a heart that is unable to perform at normal efficiency.

Many different factors may contribute to the onset of a cardiac arrhythmia. Certainly the traumatic impact of the cardiac surgical procedure itself may precipitate an arrhythmia. Prolonged cardiopulmonary bypass, interruption of coronary perfusion, ventriculotomy or atriotomy may play a role in etiology.

Patients with coronary disease are more likely to suffer a myocardial infarction in association with their surgery; in addition, of course, coronary embolism or damage to the coronary vessels in association with cardiac surgery may cause myocardial infarction. All the cardiac arrhythmias associated with the standard nonoperative myocardial infarction may occur.

Other factors which may play a role in the etiology of cardiac arrhythmias in the postoperative period include hyper- or hypokalemia, digitalis excess, surgical trauma to the SA or AV nodes and the intraventricular conduction bundles, prosthetic valve cage irritation, hypoxia, and hypotension. Hyperkalemia produces slowing of the sinus node, prolongation of the P-R interval owing to delayed A-V conduction, slowing of intraventricular conduction with widening of the QRS complex, and eventually, if severe enough, sinus arrest with nodal escape, or even ventricular standstill or fibrillation. Hypokalemia causes an increase in velocity of depolarization, but a decrease in speed of repolarization. This results in increased cardiac irritability and a tendency for the development of both supraventricular and ventricular ectopic rhythms. Hypokalemia per se occasionally causes arrhythmias, but usually a low serum potassium leads to the presence of rhythm problems that are actually the result of digitalis toxicity. They include ectopic atrial tachycardia with varying degrees of atrioventricular block disturbances and ventricular ectopic beats which may lead to bigeminy or ventricular tachycardia As mentioned previously, hyperkalemia may be effectively treated with Kayexalate enemas in addition to intravenous glucose and insulin and sodium bicarbonate. Peritoneal dialysis is not as effective as Kayexalate enemas in removing potassium but may be of some help in controlling the potassium. Hypokalemia should be treated with intravenous potassium. Digitalis excess usually may be avoided by omitting digitalis drugs a few days prior to surgery.

Surgically induced arrhythmias are usually due to injury to the SA node or its blood supply or injury to the A-V conduction bundle. A proper knowledge of the appropriate anatomy and sufficient care during the cardiac procedure, as well as careful electrocardiographic monitoring during the cardiac procedure, have markedly decreased these problems.

A better understanding of the hemodynamics of prosthetic valves and the avoidance of too large prosthetics in the mitral position has been helpful to decrease the incidence of arrhythmias from ventricular wall irritation.

Hypoxia and/or hypotension may lead to serious arrhythmias and, naturally, should be avoided.

The more common arrhythmias will be briefly discussed.

ATRIAL ARRHYTHMIAS. *Atrial premature beats* are commonly seen after cardiac surgery. They have no particular consequence and do not need treatment. Frequent atrial premature beats may progress to other atrial arrhythmias.

Atrial fibrillation is frequently seen following cardiac surgery. Many patients, particularly those with mitral valve disease of long standing or coronary artery disease are in atrial fibrillation prior to surgery. Patients who are in normal sinus rhythm prior to surgery may go into atrial fibrillation during the operation or in the postoperative period. Under these circumstances, the ventricular rate should be controlled by a digitalis preparation; a significant number of the patients will revert to normal sinus rhythm with this treatment. Patients who have been in atrial fibrillation prior to surgery and those who go into atrial fibrillation postoperatively and do not spontaneously revert, should usually undergo electrical cardioversion 6 to 12 weeks after surgery; the incidence of maintaining sinus rhythm is higher in patients who have had a short period of atrial fibrillation than in those who have had atrial fibrillation for many years. The chances of maintaining cardioversion are much better if there is a reasonable interval between surgery and the time of the electrical cardioversion. Rarely, cardioversion for atrial fibrillation must be performed early because of severe hemodynamic difficulty secondary to the atrial fibrillation. *Atrial flutter* can be a difficult problem because the ventricular rate may be quite rapid. Digitalization may slow the rate by increasing the degree of A-V block or may result in conversion to atrial fibrillation or sinus rhythm. Occasionally, uncontrolled atrial flutter may require electrical cardioversion. If the ventricular rate is difficult to control in either atrial fibrillation or flutter, the use of digitalis with the addition of a beta adrenergic blocking agent such as propranolol (10 to 20 mg. orally every 6 hours) may be very helpful. The latter agent is contraindicated, however, if congestive heart failure is present. *Paroxysmal atrial tachycardia without block* is quite uncommonly seen in the postoperative period; when it occurs it usually responds to carotid sinus massage and/or digitalization. *Paroxysmal atrial tachycardia with block* is usually a manifestation of digitalis toxicity and usually responds to potassium replacement.

NODAL RHYTHM. A nodal rhythm is frequently noted in the postoperative cardiac patient. Anesthesia, particularly halothane, may be the precipitating factor. Damage to the sinus node may also cause this problem. As the patient gets farther away from the trauma of surgery and/or the anesthetic, the nodal rhythm may disappear. A number of different drugs may correct the nodal rhythm but none are uniformly successful. Intravenous atropine (1 mg. dose) may abolish this rhythm, as may beta adrenergic drugs such as isoproterenol (1 mg. in 250 cc. D/W) or epinephrine (1 mg. in 250 cc. D/W). Electrical pacing with wires implanted on the right atrium is an excellent method of handling this problem until sinus rhythm returns. *Nodal tachycardia* is usually indicative of digitalis toxicity and should be treated with potassium.

VENTRICULAR ARRHYTHMIAS. *Ventricular ectopic beats* are common postoperatively. Reasonable criteria regarding indication for suppression of ventricular ectopic beats include a frequency of five to six per minute, multifocal beats, beats which interrupt the T wave of the previous beat, or runs of two or more ectopic ventricular beats. Intravenous lidocaine (50 mg. bolus, maximum 300 mg.) is usually effective, although this drug has a short duration of action. A continuous lidocaine drip may be effective or, alternatively, procaine amide intravenously in 100 mg. increments may be useful. Quinidine (0.2 gm. every 4 to 6 hours) or procaine amide (250 mg. every 4 hours) may be given orally or intramuscularly for long-term suppression. Propranolol (10 to 20 mg. orally every 6 hours) or Dilantin (100 mg. orally every 6 hours) may also be effective. With all these myocardial depressant drugs, there is the risk of hypotension. If ventricular irritability is due to digitalis excess, potassium replacement will be helpful. In the occasional case of drug-refractory ventricular irritability, suppression can be achieved on occasion by pacing the heart rapidly, preferably from wires in the atrium or, less ideally, from wires in the ventricle. *Ventricular tachycardia* is extremely serious and usually causes severe impairment of cardiac function. Lidocaine intravenously may successfully control this arrhythmia, but frequently electrical cardioversion is required. Antiarrhythmic agents should be given after cardioversion to avoid recurrence. Ventricular tachycardia caused by digitalis intoxication should also be treated with potassium. *Ventricular fibrillation,* of course, requires immediate precordial electrical shock and then appropriate antiarrhythmic agents to avoid recurrence.

Disorders of AV Conduction. Disorders of atrioventricular conduction may occur spontaneously in association with cardiac surgery or secondary to injury of the AV conduction system. When AV block occurs for more than a few seconds in association with intracardiac surgery, temporary ventricular epicardial electrodes should be inserted. Ventricular pacing can then be accomplished in the postoperative period should AV block recur. If the heart block remains present for more than a few weeks following surgery, a permanent pacemaker should be inserted.

Renal Complications. If there is a renal problem postoperatively, it is usually manifested by oliguria. The most common etiologic factors include a low cardiac output state secondary to cardiac dysfunction or hypovolemia, a previous period of inadequate perfusion (usually during the operation), hemoglobinuria, renal artery embolism, and pre-existing renal disease.

The determination of urine osmolarity sometimes enables distinguishing prerenal azotemia from parenchymal involvement in the postoperative patient. A highly concentrated urine with a low urine sodium would suggest a prerenal etiology such as dehydration, hypovolemia, or poor cardiac function. A marked disparity between the BUN and serum creatinine (BUN/creatinine ratio of greater than 15 to 1) would also favor prerenal azotemia.

It is frequently difficult to accurately estimate the patient's blood volume status in the postoperative period. Central venous pressure may be quite helpful, although it is not entirely reliable. Oliguria, on the basis of an inadequate blood volume, can be determined by an initial trial of increasing volume (usually giving albumin or whole blood, depending upon the hematocrit). If this maneuver improves the urine output without causing evidence of cardiac overloading, then this course should be pursued. If the urine output does not respond to this volume, then further investigation is in order. Because many cardiac patients are brought to surgery having undergone rigorous diuresis, they may be somewhat dehydrated at the time of surgery. Such a patient may well require a volume load (albumin, plasma or whole blood) to attain a satisfactory cardiac output and urine flow and/or may also be benefited by the addition of a water and electrolyte load in the immediate postoperative period.

The cardiac surgical patient is frequently peripherally vasoconstricted in the early postoperative period owing to the high level of catecholamines evoked by the stress of surgery. The systemic blood pressure may be normal with a reasonable cardiac output, but the severe peripheral vasoconstriction reduces renal perfusion. Hypothermia may accentuate the situation. Maintaining the patient at a normal or slightly elevated temperature and the administration of modest amounts of a vasodilator drug (such as Thorazine, 1 to 5 mg. intravenously) may be extremely helpful in counteracting the vasoconstriction, improving peripheral perfusion and, secondarily, urine output.

If the cardiac patient has an adequate blood volume and a satisfactory degree of hydration and vasomotor tone, then a trial with diuretics such as mannitol (25 gm.), ethacrynic acid (50 to 100 mg.) or furosemide (50 to 200 mg.) may be appropriate. If there is a urine flow response to this medication, this would be an indication that the cause of the oliguria is not primarily renal function per se. Many patients will respond favorably to this initial diuretic treatment and will have no further problems. The patient who evidences a low cardiac output state must be treated to improve the cardiac output and by so doing the renal function and urine output should also improve.

Hypotension, with or without cardiopulmonary bypass, may result in acute tubular necrosis. This is particularly true in patients who already have some renal arterial disease. It is, thus, very important to maintain adequate perfusion during cardiac surgery and cardiopulmonary bypass. Hemoglobinuria is particularly prominent in patients undergoing cardiopulmonary bypass. The longer the period of perfusion, the more likely there will be hemoglobinuria. Presumably, this is due to trauma to the red blood cells. In addition, there may be red cell incompatibility that occurs in association with multiple transfusions. Frequently, hemoglobinuria will have little effect on renal function. However, if the hemoglobinuria is severe, or if it is associated with previous renal disease, hypotension or acidosis, severe renal tubular damage may occur with resultant acute tubular necrosis. Adequate urine flow apparently dilutes the toxic effects of the hemoglobinuria, and an alkaline urine limits the formation of acid hematin. When hemoglobinuria is present, it is therefore particularly important to maintain a satisfactory perfusion; in addition, diuresis should be accomplished with mannitol and/or a diuretic agent such as ethacrynic acid, and the urine should be kept alkaline by giving sodium bicarbonate.

Renal arterial occlusion or embolism in the postoperative period is extremely rare, but must be considered. The clinical data are not specific, and it is difficult to differentiate this entity from other causes of acute tubular damage. There may be evidence of emboli elsewhere. Common findings include hematuria, oliguria or anuria. Under these circumstances, arteriography should be considered to visualize the renal arterial system. Emergency renal arterial surgery may be necessary.

If the various etiologic factors mentioned above have been properly studied and appropriate therapeutic maneuvers have not resulted in a urine output response, renal tubular damage must certainly be strongly entertained. Characteristic urine findings in acute tubular necrosis include red cell casts, inability to retain sodium and a fixed urine osmolarity (280 to 300 milliosmoles/liter). Urinary sodium is usually above 20 to 25 mEq./liter. Under these circumstances, the patient should be managed with fluid restriction, careful monitoring of serum electrolytes (particularly potassium) and judicious maintenance of optimal peripheral perfusion. Hyperkalemia should be managed with ion exchange resin enemas (Kayexalate) and intravenous glucose and insulin and sodium bicarbonate. Peritoneal dialysis is required for markedly elevated levels of blood urea nitrogen and may occasionally also be required to remove excess fluid. Peritoneal dialysis is not as effective as Kayexalate enemas in removing potassium but may also be helpful here. Hemodialysis may be necessary if peritoneal dialysis is not effective. The intravenous use of high carbohydrate, essential amino acid solutions may be useful in preventing a BUN rise by avoiding protein catabolism and allowing urea to be used in protein synthesis.

Pulmonary Problems. Pulmonary complications represent one of the major determinants regarding recovery after cardiac surgery. Most patients should have pulmonary function studies preoperatively. All patients should have pulmonary physiotherapy prior to surgery. At the very least, they should be educated as to what to expect in the postoperative period as regards pulmonary physiotherapy. Patients with significantly impaired pulmonary function can sometimes undergo improvement in lung function with a week or two of chest physiotherapy.

Except for young adults without evidence of heart failure or children with essentially normal pulmonary hemodynamics, elective postoperative ventilatory support is desirable in order to insure adequate oxygenation in the face of possible accumulation of fluid in the chest or persistent left heart failure. The length of respiratory support depends on the procedure performed and the performance of the heart and lungs. Usually 12 to 36 hours of controlled ventilation is sufficient. The respirator should be adjusted to maintain arterial pCO_2 in the normal range (35 to 45 mm. Hg). The type of respirator is less important than the quality of support provided by the personnel (physicians and nurses) and the services available from an acute care laboratory. Arterial blood gas determinations are very helpful, particularly in the very sick patient. The inspired oxygen concentration should be retained at a level which will keep the arterial pO_2 in the range of 120 to 150 mm. Hg. This level allows a margin of safety for possible acute alterations in oxygen exchange.

Possible causes for a marked deficiency of oxygenation include inadequate ventilation, primarily low tidal volume, left ventricular failure with first interstitial and finally intra-alveolar edema and pulmonary sepsis. Appreciation of the fact that a collapse of terminal airways is due principally to the use of an inappropriate ventilatory pattern or persistent left ventricular failure has placed the treatment of respiratory insufficiency on a more physiologic basis. The causes of inadequate ventilation should be corrected. Airway obstruction resulting from excessive secretion is not common with adequate humidification and chest physiotherapy, and bronchoscopy for this purpose is unusual. Patients with severe respiratory insufficiency should have their respiration controlled by a ventilator to achieve an optimal pattern of ventilation. If the patient fails to coordinate with the ventilator, then sedation and/or muscle paralysis must be initiated. Sedation is achieved with narcotics such as morphine, whereas paralysis is obtained with d-tubocurarine or gallamine. Pulmonary edema should be treated with appropriate fluid restriction, cardiotonic drugs, and diuretics. Pulmonary infection requires specific antibiotic treatment.

Occasionally, one may encounter a marked discrepancy in partial pressure of oxygen between inspired gas and arterial blood. In such cases, application of an end-expiratory pressure so that the patient's airway pressure is maintained (5 to 15 cm. of water) above atmospheric pressure at all times, has been found to produce a rapid and marked increase in functional residual capacity and an improvement in arterial oxygen tension. This finding, plus the overall success of vigorous cardiotonic therapy with careful attention to water balance, has markedly decreased postoperative respiratory problems.

Ventilatory support is feasible via an endo- or nasotracheal tube for 2 to 4 days, depending on the patient's response to therapy. After 72 hours, the likelihood of damage to the nasal septum from pressure of the nasotracheal tube or the vocal cords and larynx is markedly increased, and a tracheostomy should be carried out.

Some cases of acute respiratory failure in the postoperative period have been attributed to "the pump lung syndrome" or to "oxygen toxicity." Patients who have been treated for prolonged periods with a high concentration of inspired oxygen have demonstrated a marked reduction in pulmonary compliance and progressive arterial hypoxemia. Histologically, they show severe interstitial edema and hemorrhage, and a reduction in pulmonary surfactant has also been demonstrated. Certainly, patients should be treated with the lowest possible inspired oxygen content consistent with adequate arterial oxygenation. In addition, weaning from the respirator should be accomplished as soon as safety permits. A better understanding of fluid balance, cardiac function, and cardiopulmonary bypass perfusion has raised some doubt regarding the validity of the "pump-lung" syndrome and certainly "oxygen toxicity" is a less frequent occurrence.

Safe weaning from the respirator includes careful observation of the respiratory mechanics and observation of the clinical status of the patient as well as monitoring of arterial blood gases. If the patient's arterial pO_2 is greater than 120 mm. Hg with 40 per cent inspired oxygen, it is usually reasonable to begin weaning. In general, the patient's vital capacity should be at least 10 ml./kg. of body weight at this time. The patient may be placed on an air-oxygen mix of approximately 40 per cent O_2 and allowed to breathe spontaneously for approximately 15 minutes. If the patient's arterial blood gases are acceptable (pO_2 greater than 100 mm. Hg), weaning may be continued. If the arterial gases are marginal, it may be necessary to gradually wean the patient over hours or days, allowing the patient to breathe on his own periodically for increasing periods of time. Vigorous pulmonary physiotherapy and measures to improve cardiac function, including diuresis, may be very helpful. If the patient's arterial gases are quite satisfactory after 30 to 60 minutes of breathing on his own, it is usually possible to remove the endotracheal tube.

Post-perfusion Syndrome and Post-cardiotomy Syndrome.   A surprising number of patients following cardiac surgery suffer from either the post-perfusion syndrome or the post-cardiotomy syndrome. The post-cardiotomy syndrome usually consists of the abrupt development of fever, pericarditis, pleural effusion, and occasionally inflammatory changes in the lung itself. The white blood count may be normal or elevated; occasionally a significant number of atypical lymphocytes may be seen. It usually appears 2 to 4 weeks after cardiac surgery (range, 1 week to 3 months). Persistence of postoperative fever without a source of infection for longer than 7 days should suggest the syndrome. The cause is unknown, but is thought to be autoimmune. Treatment consists, preferably, of salicylates (300 to 600 mg. every 4 to 6 hours) for 1 week or more, or in severe, refractory cases, prednisone (5 to 10 mg. 4 times a day) for 1 week or more with gradual tapering of the drug. Relapses are common and may occur for several months and, rarely, years after surgery.

The post-perfusion syndrome usually consists of fever, malaise, splenomegaly, and a white blood cell count of 1000 to 5000/mm.[3], largely made up of atypical lymphocytes. In some cases a maculopapular rash and hepatomegaly may appear. Hemolysis and even jaundice may occasionally be noted. Commonly the syndrome develops 3 to 7 weeks after cardiopulmonary bypass and lasts 1 to 3 months. The cause is unknown. The heterophil antibody titer is negative; cytomegalic inclusion virus has been implicated in some cases. Treatment of mild cases is symptomatic, usually salicylates. In more severely affected patients, prednisone (5 to 10 mg. four times a day) for 1 to 2 weeks with gradual tapering of the drug in the subsequent weeks will control the manifestations of the disease. Relapses may occur.

As many as a third of the patients undergoing cardiopulmonary bypass suffer from one of these two conditions. Fortunately, they are almost always transitory. When this question arises, the patient should have blood cultures to rule out bacterial infection as the cause for the temperature. Other appropriate studies, such as chest x-rays and urinalysis, should be performed. If these studies are negative, the patient should be treated as mentioned above.

Embolic Complications. A major area of difficulty in association with cardiac surgery is operative and postoperative embolic complications. The usual causes include debris (usually from a damaged valve in association with valve replacement), thrombus in the heart (usually left atrial thrombus in association with mitral valve disease), air embolism at the time of intracardiac surgery, and early postoperative platelet and fibrin emboli from prosthetic valves or other intracardiac foreign surfaces.

Emboli, of course, may lodge anywhere, but the areas that are particularly critical include the coronary and cerebral circulation and occasionally the renal, mesenteric or lower extremity circulations. Air emboli for all intents and purposes have only clinical significance for the cerebral circulation. Emboli to a renal artery, a mesenteric artery, or a lower extremity artery may require operative removal. This may also be true of the coronary circulation, particularly if the occlusion is noted during the initial cardiac procedure. When the cardiac damage is noted postoperatively, the patient is ordinarily treated as any other myocardial infarction patient. Cerebral emboli represent a very important complication. Sometimes it is quite difficult to differentiate between emboli and other causes of brain anoxia, such as hypotension or hypoxia. Localizing signs favor an isolated embolus, whereas generalized neurologic signs tend to favor air embolism or general hypoxia or hypotension. When there is evidence of brain swelling, care should be taken to avoid hyperthermia. Some physicians feel that total body hypothermia to approximately 32° C. should be accomplished in order to decrease brain metabolism. Some physicians also feel that corticosteroids (20 to 40 mg. of methylprednisolone intravenously every 6 to 8 hours for 2 to 4 days) should be employed under these circumstances. It is postulated that the corticosteroids may have a beneficial effect by reducing vascular permeability and restoring the integrity of the blood-brain barrier. Some physicians also employ mannitol, an osmotic agent which is confined to the extracellular space, or urea, an osmotic agent which is selectively inhibited from rapid entry into certain cerebral cells in an effort to decrease brain swelling. The clinical benefits of these various maneuvers still remain somewhat unclear.

Infection. Postoperative infection in the cardiac surgical patient is a most serious and often catastrophic complication. As has been mentioned earlier in this chapter, most surgeons employ prophylactic antibiotics in their cardiac surgical patients because of the serious problems that are associated with postoperative infection. This is, of course, particularly true when foreign material such as a prosthetic valve is left in the heart. Usually, the prophylactic antibiotics should be discontinued after 4 or 5 days, when the usual sources of a bacteremia (operative manipulations, arterial and venous pressure lines, urinary catheters) are no longer present. It is important to discontinue these antibiotics within a reasonable period of time to avoid the problems of overgrowth by resistant organisms. Following the discontinuance of the prophylactic antibiotics, specific infections should be studied and the appropriate antibiotic instituted, depending on sensitivity determinations. It is important to control extracardiac postoperative infections so as to avoid a bacteremia and the possibility of intracardiac contamination and infection on deformed valves or prosthetic materials.

When intracardiac infection occurs, aggressive therapy is required. The organisms should be isolated by repeated blood cultures and then the appropriate antibiotic should be employed, depending on the sensitivity studies. The patient should be treated as one would treat the usual patient with bacterial endocarditis, employing high doses of antibiotics, usually by the intravenous route. Ideally, the patient should be treated for a 6 week period and then the antibiotics should be discontinued to see if the infection has been eradicated. In patients with prosthetic material in the heart, the infection is very difficult to eradicate, but in some cases antibiotic therapy alone is completely satisfactory. In patients with prosthetic valves, very commonly the infection causes disruption of the annular sutures with progressive valvular incompetence. When the hemodynamic situation becomes significant, reoperation should be undertaken with removal of the prosthetic valve and with an attempt to remove all the adjacent infected tissue. In a surprising number of instances, this form of treatment in association with appropriate, high doses of antibiotics for a prolonged period of time has resulted in cure if the offending organism is sensitive to antibiotics.

Hemolysis. Almost all patients following open heart surgery have some increased red blood cell breakdown. This is due to the mechanical trauma to the red cells caused by the extracorporeal system and also to the shortened life expectancy of transfused red cells. In addition, patients with prosthetic valves (even if the prosthesis is functioning completely normally) may have somewhat shortened red cell survival time. Patients with prosthetic valves and paravalvular leaks are well known to have an exaggerated decrease in red blood cell survival; this is thought to be due to a traumatic destruction of the red blood cells associated with the paravalvular leak and the coated foreign surface. Significant traumatic hemolysis has occasionally been seen in patients with normally functioning valvular prostheses (no paravalvular leak) and rarely in association with other foreign intracardiac surfaces (such as a prosthetic patch for closure of a ventricular septal defect). Rarely, following heart surgery, an autoimmune type of hemolytic process may occur owing to the development of red cell antibodies (Coombs positive).

All patients following cardiac surgery should have periodic monitoring of their hematocrit. It is common for the hematocrit to drop somewhat during the week to 10 days following cardiopulmonary bypass. If the hematocrit reaches a level below 30 per cent, transfusion should be given in the form of either whole blood or packed red blood cells. Otherwise, it is usually reasonable to treat the patient with oral iron (ferrous gluconate, 300 mg. orally three times a day) and folic acid (20 mg. orally daily). Usually iron and folic acid treatment for a few months results in a stable hematocrit at a satisfactory level. If the patient has a significant paravalvular leak with hemodynamic difficulties or persistent and significant hemolysis and anemia, reoperation and repair of the paravalvular leak are required.

Psychological Problems. Psychological problems are very common following cardiac surgery. The emotional stress of a life-and-death situation, the rigors of the postoperative period in an intensive care unit, and perhaps a number of other unrecognized factors result in various psychological conditions. Depression, visual and auditory hallucinations, agitation, disorientation and paranoid delusions are common problems. Although a patient who has previously had psychological problems is more likely to have such problems in the postoperative period, many patients who develop postoperative psychological difficulties have had no previous evidence of emotional troubles. The older patients and the patients who, as a group, are sickest, seem to have the highest incidence of difficulty. Treatment depends on the specific psychological problem and its severity. Depression is best handled by gentle reassurance, protection of the patient against himself, and, if severe enough, mood elevators. Hallucinations and agitation with disorientation can usually be managed by reassurance; mild sedation with drugs such as Valium may also be quite helpful. Paranoid delusions are more difficult to manage, but again, gentle reassurance and kindness are helpful. With all these psychological problems, removal from the intensive care unit when safety permits, the omission of as many painful or exhausting maneuvers as possible, allowing the patient to get a sufficient amount of sleep, and sensible reassurance are helpful. These psychological aberrations are transitory and almost always resolve in time.

REFERENCES

Amoury, R. A., Bowman, F. O., and Malm, J. R.: Endocarditis associated with intracardiac prostheses. Diagnosis, management and prophylaxis. J. Thorac. Cardiov. Surg. 51:36, 1966.

Austen, W. G.: What's new in cardiac surgery. J. Surg. Res. 10:447, 1970.

Beller, B. M., Frates, R. W. M., and Wulfsohn, N.: Cardiac pacemaking in the management of postoperative arrhythmias. Ann. Thorac. Surg. 6:68, 1968.

Bendixen, H. H., Egbert, L. D., Hedley-Whyte, J., Laver, M. B., and Pontoppidan, H.: Respiratory Care. St. Louis, C. V. Mosby Co., 1965.

Berger, R. L., Polanzak, M. L., and Ryan, T. J.: Central venous pressure and blood volume pattern following open-heart surgery. Ann. Thorac. Surg. 6:57, 1968.

Buckley, M. J., Leinbach, R. C., Kastor, J. A., Laird, J. D., Kantrowitz, A. R., Madras, P. N., Sanders, C. A., and Austen, W. G.: Hemodynamic evaluation of intra-aortic balloon pumping in man. Circulation (Supplement II) 41 and 42:130, 1970.

Christlieb, I. I., Dammann, J. F., Jr., Thung, N. S., and Muller, W. H.: Postoperative care in cardiac surgery: A frequent determinant of success or failure. Dis. Chest 44:47, 1963.

Dammann, J. F., Jr., Thung, N., Christlieb, I. I., Littlefield, J. B., and Muller, W. H.: The management of the severely ill patient after open heart surgery. J. Thorac. Cardiov. Surg. 45:80, 1963.

Delman, A. J., Robinson, G., Stein, E., Yahr, W., and Lister, J. W.: Precise determination of cardiac arrhythmias during open heart surgery by monitoring of myocardial electrograms. Amer. J. Cardiol. 21:714, 1968.

Dietzman, R. H., Ersek, R. A., Lillehei, C. W., Cootaneda, A. R., and Lillehei, R. C.: Low output syndrome: Recognition and treatment. J. Thorac. Cardiov. Surg. 57:138, 1969.

Dreifus, L. S., Rabbino, M. D., and Watanabe, Y.: Newer agents in the treatment of cardiac arrhythmias. Med. Clin. N. Amer. 48:371, 1964.

Fishman, N. H., Hutchinson, J. C., and Roe, B. B.: Controlled atrial hypertension: A method for supporting cardiac output following open-heart surgery. J. Thorac. Cardiov. Surg. 52:777, 1966.

Gaus, H., and Krivit, W.: Problems in hemostasis during open heart surgery. Epsilon aminocaproic acid as an inhibitor of plasminogen activator activity. Ann. Surg. 155:268, 1962.

Gibbon, J. H., Jr., Sabiston, D. C., Jr., and Spencer, F. C.: Surgery of the Chest. Philadelphia, W. B. Saunders Co., 1969.

Grismer, J. T., Levy, M. J., Lillehei, R. C., Indeglia, R., and Lillehei, C. W.: Renal function in acquired valvular heart disease and effects of extracorporeal circulation. Surgery 55:24, 1964.

Hazan, S. J.: Psychiatric complications following cardiac surgery. J. Thorac. Cardiov. Surg. 51:307, 1966.

Harrison, D. C., Sprouse, J. H., and Morrow, A. G.: The antiarrhythmic properties of lidocaine and procaine amide. Circulation 28:486, 1963.

Karliner, J. S.: Intravenous diphenylhydantoin sodium (Dilantin) in cardiac arrhythmias. Dis. Chest 51:256, 1967.

Kaster, J. A., Akbarian, M., Buckley, M. J., Dinsmore, R. E., Sanders, C. A., Scannell, J. G., and Austen, W. G.: Paravalvular leaks and hemolytic anemia following insertion of Starr-Edwards aortic and mitral valves. J. Thorac. Cardiov. Surg., 56:279, 1968.

Kevy, S. V., Glickman, R. M., Bernhard, W. F., Diamond, L. K., and Gross, R. E.: The pathogenesis and control of the hemorrhagic defect in open heart surgery. Surg. Gynec. & Obst. 123:313, 1966.

Linder, E., Sakai, Y., and Paton, B. P.: Electrolyte changes during dilution perfusion. Arch. Surg. 88:175, 1964.

MacLean, L. D.: Venous pressure versus blood volume. Surg. Gynec. & Obst. 118:594, 1964.

McGuinness, J. B., and Taussig, H. B.: The postpericardiotomy syndrome. Its relationship to ambulation in the presence of "benign" pericardial and pleural reaction. Circulation 26:500, 1962.

McQueen, J. D., and Jeanes, L. D.: Influence of hypothermia on intercranial hypertension. J. Neurosurg. 19:277, 1962.

Moore, F. D.: Metabolic Care of the Surgical Patient. Philadelphia, W. B. Saunders Co., 1959.

Nelson, R. M., Jenson, C. B., Peterson, C. A., and Sanders, B. C.: Effective use of prophylactic antibiotics in open heart surgery. Arch. Surg. 90:731, 1965.

Norman, J. C., McDonald, H. P., and Sloan, J.: The early and aggressive treatment of acute renal failure following cardiopulmonary bypass with continuous peritoneal dialysis. Surgery 56:1, 1964.

Phillips, L. L., Malm, J. R., and Deterling, R. A., Jr.: Coagulation defects following extracorporeal circulation. Ann. Surg. 157:317, 1963.

Rowlands, D. J., Howitt, G., and Markman, P.: Propranolol (Inderal) in disturbances of cardiac rhythm. Brit. Med. J. 1:891, 1965.

Salzman, E. W., and Britten, A.: Hemorrhage and Thrombosis. Boston, Little, Brown & Co., 1965.

Siggaard-Andersen, O.: The pH-log pCO_2 blood acid-base nomogram revised. Scand. J. Clin. Lab. Invest. 14:598, 1962.

Wheeler, E. O., Turner, J. O., and Scannell, J. G.: Fever, splenomegaly and atypical lymphocytes. A syndrome observed after cardiac surgery utilizing a pump oxygenator. N. Eng. J. Med. 266:454, 1962.

Williams, G. R., and Spencer, F. C.: The clinical use of hypothermia following cardiac arrest. Ann. Surg. 148:462, 1958.

Williams, J. F., Morrow, A. G., and Braunwald, E.: The incidence and management of medical complications following cardiac operations. Circulation 32:608, 1965.

Yeh, T. J., Brachney, E. L., Hall, D. P., and Ellison, R. G.: Renal complications of open heart surgery: Predisposing factors, prevention and management. J. Thorac. Cardiov. Surg. 47:79, 1964.

CHAPTER 16

THE STOMACH AND DUODENUM

Edward R. Woodward, M.D., F.A.C.S.

The most important principle common to all surgery of the alimentary tract is to operate on it empty and to keep it empty during the early postoperative recovery period. First, spillage and contamination are minimized should the alimentary canal be opened during surgery. Second, operative exposure is facilitated because of the smaller volume of the empty gastrointestinal tract. Third, a full alimentary canal means that there is more blood in the splanchnic bed; manipulation is tolerated less well, hemostasis is less certain, and the likelihood of shock increases sharply. Fourth, distention decreases blood flow in the gastrointestinal wall and increases the hazard of anastomotic failure. Fifth, a distended abdomen greatly increases the likelihood of postoperative pulmonary and wound complications. *Most important* of all, however, is the fact that distended smooth muscle fails to recover its normal tonus and motility over long periods. Gastrointestinal function thus fails to resume, and convalescence is correspondingly delayed.

PREOPERATIVE MANAGEMENT

Elective Uncomplicated Case. Food intake is limited to liquids the day before surgery. All oral intake is discontinued at bedtime. The bowel is emptied by either a single enema or a mild cathartic. The former should be done the afternoon or evening before surgery, since apprehension may inhibit colonic response on the day of surgery. The stomach is emptied on the day of surgery by passing a Levin tube via the nasogastric route and applying mild suction. This may be done either before or after anesthesia; the latter is preferred, since the trachea is then occluded by the anesthetist's cuffed endotracheal tube and aspiration is prevented. This method also avoids unnecessary stimulation of the patient about to be anesthetized.

Pyloric Obstruction. Obstruction of the pylorus does not constitute a surgical emergency regardless of etiology. It is important to take enough time, even several days, to adequately prepare the patient. The adequacy of preparation will in large measure determine the successful outcome of both the surgical procedure and its attendant complications. The stomach must be thoroughly decompressed. Often the stomach will contain a large volume of food debris and barium; under these circumstances a large Ewald tube is utilized initially. Lavage is performed with a large volume of normal salt solution until the stomach is cleared of all solid material. Then a nasogastric Levin tube is placed and the stomach decompressed with continuous or intermittent mild suction. The length of decompression depends upon the degree of gastric dilatation and atonicity; this will vary from a few hours to several days.

No drug or chemical has proved to be of any value in preoperative recovery of gastric tonus, and adequate decompression has no substitute. Unless the stomach is permitted to recover its tonus and motility preoperatively, and if the further insult of surgery and anesthesia is added, postoperative recovery of gastric smooth muscle function will be markedly prolonged. Acute dilatation of the stomach and aspiration pneumonitis may result. Prolonged failure of the postoperative stomach to empty sharply increases morbidity. Infectious complications in both wound and abdominal cavity are frequent, owing to intraoperative contamination by gastric content.

The period of preoperative gastric decompression is utilized to replete the patient's fluids and electrolytes by the intravenous route. The best gauge of adequacy is a progressive increase in urinary volume with a progressive fall in urinary specific gravity. Serum electrolyte determinations are useful in measuring specific ionic deficits and their correction. The greatest deficiency will be in chloride, and this is best replaced with isotonic sodium chloride. The sodium deficit is automatically replenished by the use of this solution, and the metabolic alkalosis is simultaneously corrected. pH adjustment seldom requires specific therapy. Acid salts and mineral acids such as NH_4Cl and HCl cause severe venospasm and thrombosis, and should not be utilized parenterally when $NaCl$ will correct the disturbance.

There will be a potassium deficit of clinical significance in more severe cases. It is essential that potassium repletion begin at once, since administration of non-potassium-containing fluids, particularly glucose, will aggravate hypokalemia with resultant cardiac difficulties. Ringer's solution does not contain enough potassium for treatment of hypokalemia. The deficient patient will need 80 to 120 mEq. in the first several hours; the electrocardiogram is a valuable monitor in such cases.

Surgery is delayed until fluid and electrolyte balance is returned to normal and the obstructed stomach is completely decompressed. When surgery must be performed immediately on a patient with obstruction

at any level of the alimentary canal, it is important to recognize the very
real hazard of aspiration during induction of anesthesia. Preoperative
intubation of the stomach may not be sufficient; the anesthesiologist
should be consulted regarding the advisability of preventive measures
such as endotracheal intubation under local anesthesia.

   Perforation.   Perforation of the stomach or duodenum *is* an emergency requiring surgical intervention at the earliest possible moment.
The longer a communication exists between the lumen of the upper
gastrointestinal tract and the peritoneal cavity, the greater will be the
peritoneal soiling and the more advanced the peritoneal infection. Severe deficits in fluid and electrolytes are seldom seen and immediate
surgery is ordinarily safe.

   The early shock of perforation is usually transitory. Delayed shock
is due to sepsis. Although priming doses of antibiotics should be given,
only surgical control of the perforation will alter the septic course.
Unless exudative purulent peritonitis is established, definitive surgery
for the lesion resulting in perforation is safe in most cases.

   Hemorrhage.   The patient with upper gastrointestinal tract hemorrhage is approached with three major objectives:
   1. Treatment and prevention of shock.
   2. Rapid and accurate diagnosis of the bleeding lesion.
   3. Appropriate therapy for the lesion.

   Blood is immediately withdrawn for typing and cross matching. A
large and reliable venous channel is established so that blood can be
administered in whatever volume is required to maintain the cardiovascular system in a normovolemic state. In all more severe cases, particularly with shock already present, it is prudent to have more than one
channel for intravenous administration. It is particularly useful to place
a catheter in the superior vena cava; periodic measurement of the
central venous pressure is of inestimable value in assessing the adequacy of blood replacement therapy. It also provides a route through
which large volumes of blood and other fluids can be administered
rapidly and safely. The catheter may be placed percutaneously by
subclavian or jugular vein puncture, or through a venous cutdown in
the upper extremity or neck. This technique has the added value that
dislodgment is difficult and manipulation of the patient for both diagnostic and therapeutic purposes is facilitated.

   An aggressive attitude is assumed toward immediate diagnosis.
The stomach is thoroughly lavaged with iced saline using a large bore
Ewald tube. Cold assists hemostasis by reducing blood flow, and at the
same time the lavage clears the stomach of liquid and clotted blood.
Endoscopy may be immediately performed with particular attention to
the distal esophagus for varices or ulceration. The flexible, fiberoptic
instrument can be used quickly and safely without topical anesthesia
under emergency room conditions.

   During this time a BSP test is completed. Bromsulphalein is administered when blood is withdrawn for typing, and a second blood sample is withdrawn at 45 minutes. BSP retention of less than 5 per cent usually indicates that bleeding is not from esophageal varices secondary to portal cirrhosis. Elevated BSP retention is not as helpful, owing to a high incidence of false positives.

During this period of simultaneous treatment of blood loss and assessment, as much information as possible is gleaned from history and physical examination. If a reliable diagnosis has not yet been established, it is now time to proceed with x-ray examination. This will customarily consist of an upper gastrointestinal barium contrast study. In nearly all cases it is possible to support the blood volume sufficiently so that a full study, including tilting, rotating, and compression, can be accomplished by the radiologist. In cases in which evaluation up to this point gives no clue whatever as to the etiology of the hemorrhage, selective angiography should be seriously considered instead of barium contrast. Selective injection of contrast media into the celiac axis and/or superior mesenteric artery will demonstrate the bleeding lesion when the rate of hemorrhage is as low as 0.5 cc./minute. The surgeon is provided with a "road map" so that he may rapidly and directly approach the bleeding site.

Vigorous diagnostic procedures will establish the diagnosis in most cases, and permit a logical approach to therapy. Bleeding from esophageal varices can usually be controlled with a Blakemore-Sengstaken tube. This control is often temporary and the complication rate is high. Surgical Pituitrin given by intravenous infusion lowers the portal pressure and is often accompanied by a cessation of hemorrhage from esophageal varices. By using this method, an emergency problem can sometimes be converted into an elective one. Cardiac difficulties are frequent and EKG monitoring is essential. Emergency portal-systemic shunt surgery is necessary in uncontrolled cases.

Gastric cooling may be worthwhile in diffuse gastritis and acute stress ulcer but does not have proved value in treating esophageal varices or chronic peptic ulcer. We have utilized a simple method whereby the stomach is rapidly perfused with iced saline:

A No. 18 French Levin tube is placed into the stomach by the nasogastric route and serves as the inflow tract. A large Ewald tube is placed into the stomach through the mouth and serves as the outflow tract. Saline is stored in 2 liter flasks in a refrigerator, ready for use. When infusion is begun, two flasks of saline are suspended from an IV stand and a Y tube GU set is connected to the bottles. The single line from the Y is attached to a long piece of plastic tubing which is coiled in a large stainless steel basin. The distal end of the IV tubing is connected to the Levin tube. The basin is then filled with crushed ice which is sprinkled liberally with ice cream salt. This crude heat exchanger further cools the saline, which is then infused rapidly into the stomach. Outflow from the Ewald tube is collected in another basin;

visual inspection of the intensity of red color gives a rough clue to the success of therapy. When outflow slows or stops, clots are extracted with a Toomey syringe. Surgery will be necessary in cases in which bleeding continues, but the stomach will often be found to be undistended and relatively free of clots.

Nasogastric suction through an indwelling Levin tube is useful in treating hemorrhage secondary to peptic ulcer. Acid gastric juice is removed, permitting a blood clot to occlude the ulcer base. The stomach is kept empty and decompressed in case surgery is necessary. Appearance of blood in the tube gives early warning of recurrent bleeding. Antacid therapy should not be used until it is clear that surgical intervention will not be required.

POSTOPERATIVE CARE

Temporary Gastrostomy as a Method of Gastrointestinal Tract Decompression. Temporary gastrostomy should be used when prolonged gastrointestinal tract dysfunction is anticipated, is a likely possibility, or would be particularly hazardous. It is especially useful when slow resumption of gastric emptying is expected. In vagotomy combined with a drainage operation, loss of parasympathetic augmentor influence renders the stomach particularly susceptible to acute dilatation. Several days are needed for the peripheral automatic motor mechanism to compensate. Temporary gastrostomy is useful in postoperative care of the dilated, thin-walled, atonic stomach secondary to pyloric obstruction. It can be used to advantage when prolonged distention of the alimentary canal has been present preoperatively at any level. Prolonged ileus frequently follows extensive retroperitoneal hemorrhage, dissections or infections, and temporary gastrostomy is useful.

Temporary gastrostomy is superior to, and in large measure replaces, prolonged postoperative nasogastric suction. Unlike the latter, it does not cause aspiration pneumonitis. The older the patient, the more significant this factor; in patients over 60, prolonged nasogastric suction is contraindicated because diminished pharyngeal reflexes do not protect against aspiration. More effective decompression is achieved because of the shorter length and larger size of the tube. Gastrostomy is better tolerated by the patient, with less discomfort, more cooperation, improved oral hygiene and easier physical mobilization of the patient. Nasopharyngeal and esophageal complications of nasogastric intubation, such as inflammation, erosion, necrosis and ulceration, are avoided.

Technique of temporary gastrostomy is as follows: A No. 26 French Foley catheter with a 5 cc. bag is pulled through a stab incision in the abdominal wall in the left subcostal area. The catheter is wrapped with two or three loops of freely movable omentum. This rapidly seals off the sinus tract, preventing leakage and insuring rapid closure when the tube is removed. A purse string suture is placed on the anterior wall of the stomach near the greater curvature, well proximal to the antral canal in the body of the stomach. An incision is made through the gastric wall, the catheter introduced and the balloon inflated with 5 cc. of water. The gastric wall is infolded snugly about the catheter with the purse string suture.

It is not necessary to draw the stomach flush with the abdominal wall, since the intervening catheter is covered by omentum. This prevents tenting which will interfere with adequate gastric drainage through the catheter. The slack is pulled out of the tube which is then secured to the skin with an interrupted suture. The tube leading to the Foley balloon is ligated with umbilical tape to prevent accidental deflation.

The Foley catheter may be attached to low suction, but gravity drainage has been found to be simpler and more effective. After the period of complete decompression, the catheter can be used to measure adequacy of gastric emptying. The catheter should not be removed earlier than 10 days postoperatively to insure that sealing off is adequate. The gastrostomy tube is best removed when the stomach is empty. The patient is then kept in the reclining position for 30 to 60 minutes.

Vagotomy and Drainage Procedure.   There is a slight preference for pyloroplasty over gastroenterostomy in combination with vagotomy for peptic ulcer. The postoperative management is identical.

Dissection of and manipulation around the left leaf of the diaphragm makes left lower lobe atelectasis frequent. Adequate ventilation should begin immediately in the postoperative period. Intermittent positive pressure breathing should be used freely during postanesthetic recovery. Particular attention is paid to tracheobronchial toilet. The patient is encouraged in deep breathing and coughing, with tracheal aspiration and bronchoscopy used freely. Temporary tracheostomy may be life-saving in patients with pre-existing chronic lung disease.

Temporary gastrostomy is used in all cases to prevent distention of the vagotomized stomach by swallowed air and retained secretions. The gastrostomy catheter is connected to straight drainage for three continuous days. It is clamped on the evening of the third postoperative day and gastric residual measured the next morning. If it is over 100 cc., decompression is continued one more day. If less than 100 cc., the tube is reclamped and the patient is given 30 cc. of water each hour. Residual is measured twice daily. If it continues low, fluid intake is increased on day 5 to 60 cc. of clear liquids each hour. On day 6, clear liquids are permitted *ad libitum* and intravenous administration of fluids is discontinued. Continued low gastric residual indicates a soft diet for day 7.

Since the pyloric sphincter has been ablated, the patient may be subject to "dumping." High carbohydrate liquids should be specifically prohibited until 6 weeks postoperatively. The gastrostomy tube is removed not earlier than the tenth postoperative day; this may be done at an outpatient visit. Three months afger surgery the patient is recalled for clinical evaluation, upper gastrointestinal x-ray to determine adequacy of gastric emptying, and basal gastric analysis to evaluate adequacy of vagotomy.

Esophageal Hiatal Herniorraphy. Postoperative care of the gastrointestinal tract is essentially the same whether hiatal herniorrhaphy is performed by a transthoracic or transabdominal approach. When combined with vagotomy and ancillary gastric surgery, postoperative care is the same as outlined in the previous discussion.

In hiatal herniorraphy alone, temporary gastrostomy is usually not necessary. The stomach has not been distended preoperatively and, since the vagi are left intact, tonus and motility will rapidly return. The addition of gastrostomy opens the alimentary canal, inevitably increasing the likelihood of bacterial contamination. It is preferable to use nasogastric suction for 12 to 36 hours. The patient is given nothing by mouth thereafter until auscultation of the abdomen reveals active peristalsis. The patient is then started on clear fluids, advancing to a soft diet as soon as flatus is passed.

Distal Partial Gastrectomy. Postoperative care for distal gastric resection is essentially the same whether the amount of stomach resected is large or small. The postoperative course is usually not influenced by a simultaneous vagotomy, since a relatively large sphincterless gastroenteric stoma provides gravity drainage of the remaining stomach. Therefore the propulsive motor action of the parasympathetic is not essential.

Billroth I reconstruction will not empty as rapidly, and greater caution is indicated. Since emptying is usually adequate, temporary gastrostomy is infrequently needed. It can, however, be safely performed when needed, even after extensive subtotal resection. It is important to place the catheter at some distance from the gastroenteric suture line so that the Foley balloon will not cause undue pressure or obstruction at this point. Also the gastric remnant should be left *in situ* and the relatively long segment of intraperitoneal catheter wrapped with omentum.

Ordinarily nasogastric suction is used for 12 to 36 hours. Following this the patient is given nothing by mouth until auscultation of the abdomen reveals good peristaltic activity. The patient is then begun on clear fluids and is increased to a soft diet when flatus is passed.

Dietary regulation is important. The patient is given small feedings at mealtime with an additional small serving between meals and at bedtime. Sweet liquids and highly soluble carbohydrates are prohibited as a preventive measure against "dumping." Later in convalescence the patient may experiment to test tolerance for carbohydrate. As recovery advances, the size and variety of meals are increased with a corresponding decrease in the number of feedings. Body weight is regularly recorded for several months and food intake regulated accordingly.

Proximal Partial Gastrectomy. Resection of the proximal stomach has two features which distinguish it from distal gastrectomy. First, the remaining stomach is anastomosed to esophagus which has no serosa; therefore, anastomotic sealing is less rapid and less satisfactory with a higher incidence of leak and subsequent fistula or stricture. Secondly, the residual distal stomach has its vagi severed; this creates a motility defect which requires a drainage operation, preferably pyloroplasty.

Because of these considerations, prolonged decompression is indicated. If the residual gastric pouch is large enough to permit it, temporary gastrostomy is preferred; otherwise nasogastric suction must be used. Complete decompression for a period of 4 to 7 days should be utilized. At this point we prefer to examine the anastomotic site radiographically. A water-soluble contrast material, such as Gastrografin, is preferred, although a thin barium mixture is also satisfactory. Providing that patency is demonstrated and no leak is observed, resumption of dietary intake is then regulated in the same fashion as after distal partial gastrectomy. It is necessary to watch the patients closely for 3 to 6 months so that the need for bougienage is apparent before a stricture too tight for passage is present.

Total Gastrectomy. Previously done almost solely for cancer, total gastrectomies are now done in much larger number for more benign conditions. This procedure has three relatively unique considerations. First, as in proximal gastrectomy, the anastomosis involves the non-serosa-covered esophagus with the complications of healing related thereto. Second, the storage function of the stomach is entirely ablated; this means that avoidance of a serious, chronic nutritional deficiency must be planned for from the onset. Third, absence of the stomach permits access to the esophagus of alkaline duodenal fluids, including pancreatic juice and bile. The extremely destructive potential of this fluid for esophageal mucosa renders it imperative that the operative reconstruction divert duodenal secretions away from the esophagointestinal anastomosis. This can be accomplished by enteroenterostomy, a Roux-en-Y anastomosis or jejunal interposition between esophagus and duodenum. Postoperative management must assume the presence of such a reconstruction.

Because of the likelihood of leak, a prolonged fast is indicated. Should a leak occur, the period before oral intake may be resumed can be prolonged for weeks and months. It is therefore worthwhile to consider routinely performing a temporary jejunostomy. This may be performed in the upper jejunum, using exactly the same technique as outlined above for temporary gastrostomy with the exception that a smaller Foley catheter is used (a No. 10 French with 3 cc. bag).

The patient is restrained from oral intake for 6 to 9 days. Intravenous fluid therapy is maintained until auscultation indicates intestinal peristalsis. At this time fluid therapy is changed from intravenous to intrajejunal. This is begun with isotonic fluids such as physiological saline in order to avoid "dumping" symptoms and the diarrhea of rapid transit. The tonicity of jejunal infusion is gradually increased, first using skim milk warmed to body temperature. When tolerance to this is observed, homogenized milk is used and high caloric tube feeding added gradually thereafter. Diarrhea from jejunostomy feeding can be controlled with opiates. Use 5 drops of tincture of deodorized opium (laudanum) per liter; this can be increased to 15 drops per liter if required. The synthetic alkaloid anti-diarrheal drug, Lomotil, is available in liquid form. This is not addicting and has no hypnotic properties. Substitute this for laudanum, using 10 to 15 mg. per liter of tube feeding.

The esophagointestinal reconstruction is examined radiographically on the ninth postoperative day for patency and the absence of leak. Again, a water-soluble contrast material is preferred. When oral feedings are resumed, multiple low carbohydrate feedings are given. Rapid transit interferes with iron absorption; this should be given orally if tolerated, and parenterally if not. In long-term survivors, one must remember that all intrinsic factor has been removed. After the third year vitamin B_{12} should be given parenterally every 3 months to prevent megaloblastic anemia. The patient should be watched closely for the development of stricture so that bougienage can be begun early.

REFERENCES

Baum, S., Nusbaum, M., Blakemore, W. S., and Finkelstein, A. K.: The preoperative radiographic demonstration of intra-abdominal bleeding from undetermined sites by percutaneous selective celiac and superior mesenteric arteriography. Surgery 58:797, 1965.

Schwartz, S. I., Bales, H. W., Emerson, G. L., and Mahoney, E. B.: The use of intravenous pituitrin in treatment of bleeding esophageal varices. Surgery 45:72, 1959.

CHAPTER 17

THE LIVER AND PORTAL VEIN

Seymour I. Schwartz, M.D.

Preoperative and postoperative management of patients undergoing extensive hepatic resection for trauma and neoplasms or portal-systemic shunts merits special emphasis and necessitates an appreciation of the multiple and essential functions of the liver. The liver is responsible for the synthesis of albumin and proteins required for the normal coagulation of blood. It also contributes to the maintenance of the blood sugar level by production and storage of glycogen. The liver functions as a conjugator and detoxifier of many elements that normally appear in the system and also of a wide variety of drugs that may be administered to the patient. In addition to conjugating bilirubin and other substances, the liver acts as an excretory organ responsible for their removal from the body.

EVALUATION OF LIVER FUNCTION

Nearly one-half million people in the United States presently have liver disease and there is evidence of increasing frequency. Cirrhosis with its complications constitutes the seventh major cause of death in this country.[1] Determination of liver function contributes to the evaluation of operative risk and may dictate specific preoperative and postoperative measures. So-called liver "function" tests assess the presence and degree of functional impairment and contribute to the differentiation between the major causes of jaundice but do not provide a specific pathologic diagnosis. The extreme functional reserve of the organ occasionally produces normal results in the face of significant pathology. Also, it is important to recognize that many of these tests do not measure a specific function of the liver and that other organ systems may be implicated. False positive results for each test are found in about 2.5

345

per cent of normal controls and about 10 per cent of hospital controls. False negative results for each test also occur in about 10 per cent of the cases.[2] It is appropriate to consider liver function tests according to the system studied.

Serum Proteins. The hepatic parenchymal cell is the sole synthesizer of the body's *albumin* and two proteins implicated in coagulation, namely fibrinogen and prothrombin. The degree of hypoalbuminemia provides one of the most accurate reflections of the extent of liver disease and may be used to assess the effects of therapy. Since the half-life of albumin is approximately 11 days, impaired hepatic synthesis of this protein must be present for about two weeks before significant alterations are noted. Levels below 2.8 gm./100 ml. contribute to the formation of ascites and peripheral edema by critically reducing the osmotic pressure of plasma. In general, if the serum albumin level cannot be raised above 3.0 gm./100 ml., portal-systemic shunting procedures are associated with a poor prognosis.

In contrast, the correlation between the *total protein* and disease of the liver is not good because the reduction in albumin is frequently compensated for, and even overcompensated for, by an increase in the level of the serum globulin formed in the reticuloendothelial system and by plasma cells. The main value of determining the serum protein is that it serves as an indicator of the general state of nutrition. Similarly, the albumin/globulin ratio, which has represented a popular method of evaluating liver disease, is nonspecific because it may reflect either an albumin decrease and compensatory globulin increase or a primary increase of globulin either related or unrelated to liver disease.

A variety of tests have been utilized to determine quantitative and qualitative changes in serum proteins. The *cephalin flocculation test*, which may be associated with a positive reaction within 48 hours of acute hepatic parenchymal injury and returns to normal within several days of recovery from that injury, has been replaced by evaluation of the SGOT and SGPT. The *thymol turbidity test*, which tends to parallel the severity of hepatitis with a positive reaction occurring later but persisting longer than the cephalin flocculation test, is less specific because it may be abnormal in patients with rheumatoid arthritis and other collagen disorders, infectious mononucleosis, malaria, and tuberculosis. It, too, has been replaced by enzyme evaluation.

In liver disease, a variety and multiplicity of coagulation defects may occur. In addition to reduction of platelets associated with secondary hypersplenism, changes in the ability of the liver to synthesize prothrombin and fibrinogen may have critical consequences. The two major mechanisms contributing to the deficiency of coagulation factors are (1) failure to absorb vitamin K, a fat-soluble vitamin necessary for the synthesis of prothrombin, as seen in obstructive jaundice, and (2) inability of the diseased parenchymal cell to synthesize prothrombin and fibrinogen.

The *prothrombin time,* which is dependent upon the entire prothrombin complex, including Factors II, V, and VII, is frequently abnormal in patients with hepatic parenchymal disease. Although laboratory methods are available to determine the level of individual coagulation factors, it is doubtful whether these individual assays would make bleeding more predictable than the Quick one-stage test. In general, levels of prothrombin time greater than 40 per cent of normal control are not associated with excessive bleeding. Reduction of serum *fibrinogen* from the normal level of 200 to 400 mg./100 ml. is occasionally noted in patients with marked hepatocellular disease, but significant reductions of the level of fibrinogen, i.e., below 100 mg./100 ml., occur in less than 10 per cent of patients. Another important factor implicated in bleeding accompanying surgery in patients with cirrhosis is the presence of circulating fibrinolysins in 20 per cent of patients with hepatocellular disease.

Carbohydrates and Lipids. Glycogenesis, glycogen storage, glycogenolysis, and the conversion of galactose into glucose all represent hepatic functions related to carbohydrate metabolism. Alterations in carbohydrate metabolism associated with liver disease have been demonstrated by a variety of tests, but the determinations are somewhat limited by the influence of many nonhepatic factors. Extensive hepatic disease may be accompanied by hypoglycemia. Hypoglycemic shock or insulin shock following the administration of the usual dose to a diabetic patient represents a rare but interesting observation in a patient with primary carcinoma of the liver. Amelioration of diabetes in a patient with hemochromatosis is suggestive of superimposed hepatic neoplasm. However, the more common effect of hepatic disease on carbohydrate metabolism is a deficiency of glycogenesis with a resultant hyperglycemia, occasionally glycosuria, and an abnormal *glucose tolerance test.* A specific hepatic enzyme system is responsible for the conversion of galactose into glucose.

Following the intravenous administration of galactose, its appearance in the urine coupled with an elevated blood level is seen in patients with hepatitis and active cirrhosis, whereas normal levels are noted with uncomplicated obstructive jaundice and chronic inactive cirrhosis. In the newborn, a familial deficiency in this enzyme system may account for galactosemia accompanied by jaundice which subsides when lactose is removed from the diet.

The synthesis of both phospholipids and cholesterol takes place in the parenchymal cells of the liver. Although the *serum cholesterol* level is determined by diet, activity of thyroid hormone and other organ systems, the liver represents the major organ involved in synthesis, esterification, and excretion. In the presence of parenchymal damage, both the total serum cholesterol and the percentage of the esterified fraction, which is normally about 65 per cent, decrease. Extreme depression of these levels is a particularly poor prognostic sign for patients with hepatitis or cirrhosis. Biliary obstruction is accompanied by a rise in the total cholesterol level, and the most pronounced elevations are noted with primary biliary cirrhosis and cholangiolitis following toxic reactions to phenothiazine derivatives.

Enzymes.   Several enzymes have been shown to achieve abnormal serum levels in hepatic disease. The three enzyme determinations which are most widely applied include (1) alkaline phosphatase, (2) serum glutamic oxaloacetic transaminase (SGOT), and (3) serum glutamic pyruvate transaminase (SGPT).

Four methods of assay of *alkaline phosphatase* are currently in use, and therefore expression of results should parenthetically indicate the normal values. Elevation of the alkaline phosphatase is frequently noted in patients with increased osteoblastic activity. In relation to hepatic function, the serum alkaline phosphatase provides an evaluation of the patency of the biliary duct system at all levels, since the bile represents the main vehicle for disposal of the enzyme. The test represents the best index of biliary patency. Over 90 per cent of patients with obstruction of the extrahepatic biliary tract by neoplasm and three fourths of the patients in whom the obstruction is due to calculi demonstrate an elevated serum level. In patients with bile duct obstruction, the elevation in serum alkaline phosphatase generally precedes the increase in serum bilirubin and persists for a longer period of time. An elevation also occurs with intrahepatic obstruction accompanying drug-induced lesions, biliary cirrhosis, and infiltrative parenchymal processes. The overall correlation between metastatic carcinoma to the liver and an elevated serum alkaline phosphatase is approximately 90 per cent, whereas 60 per cent of patients with primary hepatic carcinoma demonstrate a significant increase.[2]

Serum glutamic oxaloacetic transaminase (SGOT) may be elevated in patients with skeletal muscle trauma, renal infarction, pancreatitis, myocardial infarction, and liver disease. In reference to liver disease, the most marked increases accompany acute cellular damage regardless of cause, and the highest levels are seen in patients with infectious hepatitis or toxic and anoxic hepatocellular injury. The SGOT is markedly increased in patients with chronic cirrhosis or obstructive jaundice and in a significant number of cases of acute cholecystitis. The *serum glutamic pyruvate transaminase* (SGPT) is more specific to the evaluation of hepatic disease. The rise of this enzyme is greater than the SGOT in patients with viral hepatitis and other acute hepatic diseases, whereas no elevation is noted in patients with skeletal muscle or myocardial damage.

Foreign Dye Excretion.   Removal of a foreign dye from the liver is dependent upon afferent hepatic blood flow, hepatocellular function, and biliary secretion. Although 20 per cent of the *Bromsulphalein* injected intravenously is removed by extrahepatic means, measurement of the BSP retention does offer an assessment of hepatic function. Normally, less than 6 per cent of the dye is present in the blood 45 minutes after injection. The presence of jaundice produces a disproportionate determination, and fever, shock, hemorrhage, and recent surgery all may result in an increased level of retention. The test is particularly pertinent in the differential diagnosis of upper gastrointestinal bleeding, and the determination of a normal value in a patient with massive bleeding suggests that varices should not be implicated. In the nonicteric patient with hepatic disease, the BSP can be used as an indicator of functional reserve. It detects acute cellular damage, and the most marked elevations are associated with active processes such as hepatitis or active cirrhosis. Elevations in the BSP are also seen in patients with metastatic and primary carcinoma, fatty infiltration, and passive congestion. Since the rate of disappearance from the blood is constant, *hepatic blood flow* can be determined by injecting the dye at a rate that will maintain a constant blood level, and by applying the Fick principle to the blood removed from the catheterized hepatic vein.[3]

Blood Ammonia. There is great confusion concerning the nature of the material determined by the standard test. It is appreciated that no technique measures the blood ammonia level per se, because at the pH of blood less than 1 per cent of ammonia is present in solution. Elevations of blood ammonia can be related to increased intestinal absorption of nitrogenous material, including blood, shunting of portal blood around the liver, or disease of the hepatic parenchymal cell. Relationships have been demonstrated between the blood ammonia level and electroencephalographic changes and neuropsychiatric phenomena in patients with cirrhosis. However, these are not consistent. Pretreatment of a patient with nonabsorbable intestinal antibiotics, glutamic acid, or arginine negates the value of this test. It is to be stressed that any large portal-systemic shunt, e.g., paraumbilical vein to inferior vena cava, will result in a positive test even in the absence of esophagogastric varices. Levels above 120 micrograms/100 ml. have been associated with a poor prognosis following portal-systemic shunts, and ammonia has been administered postoperatively to indicate the patency of the shunt, but this technique is limited by the threat of inducing encephalopathy.

Bile Pigment Metabolism. The status of hepatic function may be evaluated by determining the levels of the bile pigments in the serum, urine and stool. The hepatic processes involved in this metabolic function include (1) the uptake of unconjugated pigment from the plasma by the parenchymal cell, (2) intracellular conjugation, (3) excretion of the aqueous solution of conjugates into the bile canaliculi, and (4) patency of intra- and extrahepatic bile ducts to permit passage of the pigment into the intestinal lumen.

The *icterus index* represents a screening colorimetric evaluation of serum compared with a chemical standard. Clinical jaundice is usually apparent at levels of 16 units. *Bilirubin* itself is normally present in the serum in concentrations up to 1.5 mg./100 ml. Most laboratories now report results as a 1-minute (prompt), direct-reacting bilirubin and total bilirubin. Elevation of the total serum bilirubin occurs in all types of jaundice, and serial determinations are of value in following the course of the disease or defining an intermittent biliary tract obstruction. The direct-reacting fraction represents conjugated bilirubin. An increase in this fraction to levels above 0.2 mg./100 ml. is indicative of hepatocellular disease or interference with flow of bile in the duct system. In uncomplicated hemolytic jaundice, this fraction is normal. In patients with jaundice secondary to obstruction of flow or hepatocellular degeneration, the ratio of prompt reacting to total bilirubin varies with the intensity of jaundice. Determination of the direct fraction is more sensitive than the total serum bilirubin as an index of early or slight hepatic damage, and a transient rise may accompany acute cholecystitis.

Normally, up to 1.2 mg./100 ml. of unconjugated bilirubin is present in the serum. Increases in this fraction accompany hemolytic processes which result in increased destruction of erythrocytes and consequent presentation to the liver of more pigment than the organ is able to clear. When the total bilirubin level is above 3 mg./100 ml. in patients with extrahepatic cholestasis, the increases in the direct and indirect reacting fractions parallel one another.

Normally, no bilirubin pigment is present in the urine. Since the unconjugated bilirubin fraction cannot pass through the glomerular filter, pure elevation of this fraction such as occurs with hemolysis is associated with an acholic urine. With an impaired excretion of bile, there is an accumulation of conjugated bilirubin in the blood; and since this is readily excreted in the urine, the urine becomes brown and foams on shaking.

The conjugated bilirubin which is excreted via the bile into the intestine is acted upon by bacteria in the colon where it is converted to *urobilinogen* (stercobilinogen). These compounds are oxidized and are responsible for the brown color of feces. Biliary obstruction decreases the fecal urobilinogen, and complete obstruction results in the absence of the compound in the stool. Hepatic parenchymal damage, such as occurs with hepatitis and cirrhosis, usually causes a reduction in fecal urobilinogen, but the extent of decrease is variable. A reduction in enteric bacteria accompanying the use of intestinal antibiotics may also be responsible for reduced pigment excretion. The urobilinogen which evolves from the action of intestinal bacteria on bilirubin is partially absorbed into the bloodstream from which it is extracted by the liver and re-excreted into the intestine or into the urine. Normally, there is only a minimal amount of urinary excretion of urobilinogen, and the levels of urinary urobilinogen parallel those of fecal urobilinogen.

Application of Liver Function Tests to Preoperative Evaluation. Normal values of the commonly employed liver function tests are presented in Table 17–1. A battery of several appropriate tests may provide

Table 17–1. NORMAL VALUES FOR HEPATIC FUNCTION TESTS*

TEST	NORMAL VALUE
Serum albumin	4.6–6.7 gm./100 ml.
Total protein	6.0–8.0 gm./100 ml.
Albumin/globulin	1.5–3.6
Cephalin flocculation	0–1+
Thymol turbidity	0–7 units
Zinc sulfate turbidity	2–20 units
Cholesterol	135–325 mg./100 ml.
Esters	65 per cent of total
Alkaline phosphatase:	
Bodansky	1.5–4.0 units
King-Armstrong	3–13 units
Shinohara-Jones-Reinhart	2.8–8.6 units
Bessey-Lowry-Brock	1.8× Bodansky units
Serum glutamic oxaloacetic transaminase	40 units
Serum glutamic pyruvic transaminase	45 units
Bromsulphalein retention	0–6 per cent at 45 minutes
Prothrombin time	90–100 per cent
Fibrinogen	200–400 mg./100 ml.
Blood "ammonia"	40–60 micrograms/100 ml.
Icterus index	3–8 units
Serum bilirubin:	
Total	Less than 1.5 mg./100 ml.
Direct	Less than 0.3 mg./100 ml.
Indirect	Less than 1.2 mg./100 ml.
Urinary bilirubin	0
Urobilinogen:	
Urinary	0.2–3.0 mg./day
Fecal	40–300 mg./day

*From Schwartz, S. I.: Surgical Diseases of the Liver. New York, McGraw-Hill Book Co., 1964.

a "profile" of liver function, which is particularly applicable in evaluating the surgical risk and prognosis of patients under consideration for elective hepatic resection or portal decompressive procedures. Since the incidence of hepatocellular carcinoma in Caucasians with cirrhosis is at least 20 times more common than in those without cirrhosis, the evaluation of hepatic function is critical prior to major hepatic resection for these tumors. Approximately 25 per cent of patients under consideration for hepatic resection demonstrate evidence of hepatic dysfunction.[4] Particular attention should be directed to the serum albumin level, the prothrombin time, and the BSP retention. This is especially important in the cirrhotic patient, because very little regeneration occurs following partial hepatectomy of the cirrhotic liver.

A variety of attempts have been made to assess the degree of hepatic dysfunction and determine the optimal timing of a portal-systemic shunt procedure in a patient with esophagogastric varices that have bled or are presently bleeding. The first correlation of surgical risk with liver function was proposed by Linton in 1951.[5] A modification was suggested by Child, who emphasized certain clinical variables,[6] and by McDermott, who devised a numerical code which represented the average of a sum of selected values for six standard liver function tests.[7] However, Jackson and associates emphasized the unreliability of standard liver function tests as criteria of morbidity or survival following portal decompressive surgery,[8] and the author's personal experience reaffirms this position.[9]

In the cirrhotic patient under consideration for a portal-systemic shunt, it is important to rule out active hepatic disease or progressive decompensation. This diagnosis may be suggested by a rising SGOT or SGPT but should be confirmed by needle biopsy of the liver. Spider angiomata are associated with a two-fold increase in postoperative mortality, and ascites that fails to respond to medical therapy is associated with an increased mortality and morbidity following shunting procedures. In the face of an improving serum albumin and prothrombin time, surgery should be deferred, but in the absence of improvement the finding of a serum albumin below 3 gm./100 ml. and a prothrombin time in the range of 30 per cent does not necessarily preclude surgery. Bromsulphalein retention of a given value affects the operative outcome less in posthepatitic patients than in patients with alcoholic cirrhosis. A markedly elevated serum bilirubin level is a poor prognostic sign but does not affect operative mortality adversely in cases of cirrhosis secondary to common duct obstruction.

Recently, hemodynamic, metabolic, and respiratory function have received deserved attention. Cirrhosis may be associated with an increased total blood volume and a hyperkinetic circulatory state. A poor prognosis has been established for patients with a combination of increased cardiac output, a high mean ejection rate, and an increased volume. Metabolic alkalosis in itself is an extremely poor prognostic sign.[10]

SPECIAL DIAGNOSTIC STUDIES

Special diagnostic studies which may be indicated in the preoperative evaluation of a patient undergoing hepatic resection or a portal-systemic shunting procedure are directed at defining the pathology within the liver, the pathologic anatomy of the arterial and portal circulations, and the pathophysiology of portal hemodynamics.

Needle Biopsy of the Liver. Percutaneous needle biopsy of the liver, performed under local anesthesia, provides an assessment of the degree of acute or chronic diffuse parenchymal disease and may demonstrate the definitive pathologic diagnosis of localized lesions. The procedure should be performed in the hospital and the patient should be screened for an abnormally prolonged prothrombin time or markedly reduced platelet count. The presence of large amounts of ascitic fluid requires paracentesis prior to biopsy but does not preclude the procedure. Percutaneous needle biopsy of the liver is attended by a small but definite risk, and an adjusted mortality of 0.086 per cent has been reported for a collective review of over 20,000 cases.[11] Hemorrhage constitutes one of the major complications; although some have suggested that the incidence is increased with metastatic malignancy, there is little to support this view.

A 96 per cent accuracy has been demonstrated in diagnosis of cirrhosis.[12] In patients with cirrhosis in whom the possibility of an active process is entertained, based on an increasing SGOT or rapidly rising serum bilirubin and increasing ascites, needle biopsy is indicated to define the state of activity prior to performing a major surgical procedure. In reference to focal lesions, such as granulomas and neoplasms, the correlation between needle biopsy and autopsy or laparotomy findings is quite high and can be improved by coupling the biopsy with external scintillation scanning to provide orientation.

Needle biopsy of the liver is particularly valuable in the investigation of jaundice of infancy and childhood, to provide a diagnosis of congenital atresia of the intrahepatic bile ducts, and to rule out the possibility of neonatal hepatitis. Also in the pediatric age group, the biopsy is diagnostic for several of the enzymatic and metabolic disorders.

Determination of Portal Pressure. In the preoperative evaluation of patients with esophagogastric varices, determination of the portal pressure indicates the degree of portal hypertension and may be helpful in differentiating between a presinusoidal and postsinusoidal obstruction. *Intrasplenic pulp manometry* provides an excellent method of determining portal pressure in that the procedure is simple, requires no special or extensive equipment, and can be performed at the patient's bedside. The procedure is contraindicated in patients with bleeding tendencies and in the presence of marked ascites, because the tamponading effect of the diaphragm is interfered with.

The presence of portal hypertension can be considered unequivocal if the splenic pulp pressure is greater than 250 mm. of saline with the zero point of the manometer at the approximate level of the portal vein. A pressure in the range of 200 and 250 mm. of saline is somewhat equivocal but usually indicates portal hypertension. The splenic pulp pressure is elevated regardless of the cause of portal hypertension, i.e., presinusoidal, postsinusoidal, or extrahepatic obstruction, and the elevated pressure may be attributed to an increase in intraperitoneal pressure, such as accompanies tense ascites. The application of splenic pulp manometry to the differential diagnosis of upper gastrointestinal bleeding has been credited with a 90 per cent accuracy in determining the presence or absence of bleeding varices in these patients.[13] A correlation has been demonstrated between the degree of pressure elevation and the extent of collateralization. However, it is to be stressed that on rare occasions bleeding varices may occur in the absence of increased portal pressure.

Portal pressure may also be determined by *occluded (wedged) hepatic vein catheterization* performed under direct fluoroscopic control. Normally, the occluded hepatic venous pressure is rarely more than 5 to 6 mm. Hg above that noted for the free hepatic vein. The occluded hepatic venous pressure is elevated in patients with postsinusoidal obstruction but normal in patients with presinusoidal intrahepatic obstruction or thrombosis of the portal vein. Thus, a combination of splenic pulp manometry and determination of the occluded hepatic venous pressure may be used to determine the level of obstruction.

Roentgenographic Studies. Evaluation of the esophagus by *barium swallow* is an important study in patients suspected of having varices and in patients with acute upper gastrointestinal bleeding in order to help differentiate between varices and peptic ulcers. However, the study has been associated with percentages of false negative results, reported to be as high as 50 per cent for elective evaluation and higher when the study is performed in an acutely bleeding patient. In recent years, with the addition of cineradiography, diagnostic accuracy has improved.

Percutaneous *splenoportography* represents the definitive roentgenographic study for demonstration of esophagogastric varices and other pathologic and anatomic features of the portal circulation. It is readily performed under local anesthesia and may be combined with splenic pulp manometry. The normal splenoportogram is one in which no collateral vessels are demonstrated (Fig. 17-1). In contrast, the demonstration of any collateral, such as the coronary vein or inferior mesenteric vein, is indicative of an abnormal circulation (Fig. 17-2). Although cavernomatous transformation of the portal vein may be defined by this diagnostic study, the absence of visualization of the portal vein in a patient with cirrhosis does not indicate thrombosis of the vessel, and it has been shown that in over 90 per cent of these instances the portal vein is patent. By properly timing the filming sequence, the portogram may be followed sequentially with a hepatogram in which there is a suffusion of dye throughout the liver. This may demonstrate intrahepatic abscesses or neoplasm. Displacement of the portal vein or its major branches or encroachment upon these vessels has been used to demonstrate extrahepatic lesions, particularly carcinoma of the head of the pancreas. Postoperatively, splenoportography may be used to determine the patency of a surgically created portal-systemic shunt.

Umbilical venography offers another method of outlining the portal venous system. In 80 per cent of the cases the obliterated umbilical vein can be isolated and dilated so that rupture of the membrane between the umbilical vein and the left portal vein can be effected. This permits injection of radiopaque material into the portal venous system, and the technique is particularly applicable when the patient has been splenectomized previously and when there is significant ascites.

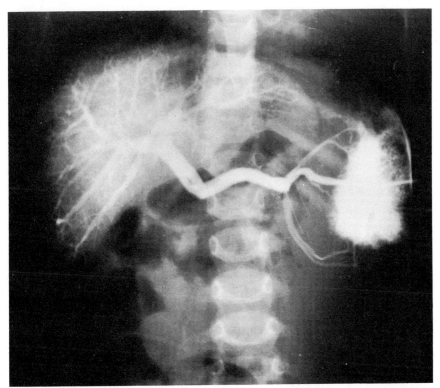

Figure 17-1. Normal splenoportogram. Note site of injection in spleen and diffusion of radiopaque material through organ. Main splenic vein and two hilar veins are visualized. Portal vein, major branches, and intrahepatic arborization can be seen. No collateral veins are present. Note radiolucency at junction of splenic and superior mesenteric veins. (From Surgical Diseases of the Liver, by S. I. Schwartz. Copyright 1964 by McGraw-Hill Book Company. Used with permission of McGraw-Hill Book Company.)

The arterial contributions to the hepatic circulation have been investigated by the injection of radiopaque media directly into the aorta or selectively into the celiac artery or the hepatic artery, using catheterization techniques. Variations from the normal *hepatic arteriogram* (Fig. 17-3) are noted in patients with cirrhosis and with large intrahepatic tumors. In cirrhosis, the intra-arterial pattern is characterized by "corkscrewing" of the fine branches, or by spreading, often straight and sparsely distributed arteries. Intrahepatic focal lesions may be associated with displacement of the major vessels, and neoplastic lesions may be diagnosed by "tumor staining" which is analogous to that found in cerebral and osseous neoplasms. *Hepatic venous angiography* may also be helpful in the assessment of the cirrhotic liver.

Radioisotope Studies. *Scintillation scanning* of the liver is a technique which may be employed as a method of evaluating liver size, shape, and position, and also of determining the presence and location of intrahepatic neoplasms or other focal lesions. The two most com-

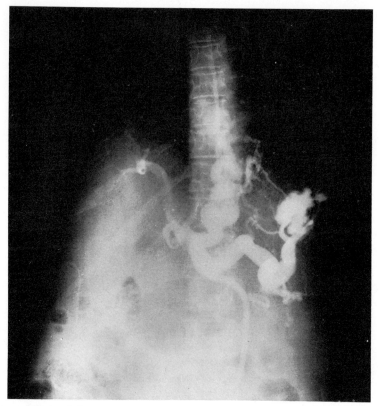

Figure 17–2. Splenoportogram: portal hypertension secondary to intrahepatic obstruction. Note large tortuous coronary vein and inferior mesenteric vein. Intrahepatic arborization is minimal. (From Surgical Diseases of the Liver, by S. I. Schwartz. Copyright 1964 by McGraw-Hill Book Company. Used with permission of McGraw-Hill Book Company.)

monly used isotopes have been radioactive gold (Au[198]), which is deposited in the cells of the reticuloendothelial system, and radioactive rose bengal (I[131]) which is absorbed and excreted by the hepatic parenchymal cells. Recently, technetium sulfur-colloid has been used with success. Scintillography is somewhat limited in that it is unable to detect lesions smaller than 2 cm., particularly those located in the posterior portion of the right lobe of the liver. Larger lesions can generally be detected by this technique. An 83 per cent correlation with autopsy or operative findings has been noted for positive scans and an 88 per cent correlation for negative scans.[14]

The technique may define a primary hepatic carcinoma superimposed upon a cirrhotic liver (Fig. 17-4) or a hepatic abscess, and has been applied as a method of localizing a lesion for needle biopsy or aspiration. In patients with diffuse hepatic disease which is mild to moderate, the scan may be within normal limits, whereas severe paren-

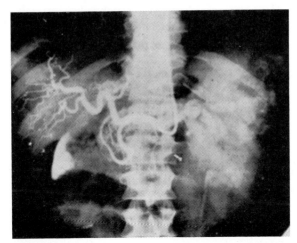

Figure 17-3. Normal hepatic arteriogram. The common hepatic artery promptly gives off the gastroduodenal, and shortly thereafter the small left hepatic and larger right hepatic artery arise. (From Bierman; *in* Abrams, H. (ed.): Angiography. Boston, Little, Brown Co., 1961, p. 644.)

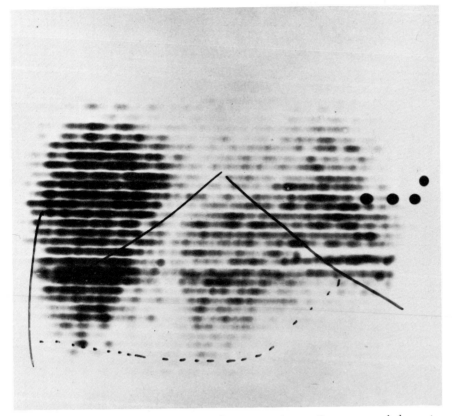

Figure 17-4. Hepatic scan: primary hepatic carcinoma. Surgery revealed massive tumor involvement of medial aspect of right lobe and of the caudate and quadrate lobes. (From Surgical Diseases of the Liver, by S. I. Schwartz. Copyright 1964 by McGraw-Hill Book Company. Used with permission of McGraw-Hill Book Company.)

chymal disease is characteristically associated with a pattern of decreased radioactivity.

Isotopic evaluation of the portal circulation by means of injecting a radioisotope directly into the spleen and simultaneously monitoring areas over the liver, the right side of the heart, and the esophagus has been used to define the dynamics of portal circulation. The system utilizes the same equipment as that employed for radioactive venography. Distinctive patterns for the normal circulation, esophagogastric varices, portal vein thrombosis, and both natural and surgically created shunts have been defined.[15] Radioactive colloidal gold or radioactive chromic phosphate may be used to estimate total liver blood flow.

Preoperative Applications of Special Diagnostic Procedures. None of the above-mentioned special diagnostic procedures are applicable to the patient with major hepatic injury requiring emergency surgery, with the exception of the angiographic techniques which may be utilized to define the bleeding site. For patients under consideration for planned hepatic resection, selective angiography may aid in outlining the extent of parenchymal involvement by the tumor and also encroachment upon the vessels entering the liver. A valuable by-product of this procedure is the definition of atypical hepatic arteries, particularly one arising from the superior mesenteric artery (17 per cent of the cases). By combining the arteriographic study with late sequential films to delineate the venous filling phase, encroachment upon the major venous system may also be defined and the need for portogram precluded. Preoperative hepatic scan may provide valuable information and helps in determining the size of the tumor.

In patients with cirrhosis under consideration for elective portal-systemic shunts, preoperative determination of the splenic pulp pressure is indicated, and splenoportography should be performed to define the pathologic anatomy. If the question is raised as to whether the block is presinusoidal or postsinusoidal, the splenic pulp pressure should be combined with occluded hepatic venous pressure. In the patient with bleeding varices and rapid progression of ascites, the possibility of a superimposed hepatoma should be considered and scintillation scan is indicated. If the possibility of an active process that precludes an operative procedure is considered, needle biopsy should be performed.

PREOPERATIVE AND POSTOPERATIVE MANAGEMENT OF THE PATIENT UNDERGOING HEPATIC RESECTION

Since the great majority of livers which sustain extensive trauma are normal and have no compromise of function, no specific preoperative preparation is required. In contrast, over 25 per cent of the patients under consideration for elective excision of a hepatic tumor demonstrate evidence of hepatic dysfunction. This may be related to the size of the tumor, the critical position of the tumor, or, more frequently, associated cirrhosis. Hepatic malignancy occurs in about 4.5 per cent of patients with Laennec's cirrhosis, and conversely almost three fourths of the cases of hepatic cell carcinoma are associated with cirrhosis. In this group, elective surgery should be delayed until maximal improvement of the patient's hepatic function has been demonstrated.

The level of serum albumin must be corrected preoperatively. This is best accomplished with concentrated albumin, 25 gm. of which provides the osmotic equivalent of 500 ml. of plasma. Albumin is a hepatitis-free product, and a salt-poor albumin is available for patients with marked sodium retention. Vitamin K is administered routinely, and the prothrombin time should be restored to a level of at least 60 per cent of normal. In the presence of liver function tests which suggest the diagnosis of obstructive jaundice, the other fat-soluble vitamins (A and D) should also be supplemented. A diet high in calories, proteins, and carbohydrates is indicated. Barbiturates and narcotics should be used only when needed and then in small doses. Long-acting barbiturates which are excreted by the kidney are safer to administer than the shorter-acting ones detoxified by the liver.

The operative procedure should be performed using an anesthetic agent which permits the administration of a high percentage of oxygen. Efforts are directed at maintaining a normal blood volume; once significant bleeding is encountered, blood should be replaced with freshly banked blood to provide coagulation factors and maintain a low ammonia level. Hypothermia and hypotensive anesthesia have been applied to protect the liver and minimize the blood loss, although the evidence for beneficial effect in this instance remains equivocal.

Postoperative management of patients undergoing a major hepatic resection is critical, particularly if cirrhosis is present, because it has been shown that the cirrhotic liver is capable of minimal, if any, regeneration. Ten per cent intravenous glucose, or preferably fructose, is continued until the patient can tolerate an oral intake. It is desirable to furnish at least 2000 calories per day by this route. Most patients undergoing a 75 to 80 per cent resection require 25 to 50 gm. of intravenous albumin daily until an adequate oral intake is achieved. Vitamin K is continued postoperatively if a response is obtained, because hemorrhagic diathesis represents one of the major postoperative complications. This disturbance is generally related, however, to a reduction of platelets in the transfused blood and a decrease in Factors V and VII in the patient with advanced hepatic dysfunction. Therapy consists of the administration of platelet packs and freshly drawn blood. Enthusiasm has been reported for the administration of epsilon aminocaproic acid to reverse fibrinolysis. It is now generally felt that this drug is rarely if ever indicated, and there is a general lack of laboratory evidence of fibrinolysis in these patients. Also, if a consumptive coagulopathy is responsible for the hypofibrinogenemic state, the administration of epsilon aminocaproic acid is potentially hazardous. Therefore, restraint in the definitive treatment of both fibrinolysis and consumptive coagulopathy is recommended, and measures designed to reverse the shock and stabilize the patient are emphasized.

Antibiotics that achieve a high biliary concentration are indicated for a period of five to seven days. Although there is experimental suggestion that cortisone improves hepatic regeneration, the drug is not employed. Following excision of 70 to 80 per cent of the liver, a normal blood ammonia level is generally maintained, but hepatic coma may be noted either immediately postoperatively or as the patient increases his oral protein intake. Efforts directed at the prevention or reversal of hepatic coma are outlined under the management of patients subjected to portal-systemic shunting procedures.

Serum proteins usually return to normal by the end of the six weeks, and fibrinogen production is only minimally impaired. Clinical jaundice is a transient phenomenon which occurs almost routinely following major hepatic resection and is accompanied by an increase in serum bilirubin, alkaline phosphatase, and BSP retention. On or about the fifth postoperative day, 95 per cent of the patients begin to show clinical and laboratory evidence of improved biliary metabolism.

Subsequent to major hepatic resection, drainage of the subphrenic and subhepatic space should be instituted routinely, and the drains should be maintained in place until the drainage has ceased, at which time they are gradually advanced. Enthusiasm has been expressed for the routine drainage of the common bile duct in order to obviate or reduce the biliary drainage from the worn-off surface of the liver. Recently, it has been shown that reduced biliary drainage is not achieved and that an increased postoperative morbidity is associated with routine T-tube drainage of the common bile duct.[16] Antacids should be given to attempt to prevent the development of stress ulceration, which often follows major hepatic resection.

PREOPERATIVE AND POSTOPERATIVE MANAGEMENT OF PATIENTS UNDERGOING PORTAL-SYSTEMIC SHUNTS

Preparation for Elective Procedures. The patient undergoing a portal-systemic shunt for portal hypertension secondary to obstruction of the extrahepatic portal venous system usually does not present a serious problem, because the liver is normal and possesses its characteristic reserve. The same generally pertains to patients with intrahepatic presinusoidal obstruction associated with schistosomal infestation or hepatic fibrosis. Performance of the same surgical procedure in the presence of cirrhosis and hepatocellular dysfunction requires critical attention to the preoperative management.

In the nonbleeding patient under consideration for an elective portacaval shunt, adequate preparation may require a period of weeks or months of hospitalization. A high caloric, high protein, low sodium diet is indicated. If the patient can tolerate it, the diet is increased up to 120 gm. of protein daily; but if protein intolerance is manifest by evidence of ammonia intoxication, the protein intake must be limited. Protein tolerance may be increased by giving nonabsorbable intestinal antibiotics. Alcohol is rigidly withheld, and antacids are administered to prevent reflux esophagitis and consequent bleeding from the varices. In anorexic patients, 10 per cent glucose or fructose is administered intravenously. Vitamins B, C, and K are administered routinely and in the presence of obstructive jaundice, the fat-soluble vitamins A and D are also added.

Transfusions may be required to achieve respectable levels of hematocrit. More frequently, hypoalbuminemia must be corrected. This is accomplished by administration of albumin concentrates.

The presence of ascites necessitates aggressive management. Therapy is centered around rigid dietary control of sodium intake, which should be restricted to 10 to 22 mEq. (0.25 to 0.5 sodium chloride) daily. In order to achieve a low sodium-high protein diet, it is frequently necessary to resort to several commercially available supplements. If bed rest and sodium restriction do not reduce the extent of ascites, diuretics are indicated. Chlorothiazide is generally used to initiate diuretic therapy, and approximately two thirds of patients with cirrhosis and ascites respond to this medication. Potassium supplements are administered because the diuresis is accompanied by a marked potassium depletion. The tendency of the drug to induce hepatic coma in patients with severe liver disease may be overcome by concomitant administration of potassium supplements and neomycin. This complication of chlorothiazide therapy is related to its action as a carbonic anhydrase inhibitor. Two gm. of the drug is administered daily until the ascites has been controlled, and the continuation of the same dose every other day following control is recommended. In patients refractory to chlorothiazide, aldosterone antagonists (100 to 300 mg./day) should be administered. Refractory cases may require more potent diuretics such as furosemide or ethacrinic acid, both of which are associated with marked potassium depletion. Ordinarily, water restriction is not necessary unless there is a dilutional hyponatremia, in which case diuresis may be achieved with an osmotic agent such as mannitol. Repeated paracentesis is ineffective and merely depletes the body of protein and contributes to the hyponatremia.

In patients with asterixis and other neuropsychiatric manifestations of portal-systemic encephalopathy, efforts should be directed at reversing the process before carrying out an operative procedure. These include reduction of protein intake and the initiation of nonabsorbable antibiotics to reduce the intestinal flora. An elective portacaval shunt is essentially contraindicated in the presence of overt or incipient hepatic coma.

Preparation of the Patient with Actively Bleeding Esophagogastric Varices. Initial efforts are directed at the control of bleeding. This should be effected as rapidly as possible in order to avoid the injurious effects of shock on hepatic function and the development of exogenous hepatic coma as a consequence of absorption of blood protein from the gastrointestinal tract. The therapeutic approaches may be divided into (1) methods which are directed at the bleeding site per se without influencing portal pressure, and (2) therapeutic agents which act indirectly by decreasing portal pressure, permitting a thrombus to form at the site of the bleeding.

Balloon tamponade has represented the most popular method of directly controlling the bleeding site, and the Sengstaken-Blakemore triple lumen tube is one of the most widely employed. After the nostrils and posterior pharynx have been anesthetized with topical anesthesia and the nostrils have been investigated for significant deviation of the septum, the tube is inserted until the tip is positioned in the posterior pharynx, and the patient then swallows the tube down to the 50 cm. mark. The gastric balloon is inflated with 50 ml. of air and the tube is then withdrawn until the gastric balloon has been engaged at the esophagogastric junction and a minimal amount of tension is maintained by taping the tube to a piece of sponge rubber around the nasal orifice or preferably by stabilization to a specially designed helmet. The esophageal balloon is then inflated to 35 or 40 mm. Hg, using an aneroid manometer to measure the effect of pressure. The stomach is then thoroughly aspirated and lavaged with iced saline solution. If bleeding continues, the esophageal balloon pressure is increased to 45 mm. Hg and the gastric balloon is then inflated with more air until a total of approximately 300 ml. has been instilled in order to compress fundal and other gastric varices. The tube is connected to suction and irrigated every 30 minutes and the pressure within the esophageal balloon should be recorded every 30 minutes and maintained at an effective level. Following control of bleeding, the esophageal balloon should be deflated after 12 hours and maintained in place. If bleeding recurs, the balloon pressure should be re-established. If no bleeding occurs for 24 hours, the tube should be totally transected to insure complete deflation and removed. In view of the complications, particularly those related to the tracheobronchial tree, constant nursing attention is required. If the patient is comatose or having marked difficulty in maintaining tracheal toilet, tracheostomy is indicated.

Recently, balloon tamponade has fallen into relative disrepute. Little change in mortality rate has been noted in poor-risk patients with bleeding varices, and reports have indicated failure to control hemorrhage in 25 to 55 per cent of the cases. Despite strict adherence to the techniques advised, aspiration, asphyxiation and ulceration at the site of tamponade have all been reported in significant numbers.

Another direct method of effecting control of bleeding is local hypothermia, using a special balloon with a long esophageal neck which permits cooling of the distal portion of the esophagus and the upper portion of the gastric fundus. The success attending this method has varied greatly. Generalized hypothermia has been suggested, but little effect is to be anticipated because the rectal temperature must be reduced to levels below 35° C. in order to achieve reduction of flow through the esophageal veins. At this critical temperature reduction fibrillation may occur, and marked shivering results in an expenditure of caloric requirements which is detrimental to liver function.

Immediate partial reduction of portal pressure may be effected in patients with tense ascites by performance of a paracentesis, because there is a direct relationship between the intraperitoneal pressure and the portal venous pressure. Drug therapy directed at portal hypertension employs Arfonad, vasopressin, or a combination of the two. Arfonad, 0.1 per cent, administered intravenously induces a predictable decrease in portal hypertension accompanied by a reduction in arterial pressure secondary to a generalized vasodilatation.

Vasopressin (posterior Pituitrin) represents the most commonly employed drug and results in an immediate 35 to 50 per cent reduction in portal pressure.[17] Twenty clinical units are administered rapidly over five to ten minutes and repeated at four hour intervals if necessary. The therapeutic action begins immediately and lasts for a period of about 90 minutes. Effectiveness of the drug should be monitored by lavage of the stomach every 15 to 20 minutes, noting the characteristics of the return. A review of the reported experience (Table 17-2) indicates that temporary control of bleeding is accomplished in about 80 per cent of

Table 17-2. EFFICACY OF VASOPRESSIN IN TEMPORARILY CONTROLLING ACUTELY BLEEDING VARICES*

AUTHOR	NUMBER OF BLEEDING EPISODES	NUMBER CONTROLLED TEMPORARILY	PER CENT SUCCESS
Merigan et al.	22	16	73
Conn and Dalessio	25	16	64
Shaldon and Sherlock	8	8	100
Orloff	63	55	88
Nusbaum et al. (selective infusion)	2	2	100
Schwartz	200	156	78
Totals	320	253	79

*From Schwartz, S. I.: Annals New York Acad. Sci. *170*:296, 1970.

the cases. Abdominal cramps are characteristic, and evacuation of the intestine is a useful by-product. Since the drug is a generalized vasoconstrictor, it is contraindicated in patients with angina or coronary artery disease. The recent findings of Nusbaum et al.[18] concerning the administration of the drug by selective arterial infusion are most attractive. This permits a continuous infusion of 0.2 mg. vasopressin/ml./min. and has resulted in persistent control and permitted elective portal-systemic shunting.

In addition to efforts directed at the control of bleeding, therapy is concerned with the correction of hypovolemia and prevention of portal-systemic encephalopathy. Hyperammonemia is best prevented by rapid removal of blood and protein from the gastrointestinal tract, using catharsis, gastric lavage, and enema. Vasopressin, in itself, induces a marked intestinal motility, and evacuation of intestinal contents is a significant by-product of this form of drug therapy. Since nitrogen-containing compounds within the intestine are converted into ammonia by the bacterial flora, a reduction in this flora, accomplished by the use of nonabsorbable antibiotics, also contributes to the prevention of hepatic coma. Potassium supplements are indicated, particularly if the patient has recently undergone diuresis. In the face of incipient or established coma, arginine and glutamic acid have been applied, but neither of these drugs has stood the test of time.

It is extremely difficult to synthesize a protocol for management of patients with bleeding varices as far as the timing of the shunt procedure is concerned, because each case must be individualized. In patients with portal vein thrombosis, particularly children, although the bleeding is frequently alarming, it rarely requires either balloon tamponade or vasopressin and is usually best treated by bed rest and transfusion. Therapy of the acute bleeding episode in these patients with extrahepatic portal vein thrombosis is one of temporizing in appreciation of the fact that decompressive procedures have a better yield in children over the age of ten. Control of coma in these patients and in patients with presinusoidal obstruction is rarely a problem, and blood replacement therapy can be accomplished with banked blood because there is no coagulation defect. In contrast, the adult cirrhotic patient with bleeding varices represents an extremely complex problem. Initial attempts to control bleeding should employ vasopressin and iced saline lavage of the stomach. If the patient is controlled with this regimen, two or three days are allowed to elapse, during which time hepatic function is evaluated and attempts are made at improvement. An elective portocaval shunt is carried out unless the hepatic function is severely compromised or if the patient demonstrates signs of incipient coma. If the patient continues to bleed massively on Pitressin therapy and has reasonable hepatic function, such as is frequently associated with presinusoidal portal hypertension, hepatic fibrosis, or schistosomiasis, an emergency portal-systemic shunt is performed, anticipating relatively good results. If the patient, particularly with Laennec's cirrhosis, continues to bleed, the course is dictated by hepatic function. With poor function—that is, a serum bilirubin greater than 3, a serum albumin less than 2, and a prothrombin time less than 20 per cent, with coma or asterixis—shunt is contraindicated and the Sengstaken-Blakemore tube is used. If the patient with alcoholic cirrhosis has reasonably good liver function tests, an emergency shunt is carried out, realizing that the mortality statistics are significantly higher than for the elective shunt.

Postoperative Management. Postoperative management of the patient who is undergoing portal-systemic decompressive procedures is essentially a continuation of preoperative considerations. If a nasogastric tube has been employed to decompress the stomach, it should be removed as soon as bowel sounds are audible. A gastrostomy tube inserted at surgery has the theoretical advantage of decreasing the incidence of atelectasis and also of esophageal ulceration and thus may be left in place for a longer period of time. Leaking from the gastrostomy site and, rarely, peritonitis have a greater tendency to develop in patients with marked ascites.

Continued postoperative bleeding is uncommon and should be treated with the administration of whole fresh blood and supplements of vitamin K. Whole blood has the advantage of providing platelets and coagulation factors, and does not have the increment of blood ammonia and potassium noted in banked blood. Ten per cent glucose or fructose is administered intravenously until the patient is able to tolerate a normal oral intake. Analgesics, which are detoxified by the liver, are used only sparingly, and hyperthermic episodes are to be avoided and treated aggressively, if necessary with a hypothermic blanket. As soon as gastric suction is discontinued and oral intake is begun, antacid medications are given to counteract the gastric hypersecretion that follows the shunting procedure. A low salt diet is maintained postoperatively, particularly if there had been preoperative ascites. Hypoalbuminemia is corrected, and in patients with marked ascites the salt-poor albumin is employed.

If asterixis or incipient coma was present preoperatively, neomycin therapy is continued postoperatively, via either the nasogastric tube or gastrostomy. When oral intake is instituted the proteins are limited and gradually increased over a period of time, assessing the patient's tolerance.

Patients developing postoperative portal-system encephalopathy may have hypokalemia alkalosis. Blood gases and serum potassium levels should be carefully monitored, and large potassium supplements are sometimes required to correct this metabolic derangement. Successful reversal of this metabolic abnormality frequently results in improvement in encephalopathy.

The so-called hepatorenal syndrome is one of the most distressing complications in patients with hepatic disease. The mechanisms are poorly understood and the effects of damaged liver on renal blood flow and renal function have been poorly defined. Therapy should be directed at the basic hepatic decompensation and maintaining fluid and electrolyte balance.

REFERENCES

1. Statistical Abstract of the United States, U.S. Bureau of the Census. Washington, D.C., U.S. Government Printing Office, 1965.
2. Schwartz, S. I.: Surgical Diseases of the Liver. New York, McGraw-Hill Book Co., 1964.
3. Bradley, S. E., Marks, P. A., Reynell, P. C., and Meltzer, J.: Circulating splanchnic blood volume in dog and man. Tr. A. Amer. Physicians 66:294, 1953.
4. Pack, G. T., and Molander, D. W.: Metabolism before and after hepatic lobectomy for cancer; studies in 23 patients. Arch. Surg. 80:685, 1960.
5. Linton, R. R.: The selection of patients for portacaval shunts. Ann. Surg. 134:433, 1951.
6. Child, C. G., III: The liver and portal hypertension; in Dunphy, J. E. (Consulting Editor): Major Problems in Clinical Surgery. Philadelphia, W. B. Saunders Co., 1964.
7. McDermott, W. V.: The double portacaval shunt in the treatment of cirrhotic ascites. Surg. Gynec. & Obst. 110:457, 1960.
8. Jackson, F. C., Christophersen, E. B., Peternel, W. W., and Kirimli, B.: Preoperative management of patients with liver disease. Surg. Clin. N. Amer. 48:907, 1968.
9. Resnicoff, S. A., and Schwartz, S. I.: Portal decompressive surgery. Arch. Surg. 97:371, 1968.
10. DelGuercio, L. R. M., Commaraswamy, R. P., Feins, N. R., Wollman, S. B., and State, D.: Pulmonary arteriovenous admixture and the hyperdynamic cardiovascular state in surgery for portal hypertension. Surgery 56:57, 1964.
11. Zamcheck, N., and Klausenstock, O.: Liver biopsy (concluded): II. The risk of needle biopsy. N. Eng. J. Med. 249:1062, 1953.
12. Braunstein, H.: Needle biopsy of the liver in cirrhosis; diagnostic efficiency as determined by postmortem sampling. Arch. Path. 62:87, 1956.
13. Panke, W. F., Rousselot, L. M., and Moreno, A. H.: Splenic pulp manometry as an emergency test in the differential diagnosis of acute upper gastrointestinal bleeding. Surg. Gynec. & Obst. 109:270, 1959.
14. Nagler, W., Bender, M. A., and Blau, M.: Radioisotope photoscanning of the liver. Gastroenterology 44:36, 1963.
15. Green, J. P., and Schwartz, S. I.: Isotopic splenoportography—a continued appraisal. Amer. J. Dig. Dis. 8:908, 1963.
16. Lucas, C. E., and Walt, A. J.: Critical decisions in liver trauma: Experience based on 604 cases. Arch. Surg. 101:277, 1970.
17. Schwartz, S. I.: Influence of vasoactive drugs on portal circulation. Annals, New York Acad. Sci. 170:296, 1970.
18. Nusbaum, M., Baum, S., Kuroda, K., and Blakemore, W. S.: Control of portal hypertension by selective mesenteric arterial drug infusion. Arch. Surg. 97:1005, 1968.

CHAPTER 18

THE BILIARY TRACT AND EXOCRINE PANCREAS

MARSHALL K. BARTLETT, M.D.

INTRODUCTION

For the purposes of this chapter it is assumed that each patient has had a careful history taken and complete physical examination performed. These are basic essentials, as in any patient who is a candidate for major surgery. It is further assumed that any leads obtained from the history or physical examination suggesting impairment of other organ systems have been appropriately pursued and that any abnormalities discovered have been evaluated as outlined in other chapters of this book. All this information must be considered in estimating the operative risk before reaching a final decision in any given case.

PREOPERATIVE EVALUATION

Chronic Cholecystitis and Cholelithiasis. For the patient requiring an elective operation for gallstones, otherwise in good general health with no significant impairment of other organ systems, relatively little preoperative evaluation is needed. The diagnosis will have been satisfactorily established by the clinical picture, supported by radiologic evidence of gallstones or of nonfunction on at least two satisfactory oral cholecystograms.

Routine blood and urine examinations should be done, together with a fasting blood sugar, blood urea nitrogen or creatinine and alkaline phosphatase. For patients over the age of 40 a chest x-ray and electrocardiogram are also carried out for additional baseline information. Blood typing is done and one unit of whole blood is matched and ready at the time of operation.

Routine use of a nasogastric tube at operation is not necessary but is often useful if the stomach is distended by swallowed air or anesthetic gases or if more than the usual postoperative ileus is expected because of an extensive inflammatory process or unusual technical difficulties.

Acute Cholecystitis. In addition to the steps outlined above, certain additional studies are valuable in the preoperative evaluation of a patient who presents with the clinical picture of acute cholecystitis.

Acute cholecystitis is usually associated with gallstones (95 per cent) and often with cystic duct obstruction caused by a stone. In other cases, certainly in those in which no stones are present, some other factor must be involved, and it may be that an irritating chemical substance in the bile or pancreatic juice is the causative agent. The process is primarily a sterile one at the onset, with edema and swelling of the gallbladder wall and increased intraluminal pressure. This may advance to impair the blood supply of the organ, with resulting gangrene and perforation. Secondary bacterial infection is common, the usual agents being staphylococcus, streptococcus, *E. coli* and related organisms from the gastrointestinal tract and occasionally clostridial organisms. Pressure from the inflammatory swelling around the common bile duct may produce enough partial obstruction so that an elevation of bilirubin as high as 5 mg./ml. will occur.

The preferred treatment of acute cholecystitis is early surgery with the hope of doing a cholecystectomy with exploration of the common bile duct if this is indicated. It is not usually necessary to operate on the patient with acute cholecystitis as an emergency. Time should be taken for careful investigation of the other organ systems, and other conditions such as appendicitis, perforated peptic ulcer, small bowel obstruction, acute pancreatitis and mesenteric thrombosis must be considered in the differential diagnosis. In addition to the history, physical examination and baseline laboratory studies suggested for patients undergoing elective cholecystectomy, the bilirubin, alkaline phosphatase, total protein with A/G ratio, amylase, lipase, SGOT and cephalin flocculation levels may give valuable information. If the patient has been vomiting, the serum electrolytes should be determined. Abdominal tap may be useful, especially in ruling out acute pancreatitis. This is particularly important, because most cases of acute pancreatitis should be treated without operation. Flat and upright abdominal films may provide valuable information, and, if the patient is not too sick, an oral or intravenous cholecystogram can be done.

While all this is going on, the patient's clinical condition must be reassessed at frequent intervals. Usually operation can be done on the day after admission, but a longer interval may be necessary to allow for careful evaluation of the patient's general condition. Operation must be done promptly if rising fever and pulse or increasing local abdominal signs indicate the possibility of cholangitis or the development of empyema. The presence of diabetes is an additional reason for early operation. During this waiting period antibiotics should be given, usually parenterally. The combination of penicillin and tetracycline offers broad coverage and relative safety.

Nasogastric suction is instituted promptly if the patient is vomiting, and in any case preoperatively. At least one unit of blood should be cross-matched and ready at the time of operation.

Jaundice. Preoperative evaluation is further complicated in the presence of jaundice because of the increased number of diagnostic possibilities. Although a detailed discussion of the differential diagnosis of jaundice[5, 15] is not within the scope of this chapter, some general comments are in order.

Hemolytic jaundice will be excluded by the history, absence of splenomegaly and appropriate blood findings, but viral hepatitis, cirrhosis and malignant obstruction must be considered, as well as biliary tract stones.

A detailed history is essential, with emphasis on the time of onset of the jaundice, the presence or absence of prodromal symptoms, ingestion of drugs or alcohol, exposure to inoculation in any form, chills and fever, itching and the character and severity of pain. On physical examination, in addition to the jaundice, particular note should be made of enlargement of the liver and spleen, spider angiomas, liver palms, purpura, peripheral edema, ascites and any evidence of hepatic coma. Abdominal tenderness and masses must be evaluated, with special attention given to the region of the gallbladder (Courvoisier's law).

Plain films and a barium study of the upper gastrointestinal tract may give useful information. As a further aid in differential diagnosis various laboratory tests of liver function are available. The functions to which these tests relate and their limitations must be appreciated to assess their value in the jaundiced patient.

Bile pigment produced in the reticuloendothelial system as a breakdown product of hemoglobin is free bilirubin, is not excreted by the kidneys and gives an *indirect van den Bergh reaction.* This is conjugated by the liver cells into bilirubin glucuronide which is normally excreted into the biliary duct system and when it reaches the intestine may be converted by bacterial action into urobilinogen. When, under abnormal conditions, conjugated bilirubin accumulates in the blood, it can be excreted by the kidneys and gives a *direct van den Bergh reaction.* Bilirubin in the serum as a result of liver cell damage should, therefore, be largely indirect by van den Bergh reaction and that caused by obstruction anywhere in the biliary canaliculi or ducts largely direct.

Normally some of the *urobilinogen* formed in the intestine is absorbed into the portal system; of this, a part is removed by the liver and some passes into the systemic circulation and may be excreted in the urine. A high urine urobilinogen (over 3.0 Ehrlich units) in a patient who is passing clay-colored stools may be a valuable test because it suggests that the liver cells cannot handle even the small amounts of urobilinogen absorbed from the intestine under these circumstances and so points to severe cellular damage rather than obstruction.

Total protein and the *albumin-globulin ratio* may give some further information as to liver cell damage as this tends to decrease albumin and increase globulin production. The output of certain other proteins such as *prothrombin* is also reduced by liver cell damage. The *transaminases* by contrast appear in the plasma in increased amounts with liver cell injury and may give useful information.

The *cephalin flocculation* test is another useful and relatively delicate index of impaired liver cell function when it is strongly positive (3 or 4 plus in 48 hours).

The serum level of *alkaline phosphatase* does not normally rise appreciably with parenchymal damage to the liver but will go up in the presence of obstruction to biliary outflow and constitutes another valuable index of liver cell function. Increasing knowledge of the Australia antigen offers the possibility of a new and more accurate means of identifying viral hepatitis and possibly of distinguishing between infectious and serum hepatitis.[1, 7]

If the nature of the jaundice still remains uncertain, there are several rather more complicated procedures which may be carried out.

DUODENAL DRAINAGE. The presence of cholesterol or calcium bilirubinate crystals in the sediment from the duodenal aspirate predicts the presence of stones in the biliary tree with considerable accuracy. The test requires careful placement of the tip of the tube in the duodenum by fluoroscopy and careful hand aspiration of the tube to save duodenal and discard gastric fluid before and during stimulation with magnesium sulfate.

NEEDLE BIOPSY OF THE LIVER. Needle biopsy will sometimes produce a definite diagnosis in obscure cases. At other times the microscopic picture will be much less conclusive. The risk of the test is increased somewhat in the presence of obstruction because of the danger of bile leakage from the puncture site.

PERCUTANEOUS TRANSHEPATIC CHOLANGIOGRAPHY. This method finds a useful application occasionally as a means of localizing the point of obstruction in the biliary tree.[13] Obviously some risk of bile leakage from the puncture site is involved, and the test is best done immediately before operation.

When the picture is still obscure in spite of all appropriate tests and examinations, it may be best to defer the decision until some change in the clinical picture or laboratory pattern occurs to clarify the situation. Here the risk of an unnecessary operation on a patient with liver cell damage, which may be considerable, must be balanced against that of increasing damage from back pressure in the biliary tree. Usually this is quite well tolerated for the necessary period of time, and the risk of delay is less than that of a premature decision.

Cholangitis. Cholangitis is usually characterized by chills and spiking fever. There is almost always some obstructing lesion in the biliary tree, most commonly a stone or occasionally a postoperative stricture, rarely a malignant obstruction. The infection may progress rapidly to an overwhelming bacteremia, usually caused by gram-negative organisms, with prostration, cyanosis, and hypotension. Decompression of the biliary tree must be done in such severe cases, preceded by vigorous resuscitation with fluids, colloids, antibiotics and cardiorespiratory support as indicated. The most effective antibiotic combination is penicillin and chloramphenicol in large doses. The effectiveness of the latter drug under these circumstances more than offsets its well-recognized hazards. Adequate blood studies must, of course, be carried out during its use.

In milder cases the infection may be controlled so that a more leisurely approach can be made to the problem of the biliary tree. Not infrequently, however, the situation is critical, and decompression of the common bile duct is an essential step in treatment.

Recurrent Pancreatitis. The patient with recurrent bouts of pancreatitis, for whom an operation in an interval between attacks is planned, presents a preoperative problem similar to that of a patient with chromic cholecystitis and cholelithiasis. These two conditions do, of course, frequently occur together. The diagnosis will have been established during previous attacks by the clinical picture and by appropriate elevation of serum amylase and lipase or in the urinary amylase, if this is preferred. In doubtful cases an evocative test of the pancreas with morphine and prostigmine may give useful information by producing an attack of the patient's usual pain or an elevation of serum amylase or lipase or both.

As in patients with chronic cholecystitis and cholelithiasis, routine blood and urine examinations should be done, together with a fasting blood sugar, blood urea nitrogen or creatinine and an aklaline phosphatase. Baseline values of serum amylase and lipase should also be included. Patients over 40 years of age should have a chest x-ray and electrocardiogram done, and a unit of blood should be matched and ready at the time of operation. The use of a nasogastric tube is advisable during and after operation, particularly if the duodenum is opened or extensive manipulation of the pancreas is involved.

Acute Pancreatitis. As has been stated earlier in this chapter, most patients with acute pancreatitis should be treated by vigorous supportive measures and without operation. In certain selected patients whose acute attacks will not subside in spite of prolonged treatment[12] or who are critically sick with severe acute necrotizing pancreatitis and are deteriorating in spite of all available supportive measures, an operation may make the acute process subside, and in the latter group salvage a patient who seems in an otherwise almost hopeless situation.[9]

Acute pancreatitis is usually distinguished from acute cholecystitis and other acute upper abdominal conditions which may give a similar clinical picture by elevation of the serum amylase and lipase or by the enzyme levels in fluid obtained by abdominal tap.

In addition to the blood chemical values appropriate for patients with recurrent pancreatitis, a reduced serum calcium level may provide some clue as to the severity of the acute pancreatitis. Serum electrolytes should be determined as a guide to replacement needs. Arterial blood gases are valuable if respiratory or circulatory failure is suspected in severe cases.

With the working diagnosis of acute pancreatitis established, measures should be instituted to reduce stimulation to the pancreas and to protect the patient from secondary bacterial infection. Nasogastric suction should be started and nothing should be given by mouth. This will reduce the amount of gastric content that will pass into the duodenum and stimulate the pancreas through the secretin mechanism. Adequate fluid and electrolyte replacement will be necessary, and in all but mild cases the loss of plasma and blood into the peritoneal cavity and retroperitoneal tissues will require the replacement of considerable colloid. The monitoring of central venous pressure is an invaluable guide to the adequacy of fluid and colloid replacement in these sick patients.

Vagal stimulation of the pancreas should be reduced by the administration of anticholinergic drugs in adequate amounts, and efforts should be made to prevent secondary bacterial infection by the parenteral administration of suitable antibiotics. The combination of penicillin and tetracycline offers broad coverage with relative safety.

In cases of severe necrotizing pancreatitis, pressor drugs may be necessary for circulatory support, even after adequate volume replacement and endotracheal intubation with assisted ventilation may be required for respiratory failure.

If operation is undertaken in such critically sick patients, all areas of necrotic tissue should be drained and the biliary tree and gastrointestinal tract should both be decompressed.[9] The same vigorous supportive measures used preoperatively must be continued after operation.

POSTOPERATIVE MANAGEMENT

General.   Postoperatively, vital signs are monitored as long as indicated by the patient's clinical progress. For the good risk patient having an elective operation on the biliary tree or pancreas this will involve observing the temperature, pulse, blood pressure and respirations at frequent intervals for a few hours, and then at longer intervals, being sure that the patient voids or is catheterized before the bladder becomes overdistended. For a sicker patient who has required considerable colloid, fluid and electrolyte replacement, a central venous pressure monitor, hourly urinary output by indwelling catheter and serum electrolyte determinations are essential to the intelligent conduct of the case. Cardiopulmonary conditions may require a cardiac monitor, assisted ventilation with an intratracheal tube or tracheostomy and frequent determinations of arterial blood gases. Antibiotics used preoperatively to control infection must be continued postoperatively for an appropriate period which will be governed by clinical progress. Changes in the choice of drugs may be dictated by information obtained from cultures taken at operation.

For the first few days after operation the patient is given nothing by mouth. The routine use of a nasogastric tube at operation is not necessary but is often useful if the stomach is distended by swallowed air or anesthetic gases or if more than the usual postoperative ileus is expected owing to an extensive inflammatory process or unusual technical difficulties. If nasogastric suction is instituted, it should be continued postoperatively. If prolonged gastric drainage is anticipated, in seriously sick or particularly in older patients or those with any pulmonary problem, a gastrostomy should be done to avoid the hazards inherent in nasogastric suction. Oral fluids are withheld until active peristalsis is present or until gas is passed by rectum. This requires intravenous fluids and electrolyte administration, which must be adjusted to include nasogastric and T-tube losses.

With the resumption of normal gastrointestinal function the diet is gradually increased. The regular house diet can usually be tolerated at the end of a week. There is no reason to maintain a low fat intake other than obesity or personal prejudice.

The drain which was left down to the region of the cystic duct stump can usually be removed at the end of a week after operation. The T-tube, if present, is then clamped, and if this is well tolerated for 24 hours, it is removed. A cholangiogram should be done before the T-tube is removed, even though a negative examination was obtained on the operating table.

In addition to these general principles of management, a variety of complications directly related to the operation on the biliary tree must be recognized and treated if any should occur.

Hemorrhage. Hemorrhage occurring during operations on the biliary tree usually results from injury to the cystic artery. The anatomic variations of this artery have been carefully studied and documented.[3] They must be thoroughly understood and carefully searched for in every case.

The cystic artery will have divided into its inferior and superior branches before reaching the gallbladder wall, or these will be two separate arteries in about 50 per cent of cases. These common or separate trunks usually arise from the right hepatic, which may pass under the common hepatic duct (65 per cent) or over the duct (35 per cent). Occasionally one or both of the branches to the gallbladder may come from the main hepatic or even from the gastroduodenal or superior mesenteric arteries.

If bleeding occurs from an injured cystic artery, it should be controlled by pressure on the hepatic artery between the thumb and a finger in the foramen of Winslow, and not by efforts to clamp the bleeding vessel blindly in a field obscured by blood. With the bleeding controlled, the point of bleeding can be accurately identified and carefully ligated.

Hemorrhage after operation is usually arterial in origin, either from a branch of the cystic artery or a vessel in the liver bed. Less commonly it may be from a small vessel overlying the common duct or from an injury to the portal vein or vena cava. If this occurs, it is usually soon after operation; changes will appear in the vital signs with tachycardia and hypotension, and the patient will be cold, perspiring, restless and apprehensive. Blood replacement will give only temporary improvement. Postoperative hemorrhage of significant amount should be treated by prompt reoperation. Such bleeding may not be accompanied by the appearance of large amounts of blood from the drain site in the right upper quadrant, and waiting for this evidence to confirm the presence of hemorrhage will cause unnecessary delay in diagnosis and treatment.

Common Duct Injury. Common duct injury is a real surgical tragedy, both because it should be preventable and because repair of the resulting stricture is difficult and the result not always satisfactory.[2]

It is often impossible to determine the exact mechanism of the injury because it will have occurred in the course of an operation which seemed entirely uneventful to the surgeon. Judging from available information and the findings at secondary operations, there are two principal situations which predispose to injury of the common duct. The first is an inadvertent injury to the cystic artery and efforts to clamp the retracted bleeding vessel. The second results from failure to correctly identify the junction of the cystic duct with the common and common hepatic ducts. This may be extremely difficult because of adhesions between the cystic duct or even the ampulla of the gallbladder and the common hepatic duct. The surgeon should not commit himself to removing the gallbladder until these three structures are clearly identified to his complete satisfaction. If this is not possible, a cholecystostomy should be done.

If injury to the common duct is recognized at operation, it should be repaired at once. A careful end-to-end suture can usually be done without tension if no portion of the duct has been excised. If too great a defect has been created, a choledochoduodenostomy or choledochojejunostomy (Roux-en-Y) should be done.

If the injury is unrecognized at operation it may result in the prompt development of increasing jaundice or profuse bile drainage, or the stricture may develop gradually and the onset of jaundice may be delayed for weeks or even months.

When the presence of such an injury is recognized, it should be repaired as soon as the patient has recovered sufficiently from the previous operation. The choice of procedures will be the same as those given above for immediate repair. If the upper and lower ends of the injured duct can be identified and are of adequate size so that a good approximation is possible without tension, an end-to-end anastomosis can be done. Otherwise, an anastomosis between the proximal common hepatic duct stump and either the duodenum or a Roux-en-Y loop of jejunum should be done. If no proximal duct can be identified at the hilum, the intrahepatic duct system can be exposed by incising the anterior surface of the liver in the plane between the right and left lobes.[14]

The success of this anastomosis will depend considerably on the degree to which all scar can be excised and normal tissue made available for suture. If good normal tissue is available and the lumen is of normal size, no splinting against restricture is necessary, although temporary decompression by catheter or T-tube may be used if desired. If scar and inflammation are still present in the tissues, splinting of the anastamosis for at least several months is important. All the substances available to date for use as a splint will eventually become plugged by bile salt deposits. Rubber T-tubes will usually remain patent for some months and can then be removed without an additional operation. When longer splinting is desirable, a tube of Vitallium or plastic may be used. When these become plugged they must be removed surgically, but this may not occur for several years.

Hepatic Artery Injury. The position of the hepatic artery and its branches in relation to the common and cystic ducts and their many anatomic variations make them vulnerable to injury during operations on the biliary tract.[11] This is particularly true when the right hepatic artery lies anterior to the common duct or passes behind the common duct and then parallels the cystic duct before giving off a short cystic artery and swinging upward into the liver.

If injury to the hepatic artery or its right or left branches occurs, the resulting bleeding should be controlled by digital pressure on the portal triad until the proximal and distal stumps can be identified and controlled by suitable arterial clamps and a direct anastomosis carried out. If a sufficient length of artery has been destroyed to prevent direct end-to-end anastomosis, the defect should be bridged by a vein graft.

The value of the use of antibiotics following hepatic artery injury is not clearly established, but it is probably wise to start prophylactic antibiotic therapy whenever hepatic arterial flow has been interrupted. Because of the possibility of clostridial infection this should include large doses of penicillin.

Acute Pancreatitis. Acute pancreatitis developing after surgery on the biliary tract is a serious complication and carries a considerable mortality. It is more apt to occur when a common duct exploration has been done with an attempt to pass instruments into the duodenum than after simple cholecystectomy. In our experience pancreatitis is one of the main factors contributing to the increased risk that accompanies common duct exploration.

Exploration of the common bile duct should not be done without adequate indications. Only gentle instrumentation should be done, with efforts directed at calibrating the size of the lower end of the duct and not dilating it. If there is doubt about the situation, the papilla of Vater should be exposed transduodenally and a sphincteroplasty done if necessary.

Acute postoperative pancreatitis should be suspected if there is excessive pain or fever and tachycardia or a persistent ileus. Serum amylase and lipase determinations may be useful in confirming the diagnosis. Vigorous treatment should be instituted promptly with nasogastric suction, anticholinergic drugs, replacement of fluids, electrolytes, plasma and blood and appropriate antibiotics.

For patients who are operated on to control an acute pancreatitis, all appropriate supportive measures will have been used preoperatively and must be continued after operation.

Subhepatic Collection of Bile, Blood and Lymph. This, in varying proportions, constitutes perhaps the most common complication of biliary tract surgery. Secondary infection is a frequent occurrence.

The presence of a subhepatic collection which has not been absorbed or evacuated through an appropriately placed drain should be suspected if the patient runs an unexplained fever after operation. Pain and tenderness may be entirely absent, and the excursion of the diaphragm may not be limited unless there is also a subphrenic collection. Some degree of persistent ileus may occur. If gas-forming organisms are present, bubbles of gas may be demonstrated on films of the abdomen.

If a subhepatic collection is suspected and the drain is still present in the right upper quadrant, it should not be removed because it may offer a tract for spontaneous drainage of the collection. If the drain has been removed, the sinus may be gently probed in the hope of evacuating the collection. Careful search must be made for other causes of fever in the wound, lungs and urinary tract and for evidence of phlebitis. A short trial of antibiotics is usually justified. The collection may gradually absorb, may drain spontaneously or may require formal drainage by operation.

Collections in the subphrenic spaces are less common but are often easier to detect, because pleural effusion is frequently present and diaphragmatic excursion is limited. Once established, these will usually require surgical drainage.

Biliary Fistula. Several different conditions will produce a persistent postoperative biliary fistula. When a cholecystostomy has been done, persistent drainage of small amounts of bile and mucus suggests a residual stone in the gallbladder with intermittent obstruction to outflow from the gallbladder. Profuse bile drainage suggests common duct obstruction below the level of the cystic duct. This is usually due to a stone. Scarring and tumor are less common causes. Injection of radio-paque material through the sinus will usually lead to a correct diagnosis.

Drainage of some bile following cholecystectomy is not uncommon. It is usually scanty in amount and comes from the small accessory bile radicles in the ballbladder bed or small tears in the liver substance. This will usually stop in a few days. More voluminous bile drainage suggests an inadequately ligated cystic duct stump, but this too usually stops spontaneously after some days. If profuse drainage continues, common duct obstruction must be suspected and appropriate diagnostic studies carried out.

Profuse T-tube drainage following choledochostomy likewise suggests common duct obstruction and a cholangiogram through the T-tube will usually make the diagnosis. The obstruction may be due to postoperative edema, residual stone, tumor or stenosis and, except for the first of these, will require surgical correction.

A total biliary fistula with a loss of 800 to 1500 ml. of bile in 24 hours involves substantial electrolyte losses, and both fluid and electrolytes must be quantitatively replaced. If such losses persist, consideration must be given to the prompt surgical correction of the underlying condition. If the patient's condition is not satisfactory for operation, some means of replacing the bile into the gastrointestinal tract must be devised. Some patients can be persuaded to drink bile disguised in fruit juice, but more often a small indwelling nasogastric tube or feeding jejunostomy will be necessary. With the bile being refed, any necessary length of time can be spent in improving the patient's condition in preparation for reoperation.

Cholangitis. If the patient has had cholangitis before operation, treatment should be continued postoperatively. Changes in the choice of antibiotics may be indicated by the results of bile cultures obtained at operation.

Occasionally a patient who has not manifested the signs of cholangitis before operation will develop it postoperatively, and if it is severe the same vigorous program of management is indicated as described earlier in this chapter. Usually, in such cases, the common bile duct will have been explored and drained, so decompression will have been established and bile cultures will be available to guide the antibiotic therapy.

Bile Peritonitis. Occasionally bile leaking from small tears in the liver substance, from small accessory biliary radicles in the gallbladder bed or from an improperly ligated cystic duct stump will not be walled off or drained out through the drain left in the right upper quadrant, and generalized bile peritonitis will occur. This will usually happen in the first 24 to 48 hours after operation, but at times the delay may be longer.

Bile peritonitis should be suspected if the patient has increasing abdominal pain and spasm, fever, tachycardia and hypotension. An abdominal tap may clinch the diagnosis but is only of value if it is positive. This is a serious complication and successful management requires prompt recognition. Re-exploration of the abdomen with evacuation of the bile, correction of the source of leak, if possible, and adequate drainage of the area should be done as soon as proper replacement of fluids, electrolytes and colloid has been carried out.

Residual Common Duct Stones. In spite of the best methods and techniques available, the problem of retained stones in the biliary tree after operation has not been solved. The reported incidence varies from 1 to 20 per cent, with the average about 10 per cent. Errors of judgment, with failure to recognize and heed the indications for common duct exploration, are less common than errors of technique, with failure to remove all the stones present in the duct which is explored, as a cause of retained stones. Intraoperative cholangiography has undoubtedly reduced the frequency of this error, but in spite of its routine use there was an incidence of 3.5 per cent proved and 3.5 per cent probable retained stones in a recent large series.[6]

Even though a normal postexploration cholangiogram is obtained at operation, the examination should be repeated before the T-tube is removed. It is usually at this time that the retained stone or stones are discovered and the question as to the best method of treatment comes up.

Retained stones may require removal, may pass spontaneously or may remain dormant and asymptomatic for long periods of time. They present a problem with many variable factors and careful individual evaluation is essential, but in general about 75 per cent of retained stones will sooner or later require removal.

If the stone is obstructing the distal common duct and the patient has a total biliary fistula, reoperation should be done as soon as the patient's general condition warrants it. If this involves a long interval, refeeding the bile drainage is important.

If the retained stone lies above the T-tube, and the common duct is not sufficiently dilated to let it pass to the lower end of the duct, any proposed program, other than reoperation, must include removal of the tube.

With a retained stone in the lower end of the common duct which is of a reasonable size in relation to the size of the papilla, as calibrated at operation, and if clamping the T-tube produces no ill effects, the patient may be sent home for a period of weeks. The T-tube should be opened for an hour or two each day and the cholangiogram should be repeated after a reasonable interval, usually four to six weeks. If the stone has not passed in three months, reoperation is in order unless contraindicated by the patient's general condition.

If the symptoms and signs suggesting residual stones appear after the T-tube has been removed, or if the common duct was not explored at the first operation, prompt reoperation is usually indicated. In doubtful cases confirmatory evidence may be obtained by intravenous cholangiogram or duodenal drainage or both.

Successful efforts at nonoperative manipulation of residual stones through the sinus provided by the T-tube have been reported recently but have not as yet had an extensive trial.[8-10] Operative removal of residual stones is the treatment of choice for most patients at present.

REFERENCES

1. Blumberg, B. S., et al.: Current concepts: Australia antigen and hepatitis. N. Eng. J. Med. 283:349, 1970.
2. Cattell, R. B., et al.: General considerations in the management of benign stricture of the bile duct. N. Eng. J. Med. 261:929, 1959.
3. Dowdy, G. S., et al.: Surgical anatomy of the pancreatobiliary ductal system. Arch. Surg. 84:229, 1962.
4. Egbert, L. D., et al.: Reduction of postoperative pain by encouragement and instruction of patients: A study of doctor-patient rapport. N. Eng. J. Med. 270:825, 1964.
5. Ingelfinger, F. J.: Differential diagnosis of jaundice. Disease-a-month. Chicago, Year Book Publishers, Inc., November 1958.
6. Jolly, P. C., et al.: Operative cholangiography: A case for its routine use. Ann. Surg. 168:551, 1968.
7. Krugman, S., et al.: Viral hepatitis: New light on an old disease. J.A.M.A. 212:1019, 1970.
8. Lamis, P. A., et al.: Retained common duct stones: A new nonoperative technique for treatment. Surgery 66:291, 1969.
9. Lawson, D. W., et al.: Surgical treatment of acute necrotizing pancreatitis. Ann. Surg. 172:605, 1970.
10. Mazzariello, R.: Removal of residual biliary tract calculi without reoperation. Surgery 67:566, 1970.
11. Michaels, N. A.: The hepatic, cystic and retroduodenal arteries and their relation to the biliary ducts. Ann. Surg. 133:503, 1951.
12. Salzman, E. W., et al.: Pancreatic duct exploration in selected cases of acute pancreatitis. Ann. Surg. 158:859, 1963.
13. Thorbjarnason, B., et al.: Percutaneous transhepatic cholangiography. Ann. Surg. 165:33, 1967.
14. Waddell, W. R.: Exposure of intrahepatic bile ducts through interlobal fissure. Surg. Gynec. & Obst. 124:491, 1967.
15. Zimmerman, H. J.: Differential diagnosis of jaundice. Med. Clin. N. Amer. 52:1417, 1968.

CHAPTER 19

SMALL INTESTINAL PROBLEMS

W. Dean Warren, M.D., F.A.C.S.

NONOBSTRUCTIVE SMALL INTESTINAL DISEASE

Diseases of the small intestine which require surgical intervention present several specific problems which must be well understood to allow optimal pre- and postoperative care. The most important clinical entity, obstruction of the small bowel, will be considered in detail in the latter part of this chapter. Other problems of great importance in surgery of the small intestine include (1) fistulous drainage of large volumes of intestinal contents, necessitating careful fluid and electrolyte replacement and meticulous wound management; (2) the treatment of prevention of severe nutritional deficiencies secondary to primary small bowel disease or high intestinal fistulae; and (3) the control of intra-abdominal sepsis when the source and location of the septic process may be extremely difficult to delineate.

Some specific types of nonobstructive small bowel disease will be considered individually, but the basic problems are remarkably similar.

Regional Enteritis

Patients with regional enteritis often present with intestinal obstruction, and the general management of these patients is summarized later. However, if the diagnosis of obstruction secondary to regional enteritis is well established, in contrast to most other types of small bowel obstruction, early operation should usually be avoided. The principal reasons for this are the comparatively smaller chance of gangrenous small bowel and the probability that a resection of or anastomosis involving the colon will be required to relieve the obstruction. A long tube passed into the small intestine will provide decompression and allow subsidence of the edema and inflammatory changes in the proximal small bowel. When this is accomplished, several days or more may be utilized to prepare adequately for the operative procedure. An "elective" procedure decreases the hazards of surgery and provides greater freedom in choosing the type of operation. However, many patients require surgery because of failure to respond to a medical regimen or because of complications such as perforation and fistula formation. Under these circumstances a complex problem seen frequently is progressive nutritional deficit accompanied by intra-abdominal sepsis. If at all possible, these complications should be controlled prior to definitive surgery. When an abscess can be demonstrated, drainage is indicated, although development of an enterocutaneous fistula is probable. When abscess formation cannot be defined, systemic antibiotic therapy with modification of intestinal alimentation is required. In some instances cessation of oral alimentation and institution of gastrointestinal suction to place the small bowel at maximal rest will accelerate greatly the regression of the inflammatory process.

When sepsis is controlled, definitive improvement in nutrition can be expected by the improved techniques of intravenous hyperalimentation or the use of the so-called elemental diet. Each of these modes of therapy has the important characteristic of markedly lowering the volume of intestinal contents while providing an intake of sufficient calories and nutriments to allow positive nitrogen balance and actual weight gain under most circumstances. A period of three or four weeks of such treatment will frequently change the character of the operation, allowing a definitive procedure with markedly reduced risk of sepsis or suture line leakage. The details of intravenous hyperalimentation and the elemental diet, given in Chapter 4, are of extreme importance to physicians managing patients with complex small bowel disease. Meticulous attention to the details of these procedures is vital to the successful management of the seriously ill patient.

Preoperatively one must consider certain other problems that may arise in patients treated for chronic regional enteritis. If the condition of the patient permits, radiographic study is usually indicated to search for diseased bowel other than that seen typically in the terminal ileum. This may occur anywhere in the gastrointestinal tract, and study of the colon as well as the upper gastrointestinal area should be accomplished.

An intravenous pyelogram should also be obtained preoperatively because of the high incidence of obstruction to the right ureter, often requiring operative decompression by ureterolysis.

As an ileal or jejunal anastomosis to the colon is generally performed, preparation of the large bowel is indicated. The principal goal, thorough cleansing of the colon, is accomplished by restricting the diet to clear liquids for two to three days prior to operation and the use of oral catharsis and enemas. Utilization of intestinal antibiotics to suppress the bacterial flora is controversial, but is generally thought to be of value.

Postoperatively, careful attention should be directed toward prevention of distention of the stomach and small bowel and the prevention of sepsis. The "prophylactic" use of systemic antibiotics, started
the evening before or the morning of operation, is indicated in these
patients and will help to lower the incidence of postoperative infection.

When constant corticosteroid therapy has been utilized preoperatively, additional supportive therapy is required. An appropriate regimen
of supplemental corticosteroid administration is outlined in an earlier
chapter. In general, a full maintenance dose begun the day prior to
surgery and continued for 24 to 48 hours is gradually decreased over
several days or weeks.

Small Intestinal Fistulae

Fistulae from the proximal jejunum create far greater problems
than fistulae at the distal end of the small bowel. The greater loss of
fluid and electrolytes and the diminished absorptive surface proximal
to the fistulae are factors of great importance. In such patients intravenous hyperalimentation may be of tremendous value, often allowing
control or even closure of fistulae while maintaining adequate nutrition. Proximal intestinal fistulae may occur with primary disease of the
small bowel, such as regional enteritis, but more frequently are seen as
a result of either operative or nonoperative trauma. The latter are
frequently associated with multiple, intra-abdominal injuries, postoperative sepsis and ultimate drainage of an abscess creating an enterocutaneous fistula. Once the diagnosis of small bowel fistulae is suspected,
efforts to delineate the site and nature of the lesion should be begun.
Standard techniques include gastrointestinal radiography and the oral
administration of an appropriate marker with careful observation for its
appearance in drainage from the wound. Frequently these procedures
will not be necessary because of the characteristic nature of the fistulous drainage combined with excoriation and irritation of the surrounding skin. Of great value in the diagnosis of the length and location of
the fistula is radiographic examination of injection of the fistulous tract.
This technique may also be of help in localizing areas of incompletely
drained abscesses, a frequent cause of continuing sepsis. Adequate
drainage of such areas is most desirable and often leads to a marked
improvement in the patient's condition. With control of systemic toxicity and a carefully planned regimen of intravenous hyperalimentation,
a positive nitrogen balance and a gain in weight and strength may be
anticipated. If there are a few feet of relatively normal bowel proximal
to a fistula, an "elemental" diet delivered into the stomach by a small
feeding tube can achieve the nutritional goals with somewhat less risk
than the intravenous route.

Another problem of the high volume fistula is the accurate assessment of the fluid and electrolyte loss. This is particularly difficult if multiple fistulous tracts open onto the abdominal wall with collection of all drainage being virtually impossible. Under such circumstances daily body weights and electrolyte determinations are desirable to give reliable estimates of the needs of intravenous or oral replacements. Occasionally there is difficulty with severe excoriation and inflammation of the skin around such a fistula, and several different techniques have been utilized in an attempt to facilitate management of this problem. One of the simplest devices is the use of a temporary ileostomy bag with the adherent facing carefully patterned to closely surround the opening of the fistula. Also of value is the use of a large sump catheter to occlude the tract superficially while evacuating the drainage fluid by suction. In many patients this fistulous drainage occurs within a large, opened area of an abdominal incision without the nature or number of the fistulae being apparent. In such situations it is frequently helpful to institute sump suction through a catheter lying at the dependent portion of the open wound while dripping a buffered saline solution onto the upper angle.

Ideally surgical intervention should be undertaken only when there has been control of intra-abdominal sepsis and achievement of adequate nutritional status with no evidence of spontaneous closure of the fistula. With the newer methods for control of the nutritional problem, the operative procedures can be safely delayed in most instances, even with a very high volume fistula. This allows for careful attention to the details of general preoperative preparation such as restoration of blood volume and red cell mass, improvement in pulmonary toilet, and so forth. The most difficult problem arises in patients with severe sepsis. Constant search for an abscess must be undertaken, including careful clinical evaluation, gastrointestinal radiography, radiography of fistulous tracts, liver-lung scans, and intravenous pyelography. Drainage of an abscess can achieve a dramatic improvement in an apparently moribund patient. Conversely, inability to control sepsis is the most frequent cause of death in this group of patients.

TRAUMA

The preoperative preparation of a patient suspected of having an injury to the small bowel is generally modified by the possibility of other injuries that are of more immediate threat to the patient. A complete consideration of this problem is included in Chapter 30. From the standpoint of injury to the small bowel itself there are two primary steps to be instituted as soon as practicable. The first is decompression of the stomach with nasogastric suction. This helps to reduce peritoneal soiling, but is most important in minimizing the danger of aspiration of gastric contents during the induction of anesthesia. The second step is the early systemic administration of broad-spectrum antibiotics. Although the bacterial flora of the normal small bowel are relatively few, sepsis remains the greatest threat to the patient. If there are multiple injuries (e.g., gunshot wound) to the bowel, it is usually wise to decompress the small intestine by a tube inserted via a gastrostomy or jejunostomy at the time of surgery. Extensive irrigation of the peritoneal cavity with several liters of normal saline solution helps to reduce the potential hazards of the chemical and/or bacterial peritonitis.

Postoperatively, every effort should be extended to prevent intestinal distention as the traumatized bowel is especially prone to suture line complications. The possibility of leakage of an anastomosis with single or multiple abscess formation is a constant threat. Intravenous alimentation with continuous gastrointestinal suction is usually indicated for several days. Antibiotic therapy should be continued for at least 48 to 72 hours postoperatively.

TUMORS

Tumors of the small intestine are relatively uncommon, and are frequently diagnosed with difficulty. The occurrence of incomplete bowel obstruction or gastrointestinal bleeding without an easily demonstrable source should raise the question of the presence of a small bowel neoplasm. A carefully performed barium study of the small intestine is the basic diagnostic tool in these circumstances, but is frequently inconclusive. A valuable technique in cases with bleeding is selective superior mesenteric arteriography. A number of centers have reported markedly improved results in locating the site of bleeding in the small bowel and frequently establish the nature of the lesion. This is particularly valuable when the tumor may be difficult to identify at operation, the classic example being hemangiomata of the small bowel.

SMALL INTESTINAL OBSTRUCTION

Obstruction of the small intestine continues to be one of the leading causes for emergent surgical procedures. Its significance is further emphasized by a continuing mortality of about 10 per cent. Advanced age, associated disease and patient delay are important factors, but a significant fraction remains in which a remediable or preventable condition leads to death. Principal pitfalls for the surgeon are (1) delay in establishing the diagnosis, (2) failure to appreciate the presence of gangrenous bowel, and (3) failure to anticipate or treat vigorously the three specific complications of aspiration pneumonitis, losses of body fluids and sepsis.

PATHOPHYSIOLOGY OF SMALL INTESTINAL OBSTRUCTION

Simple Mechanical Obstructions. This condition is characterized by obstruction of the bowel without impairment of blood supply. In the adult patient, adhesive bands are the most common causative agent, followed by tumors, foreign bodies and inflammatory lesions. The essential physiologic deficits are:

FLUID AND ELECTROLYTE LOSS. Losses of fluids occur through vomiting, sequestration into the lumen of the stomach and bowel, and edema of the bowel wall. In simple obstructions the loss of 3 to 4 liters of electrolyte-rich fluid frequently occurs during the first 24 hours, causing a reduction in the volume of extracellular fluid. As there is little plasma protein or erythrocyte loss early, an elevated hematocrit is frequently encountered. The acute reduction in circulating plasma volume initiates a compensating movement of interstitial fluid into the intravascular compartment. In long-standing cases, the signs of loss of tissue fluid (decreased skin turgor) emphasize the large total volume of fluids functionally lost to the body. In certain instances, additional losses of sodium, chloride or potassium ions may occur (see Chapter 3).

DISTENTION OF THE BOWEL. Distention of the proximal intestine occurs in most cases and is of significance for two reasons. First, the fluid sequestration is accelerated, and, second, the large intestinal volume may seriously restrict diaphragmatic movements, a serious complication in patients with pulmonary disease.

Strangulating Mechanical Obstruction. This term implies a mechanical intestinal obstruction associated with impairment of the vascular supply of the bowel. The group of patients with this condition is exceedingly important for it contains most of the instances in which preventable fatalities occur. The usual etiology is either postoperative adhesions or incarceration of an external hernia. In either instance, a closed loop obstruction occurs and intestinal contents within the loop can pass neither proximally nor distally. As the loop becomes severely distended the intramural pressure impedes capillary perfusion, initiating gangrenous degeneration.

In addition to the usual fluid losses, there may be a marked loss of red cell mass into the obstructed loop, frequently of a severity that requires preoperative transfusion. However, the most significant difference from simple obstruction is the lethal nature of the contents of the strangulated loop. Although debate continues about the nature of the toxic material, it is clear that bacteria are necessary for its production. Systemic absorption occurs from the peritoneal cavity as the fluid seeps through a deteriorating bowel wall. If absorption of this toxic fluid continues, peripheral vascular collapse occurs; this is the major cause of death related directly to intestinal obstruction.

Primary Vascular Obstruction. Sudden occlusion of superior mesenteric vessels by embolus or thrombosis usually leads to a gangrenous obstruction of the small intestine. Although lumen patency is frequently maintained, the loss of peristaltic activity through the involved bowel results in an obstruction which can produce all the aforementioned physiologic changes. It differs somewhat from closed loop strangulation in that bowel necrosis often occurs much earlier and prompt surgical therapy is required if survival is to be obtained.

Paralytic Ileus. This term implies a functional obstruction caused by cessation of peristalsis. This is most often seen following operative manipulation of the intestine, neurologic injury, retroperitoneal hemorrhage, or trauma and intraperitoneal sepsis. Strangulation is rare and if the diagnosis is well founded, nonoperative treatment is indicated.

DIAGNOSIS

The differential diagnosis can be difficult, and represents one of the points at which physician error is apt to occur. This is particularly important because a wrong diagnosis (such as acute pancreatitis) may obscure the significance of the clinical signs generally indicative of gangrenous bowel.

The usual features of intestinal obstruction are well known and include nausea and vomiting, crampy abdominal pain, hyperperistalsis, obstipation and abdominal distention. The most important diagnostic problem is the detection or suspicion of nonviable bowel, which carries a fatality rate four times that of simple obstruction. Delay in diagnosis correlates closely with increasing mortality, yet in one third of patients with this complication it was not seriously considered on admission to the hospital. The following clinical points serve to accentuate the suspicion of strangulation, but there is no test or combination thereof that can completely rule out the presence of nonviable intestine.

1. *Pain:* Progresses more rapidly after onset than with simple obstruction and may become severe and continuous.

2. *Tenderness:* Definite tenderness, particularly if localized.

3. *Mass:* Palpable mass may be present with closed loop obstruction.

4. *Shock:* Onset of shock-like picture prior to extensive fluid loss.

5. *Fever:* Frequently present.

6. *Leukocytosis:* Frequently present and progressive with shift to the left.

7. *Peritoneal irritation:* Abdominal guarding or spasm may be present.

8. *X-ray:* Not to be relied upon to rule out gangrene. Pseudotumor of closed loop obstruction is sometimes demonstrable.

PREOPERATIVE PREPARATION OF THE PATIENT

Once a tentative diagnosis of intestinal obstruction is made, a vigorous program should be undertaken to prepare the patient for a possible operation. In a good-risk patient, the major hazard is the presence of strangulation, and surgical exploration should be undertaken unless definite contraindications arise. Only in the patient with coexistent disease so serious that the operative risk outweighs the potential hazard of gangrenous bowel is definitive nonoperative therapy generally undertaken. Factors that create exceptions to this rule include obstructions in the early postoperative period and a history of many previous obstructions.

In most patients with intestinal obstruction, adequate preparation for operation can be accomplished within 3 to 4 hours. In the exceptionally ill patient with a complicated problem, occasionally 6 to 8 hours may be required.

Fluid Replacement. An initial blood sample is drawn for complete blood count, cross-match and baseline chemistries, which should include a BUN, serum sodium, potassium chloride and CO_2 and other determinations indicated by specific problems. The volume of fluids needed for replacement cannot be accurately calculated, but for the patient with moderate distention of several small bowel loops 2000 to 3000 ml. of a salt-containing solution is usually needed. The major indicator as to efficacy of fluid therapy is the clinical response of the patient; the importance of careful observation of the pulse, blood pressure and urinary output cannot be overemphasized. Monitoring the central venous pressure may be of considerable help when cardiovascular disease is present.

In patients with simple mechanical obstruction, transfusion is rarely necessary prior to operation. However, in patients with a long closed loop obstruction, large amounts of blood can be lost into the loop and preoperative transfusion with blood or plasma is frequently indicated.

The type of fluid to be administered varies somewhat with the level of obstruction. In very high jejunal obstruction, a pattern may be seen which closely resembles gastric obstruction with excessive loss of chloride and potassium. In these instances, there may be severe hypochloremic, hypokalemic alkalosis; replacement should be with normal saline and supplemental potassium. In the usual small bowel obstruction, however, the fluid of choice is Hartmann's solution (or lactated Ringer's) with a potassium supplement. This fluid is particularly advantageous because (1) it more nearly approximates the physiologic losses and (2) it is hypotonic, thus lessening the metabolic load on the kidney and obviating the need for dextrose/water infusion.

The final determination of the adequacy of fluid replacement again should be based on both clinical and laboratory findings. Only in rare instances is there ever justification for submitting a patient to a major surgical procedure before stabilization of the cardiovascular system has been achieved.

Decompression of the Gastrointestinal Tract. There continues to be disagreement as to the type of gastrointestinal obstruction. If early operative intervention is planned, the major functions of the tube are to decompress the stomach completely and to minimize the danger of aspiration during the induction of general anesthesia. In the past, aspiration pneumonitis was one of the major causes of death in patients undergoing operation for intestinal obstruction. It should be noted that passage of a long tube into the small intestine may fail to maintain decompression of the stomach. In these instances additional gastric aspiration may be needed.

When clinical findings indicate absence of gangrenous obstruction and there is serious coexistent disease, delay of operation may be exceedingly desirable. In such instances, intestinal decompression with a long tube is the keystone of therapy. To facilitate passage of the long tube, the balloon should be partially filled with a liquid (either water or mercury) to give a bolus which will stimulate passage through the gastrointestinal tract. The balloon may be maneuvered to the pylorus under fluoroscopic control and the patient positioned to facilitate its passage into the intestine. With successful intubation, beginning regression of the distention can be anticipated within a few hours, and in the absence of gangrenous bowel, the emergent nature of the obstruction changes. With the use of either a gastric or an intestinal tube, it is important that *continued function* of the tube be established by appropriate irrigations and aspiration.

Treatment of Potential or Established Sepsis. From experimental data and from the limited information that can be obtained from clinical studies, it is becoming increasingly apparent that the prophylactic use of antibiotics is of value in delaying or preventing the consequences of strangulation obstruction and in lessening the chance of postoperative sepsis. Once the diagnosis of intestinal obstruction is established, intravenous wide-spectrum antibiotic therapy should be begun. This is most important in those patients for whom nonoperative therapy is indicated or whose preoperative preparation will require several hours.

Treatment of Associated Problems. Chief among these are diseases of the cardiovascular system, particularly cardiac failure. If necessary, vigorous treatment for incipient or frank heart failure may be carried out with marked improvement of the patient within 6 to 8 hours. This would include rapid digitalization as well as the use of appropriate techniques for the relief of pulmonary edema. These problems are usually encountered in patients suffering from an acute embolic infarction of the bowel, and rapid surgical intervention is necessary. Occasionally, problems of other types, such as diabetic acidosis, may be encountered and require several hours of intensive treatment.

OPERATIVE PROCEDURES

The choice of incision is governed by the nature and location of the lesion causing the obstruction; a single type of incision should not be made to fit all patients. In a patient in whom an adhesion in the pelvis is the most likely obstructing lesion, a different incision should be used from that for an embolectomy of the superior mesenteric artery.

Operative decompression of the intestine is frequently indicated because of severe bowel distention. This can be accomplished by several means, the simplest of which is the introduction of a long sump-type suction tip with threading of the bowel over this instrument. In this way the entire small bowel may be decompressed with just one or two enterostomies. Decompression of the bowel lessens the problem of postoperative absorption of unknown amounts of fluid, facilitates respiratory care, and aids in obtaining an optimal wound closure—all of which are potential sources of postoperative problems.

POSTOPERATIVE CARE

Careful regulation of fluid therapy is mandatory in the postoperative period. In a critically ill patient, the monitoring of central venous pressure, as well as pulse, blood pressure and urinary output, is helpful in assessing the optimal rate and volume for fluid replacement. Accurate records of all intake and output are essential. In complex cases of long standing, particularly if oliguria is a problem, daily body weights are needed to follow total body water. Aliquots of output (urine and gastric drainage) may be analyzed for electrolyte content and accurate replacement accomplished. Frequent and sometimes daily determinations of serum Na, K, Cl, CO_2 and urea are necessary in the seriously ill. As losses of salt-rich fluids are often underestimated, large amounts of salt-free fluids should *not* be given in the early postoperative period. This has the usual effect of producing hyponatremia which may aggravate an existing renal malfunction.

Gastrointestinal decompression should be continued for protection of intestinal and abdominal incisions and is very important in attempting to avoid serious pulmonary complications. Within 48 to 72 hours gastrointestinal function is usually regained, but the tube should be removed only when evidence of *effective* function is established by the passage of stool or flatus. In the case of a long intestinal tube, a test of oral intake with the tube clamped is often wise because of the difficulty of replacement should the tube again be needed.

Particular attention should be devoted to the respiratory system, a major site of serious complications, especially in the elderly patient. Careful endotracheal suction is frequently needed in addition to intermittent positive pressure breathing and other adjuncts for the care of the patient with pulmonary disease. Antibiotics should usually be continued in the early postoperative period.

REFERENCES

Colcock, B. P., and Fortin, C.: Surgical treatment of regional enteritis: Review of 85 cases. Ann. Surg. *161*:812, 1965.

Davis, S. E., and Sperling, L.: Obstruction of the small intestine. Arch. Surg. *99*:424, 1969.

Dudrick, S. J., Wilmore, D. W., Vars, H. M., and Rhoads, J. E.: Can intravenous feeding as the sole means of nutrition support growth in the child and restore weight loss in an adult? Ann. Surg. *169*:974, 1969.

Enker, W. E., and Block, G. E.: Occult obstructive uropathy complicating Crohn's disease. Arch. Surg. *101*:319, 1970.

Johnson, C. L., and McIlrath, D. C.: Management of patients with enterocutaneous fistulae. Surg. Clin. N. Amer. *49*:967, 1969.

Moore, F. D.: Metabolic Care of the Surgical Patient. Philadelphia, W. B. Saunders Co., 1959.

Schwartz, S. I.: Principles of Surgery. New York, McGraw-Hill, 1969.

Shannon, R.: Strangulating intestinal obstruction. A review of 115 cases. Austr. N. Z. J. Surg. *38*:21, 1968.

Silen, W., Hein, M., and Goldman, L.: Strangulation obstruction of the small intestine. Arch. Surg. *85*:137, 1962.

Stevens, R. V., and Randall, H. T.: Use of a concentrated, balanced liquid elemental diet for nutritional management of catabolic states. Ann. Surg. *170*:642, 1969.

CHAPTER 20

THE CARE OF INTESTINAL STOMAS

Rupert B. Turnbull, Jr., M.D., F.A.C.S.

The objective of this chapter is threefold: (1) to describe improved methods of stomal care and rehabilitation of stomal patients, (2) to direct attention to the availability of new and improved equipment and drugs for stomal care, and (3) to provide a specific guide for the care of the various types of intestinal stomas.

IMPROVED METHODS OF STOMAL CARE

The postoperative care of stomas begins on the day of surgery, the principal role being played by the operating surgeon. The stoma is placed on the abdominal wall at a site *known* to be suitable for the wearing of a collecting device. The surgical technique and the ideal placement of all intestinal stomas can be found in the *Atlas of Intestinal Stomas* (C. V. Mosby Company, 1967).

The operating surgeon may wish to care for the stomas he makes, but consistent and expert management of the stoma and the stomal patient is available in most medical centers from members of the American Association of Enterostomal Therapists.* Their function is to advise or counsel the patient preoperatively if the surgeon desires. During the postoperative phase in the hospital, the patient is visited and the stoma is cared for on a daily basis. The pouch is changed as often as indicated and the peristomal skin is observed and cared for in such a manner as to protect it so that a permanent appliance can be fitted on the tenth postoperative day. During the hospital stay, the daily

---

*For a complete list of members, write Mrs. Norma Gill, Secretary, American Association of Enterostomal Therapists, Cleveland Clinic Foundation.

visit by the surgeon and the expertise and daily counseling by the enterostomal therapist account for the rapid emotional and sociophysical rehabilitation of stomal patients.

Following hospital discharge, the trained therapist must continue to see the patient. The ileostomy decreases in diameter at the base and must be calibrated in three weeks and a new mounting ring with an appropriate aperture ordered from a manufacturer. The peristomal skin must never be exposed to the corrosive action of liquid stool or the constant wetting of urine from the ileal conduit.

The colostomy patient needs less follow-up care after discharge from the hospital. He has been instructed in irrigating techniques and supplied with a suitable irrigating apparatus. He has already irrigated his colon on two or three occasions with a therapist standing by, has been given a diet to follow temporarily and has been supplied with a stool deodorant and "safety" pouches.

EQUIPMENT FOR THE CARE OF INTESTINAL STOMAS

American manufacturers have contributed a great deal to the postoperative care and social rehabilitation of the stomal patient. Drug companies have particularly made available antidiarrheal agents and bowel deodorants useful to colostomy and ileostomy patients. Equipment manufacturers have produced a line of odorless pouches for the ileostomy patient and compact enema equipment for the management of the temporary or permanent colostomy.

Equipment for operative and immediate postoperative use is ideally kept in stock in hospitals where stomas are made. A list of this equipment and some drugs and drug companies are listed in the appended *manufacturers' index* and may readily be referred to by the reader. As each manufacturer or drug is referred to, the reference marker[M] will appear. An attached number will locate the item in the *manufacturers' index*; thus a reference to karaya washers[M2, M3, M5] will locate this item in the manufacturers' index. If more than one item is suitable, additional numbers will appear.

THE HOSPITAL CARE OF INTESTINAL STOMAS

Ileostomy (Colectomy for Ulcerative Colitis or Polyposis). The ideal location of any ileostomy has been described in the second paragraph. Care of the stoma and the skin around it starts in the operating room. The integrity of the skin around the stoma must be maintained; i.e., the cornified layer of the skin must not be disrupted. As soon as the stoma has been made, wipe the skin dry and spray the entire abdomen with a *protective spray*,[M13, M14] Cut a suitable aperture in an *oval karaya*

SUGGESTED EQUIPMENT FOR HOSPITAL CARE OF ILEOSTOMY

QUANTITY		INDEX AND ITEM
10	Postoperative disposable pouches	M3, M5, M10
10	Oval karaya washers	M5
1	Protective skin spray	M10, M13, M14
2	Binder clip or rubber bands	
6	Rolls microporous tape 1½ inches width	M4

washer,[M5] use this washer on the skin and apply the pouch over it.[M5] Now, tape[M4] the periphery of the pouch and the underlying *oval washer* to the skin. A *binder clip* will secure the end of the pouch.

When the ileostomy begins to function, it may be necessary to apply a new pouch every other day. Frequent emptying of the pouch by the nursing staff will prevent leakage resulting from overfilling. At every change of pouch, the abdominal skin is again coated with protective spray.

Fitting the Permanent Pouch. On the tenth postoperative day, the transparent pouch is removed and the diameter of the ileostomy is measured at the base. A permanent pouch and accessories are ordered. A number of manufacturers[M1 to M10] make suitable equipment. If the patient is held over in the hospital, or if there is excessive edema of the ileac stoma, it is wise to defer ordering permanent equipment. One particular appliance[M3] is useful during the waiting period.

SUGGESTED PERMANENT ILEOSTOMY EQUIPMENT (THE MARLEN COMPANY)[M5]

Instructions for the patient:
In your box you will find the following equipment:

2 Oval convex faceplates (hard or flexible, adult size).

10 Odor ban pouches, large, medium or small, with flap to pull pouch on disc (opaque preferred).

3 Rings (black ring to seal pouch to faceplate).

2 Packages of adhesive discs to hold pouch to oval washers or to skin.

2 Packages of small karaya washers. The aperture is smaller in the washer than in the adhesive disc.

1 Package stoma guide strips—to guide appliance over stoma. (Paper strip dissolves in pouch.) See diagrams for use.

1 Brush to scrub appliance (do not take pouch apart to clean).

1 Hanger—to hang appliance up to dry.

1 Bottle deodorizer—instructions on bottle.

1 Closure clip—you may use this closure clip or the black binder clip.

1 Belt (we prefer you do not wear the belt, but if you do use it, leave it loose about the waist).

1 Can solvent[M5, M7] to cleanse the skin.

1 Package of oval skin shields.[M5]

METHOD OF APPLICATION OF PERMANENT POUCH

Mount the faceplate on the pouch. Seal with the O-ring. Cut an appropriate opening in the oval skin shield[M5] and after cleansing the peristomal skin with solvent,[M5, M7] press the oval shield down over the stoma and onto the skin. Now apply a small karaya washer (item No. 5) over the stoma, stretching the aperture so that it will contract against the stoma after it seals to the oval shield. Now activate a double-sided adhesive disc (Fig. 20–1). Apply it to the faceplate of the pouch and then activate the exposed surface (Fig. 20–2). A stoma guide strip (Fig. 20–3,*A*) is coiled and put in the aperture in the faceplate (Fig. 20–3,*B*) to act as a guide for centering the stoma when applying the pouch (Fig. 20–4).

We prefer that you do not use the belt but rather fix the faceplate to the skin with strips of microporous paper tape.[M4]

You will note that the skin around your ileostomy is protected from damage by the use of the oval skin shields as an adhesive seal. If you find that leakage occurs because the oval shield is not sticky enough, do not use it. Paint the skin with skin prep,[M10] let it dry, and then apply the pouch as shown in Figures 20-1 to 20-4, allowing the adhesive discs to seal the faceplate to the skin. The small karaya washers[M5] must always be used.

General Considerations. Baths are encouraged. Remove the pouch if the ileostomy is not too active. You can also shower and bathe with it on. Water is beneficial to the skin. You can wear your pouch up to five days if it does not leak. Should it break loose from the skin, start all over again and put it back on.

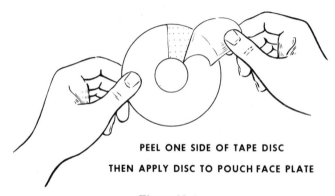

PEEL ONE SIDE OF TAPE DISC

THEN APPLY DISC TO POUCH FACE PLATE

Figure 20-1.

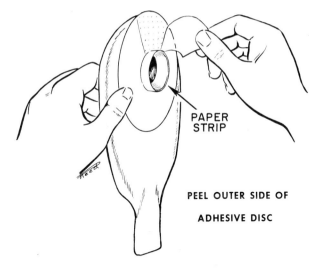

PAPER
STRIP

PEEL OUTER SIDE OF

ADHESIVE DISC

Figure 20-2.

A Marlen Odorban pouch[M5] will last about two weeks. Replace it with a new one when it becomes discolored. Other excellent pouches[M1, M3, M7, M9] are available and the wearer may wish to try them.

To remove the pouch, pull it away from the skin if the oval skin shield is used. If adhesive discs are used next to the skin, dissolve the faceplate off the skin by allowing the solvent to drip (eye dropper) between the skin and the faceplate. Pulling the faceplate away without solvent will pull hairs, causing infection, and will strip away the outer layers of the skin, causing ulcers to appear or yeast to grow. When there is skin irritation or damage, we suggest prolonged baths; spray the skin with a cortisone spray[M13] and dust the skin lightly with antiyeast powder,[M13] before returning to the application of the pouch with oval skin shields.[M5]

Special Problems. Occasionally, the peristomal skin reacts to gum karaya washers or to some other agent, becoming moist, shiny and red, and no pouch will adhere to it. The only truly suitable pouch is one that does not need to seal to the skin to act as a collecting device. This is the Perry Model 51 with rubber sleeve.[M8] This pouch consists of the following parts:

Polyethylene clear plastic pouches
Plastic bushings
Laminated paper skin protectors
Rubber sleeves
Belts (2)
Belt ring

To assemble the Perry Model 51, insert the plastic bushing into the

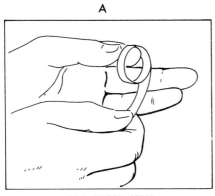

A

COIL PAPER STRIP

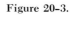

Figure 20–3.

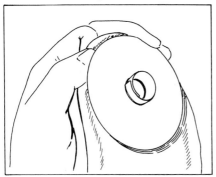

B

TUCK STRIP INTO DISC

Figure 20–4.

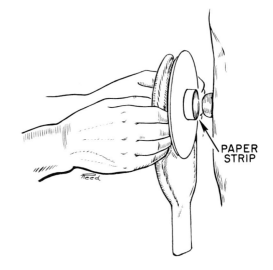

PAPER STRIP

APPLY POUCH

hole of the pouch. Put the small side of the bushing in, and handle the pouch by its thin plastic flange so as not to tear it. Spin the flange to be certain it is seated in the pouch aperture. Put a rubber sleeve on the bushing and push the sleeve into the pouch through the bushing. Pull the mounting ring up over the pouch and apply the pouch, allowing the ileostomy to project through the sleeve into the plastic pouch. The sleeve must come to the very end of the ileostomy and should not be shorter than the ileostomy.

Moisten a paper protector pad with aluminum acetate solution,[M15] and apply it over the stoma, hard surface next to the skin; then apply the pouch and fasten the two belts to the four posts on the mounting ring. Tighten the belts, with one across the buttocks and the other in the belt line. When fitting the rubber sleeve over the stoma, remember that it must not constrict or squeeze the stoma, nor must it be loose or it will leak. It must merely "touch" the stoma (the so-called "touch fit"). The prerequisite to wearing this pouch is that the stoma must be long enough to protrude. A skin-level stoma will not accommodate the pouch.

After 4 or 5 days of moist dressings (aluminum acetate[M15] solution on paper protectors) on the weeping peristomal skin, the skin reaction usually subsides and an adhesive pouch may once again be worn.

The Hollister[M3] ileostomy pouch is particularly suited as an ileostomy collecting device for use under the conditions described above, providing that the patient's skin does not react to gum karaya. This simple one-piece pouch is readily worn. Very little of it touches the peristomal skin.

CARE OF THE ILEAL CONDUIT ILEOSTOMY

Marlen[M5] equipment has been the most satisfactory and most available, although other manufacturers produce suitable articles of use for the urinary ileostomy. Figures 20-5 to 20-10 illustrate postoperative and permanent children's equipment. Vinyl pouches are durable and odorless compared to rubber products.

POSTOPERATIVE EQUIPMENT (IN THE HOSPITAL)

Equipment:
- 2 Packages tape-backed postoperative urinary pouches[M5, M10] with valve fittings (Fig. 20-10). Sizes: adult, child, infant.
- 1 Can solvent.[M5, M7]
- 2 Rolls of 1½ inch micropore tape.[M4]
- 1 Box Protex Powder pads (optional).[M5]
- 2 Bottles of United Skin Prep.[M10]

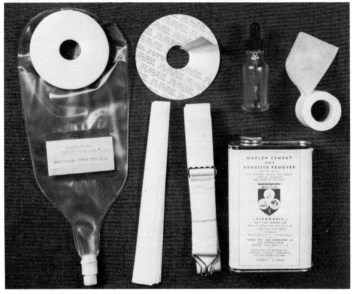

Figure 20–5. Marlen^{M5} adult equipment for ileal conduit. Vinyl pouch with valve, adhesive disc, belts, solvent and paper tape.

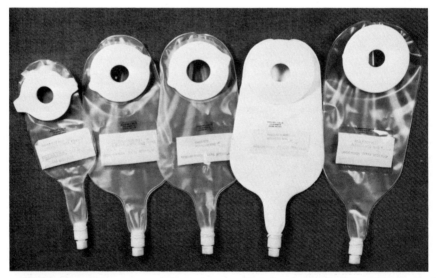

Figure 20–6. Permanent adult equipment. Variation in Marlen^{M5} pouches for ileal (ileostomy) conduits.

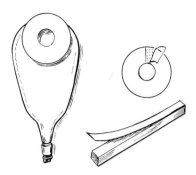

Figure 20-7. Basic permanent equipment for the ileal conduit ileostomy. Vinyl pouch, adhesive discs, soluble paper strips.

What to Do

THE STOMA. Clean the skin around the stoma with cotton, moist with solvent. Wipe dry; paint the skin around the stoma with skin prep,[M10] and allow it to dry.

THE POUCH. Cut an opening in the pouch 1/8 inch larger than the stoma base. Peel the back off the tape surface and apply this tacky side over the ileostomy, centering the stoma in the middle of the hole. Press the tacky edges of the pouch to the skin around the stoma. Put a strip of micropore tape[M4] across the top and bottom and both sides to hold it in place.

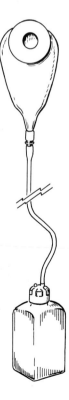

Figure 20-8. Ileostomy pouch with night drain assembly,[M5] essential for children.

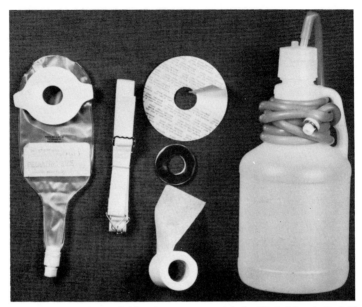

Figure 20–9. Permanent children's equipment. Marlen[M5] children's ileal (ileostomy) conduit. Note pouch, belt, adhesive discs, protex washers, paper tape and night drain assembly.

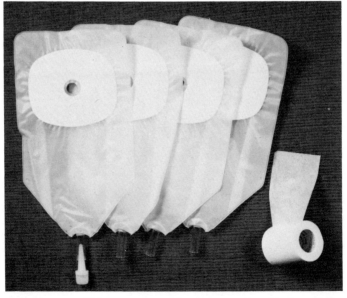

Figure 20–10. United[M10] postoperative ileostomy pouches (ileal conduit) and micropore paper tape.

To EMPTY POUCH. Pull the valve fitting down to open. To close the valve, push it back in. The valve may be opened and then attached to a night drain or bedside container, attaching a connector adapter (Figs. 20-8 and 20-9).

Ten days after surgery, the ileostomy is calibrated at the base because the manufacturer will need to know the size of the aperture in the faceplate. Oval, convex faceplates will be suitable for both adults and children. They have the same dimensions. Permanent equipment is ordered ten days after surgery.

THE PERMANENT POUCH

Marlen[M5] *Equipment:*
In your box of equipment are the following items:
- 2 Faceplates* (convex, hard); child size is preferable for adults.
- 10 Clear pouches large, medium or small, with flap to pull pouch onto the disc.
- 3 O-rings (black ring to hold pouch securely on faceplate).
- 2 Packages of adhesive tape discs.
- 1 Brush, to scrub the appliance (do not take off the faceplate to clean pouch).
  Stoma strip guides (dissolvable paper strips)
- 1 Bottle of deodorizer—instructions are on the bottle.
- 2 Urinary fittings (pouches with fittings already attached can be ordered from Marlen Manufacturing Company).
- 2 Packages of rubber bands.
- 1 Plastic hanger—to hang appliance up to dry.
- 1 Belt—optional for adults, but we prefer that adults not use a belt. Belts are needed for children (Fig. 20-2).

Application of Pouch. Cleanse the peristomal skin with water. Dry it and paint it with United skin prep.[M10] When dry, apply the pouch with an adhesive disc and center it over the stoma with a dissolvable paper strip[M5] in the faceplate aperture as already described. Tape the faceplate to the skin on all sides. The belt is optional. The pouch may be worn as long as it does not leak. The night drain may be useful, particularly in children with a high urinary output.

To Remove the Pouch

Equipment:
Eye dropper and 1 oz. bottle Solvent[M5, M7]

To remove the pouch, push the skin away from the upper edge of the disc, and from the eyedropper allow a few drops of solvent to drip

---

*Sizes of pouches: Infant, child, regular, large; opaque white, pink and blue pouches are available.

between the disc and the skin until it loosens the pouch so that it will come off easily.

Special Problems. The mucosa of the ileostomy in children occasionally reacts to vinyl. This is a hemorrhagic mucosal reaction, and blood exudes from the mucosa to produce bloody urine in the pouch. Ten minutes after the vinyl pouch is removed, the bleeding stops. A polyethylene pouch[M1, M10] substitute usually solves the problem.

In some children, the end of the stoma becomes white and tufted in appearance and bleeds. Urine crystals can be seen deposited on the mucosa and are responsible. The crystals are dissolved away by putting several ounces of table vinegar in the pouch at bedtime.

Another cause of bleeding from the stoma is the deposition of urine crystals inside the pouch where the end of the ileostomy is "sandpapered" by the rough crystalline surface. Crystals can be removed by soaking the inside of the pouch in vinegar.

FOLLOW-UP STOMA CARE

The base of the ileostomy should be calibrated intermittently for two years, particularly in children. The stoma shrinks progressively during that time, and unless smaller apertures in the faceplate are provided, the peristomal skin is exposed and wet. It becomes water soaked and a peristomal pseudoepitheliomatous hyperplasia develops to such an extent and is so painful that the child cannot attend school. In neglected cases, the problem is solved by the refitting of a small aperture faceplate. In two or three days, the raised skin has flattened under the new faceplate and the problem is solved. Final advice to the patient with the ileal conduit ileostomy: *Do not take your pouch off the faceplate until you are ready to discard the pouch.* Pouches last about two weeks. Be sure to save the faceplate, O-ring and urinary fitting for the new pouch.

CLEANING THE APPLIANCE

Equipment:
A basin of water
Any liquid detergent
Deodorizer[M5]
Nylon brush[M5]
Urinary crystal solvent[M5]

What to Do. Pull the adhesive disc off the faceplate. Clean the faceplate with solvent. Immerse the pouch in a basin of water to which detergent has been added and scrub it inside with the brush, rinsing it out with clear tepid water or adding a little detergent. Soak the appliance for five or ten minutes in deodorizer, and then hang the appliance up to dry on the plastic hanger. Discard vinyl pouches[M5] after 14 days' wear (average). If crystals form in the pouch, soak it in vinegar or urinary crystal solvent[M5] solution for 15 minutes before deodorizing the pouch.

Hints. A child should always use a night drain[M5] (Fig. 20–9). Wrap an Ace bandage around the right leg first, then wrap the spout of the pouch on the leg with the Ace bandage to hold it. The bandage will keep the appliance from twisting with the night drain. An alternate plan is to have the tubing go down inside the leg of the sleeper and out through the foot or through an opening made in the pajama leg near the ankle. A night drain is optional for adults. To dispel the urine odor, drink cranberry juice; this is helpful. Asparagus causes odor; avoid it.

CARE OF THE PERMANENT COLOSTOMY

This communication to the colostomy patient (permanent end colostomy) will present a method of control by an irrigating technique. The habits of the colon are discussed and suitable irrigating equipment is suggested.

Hospital Care. A plastic pouch[M3, M5] is applied over the newly constructed end colostomy. There will be passage of gas and possibly a small bowel movement on the fourth postoperative day. Pouches are replaced as necessary to keep the patient clean. As diet is started, bismuth subgallate tablets[M11] are given before each meal and at bedtime as a bowel deodorant. Loose bowel movements are controlled by Lomotil tablets,[M12] usually one before each meal; fruit and juices are avoided.

Beginning on the tenth postoperative day, the patient is instructed in an irrigating technique and supervised at three irrigating sessions by the enterostomal therapist who supplies the patient with colostomy irrigating equipment and small coloplast[M2] polyethylene safety pouches to wear on a daily basis.

Every colostomy patient is instructed in the care of the stoma while in the hospital. The following printed material is given to the colostomy patient by the enterostomal therapist who personally instructs each patient.

INSTRUCTIONS TO THE PATIENT

The objective of this pamphlet is to teach you to empty the colon completely by an enema. In most adults, the colon when emptied completely does not fill for two days. Therefore, if the emptying is complete, you could expect to have no movement except during enemas that are given every second day. In some patients, the colon fills rapidly, and it is therefore necessary to irrigate the colon every day. We shall help you to decide how often you might irrigate the colon.

Some patients have an "irritable" colon. An irritable colon has cramps and excessive gas formation, and the bowel movements are not always predictable; a movement may occur at any time, particularly after meals, or there may be constipation and no movements. This unpredictable pattern of movements may be a lifelong habit. For such a person, irrigation may not be the best way to manage the colostomy. Perhaps you belong to this group of patients, and you should not irrigate your colostomy. Perhaps you should allow the bowel to move spontaneously; this may occur at fairly regular intervals. Whether or not you are going to control your bowel movements by irrigation will depend on the type of colon you have. However, while you are in the hospital, we are going to acquaint you with the technique of irrigation. You will be using a special apparatus.[M2, M5]

IRRIGATING THE COLOSTOMY

1. Put on the plastic irrigating sleeve, centering the stoma in the middle of the metal ring, and fasten the belt.

2. Fill the water reservoir with 1 quart of warm water and hang it about 5 feet from the floor on a hook (if you are not at home, a hook can be fashioned from a wire coat hanger). Remove all air from the tubing by releasing the shutoff valve and allowing water to run from the bag through the hose and out the tip of the catheter. Lubricate the end of the catheter.

3. Insert your finger into the colostomy and determine in what direction you will be inserting the catheter. Cautiously insert the catheter into the colostomy for 2 inches.

To clean out the lower 5 or 6 inches of colon, never force the catheter into the colostomy but push it gently, feeling your way along with the water running briskly.

4. Refill the enema bag with a quart of water, or more if you wish. After filling the tubing with water, insert the irrigating catheter again. Push the shield or dam tightly against the colostomy so that the water will not leak around the tubing. Allow the water to run slowly. If a cramp develops, stop the flow of water until the cramp passes and then allow more water to flow. Most people can take a little less than a quart of water, but some can take more. When the enema is completed, remove the catheter, and fasten the top of the irrigating sleeve with clips. Note that it is important to get as much water as possible into the colon at the time of irrigation, because this will stimulate the colon to contract and to empty. Too little water gives too little "returns."

Most patients wait about 15 minutes with the plastic drainage sleeve in the toilet. Some of the water will have returned by this time. Fold the bottom of the sleeve up against the top of the apparatus and fasten with clips so that you can leave the bathroom. During the 45 minutes following this first irrigation, most of the water will return.

5. About 45 minutes after you have completed the irrigation, apply the colostomy cap that is in your set. Put some facial tissues inside the cap and place it over the colostomy to catch any extra returns of mucus or water. Now apply a coloplast "safety" pouch[M2] over your colostomy.

Discussion. If you allow the water to run too rapidly into your colon, or if you use too much water, or if the water is too cold, you may feel faint and become sweaty or dizzy. Sometimes vomiting results.

Occasionally, after the water has been run into the colon it will not come out until three or four hours later, and then only in small amounts repeatedly. This means you have an irritable colon. Remember that the colon may only be irritable when you are irritable or apprehensive or worried. It may act normally at other times. We will give you medications to alleviate this condition should it become necessary.

If all the water put into the colon does not return, do not be alarmed, because this water is simply absorbed and in the ensuing hours the bladder will fill and empty more frequently.

You must be careful never to force the catheter up into the colon against an obstacle. You could perforate the colon and cause peritonitis. The colon has no nerves, and consequently perforation does not always produce immediate pain. However, should severe pain develop after a difficult catheter passage, call your own doctor on the telephone. Fortunately, perforations are rare. To prevent this catastrophe you are given a French 24 Foley catheter to use for irrigation. Note that its end is quite soft.

Remember that the entire irrigation procedure is simply a thorough cleansing enema, and some time is required to empty the colon. Do not forget that it takes water to get water. After irrigation the colon must be completely empty or you will surely have unwanted additional bowel movements. Do not be discouraged if you do not promptly learn how to irrigate the colon, as it takes several weeks before one can be considered expert.

VARIATIONS IN IRRIGATING TECHNIQUE

The method of irrigation described above is presented only as a guide; your irrigating technique should be individualized. For example, you may want to start with a pint of water and repeat the insertion of a pint after each return. Or perhaps you would like to use more than a quart of water for the first irrigation, or possibly you would like to put a quart—or pint—in repeatedly following each return. These are some of the variations in techniques.

Occasionally salt or soda may be added to the irrigating water. Some patients add a tablespoonful of salt to each quart of irrigating water.

DIET

You have been supplied with a diet sheet that should be followed for about six weeks after your discharge from the hospital. The diet simply omits foods that cause gas (peas, beans, cabbage, fish) or frequent bowel movements (fruit, fruit juice and vegetables such as green spinach and tomatoes). There may be some other foods that you personally should avoid—you will already be aware of these foods.

Six weeks after your discharge from the hospital, you should return to what you consider a normal diet. You will find that some foods still cause diarrhea or gas, and you may have to omit them permanently.

BATHING

You may take a bath or a shower at any time. The colostomy can be submerged. Do not be alarmed if there is a little bleeding around the edges from time to time. This is natural. Do not try to sterilize the skin around the colostomy with iodine, alcohol, or antiseptic solutions. Treat it as any other part of the body with soap and water. Do not use sterile dressings.

SAFETY POUCHES

We encourage you to wear a small coloplast safety pouch[M2, M6] over your colostomy. This will protect your clothes from mucus or any sudden discharge of stool or enema water.

MANUFACTURERS' INDEX

Reference Number:

1. Atlantic Surgical Company
   1834 Lansdowne
   Merrick, New York 11566   Telephone: (516) TN 8-4545

2. John Greer Company
   5335 College Avenue
   Oakland, California 94618   Telephone: (415) 652-2213

3. Hollister Company, Inc.
   211 E. Chicago Avenue
   Chicago, Illinois 60611   Telephone: (312) 642-2001

4. 3 M Company
   Medical Products Division
   2501 Hudson Road
   St. Paul, Minnesota

5. Marlen Manufacturing &
    Development Company
    5150 Richmond Road
    Bedford, Ohio 44146   Telephone: (216) 292–7060

6. Marsan Manufacturing Co.
    5924 S. Pulaski Road
    Chicago, Illinois 60629   Telephone: (812) RE 5–7461

7. Perma Type Company, Inc.
    P.O. Box 175
    Farmington, Connecticut 06032   Telephone: (203) 521–2244

8. Perry Products
    3803 E. Lake Street
    Minneapolis, Minnesota   Telephone: (612) 722–4783

9. The Torbot Company
    1185 Jefferson Boulevard
    Warwick, Rhode Island 02886   Telephone: (401) 739–2241

10. United Surgical Supplies Co., Inc.
    11775 Starkey Road
    Largo, Florida   Telephone: (813) 392–1261

DRUGS

11. Devrom (bismuth subgallate)

    The Parthenon Company, Inc.
    P.O. Box 11274
    Salt Lake City, Utah 84111   Telephone: (801) 467–4305

12. Lomotil tablets
    Searle Company
    P.O. Box 5110
    Chicago, Illinois 60680

13. Rezifilm, Mycostatin Powder-Kenalog spray
    E. R. Squibb & Sons
    745 Fifth Avenue
    New York, New York 10022

14. Vidrape Adhesive Spray (sterile/tinted)
    Parke, Davis & Company
    Detroit, Michigan 48232

15. Domeboro tablets
    Dome Laboratories
    400 Morgan Lane
    West Haven, Connecticut 06516

TEMPORARY COLOSTOMY DIET

Foods Included	*Foods Excluded*
Cereals	Fruits

Foods Included	*Foods Excluded*
Cream of Wheat, farina, Wheatena, barley, oatmeal, corn flakes, Puffed Rice, Puffed Wheat, Rice Krispies, Shredded Wheat, Muffets.	Fruits in any form, cooked or raw. All fruit juices except nectars.

Breads

<table>
<tr><td>White, refined whole wheat, graham or rye, simple wafers or crackers, arrowroot crackers, melba toast, zwieback, Holland rusk, rolls, muffins, baking powder biscuits, waffles, pancakes.</td><td>Cereals

Those containing bran, such as All bran, 40 per cent Bran Flakes.

Cracked wheat bread; bread, muffins or rolls made with bran; bread or rolls with nuts, dried fruits such as raisins. Muffins made with fruit such as blueberry muffins.</td></tr>
</table>

Eggs

Soft boiled or hard boiled, poached, scrambled, omelet, fried, creamed, or as soufflé.

Soups

Cream soups made of rice, potato, or allowed vegetables. Clear broth or broth with noodles or rice. Strained broth from soups made with vegetables such as corn or mushrooms.	Whole vegetable soups made with other than allowed vegetables. Vegetable juices: V-8, tomato, carrot. Oil and vinegar and cheese salad dressings.

Meats

Beef, lamb, veal, pork, ham, liver, sweetbreads, bacon, domestic rabbit, loose sausage, luncheon meats, chicken, squab, turkey, duck, goose, oysters. Fresh, smoked or canned fish. Meats may be fried, boiled, broiled, or roasted.

Potatoes etc.	Potato skins.
White potatoes—baked, mashed, boiled, creamed, escalloped, or fried, sweet potatoes, spaghetti, noodles, macaroni, rice, hominy.	

Vegetables (cooked),

Asparagus tips, celery hearts, cauliflower tips, squash (no seeds or skins), rutabagas, turnips, puréed beets and carrots. Crisp tender lettuce is the only raw vegetable permitted.	Salads except tender lettuce. Green vegetables such as broccoli, Brussels sprouts, peas, spinach, tomatoes, corn, cabbage, string beans, wax beans, green lima beans, mushrooms, or dried beans. (All these vegetables may be used in puréed form, but produce gas.)

Foods Included	*Foods Excluded*

Desserts

Custards, puddings, plain cakes and cookies, ice cream, gelatin desserts; pastries such as cream puffs; pies such as custard or chocolate cream.

Any dessert containing fruits, nuts, or coconut, such as fruit cake, fruit pies, mincemeat pie, raisin pie, sherbets, fruit whips, coconut cookies.

Beverages

Coffee, tea, Sanka, Kaffe Hag, Postum, milk, milk beverages such as milkshakes, eggnogs and malted milks. Carbonated beverages. Wines and hard liquors are also permitted.

Miscellaneous

Cheese may be used as desired. Any fats as butter, margarine, oils, cooking fats. Smooth peanut butter. Potato chips, pretzels. All seasonings and condiments such as catsup and mustard. Jellies, honey, syrups, molasses and candies. Gravies and white sauce, mayonnaise.

Popcorn. Relishes made of raw vegetables such as piccalilli or pepper hash. Jams and marmalades. Pickles, olives and nuts. Any other foods which you may find will cause diarrhea.

NOTE: The colostomy diet is one of personal management. This diet is a guide in that it shows you which foods are most likely to be tolerated and which ones are not.

SAMPLE MENU

Breakfast:
Cereal
Cream of Wheat

Egg
Poached egg with bacon

Bread
Toast with butter and jelly

Beverage
Coffee, cream and sugar

Luncheon:
Meat or substitute
Cheese soufflé

Potato
Baked potato

Vegetable
Buttered asparagus tips

Bread
Whole wheat bread and butter

Dessert
Ice cream

Beverage
Milk, coffee, or tea, as desired

Dinner:
Soup
Chicken rice soup

Meat
Roast beef with gravy

Potato
Mashed potatoes

Vegetable
Puréed beets (buttered)

Dessert
Plain cake

Beverage
As desired

CHAPTER 21

THE COLON AND RECTUM

Claude E. Welch, M.D., F.A.C.S.

PREOPERATIVE CARE

Pre- and postoperative care of patients who have surgery for colonic or major rectal lesions will vary considerably, depending upon the underlying diagnosis and the presence or absence of complicating factors. The important diseases to be included are tumors, diverticulitis, ulcerative colitis, and volvulus. Less common are traumatic wounds, vascular lesions that vary from bleeding to thrombosis, and rectal prolapse. "Minor" rectal surgery, such as that for hemorrhoids, fistulas, or abscesses, will be discussed later.

In general terms, the major cases may be separated into two large groups; the first includes those with elective operations, and the second those who must have operations before optimal preparation may be possible or as an emergency. In this section attention will be given first to these large general groups, following which comments will be made about specific diseases.

Preoperative Preparation for Elective Procedures on the Colon or Rectum

In these cases opportunity is given for the correction of preoperative abnormalities and the preparation of an empty colon. Whether or not all these preparations need to be carried out in the hospital is questionable. Certainly it is convenient to allow four or five days for this purpose, but economic considerations make it increasingly difficult for a patient to spend more than 48 hours in a hospital prior to operation, so that many of these details may be completed before entry.

The preoperative work-up should include a complete history and

411

physical examination, sigmoidoscopy, pelvic examination in females, barium enema, and urine and blood examinations. Nearly all patients should have an electrocardiogram and x-ray of the chest. Other x-ray studies that are valuable include an intravenous pyelogram whenever there is a lesion near the ureter. Cystoscopy may be required in case there is a suggestion of involvement of the bladder by tumor or fistula.

A number of blood chemistry determinations are necessary in special cases. Potassium levels are particularly important when the patient has had diarrhea from either colitis or a large villous tumor. Furthermore, if a patient is receiving digitalis, the potassium must be kept in a normal range if serious cardiac arrhythmias are to be avoided. Sodium and chloride levels rarely need correction. The prothrombin time may be high in some patients with protracted diarrhea or sepsis; correction is easily obtained in the absence of liver disease by daily intravenous injections of 10 mg. of Hykinone. The serum albumin may be low in patients with ulcerative colitis; daily intravenous injections of 25 gm. of human albumin should be given to bring the level to normal. The blood urea nitrogen (BUN) may be high in some patients and require either catheter drainage of an obstructed urinary tract or appropriate fluids and diuretics if renal function is poor.

In certain instances the patient may have been on cortisone for protracted periods of time. Relatively large doses then must be given prior to, during, and immediately after operation. Our usual method is to give 100 mg. of hydrocortisone intravenously the evening before operation, 100 mg. on the morning of operation, 100 mg. during the course of operation, and 100 mg. later in the same 24-hour period. The dosage is continued at a lower level for the next few days and then gradually cut down to zero in the course of the next 7 to 14 days, substituting prednisone at appropriately adjusted doses as soon as oral intake is feasible.

Many other patients will have been on antihypertensive drugs. Special attention must be given to these patients because they are very prone to show a marked fall in blood pressure during or immediately after operation.

Anemia is the most common abnormality that requires preoperative correction. If a patient has a hematocrit below 35, preoperative transfusions are far more valuable than blood given coincidentally with the operative procedure and will provide a far more stable anesthesia.

The respiratory tract should be investigated carefully. If there is any problem with emphysema or ventilatory insufficiency, pulmonary therapists are introduced as soon as possible and exercises and therapy initiated. If the patients can be made to breathe correctly before operation, they are more likely to be able to continue in the painful postoperative phase.

The local preparation of the colon is designed to produce a clean, empty bowel as free as possible from pathogenic organisms. Although everyone agrees upon the necessity of mechanical preparation, there is no consensus about the use of preoperative antibiotics.

Preferably the patient is put on a low-roughage or liquid diet for three days preoperatively. A mild laxative such as 6 oz. of citrate of magnesia is given daily. Enemas likewise are given daily, with the last one on the night before operation. Barium enemas should be avoided in the last few preoperative days, because they irritate the bowel and if not emptied completely may lead to postoperative barium impaction. With this routine the bowel on the day of operation should be mechanically clean, dry and quiet.

Despite the enormous amount of work that has been done on the antibiotic preparation of the colon and the very clear conclusion from laboratory experiments that control of sepsis can be achieved in such a way, most surgeons now pay relatively little attention to this factor. The unfortunate emergence of staphylococcus enterocolitis a number of years ago with the direct implication of broad-spectrum antibiotics as the causative agent led many surgeons to abandon them. In this brief outline it would be impossible to review the evidence or cite various opinions. However, since this is a personal statement the author will indicate his preference.

I continue to use a four- or five-day preparation of the colon with phthalylsulfathiazole (Sulfathalidine) in a dosage of 2 grams four times daily. This is given in the expectation that no antibiotics will be given postoperatively except for special complications such as pneumonia. In all probability this method of preparation offers very little when the right colon is resected; on the other hand, with low anterior resections theoretically it should be of more value. The clinical studies of Herter and Slanetz would bear out this impression; they were able to find no advantage from preoperative antibiotics in colon surgery except in this one group. Cohn has presented very persuasive arguments for the routine preparation of the colon with kanamycin (1 gm. every hour for four hours, then every six hours for a total of 72 hours).

The immediate preoperative preparation of the patient is carried out on the morning of the procedure. Appropriate shaving at this time rather than on the night before prevents minor skin and hair follicle irritation. A Foley catheter is inserted routinely preoperatively to monitor urinary output and to keep the bladder out of the operative field. A Levin tube is usually passed by the anesthesiologist after the patient is asleep. All patients are monitored during the operation by blood pressure and pulse. A central venous catheter is inserted in poor risk patients or in those in whom a large blood loss is to be expected. Electrocardiograph monitors are often wise. Direct arterial catheterizations are indicated for extensive operations, such as exenterations, in which the frequent determination of blood gases is essential during the operation and immediately thereafter. Elastic stockings are applied prior to the operation.

PREOPERATIVE PREPARATION FOR URGENT OR EMERGENCY OPERATIONS

Such operations make it impossible to carry out careful preparation of the colon. In certain instances there will be no evidence of obstruction or perforation, and in them a rapid preparation may be obtained by the administration of 2 oz. of castor oil on the night prior to operation and the oral administration of 8 gm. of neomycin in divided doses of 2 gm. each during the 12 hours prior to the operative procedure. This will produce an empty bowel that is relatively sterile.

In other instances it will be necessary to operate on a patient as an emergency. Perforation of the colon with general peritonitis will demand vigorous volume replacement, particularly by albumin or plasma, and antibiotics. Our present preference is for large doses of penicillin (up to 10 million units daily) and of chloramphenicol (2 gm. daily) by the intravenous route. Although the latter drug is controversial, the seriousness of the illness calls for its use. Massive hemorrhage will require adequate blood replacement. In both instances it is particularly necessary to monitor the central venous pressure and, if possible, to obtain a urine flow of at least 30 to 40 cc./hour.

Acute colonic obstruction requires urgent operation with comparatively little preparation. If a sigmoid volvulus is the cause, it may be possible to secure decompression by means of a long rectal tube inserted through a sigmoidoscope; in any case a long tube is placed in the rectum to aid in evacuation of the bowel at the time of operation.

POSTOPERATIVE CARE

RESECTIONS OF THE COLON

After a resection and anastomosis for a carcinoma of the colon, the usual postoperative course is smooth. The main problem is that there is always a period of ileus that lasts for a few days. This requires some type of intestinal decompression. My personal preference is for the use of a Levin tube that is maintained until peristaltic sounds are active and some gas has escaped by rectum. Other surgeons prefer a gastrostomy or a cecostomy. Gastrostomy catheters are tolerated better by the patient than Levin tubes but do have the disadvantage that occasionally there may be bleeding from the gastric incision or sepsis owing to some leakage from the opening made for the catheter. A cecostomy catheter is employed by some surgeons after all anastomoses of the left colon. As a routine measure I abandoned this type some 20 years ago chiefly on the basis that it was not necessary in the uncomplicated case and that it sometimes led to a rather persistent fistula and sometimes to a hernia that required secondary operation. On the other hand, such authorities as Sir Naughton Morgan believe very firmly in its routine use; certainly it introduces an additional safety factor and tends to reduce intracolonic tension and prevent anastomotic leaks.

Thus, the usual care after colon resection and anastomosis involves intestinal decompression for four to five days by a Levin tube, intravenous fluids for that period, and then gradual progression to a low-residue diet. The Foley catheter that was inserted into the bladder prior to operation is retained for four to five days. Elastic stockings are put on at the time of the operative procedure. Ambulation is started the day after operation. Antibiotics are not used postoperatively except on special indication. No anticoagulants are employed. Enemas and laxatives are avoided; however, in certain instances if ileus is prolonged after resection of the right colon, small saline instillations in the rectum may be employed after a few days.

The important complications that occur after colon resections include leaking anastomoses, residual abscesses, and intestinal obstruction. Less common are bleeding from the suture line and urinary retention. Thromboembolic manifestations, formerly quite common, now seem to be most unusual.

Leakage from an anastomosis is a rather common occurrence. It seems probable that if barium enema studies were made of sigmoid anastomoses a week after operation, nearly 90 per cent of the patients would show a trivial leak. Fortunately such leaks are of only academic importance. However, in about 10 per cent of the patients there will be a leak that is sufficient to cause clinical symptoms, and in about 5 per cent enough to require active therapy. Leakage is dependent upon several factors. The most important is an anastomosis that is too narrow, either because of the manner in which it was formed or because of postoperative edema or fluid collection around the bowel so that obstruction leads to increased intracolonic tension and perforation. Lack of adequate blood supply or of tension on the anastomosis are also important features. I personally believe that everting anastomoses are more liable to leak than inverting. Inverting anastomoses, however, must be made with great care. Personally I prefer a two-layer anastomosis with an inner layer of interrupted 3-0 chromic catgut and an outer layer of interrupted No. 20 cotton. Silk is used in place of cotton if the suture line is low in the pelvis. With these techniques leaks from anastomoses after resection of the right colon are very rare. Essentially the main problems are those that occur in association with low anterior resections or those in which the anastomosis has been made in a peritoneal cavity previously contaminated by peritonitis or by an abscess. Leakage after right colon anastomoses therefore can nearly always be handled conservatively. However, if there is leakage after a low anterior resection, a transverse colostomy should be carried out. Any attempt to revise the anastomosis or to effect a resuture will be meddlesome and do more harm than good. However, if the colostomy does not relieve the situation rapidly, drainage of the pelvic abscess through an anterior approach may be necessary.

It is important to recognize that if an anastomosis is not technically perfect, it should be protected by a concomitant transverse colostomy or cecostomy.

Postoperative bleeding can produce a number of problems. It is uncommon on the right side, and for this reason there is very little reason to drain the right gutter after such resections. On the left side if there has been a resection of the splenic flexure, there may be bleeding from perisplenic adhesions. In obese patients it is often wise to drain this area primarily. The main problems occur, however, with the low anterior resections. Here our preference is to insert a sump catheter deep into the pelvis at the time of the resection because a pelvic hematoma is an important cause of compression of an anastomosis with obstruction and then leakage. Many surgeons prefer to irrigate the catheter frequently with antibiotics, such as kanamycin solution. The important feature, however, seems to be the removal of any loculated blood. The suction catheter is left in as long as there is drainage. This means it usually can be removed in about four or five days.

Intestinal obstruction furnishes one of the most important complications after resections. Although it is usually due to adhesive bands and plastic adhesions, a much more serious type can occur if a loop of bowel forces its way through a mesenteric trap, around a colostomy, or through a newly constituted pelvic floor. After certain operations on the colon it is impossible to close off all interstices. For example, if the colon has been resected from the distal transverse down to the upper rectum, the lesser omental sac is open and furnishes an opening into which small bowel may intrude. If the small bowel should then pass through the foramen of Winslow from left to right, a strangulating obstruction can be produced. Furthermore, after a left colectomy it is often very difficult to close the mesenteric trap, particularly when the ligament of Treitz is high. Every attempt, however, should be made to do this because herniation in this area is not uncommon. It is well to remember that a wide trap is less likely to produce trouble than one that is inadequately closed. However, even the wide ones can furnish a locus for difficulty. After right colon resections there is no difficulty in closing the mesentery, so that this complication should never occur. If there has been a colostomy or ileostomy, there is a potential trap located lateral to the stoma and this furnishes another site for strangulating obstruction.

In all these instances the surgeon must be aware of this possibility of strangulation, and if the patient has intestinal obstruction together with pain and tenderness in a localized area this diagnosis must be entertained. Usually in these instances peristalsis that was active becomes very quiet. On the other hand, if true obstructive peristalsis is present, the chances are in favor of a nonstrangulating obstruction either from adhesions or bands or perhaps because of a defect in the pelvic floor.

The most difficult problem for the surgeon under these circumstances is to distinguish between a simple paralytic ileus and an actual obstruction. If peristalsis is diminished and the abdomen nontender, paralytic ileus is more likely. In other instances acute mechanical obstruction, either nonstrangulating or strangulating, must be considered strongly. Plain x-rays are of some help but are often very difficult to interpret in this early postoperative phase. Serial plates, however, if not contraindicated by evidence of strangulation, will indicate progression or improvement of the situation. In regional uses, Gastrografin by mouth may clarify the situation.

Because of the high incidence of strangulation in these patients, we are strongly inclined toward operation in any questionable case. We have essentially abandoned long tubes in the treatment of intestinal obstruction and would rely upon Levin tube intubation and reoperation when necessary.

The various *septic complications* that occur after colon resection are essentially all due to leaking anastomoses or to infected hematomas. If they can be avoided, the incidence of residual abscesses becomes very low. Subdiaphragmatic abscesses and pelvic abscesses are essentially the only ones that will require formal drainage. Others do tend to gravitate to the wound and later discharge through it.

Wound sepsis usually requires only a short opening through the incision and evacuation of old blood clot and pus. In some instances the infection may be much more severe and dangerous. Diabetics are especially prone to advancing infections that will require wide opening of the wound down to the fascia. Rarely, pyogenic gangrene may occur; this requires complete excision of the wound and later skin grafts.

The question always arises as to whether or not residual sepsis could be reduced by the use of antibiotic therapy. At the present moment it must be concluded that this problem has not been solved satisfactorily by any studies. Burke's carefully controlled laboratory experiments would indicate that prophylactic antibiotics given prior to operation, at the time of the operation, and immediately postoperatively are of value. Clinical studies are suggestive; for example, Noon et al. found a reduction in postoperative septic complications from 20 to 8 per cent by the use of antibiotics at the time of operation and postoperatively. On the other hand, postoperative antibiotics enhance the dangers from staphylococcus enterocolitis. Personally I do not use postoperative antibiotics as a routine but employ them only for therapeutic indications such as a definite residual infection or pneumonitis. Accurate, well-controlled clinical studies are urgently needed to settle this problem.

Urinary retention is a very common complication in males, particularly after operations on the lower part of the colon. A preoperative urine culture is useful. Since it is much safer to prevent urinary sepsis than to gain control once it has occurred, we prefer to insert a Foley catheter prior to operation in these patients and to leave it in place until it is quite certain that the patient will void. This usually means that patients retain a catheter for about four to five days. If repeated catheterizations can be avoided and the patient is kept on sterile closed drainage, the chances of a urinary tract infection become very low.

Thromboembolism is a threat in the postoperative period. Exercises of the legs are begun as soon as the patient is awake. Early ambulation (usually on the first postoperative day), the use of supportive stockings, better replacement of blood and fluids, and better anesthesia may help to reduce the incidence. A number of years ago prophylactic anticoagulants were employed in these patients. In some institutions this is used on high-risk patients; in others it is used only in patients who have had previous problems with deep thrombophlebitis or with venous disease of the legs.

PROBLEMS ASSOCIATED WITH INTESTINAL STOMAS

Since these are considered in detail elsewhere, only brief mention will be given to them here.

Ileostomies. Most of the problems associated with ileostomies can be avoided if proper technique is employed in the original formation. Peri-ileostomy hernias are avoided by careful closure of the trap lateral to the stoma. This closure likewise essentially prevents ileostomy prolapse. The Brooke technique of fashioning a stoma has entirely eliminated the problems of intestinal obstruction resulting from the obstructing serositis that follows the formation of an unmature ileostomy. Herniation of a loop of adjacent ileum about the ileostomy through the abdominal wall can be avoided by making the incision in the abdominal wall of the proper size. Retraction of the ileostomy with skin irritation can be avoided by making the ileostomy of a proper length.

Consequently, after attention to all these details the care of the postoperative stoma is now a very simple matter. As soon as the stoma is made on the operating table a temporary ileostomy bag is applied. Within two weeks it is possible to apply a permanent bag. In the early postoperative days the main problems that occur are those secondary to skin irritation from adhesive. Fortunately karaya powder will answer most of these problems. In other instances the use of a karaya gum seal, such as is afforded by the Hollister bags, will be necessary.

Colostomies. *Transverse colostomies* are subject to a number of complications that include prolapse and herniation of a loop of small bowel about the stoma. In addition, a loop colostomy may not defunction the bowel completely, so that fecal matter may spill over into the left side and loop colostomies may have to be converted to divided colostomies. A significant amount of prolapse in the early postoperative phase may require an early secondary operation with resection of the involved loop. However, in general terms serious prolapse is quite uncommon and minor degrees of prolapse can be tolerated without any particular difficulty. Retraction is uncommon with a transverse colostomy, although occasionally there will have been such a short mesentery of the transverse colon or so much previous abdominal inflammation that this does occur; operative revision will likewise be necessary for it.

End-sigmoid colostomies are much less likely to prolapse than transverse colostomies. They are more subject to retraction, and if the mucosa does retract below the skin margin, secondary stenosis may occur. This is not prominent in the early postoperative days but may require operative revision within a matter of a few weeks. As this time the stoma can be elevated adequately and the stenosis relieved. Strangulation of a loop of small bowel about a sigmoid colostomy has already been mentioned. Late herniations of small bowel about sigmoid colostomies into the abdominal wall are extremely common. If the patient is obese, prevention of these hernias or a cure once they have occurred is, I think, nearly impossible. Even a transplantation of the stoma to another area of the abdominal wall is likely to be followed by recurrence.

POSTOPERATIVE DIETS

In the usual care, water is given by mouth on the fourth day, with gradual progression to a soft, solid diet in the next three or four days. Thereafter the patient is kept on a low-roughage diet for a month after the resection. This diet restricts the intake of raw fruits and such vegetables as celery and lettuce. If the patient's bowel habit is fairly normal at the end of the month all restrictions may be removed.

After resections of the right colon, diarrhea may be severe and present for months or years. A low-roughage diet then must be continued. The addition of Lomotil (1 or 2 tablets three times daily) is often helpful. Paregoric (1 teaspoonful three times daily) or deodorized tincture of opium (5 to 10 drops three times daily) is more effective. Patients with colostomies require a constipating diet; the habitual use of cheese and the avoidance of high roughage, fruit or juices, and milk will be helpful.

If the patient has been constipated prior to a left colon resection, the same symptoms may return postoperatively. The usual measures are available. Colace or Metamucil and prune juice are valuable as the primary remedies, although stronger laxatives may be necessary in some instances.

SPECIFIC DISEASES

Ulcerative Colitis. Patients with ulcerative colitis or Crohn's disease of the colon are often poor risks because of malnutrition and long preceding courses of cortisone therapy. For these reasons they tolerate operations poorly and often heal slowly with numerous complications. Preoperative replacement of blood and correction of low serum albumin is desirable. When a perforation of the colon has occurred preoperatively, or if the colon at the time of operation is found to be densely adherent, it is well to start large doses of intravenous antibiotics prior to the dissection.

Toxic dilatation of the colon is an uncommon but grave emergency. Our policy is to institute a course of intensive cortisone or ACTH therapy. Unless there is dramatic improvement in 48 hours—which time is devoted to vigorous replacement therapy as well—operation is carried out. A discussion of the operation to be employed is beyond the scope of this paper; however, since most surgeons prefer subtotal or total colectomy, it is obvious that provisions must be made for a difficult and dangerous procedure, and that all measures mentioned above must be used.

Postoperatively, if the patient has been on long cortisone support, this must be continued for several weeks after operation. Appropriate measures must be taken to avoid wound dehiscence. Secondary abscesses, especially in the pelvis, are common and may be difficult to detect. The astonishingly slow healing of perineal wounds after rectal resection for this disease has been noted above.

Cancer of the Colon. The elective treatment of cancer of the colon has been considered in detail above. A few special problems deserve additional comment.

Acute obstruction caused by cancer of the colon can be very serious if the ileocecal valve is competent, for a closed loop is produced and perforation can occur rapidly. For this reason early operation is mandatory. As mentioned above, the procedures of transverse colostomy, or, in some cases, cecostomy, will relieve the obstructed left colon in a simple fashion. Local anesthesia can be used in the very ill patient. In the right colon, however, the proper operation is a one-stage resection and anastomosis. These patients must be prepared rapidly for a major procedure, with provision for adequate blood, plasma and electrolyte replacement.

The situation is critical when the patient has an acute perforation of the colon with general peritonitis. Here the preferable operation is a resection of the perforated segment. Whether or not an immediate anastomosis should be done in such cases must depend upon the operative findings. At any rate, such patients will be extremely ill. Central venous pressure and direct arterial lines are necessary for accurate monitoring. If the CVP is near 0, it should be brought up to 5 or 6 cm. of water prior to operation.

It must be remembered that patients with peritonitis are particularly vulnerable to pulmonary complications because of the combination of shock, infection, and elevated diaphragms, and perhaps to some unidentified factor in circulating blood, as outlined by Clowes et al. Therefore, these monitors must be continued for a least three to four days after operation. If the CVP rises to a high level, such as 15 to 20 cm. of water, and the PaO_2 falls concomitantly, pulmonary congestion is certain even though the physical examination and x-ray indicate that the lungs are normal. Small repeated doses of Lasix are essential. Ethyl ethacrinic acid is also effective but may lead to deafness even in small doses.

Diverticulitis. Postoperative problems that accompany the surgical treatment of diverticulitis are numerous. Many of them can be avoided if staged procedures are used for patients who have emergency operations for perforation, obstruction, or large inflammatory masses. However, even after elective resection the course is not always smooth. Intestinal obstruction, anastomotic leaks, residual abscesses, refistulization into the bladder at the site of a previous fistula, and late anastomotic stenosis may be cited as examples.

It is impossible to discuss the treatment of all these complications in a brief summary. However, it may be said that if an elective resection for diverticulitis has proved to be difficult and the anastomosis is less than satisfactory, then a concomitant transverse colostomy should be made at the time of the original operation. By the same token, if anastomotic problems appear a few days after a one-stage resection and anastomosis of the sigmoid colon, an early transverse colostomy is essential. The postoperative course is bound to be slow. Complete defunction of the colon will be necessary for several weeks. Colostomy closure is deferred until barium enema studies show an intact, nonobstructed anastomosis.

The problems attendant upon perforated diverticulitis with general peritonitis are very serious. Massive doses of antibiotics, accurate replacement of blood, plasma, and electrolytes, and special care of the ventilatory tract are essential.

Acute massive hemorrhage can progress to the point of exsanguination, particularly in old patients. Since the preferable operation is often subtotal colectomy, rapid preparation must be made for an extensive emergency procedure.

Volvulus. Volvulus of the colon leads rapidly to circulatory impairment and gangrene in many cases. However, if the sigmoid is involved and deflation can be secured with the sigmoidoscope and rectal tube, laparotomy is deferred, providing that the patient has no signs of vascular occlusion. Volvulus of the cecum requires rapid preparation and immediate operation.

Rectal Prolapse. *Massive rectal prolapse* is never an emergency. Selection of the type of operation to be employed may be difficult, since many of these people are old. However, time for adequate elective operation is always available. Temporary reduction of the prolapse meanwhile may be maintained by tight compressive bandages.

RESECTIONS OF THE RECTUM

Several special postoperative problems occur after resections for cancer of the rectum. The most important are intestinal obstruction, bleeding from the perineal wound, and urinary retention. The most serious is that of intestinal obstruction. It may be due to adhesions (posteriorly in the low pelvis), to strangulation of a loop of small intestine lateral to the colostomy, or to prolapse of a loop of small bowel through the newly constituted pelvic floor.

I firmly believe that the lowest incidence of intestinal obstruction will be obtained if a lateral colostomy is made and the trap lateral to it is closed; furthermore the pelvic peritoneum should be closed in two layers and the retroperitoneal space drained widely through the perineum. Some surgeons have left the peritoneum wide open and inserted a Mikulicz pack through the perineum against the small bowel. Others leave the peritoneum open, close the perineal skin, and evacuate any hematoma by suction.

Because prolapse of a loop of intestine lateral to the stoma or through the peritoneal floor produces a strangulating obstruction, early reoperation is desirable whenever the diagnosis of intestinal obstruction is made after a combined abdominoperineal resection. In questionable cases radiologic studies with Gastrografin may make the diagnosis clear.

Urinary retention is apt to be very serious after a combined abdominoperineal resection. If the operation has been done for cancer in males, one may expect that spontaneous voiding will essentially never be regained before ten to twelve days. Nearly a quarter of all patients will require prolonged urinary tract drainage, and this must often be combined with a transurethral resection. Catheter drainage is continued until the residual urine is under 100 cc.

Secondary abscesses in the retroperitoneal area can be avoided by wide drainage. Wide drainage is particularly desirable in patients who have had resections of the rectum for ulcerative colitis in which there is a great deal of perirectal inflammation. Primary closure with suction drainage in the hands of those who have attempted it has not led to good results.

The slowly healing perineal incision after rectal resections for ulcerative colitis furnishes one of the greatest problems for the surgeon. There has been no way to eliminate this complication. Eventually these incisions will close, but it may take five years or so in recalcitrant cases. Repeated curettages and irrigations with antibiotic and fungicidal solutions may be helpful.

"Minor" Surgical Procedures on the Rectum

Hemorrhoids and minor degrees of prolapse require special consideration. Preoperatively the colon should be emptied, preferably by an enema on the morning of operation. Though most of the incisions after hemorrhoidectomy heal nicely, there is no point in inviting disaster by operating on a patient with acute diarrhea or with an acute extensive thrombosis. These should be controlled with appropriate measures so that the operative field is as free of edema and as noninfected as possible.

Postoperatively, the usual patient is given Demerol, 100 mg. every three hours as necessary, deodorized tincture of opium, 10 mg. three times daily, and a liquid diet. Warm perineal packs are very comforting and are started two to three days after operation. On the third postoperative evening a mild laxative such as milk of magnesia is given. On the following morning, if there is no bowel movement, an oil retention followed by a tap water enema is given. Thereafter the patient is discharged from the hospital. The mild discomfort that he has thereafter can be reduced by witch hazel compresses ("Tucks") or ointment. The first digital examination is made in the office about ten days after operation.

The important complications of hemorrhoidectomy are undue pain, hemorrhage, infection, and residual skin tags. Pain can essentially be eliminated by the use of long-lasting local anesthetics in an oil base; however, since these injections may produce local abscesses, they have been eliminated. However, a perineal procaine injection at the time of operation can reduce the need for excessive amounts of analgesics in the early postoperative period. Nevertheless, the postoperative patient may require generous analgesics so that morphine or Pantopon in large doses may be required in the first 48 hours.

Infection, though uncommon, can be very serious. Pylephlebitis has been reported, and local abscesses may lead to a fistula. Broad-spectrum antibiotics are indicated if there is a rise in temperature associated with local signs of inflammation. A local abscess in the hemorrhoidal bed may require internal drainage.

Although hemorrhage should never be of serious significance, it can be extremely troublesome if there is an associated proctitis. Secondary suture is usually necessary. If this fails, packing of the rectal ampulla with Gelfoam and gauze is required. Minor bleeding about seven days after operation is not uncommon as the gut sutures disintegrate; spontaneous cessation is the rule.

Urinary retention is common postoperatively, particularly in males. It is advisable to deflate the bladder with an inlying Foley catheter and closed drainage before overdistention occurs.

Residual skin tags are not uncommon. They are bothersome from the point of view of cleanliness. They tend to diminish in size with time. At the end of six months if they are still prominent they may be removed in the office under Novocain anesthesia.

Anal fissures, fistulas, and perianal abscesses pose essentially the same problem in pre- and postoperative care. Any packs that are inserted in these incisions are usually removed in three days after several sitz baths. Postoperative examinations must be frequent enough to insure healing from the depths of the operative incision and to avoid skin bridging over the top.

The complications of postoperative stenosis and of fecal incontinence that follow any of these operations are nearly always due to operative technique rather than to the original diseases. Posthemorrhoidectomy stenosis often follows the Whitehead operation and may occur after any operation in which too wide an excision of mucous membrane and skin is carried out. Any operation in which the external or internal sphincter is cut may lead to incontinence; hence this maneuver is avoided except when necessary to cure the disease.

REFERENCES

Burke, J. F.: Effective period of preventive antibiotic action in experimental incisions and dermal lesions. Surgery 50:161, 1961.

Clowes, G. H A., Jr., Vucinic, M., and Weidner, M. G.: Circulatory and metabolic alterations associated with survival or death in peritonitis: Clinical analysis of 25 cases. Ann. Surg. 163:866, 1966.

Cohn, I., Jr.: Value of antibiotic preparation of large bowel; in Ingelfinger, F. J., Relman, A. S., and Finland, M. (eds.): Controversy in Internal Medicine. Philadelphia, W. B. Saunders Co.., 1966.

Cohn, I., Jr.: Intestinal antisepsis. Surg. Gynec. & Obst. 130:1006, 1970.

Hedberg, S. E., and Welch, C. E.: Suppurative peritonitis with major abscesses; in Hardy, J. D. (ed.): Critical Surgical Illness. Philadelphia, W. B. Saunders Co., 1971.

Herter, F. P., and Slanetz, C. A.: Influence of antibiotic preparation of bowel on complications after colon resection. Am. J. Surg. 113:165, 1967.

Noon, G. P., Beall, A. C., Jr., Jordan, G. L., Jr., Riggs, S., and De Bakey, M. E.: Clinical evaluation of peritoneal irrigation with antibiotic solution. Surgery 62:73, 1967.

Parks, A. G.: New concepts in hemorrhoidectomy; in Welch, C. E. (ed.): Advances in Surgery, Vol. 5. Chicago, Year Book Medical Publishers, Inc., 1971.

Tyson, R. R., and Spaulding, E. H.: Antibiotic preparation of bowel—a chimera; in Ingelfinger, F. J., Relman, A. S., and Finland, M. (eds.): Controversy in Internal Medicine. Philadelphia, W. B. Saunders Co., 1966.

CHAPTER 22

THE GYNECOLOGIC PATIENT

HOWARD ULFELDER, M.D., F.A.C.S.

Gynecologic surgery has the reputation of being less difficult, safer, and better tolerated than the average. Because neither the genital organs nor their neighboring pelvic structures are immediately vital to the patient's continued survival, this may in one sense be correct. And it is certainly true that women appraise the discomforts and risks of operation more realistically than do men. These facts notwithstanding, gynecologic surgery is endowed with no special immunity from the risks of surgery in general; to embark on it with any other understanding is unfair to the patient in both the moral and legal senses of the word.

The initial appraisal of a patient establishes the need for surgical treatment and then goes on to evaluate accurately all anatomic, endocrine and functional deficiencies and such other items as may be necessary to calculate the risks of confinement to hospital and to bed, and of exposure to anesthesia, surgical trauma, and the customary drugs used in these circumstances. Major curtailment of studies will sometimes be dictated in situations in which delay appears to be hazardous, but this should never be condoned for reasons of expense or inconvenience, or in an effort to minimize to the patient the procedure contemplated. The emotional implications of all surgery, indeed of all illness, have long been clearly recognized. Nowhere are these psychic overtones more audible than in gynecologic surgery. Experience suggests that a stance on the part of the physician which clearly conveys reassurance, concern, honesty, and kindness is most effective in this regard. One should avoid both intimacy, always treacherous, and compassion, that sadly overstressed quality which can be legitimately claimed only by one's closest relatives and the occasional mystic.

425

INDICATIONS FOR OPERATIONS

Simple curettage of the uterine cavity and biopsy of the cervix is one of the most common operating room procedures in the world. Indications may be diagnostic or therapeutic, often both. The easy access to uterus, cervix, and vagina which the normal anatomy offers makes it possible to investigate with safety and certainty all cases of unusual discharge or bleeding, erosion or ulceration, gross menstrual irregularity, hemorrhage, or of cytological suspicion. When the indications are equivocal, and when hospitalization seems more costly in time and money than the circumstances would justify, a less comprehensive but eminently satisfactory evaluation can be made by endometrial sampling, Schiller testing and cervix biopsy done without anesthesia in the office examing room. Even when the indications are for hospitalization, these office findings will often enable one to complete studies in hospital quickly and efficiently by pointing the way to the probable ultimate cause of symptoms.

Surgery today is the treatment of choice for most pelvic neoplasms, cystic or solid, particularly when they are producing symptoms or suggest the possibility of malignant disease. Surgery is indicated for the control of hemorrhage, internal or external, and to eradicate infection when it manifests itself as undrained abscess or unresolving adnexal mass. Surgery may be invoked to correct anatomic aberrations, sometimes congenital, sometimes acquired and producing deformity, infertility, or weakness with herniation. Finally surgery may be necessary to deal with a variety of the complications of pregnancy.

PROCEDURES BEFORE ADMISSION TO HOSPITAL

Often the indications for an elective operation may be clear and unequivocal. Nevertheless, there are several excellent reasons why much of the preliminary study is better accomplished before the patient enters the hospital. These are first of all financial and secondly psychological (in recognition of the fact that it gives the patient time to assimilate and accept the recommendations of the physician). Finally, this preadmission interval may be of direct benefit to both patient and physician by bringing to light important facts which might be overlooked or underrated during the pressure of preparation for surgery after hospitalization.

No single item of past history, for example, is likely to be more helpful than the findings and procedures of previous operations. The time needed to acquire this information is often much longer than anticipated, and one is tempted again and again to proceed without these facts. Time also is needed to summon and review x-rays, laboratory reports, and the pathological and cytological slides on which present and future decisions must be based. Known allergies and untoward reactions to previous medications, as well as a complete list of recent and current drugs taken by the patient, may truly be of lifesaving importance to her during and after operation.

Both the patient and her husband must understand the diagnosis and the nature of the surgery contemplated and be able to discuss its possible effect on fertility, coitus, and the menopause. Their true physical marital relationship and their hopes for future childbearing must be clearly understood. The timing of operation in relation to the menstrual cycle, the length of hospital stay and its costs are all legitimate points for inquiry and demand serious and honest replies.

Pre-admission blood chemistries and urine and hematologic analysis will vary from one case to the next. The customary warning to medical students to be watchful for the unsuspected presence of lues, tuberculosis, or blood dyscrasia must, in gynecology, also include unsuspected pregnancy. Here too, timing is a consideration since some studies take longer, and some, if abnormal, will suggest additional procedures. Thoroughness must be tempered with constant concern for avoidance of the unnecessary, not only for thrift's sake but also in recognition that no unit in our medical care system is more grossly overutilized than the clinical laboratory.

PREOPERATIVE HOSPITAL CARE

Surgery exposes the organism to injury: incisive, contusive, bacterial, chemical, and psychological. The tolerable range of insult varies widely, and this compels us to keep all trauma to the absolute minimum. Anticipation of the untoward event is the hallmark of the surgeon whose patients "always do well," and this practice had better by far be learned by attention to precept than by tragic personal experience.

Anesthesia. Whenever possible, the anesthesiologist should see the patient and her record preoperatively; if any unusual features exist, such consultation is mandatory. An adequate pulmonary vital capacity and a free, dry airway must be obtained in all cases no matter what method of anesthesia is planned, and the physicians must know to what extent these may be compromised by chronic parenchymal pulmonary or bronchial disease, by skeletal deformity or rigidity, by such habits as smoking or by upper gastrointestinal obstruction with the stomach not empty despite fasting.

Known intolerance to certain classes of drugs, sensitivities or physiologic deficiencies which modify the patient's ability to accept medication in customary dosage must be known to the anesthesiologist. Excessive and habitual consumption of alcohol, even without demonstrable liver damage, will modify the patient's responses sufficiently to interfere with satisfactory anesthesia and surgery if not appreciated ahead of time.

Blood Loss. Gynecologic surgery, particularly by the vaginal approach, often does not lend itself to meticulous technical hemostasis. It is required, therefore, in all cases that preoperative serum iron and hemoglobin levels and blood volumes be up to normal. Compatible blood for transfusion should be on the hospital premises near the operating room before operation begins. Any suspicion of bone marrow disease or of bleeding diathesis must be investigated.

Infection. The field of gynecologic surgery is usually contaminated with microorganisms which experience has shown cannot be eradicated by any amount of antibiotic preparation or mechanical cleansing. In the patient with recent sepsis or with active ulceration of vagina or cervix, cultures must be made a sufficient time before surgery to detect the presence of pathogenic organisms and to defend the patient with appropriate measures. In the usual clean case, as in surgery in other sites, sepsis will not complicate recovery unless hematoma or a devitalized clump of tissue lies fallow in the depths of the wound.

It is always a mistake to perform hysterectomy in the presence of necrotic tissue in the cervix. Pelvic abscess, wound abscess or peritonitis will follow with predictable regularity, and it is this sequence of events that for many years discouraged surgery for cancer of the cervix. In similar fashion the recently conized cervix is an indication for delay; and hysterectomy for prolapsed and gangrenous submucous fibroid is to all intents impossible without septic complications unless the necrotic fibroid is removed from below at a separate and preceding operation.

The indications for preoperative antibiotic therapy are the same as those for general surgery. It is not demonstrably of benefit unless pathogenic organisms are already present or when gross contamination with bowel flora is anticipated.

Urinary Tract. Whenever the patient's complaints include urinary dysfunction it is advisable to determine preoperatively if the urine is infected, whether the bladder fills and empties normally, and the efficiency of bladder neck control. Studies in this direction vary from the simplest to the most complex and must include consultation with a urologist when diagnosis and treatment are not manifest and straightforward. The goal is to identify associated or independent urinary tract disease and its implications for the proper management of the gynecologic problem.

Intestinal Tract. Special preparation is indicated only when the surgeon suspects the possibility that the bowel will need to be entered during the course of operation. In this case the procedure will follow the plan outlined in this manual in the chapters on intestinal surgery.

Otherwise, ordinary considerations only should be our guide, designed chiefly to send the patient to the operating room with the stomach empty and the intestines clean of bulky contents and collapsed.

Psychologic Preparation. Usually the patient's unquestioning faith in her doctors outweighs the need for other, more subtle forms of psychologic preoperative support. Ordinary consideration dictates that the surgeon not make himself so inaccessible that the patient and her family interpret his attitude as unfeeling or disinterested. The nature of the disorder and the surgery anticipated, its immediate and remote effects, and many other pertinent matters will usually need further discussion.

The possibility of cancer often presents itself urgently at this time, even when the indications are completely absent, and the physician's handling of this question may be setting the stage and tone for his most important future dealings with the patient and her family. The hospital environment must be supportive and efficient, and attention focused on the need to inspire the patient with relaxed confidence, with the help of sedatives if necessary.

CARE OF THE PATIENT IN THE OPERATING ROOM

Measures to Protect the Patient. Everyone concerned with the handling of the patient in the operating room needs to be reminded from time to time that she is insensible and unresponsive while under anesthesia. Even so simple an affair as cutting the adhesive strap that has held an armboard in place has resulted in lacerations when skin folds raised by the adherent were unwittingly caught by the scissors.

Prolonged holding of the patient in an awkward position, particularly if joints are hyperflexed or overextended, must be avoided. In gynecology the lithotomy position is always used during the initial examination and catheterization and is the preferred position for the patient during vaginal operation. It is advisable to plan the disposition of the patient on the table before anesthesia is induced to avoid unnecessary lifting and moving or rearrangements of the mattress sections on the operating table.

Most leg holders nowadays are designed to maintain the thighs flexed and abducted by slings which clasp only the feet and ankles. This avoids prolonged pressure from metal parts on the calves or popliteal areas.

As a general rule the intravenous running during gynecologic surgery cannot be located in a leg vein and there are obvious reasons why it should not be. The arm with the needle in it should be extended on a board, although some surgeons find this cramps their space a bit. Leaving the arm at the patient's side under the drapes not only makes the site of injection invisible and inaccessible but also tends to tug on the roots of the branchial plexus on that side, particularly when the table is inclined and the patient's head is bent or turned sharply the other way. For similar reasons most surgeons have abandoned trying to use shoulder braces even in extreme Trendelenburg position.

For laparotomy the abdomen and pubes will have been recently washed and shaved. Although depilatories offer the theoretical advantage of avoiding skin damage and the contamination with bacteria from these tiny wounds, no product has yet appeared which is completely effective, bland, and acceptable to both patients and nurses. In the operating room the area of incision will be prepared and draped as carefully as for any sterile procedure; the adherent transparent drapes now widely available mold themselves admirably to this location.

In the lithotomy position, solutions used to prepare the skin and vagina will run down the intergluteal fold and puddle between the sacrum and the mattress. Annoying blistering or even ulceration of the skin can result unless solutions are selected with care and a temporary towel, placed under the patient at the start, is removed when the cleansing is concluded.

Measures to Facilitate the Surgery. The usual position of the patient for pelvic laparotomy is flat on her back with the table flexed slightly at her knees. This helps relax the rectus abdominis muscles and keeps the foot of the table lower when it is placed in Trendelenburg position. For vaginal surgery, the lithotomy position usually offers the best exposure, but occasionally the knee-chest position gives easier access. When both abdominal and perineal exposure is desirable, it is possible with proper equipment to position and drape the patient with hips slightly flexed and widely abducted.

There is a widespread tendency today to send patients to the operating room with indwelling catheters and immediately proceed with laparotomy. The advantages cannot outweigh the loss of information which is available when pelvic and rectal examination is done under anesthesia and if curettage is performed. These are particularly useful in cases in which the uterus is to be spared. Similarly at laparotomy, when the peritoneum is first opened in clean cases, gentle exploration of all the accessible abdominal space may disclose facts of major significance not discoverable in any other way.

Extended surgical procedures for the care of pelvic cancer or of complicated fistulas are well established and must be recognized for the physical demand they make of both patient and surgeon. The sum total of benefits accruing from attention to every small detail will, in operations like these which extend in their definitive stage over a period of hours, contribute heavily to the outcome. The position of the lights, the height of the operating table, the immediate availability of unusual instruments or supplies, yes, even the relationship between the surgeon and his assistant or anesthetist, are items for consideration in this situation.

The Recovery Room. No recent innovation has helped the surgical patient more than her postoperative sojourn in a well-staffed, well-equipped recovery room. The gynecologic patient is just as likely to develop sudden airway obstruction, cardiac arrhythmia, and a host of lesser problems in which prompt recognition and aggressive resuscitation can completely and quickly restore the normal state of affairs.

Our patients are more likely than others to show an unexpected drop in blood pressure postoperatively. This may reflect misjudgment of the amount of blood loss and underreplacement, but often it is not associated with sweating or a faster pulse rate. In this case it is quite likely to follow surgery in the lithotomy position and may be avoided if the legs are wrapped before being brought down out of stirrups and if they are lowered in stages rather than abruptly.

As the patient is transferred to the recovery room, both written orders and verbal explanations must clearly indicate the nature of the case and its special problems, the likelihood of shock, of overt or occult bleeding or of other discharge. All tubes and drains should be identified and their proper functioning checked after the patient is settled in bed. Special note must be taken of those which must never be allowed to obstruct or the reverse. In unusual or complex circumstances one of the surgical team will do well to recheck these points and the patient's general condition within a short time.

When at the conclusion of an operation the condition of the patient is so critical that it seems wiser not to move her, or when the probability of immediate re-exploration is high, it is customary to leave her on the operating table. This can be moved to the recovery room or intensive care unit if one is adjacent.

It should be remembered that many women recall their stay in the recovery room with horror. Apparently the sights and sounds accentuate the feeling of helplessness which bothers everyone as consciousness is regained. For this reason, among others, stay in the recovery room should end as soon as condition permits.

POSTOPERATIVE CARE OF THE GYNECOLOGIC PATIENT

Care of the Wound. Clean wounds, closed without drainage, appear to be most comfortable with no dressing over them at all. The gauze applied in the operating room can be removed and left off the next day. With stay sutures or superficial drains, this may be too messy and with deep drains or sump tubing the volume of drainage makes some form of absorbent dressing always necessary. When suction catheters are used to keep subcutaneous or retroperitoneal pockets empty, it may work out best if the patient reclines without dressings under a cradle which keeps the bedding away from her body below the chest. This permits inspection of the wound whenever desired and lets atmospheric pressure work evenly to keep skin flaps in place.

Care of the Bladder.   Postoperative dysfunction is completely unpredictable but must be anticipated, particularly after surgery from the vaginal approach. Our prime concern is to prevent episodes of overdistention by the use of catheterization, either indwelling or as needed. The choice in each case will depend on the operation, the personality of the patient and her tolerance for discomfort, and perhaps more than anything on the quantity and quality of nursing care available.

No regimen ever described proposing to hasten re-establishment of normal emptying has stood the test of time, nor has any treatment other than extended constant drainage been necessary in the infrequent situation in which initiation of spontaneous voiding is delayed far beyond the normal interval. It is today a simple matter to send the patient home with a Foley catheter in her bladder connected to an inconspicuous thigh urinal bag of plastic with instructions to cut the catheter and let it slide out about four hours before she is due to be seen in the office two or three weeks after discharge. In this way her ability to void without difficulty, or a residual over 50 to 75 ml., can be checked at that time and the catheter left out if this is the case.

Attention in recent years has again been focused on the risks of catheterization. Certainly one must have good reasons for any catheterization and when it is repeated or constant some form of urinary tract antibiotic should be given for at least a week after it is discontinued. Another approach to the question is offered by the use of percutaneous suprapubic cystostomy for continuous bladder decompression. Modern siliconized plastic tubing such as that used for infant feeding catheters can be passed into the bladder through a large bore (No. 17) needle plunged directly into the fluid-filled organ. The needle is withdrawn and the catheter fixed to the skin with little chance of kinking or obstructing. Antiseptic care of the puncture site and the connecting points in the drainage system almost guarantees that bacterial contamination of the urine will not occur, at least over the course of a week or so. Another advantage is that voluntary voiding can be tested and the residual measured without removing the catheter until it can be dispensed with altogether.

Sepsis, Thrombosis and Embolism.   These are the major preventable complications. They will occur least often to the patient of the surgeon who constantly monitors his own technique for gentleness, hemostasis and thoroughness of debridement. Most important is his awareness that complications can and will occur and that the only serious error he can make is to refuse to recognize the early signs and symptoms and to delay proper treatment.

There is no doubt that the encouragement of active physical exercise with deep breathing, turning in bed and standing up or walking, together with the use of foot boards, elastic stockings and anticoagulant drugs in selected cases, has reduced the incidence of venous thrombosis and embolism.

Stages of Recovery. Wound pain, thirst, nausea and apprehension are the major preoccupations for the first few hours after surgery. By the next day it is usually possible in gynecologic patients to substitute sedatives for some opiates and to allow sips of clear liquids. Although the majority can move up the diet scale quite rapidly thereafter as everyone's anxiety to end intravenous supplementation goads them along, it is advisable in all to withhold full oral nourishment until peristaltic sounds are normal and distention has subsided. Evacuation of the colon usually resumes spontaneously about four or five days after surgery, but it simplifies matters if mild catharsis or a small enema is used the first time.

The choice of time and procedure for removal of sutures is the prerogative of each surgeon, and so is the length of time before discharge from the hospital. Most people, once their discomfort subsides and their self-confidence returns, are anxious to return to the security of their normal routine.

Program After Leaving the Hospital. The surgeon's responsibility to his patient does not end until she is back in full harness (often quite literally true). Her instructions when leaving the hospital must define the rate of resumption of activities with specific dates for going up and down stairs, driving a car and having intercourse. She must be told whether to wear a girdle, if douching is permitted, what to do if constipated, when vaginal discharge may be expected and, if menstruation will resume, when this will be and when conception is a possibility. Finally, a date must be set for a postoperative office examination by a doctor familiar with her hospital course and able to make a final appraisal as she resumes her full normal life pattern.

REFERENCES

Parsons, L., and Ulfelder, H.: An Atlas of Pelvic Operations. 2nd Ed. Philadelphia, W. B. Saunders Co., 1968, 448 pp.

Te Linde, R. W., and Mattingly, R. F.: Operative Gynecology. 4th Ed. Philadelphia, J. B. Lippincott, 1970, 874 pp.

CHAPTER 23

THE SPLEEN AND ITS DISORDERS

Walter F. Ballinger, M.D.

INTRODUCTION

Knowledge of splenic disorders has become of increasing importance to the modern-day surgeon. As the indications for splenectomy have extended, primarily for hematologic disease, more and more surgeons are required to have an understanding of these indications. The disorders of the spleen that may respond well to splenectomy are (1) certain hematologic diseases, (2) rupture, (3) cysts, (4) torsion of an ectopic spleen, (5) splenic artery aneurysms, (6) abscesses and (7) primary neoplasms. Hematologic diseases and rupture of the spleen account for over 95 per cent of all splenectomies.

ANATOMY, PHYSIOLOGY AND PATHOPHYSIOLOGY

The normal adult spleen is a highly vascularized organ, composed of a specialized capillary bed interposed between the splenic artery and the portal venous system. The splenic pulp is composed of the red pulp, which contains splenic cords and sinuses, and the white pulp, which consists of aggregations of lymphocytes, plasma cells and macrophages, together with a variety of other cells which are distributed throughout a reticular network. There is an ill-defined marginal zone between the red and white pulp which may contain many or no cellular elements of blood. Foreign materials are preferentially sequestered in this area.

Approximately 350 liters of blood flow through the human adult spleen per day by a variety of different pathways. Normal cells usually pass quickly through the organ, whereas abnormal cells, or normal cells in an abnormal stream, may be sequestered or removed from the circulation. Under normal conditions, only a few cells are filtered, probably reflecting the efficiency with which the normal bone marrow produces cells of standard size and shape. After splenectomy, the appearance of a considerable number of abnormal cells or cellular elements, such as target cells, siderocytes, Heinz bodies and Howell-Jolly bodies, attests to the filtering function of the normal spleen. Postsplenectomy thrombocytosis is also a regularly occurring phenomenon seen following removal of an abnormal or a normal spleen. The platelet count will start to rise a few days after splenectomy and may reach one million cells or more per cubic millimeter. A modest temporary leukocytosis is also observed after splenectomy. It is primarily due to an increased number of lymphocytes and appears to be higher and more prolonged than after other surgical procedures. It is of no known clinical significance, except that it may confuse the picture in a postoperative infection. Changes in the physical structure or surface composition of blood elements, such as occurs in congenital hemolytic anemia, will greatly impede their transit through the spleen. The sequestration of cells does not necessarily mean their destruction. However, the delay in transit gives the reticuloendothelial tissue time to phagocytize abnormal blood elements, aged cells, abnormal cellular granules, and foreign matter, and to further age cells with a weakened membrane.

The reticuloendothelial cells in the adult spleen are involved in the normal production of monocytes, lymphocytes and plasma cells. Hematopoiesis of the other blood elements occurs in the fetal spleen, but normally stops between the sixth and eighth months of gestation. Apparently, after that, hematopoietic stem cells remain in the spleen in a dormant state, but can be reactivated after a prolonged and intense demand for blood cell formation. This extramedullary hematopoiesis is apparently carried out in a less favorable environment than in the bone marrow, because there is often cell death in situ and premature release of early erythroid and myeloid cells. The mature cells are characterized by a great deal of anisocytosis and poikilocytosis. Megakaryocyte fragments and giant platelets are often observed. However, it is possible that this dyshematopoiesis is related to the underlying disease process, rather than to extramedullary hematopoiesis, per se. Thus, for example, in myeloid metaplasia, the abnormal proliferation of the primitive mesenchymal precursors from which the hematopoietic system takes origin, leads to an overgrowth of connective tissue in the bone marrow and reactivation of marrow stem cells in the spleen and liver and might explain the close association of polycythemia vera, myeloid metaplasia and myelogenous leukemia.

Antibodies are normally produced by cells within the spleen. Splenectomy can lead to a slight temporary reduction in antibody formation. In acquired hemolytic anemia, splenic neutropenia and idiopathic thrombocytopenic purpura, antibodies to specific cellular elements are produced. Splenectomy then will not only remove an organ designed to sequester antibody-coated cells, but will also reduce antibody production, at least temporarily.

HYPERSPLENISM

Hypersplenism is the inappropriate sequestration and destruction of blood elements, with reduction in circulating red blood cells, white blood cells or platelets. Primary hypersplenism includes a group of diseases in which the spleen becomes hypertrophic in response to a sustained and heavy workload (Table 23-1). In these conditions, the abnormal cells or platelets are removed so efficiently that the resulting cytopenia becomes of greater concern than the presence of the abnormal cells. Secondary hypersplenism includes a group of diseases (Table 23-1) in which an enlarged spleen leads to increased destruction of normal or abnormal blood cells or platelets. Secondary hypersplenism can thus be caused by primary hypersplenism, by inflammation, by congestion, by ingestion of macromolecular colloids, or by infiltration of normal or abnormal cells. It must be emphasized that splenomegaly is not always associated with hypersplenism (e.g., splenic cysts or some cases of infectious mononucleosis) and conversely, pancytopenia may be associated with splenomegaly without being caused by it (e.g., bone marrow failure with secondary extramedullary hematopoiesis). Many diseases involve both bone marrow and spleen, and it is of importance in patients with cytopenia and splenomegaly to establish a diagnosis of hypersplenism and adequately evaluate bone marrow function before splenectomy is considered.

Diagnostic Evaluation of Hypersplenism. The decision to perform a therapeutic splenectomy depends upon an accurate assessment of both the size of the spleen and the degree of hypersplenism. An

Table 23-1. CLASSIFICATION OF POTENTIAL
HYPERSPLENIC DISORDERS

I. *Primary Hypersplenism*
  A. Congenital hemolytic anemia: Hereditary spherocytosis or elliptocytosis, pyruvate-kinase deficiency, hemoglobinopathies, thalassemia, porphyria hematopoietica
  B. Acquired hemolytic anemia
  C. Idiopathic thrombocytopenic purpura
  D. Primary splenic neutropenia
  E. Primary splenic pancytopenia

II. *Secondary Hypersplenism*
  A. Inflammation
    1. Acute: Typhoid, rubella, chickenpox, septicemia, etc.
    2. Chronic: Malaria, tuberculosis, sarcoidosis, syphilis, parasitic and fungal diseases, "collagen" diseases, etc.
  B. Congestion: Cirrhosis, congestive heart failure, portal or splenic vein obstruction
  C. Ingestion: Amyloidosis, Gaucher's disease, etc.
  D. Infiltration
    1. "Benign": Mononucleosis, compensatory hematopoiesis
    2. "Neoplastic": Lymphoma (Hodgkin's disease), leukemia, agnogenic myeloid metaplasia, etc.

---

enlarged spleen can usually be demonstrated by careful physical examination, x-ray examination or radioisotopic scanning. Splenomegaly can result in significant dullness to percussion at or above the left ninth intercostal space. Bimanual examination, with the left side of the patient tilted upward, will often differentiate between an enlarged spleen (with its typical notch) from the left lobe of the liver, a pancreatic cyst or a large left kidney. On flat film of the abdomen, the splenic shadow can often be visualized immediately below the left leaf of the diaphragm, medially bordering on the fundus of the stomach and with its lower pole impinging on the colon. Thus, enlargement of the spleen results in displacement of the stomach medially and downward, and of the colon air bubble posteriorly and inferiorly. The outline of the spleen can be accentuated by introducing air or contrast material into the stomach or colon. Tomograms may also be of assistance in outlining an atypical spleen, but are seldom necessary. Two methods for radioisotopic scanning are currently in use. In the older method, erythrocytes are heated to 50° C. for one hour and tagged with Cr^{51}. The heated red blood cells become spheroid and are trapped and destroyed by the spleen, which is then selectively visualized by scintillation scanning. A less selective method, but one giving equally good results (Fig. 23-1), employs a sulfur colloid linked to In^{113m} or to $Te,^{99m}$ which is picked up by the reticuloendothelial system, predominantly in the liver and spleen. A third method used labeled Rh-positive cells coated with anti-Rh antibodies, but is seldom used today in the determination of splenic size.

Functional abnormalities in hypersplenism may be revealed in the peripheral blood by anemia, leukopenia or thrombocytopenia. However,

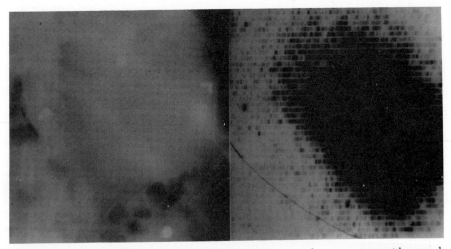

Figure 23-1. A splenic scan demonstrating splenomegaly in a patient with secondary hypersplenism.

the circulating red cells, white cells or platelets can remain at normal levels indefinitely, because the bone marrow can increase its rate of hematopoiesis by a factor of six to ten times, as long as the metabolic requirements are met. The peripheral blood smear may show characteristic abnormalities such as spherocytes, elliptocytes or target cells.

The increased destruction of red cells that occurs in hemolytic anemia usually results in a compensatory rise in the rate of erythrocyte production, as evidenced by increases in the reticulocyte count, the erythroid-myeloid ratio in the bone marrow and the turnover of iron. There are frequently elevations of the serum bilirubin and fecal urobilinogen, and gallstones are common. In acquired hemolytic anemia, the Coombs test is positive, indicating abnormal protein coating of the red cells that may or may not be due to true autoantibodies. The autohemolysis test is important in identifying pyruvate kinase hemolytic anemia. For this disorder, glucose will not abolish autohemolysis, but ATP will.

Splenic sequestration and destruction of red blood cells can be evaluated indirectly, by measuring the rate of cellular destruction or the degree of compensatory production, and can be evaluated directly by measuring splenic sequestration of labeled cells. Transfusion requirements will give a rough but useful estimate of the rate of red cell destruction. Since the adult human loses approximately 20 ml. of red cells per day under normal conditions, in 10 days he will have lost approximately 200 ml. of erythrocytes. Thus, if the transfusion requirements are in excess of 1 unit of blood every 10 days, it can be assumed that the patient has a shortened red cell life span with accelerated destruction. A more sophisticated measurement of the rate of disappearance of red cells from the circulation and the sequestration of these cells in the spleen, utilizes Cr^{51} tagged erythrocytes. A measured half-life of less than 20 to 25 days is considered an accelerated rate of red cell destruction. The relative role of the spleen in this destruction of erythrocytes can be further assessed by daily scanning over the spleen and liver. A selective rise in the ratio of radioactivity in the spleen as compared to the liver suggests significant splenic sequestration. With this technique, a satisfactory result from splenectomy may be predicted with a degree of accuracy approaching 90 per cent in situations in which the half life of Cr^{51} labeled erythrocytes is below 50 per cent of normal (less than 15 days) and there is a progressive rise in the spleen: liver ratio.[1]

In most categories of hemolytic anemia, splenectomy is not indicated unless hypersplenism is functionally incapacitating or progressive on medical management. If steroids, for example, do not maintain an adequate remission in acquired hemolytic anemia, then splenectomy is indicated. However, in hereditary spherocytosis with evident hypersplenism, splenectomy should be considered much earlier in the course of the disease, even with compensated hemolytic anemia, owing to the high incidence of aplastic crises and gallstones. The only exception occurs when the diagnosis is made very early in life, and then delay until the third or fourth year is preferable. Splenectomy is almost invariably beneficial, even though the basic cellular defect is not corrected. Cholecystectomy may be performed when gallstones are present.

At the present time, there are no satisfactory clinical methods for measuring shortened half-lives of leukocytes. Determination of platelet survival time has also had limited practical clinical application. Platelet life spans, however, have been measured using a Cr^{51} tag, and a shortened platelet life span has been demonstrated in many cases of idiopathic thrombocytopenic purpura in relapse.[2] The most reliable methods of determining hypersplenic thrombocytopenia, such as in idiopathic thrombocytopenic purpura, remain in the clinical evaluation and bone marrow biopsy, which disclose a compensatory increase in immature megakaryocytes. Platelet agglutinin and complement-fixing antibodies have been demonstrated in a large proportion of tested cases of ITP, but these tests are of limited clinical value at the present time. There is also some question about whether or not these antibodies are true autoantibodies or rather antibodies directed at foreign antigens, which form an antigen-antibody complex that absorbs to the surface of the platelets.

In most cases of idiopathic thrombocytopenic purpura, the initial therapy is corticosteroids for two weeks to several months. Azathioprine has also been of some benefit. If remission does not result, splenectomy is indicated. Initial response to splenectomy is unquestionably good in over 85 per cent of patients, with platelet counts rising within 24 to 48 hours. In spite of the immediate gratifying response to splenectomy, the platelet "antibodies" are often still present following removal of the spleen. Relapse occurs in 20 to 40 per cent of patients following splenectomy. Rarely can this relapse be attributed to accessory spleens. Nevertheless, they should be searched for by scanning techniques. In my experience, the patients with a good steroid response will uniformly have a good splenectomy response. Those with no steroid response at all will respond poorly to splenectomy. An important indication for splenectomy is to reduce or obviate steroid requirements.

In thrombotic thrombocytopenic purpura, corticosteroids give few remissions, which are usually not sustained. Splenectomy may be indicated early in the course of the disease, particularly if there is evidence of neurologic involvement. The results are far from universally successful, but patients treated with combinations of steroids and splenectomy seem to do better than those treated with either mode of therapy alone. It is sometimes possible to wean patients from steroids at variable periods after splenectomy.

Splenic neutropenia is a rare condition, characterized by splenomegaly, hyperplastic bone marrow and leukopenia. Pancytopenia may also occur in this form of hypersplenism. The treatment of choice is splenectomy, which usually results in a rapid return to normal of the number of circulating cellular elements of the blood.

Although the multiple causes of secondary hypersplenism (Table 23-1) are usually best treated by medical management, splenectomy may be indicated for clinically significant splenic hyperfunction or for greatly enlarged spleens, resulting in discomfort from impaired respiration or rupture. For example, cellular infiltration in leukemias or lymphomas can lead to secondary hypersplenism of a clinically significant degree. Occasionally, splenectomy will be of palliative benefit in decreasing the transfusion requirements or making radiotherapy, or perhaps chemotherapy, technically easier.

Recently, exploratory laparotomy, splenectomy, para-aortic lymph node biopsy and liver biopsy have been advocated as helpful adjuncts to the staging of Hodgkin's disease.[3] With the rapidly improving prognosis of patients in the later stages of Hodgkin's disease, by the use of aggressive radiotherapy and chemotherapy, accurate staging has become essential. Recent evidence suggests that as high as 40 to 50 per cent of patients with Hodgkin's disease are restaged following diagnos-

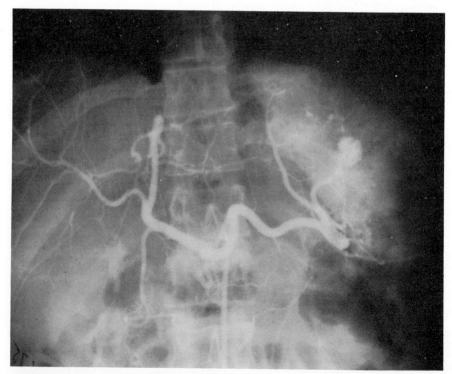

Figure 23–2. A selective celiac arteriogram demonstrating a subcapsular hematoma following blunt trauma to the abdomen.

tic laparotomy. The eventual benefits and proper use of this procedure remain to be clarified, and at present it should be utilized only in carefully selected individuals.

Rupture of the spleen, whether traumatic or spontaneous, is an indication for splenectomy. If there is any doubt about the diagnosis, careful, repeated clinical evaluation is mandatory. X-ray examination is usually not helpful, but plain films of the abdomen should be obtained. On occasion, positive roentgenologic findings will include a decrease in the left psoas shadow or kidney outline, compression of the stomach bubble medially, depression of the left colon inferiorly, or grossly enlarged spleen without a sharp splenic outline. The presence of rib fractures can be helpful and is said to occur in 20 per cent of splenic injuries. Hematuria, in association with fractures of the left rib cage, usually means that the spleen is also damaged. Arteriograms, with injections into the splenic artery, can be quite useful in difficult diagnostic cases (Fig. 23-2), but are seldom needed. Splenic scanning (Fig. 23-3) can also demonstrate subcapsular hematomas. The yield, however, is often low and, once again, is seldom needed.

Cysts, abscesses and primary neoplasms of the spleen, as well as torsion of an ectopic spleen and splenic artery aneurysm, are rare disorders frequently diagnosed only at the time of laparotomy. Splenectomy is indicated and often curative.

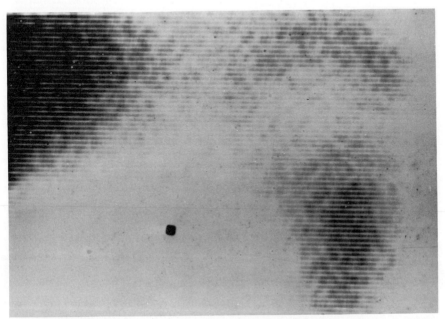

Figure 23–3. A splenic scan done one week after minor abdominal trauma, demonstrating a subcapsular hematoma in the midportion of the spleen.

At the present time, only rupture of the spleen or splenic artery aneurysm requires emergency splenectomy. In all other instances, the patient should be completely evaluated and prepared as needed with fresh blood transfusions, steroids if indicated and platelet packs, if the platelet count is below 10,000 to 30,000. Platelets should be given during the operative procedure after the splenic artery has been clamped to preserve as many of the transfused platelets as possible.

Hemorrhage, atelectasis and wound or subphrenic abscesses are the most frequent complications of splenectomy. They can usually be avoided by careful operative technique and postoperative management, including frequent coughing, positive pressure breathing, and nasotracheal aspiration. Plasma, blood or lymph with elevated amylase content occasionally collects under the left hemidiaphragm following difficult splenectomies. These collections may become manifest with the signs and symptoms of subphrenic abscess and require surgical drainage. Left pleural effusion and splinting of the diaphragm, which are not infrequent following splenectomy, do not necessarily signify an abscess. If they do not clear rapidly after several days, however, or if other roentgenologic or clinical manifestations of abscess appear, drainage is mandatory. Rarely, injury to the greater curvature of the stomach or to the pancreas can occur during splenectomy, and may present severe complications.

Thrombocytosis, which usually occurs following splenectomy, rarely results in thrombotic disease with ischemic complications, in spite of platelet counts as high as a million or more. In most instances, prophylactic anticoagulation is not indicated even with such severe thrombocytosis unless the patient has had previous thrombotic or embolic episodes. The only exceptions to this may be in polycythemia vera and agnogenic myeloid metaplasia when the platelet count rises to one and a half to two million, in which case thrombosis is not infrequent. Even in these instances, however, thrombocytophoresis is probably a better prophylactic approach than anticoagulation.

Splenectomy usually presents few technical difficulties. Exposure is adequate through a midline, left paramedian, or subcostal incision. The operative procedure can be quite difficult when the spleen is very large (e.g., lymphoma). Drainage of the left subphrenic space is usually not necessary. Careful technique and meticulous hemostasis are preferable to routine drainage. Occasionally, with extensive dissection of dense adhesions or severe clotting abnormalities, the splenic fossa should be drained through an anterolateral stab wound. If the pancreas is damaged during splenectomy, drainage, preferably with a sump drain, is almost always indicated.

From the surgeon's viewpoint, then, the main difficulties with splenectomy usually arise in the diagnostic evaluation to determine the indications for splenectomy and the appropriate timing of it. The informed surgeon is better equipped to assist the hematologist in this evaluation, and thus provide more than just a technical service.

REFERENCES

1. Goldberg, A., Hutchison, M. E., and MacDonald, E.: Radiochromium in the selection of patients with haemolytic anaemia for splenectomy. Lancet 1:109, 1966.
2. Baldini, W.: Idiopathic thrombocytopenic purpura. N. Eng. J. Med. 274:1245, 1966.
3. Glatstein, E., Guernsey, J. M., Rosenberg, S. A., and Kaplan, H. S.: The value of laparotomy and splenectomy in the staging of Hodgkin's disease. Cancer 24:709, 1969.

CHAPTER 24

SURGERY OF THE PERIPHERAL ARTERIES: Principles of Preoperative, Intraoperative, and Postoperative Management

D. EMERICK SZILAGYI, M.D., F.A.C.S.

Introduction. In order to establish the scope of this chapter, it is necessary to define the term "peripheral arterial surgery." A number of definitions have been in vogue, but for the purposes of this survey peripheral arterial surgery is taken to be the treatment by reconstructive means of the diseases of the extracranial and extrathoracic sectors of the arterial tree. In addition to lesions of the arteries of the limbs, this definition also encompasses those of the extracranial cerebral and intra-abdominal visceral arteries.

Operations for lesions of atherosclerotic origin make up over 90 per cent of all surgical procedures for arterial disease. The remainder comprise arterial lesions of the acute variety, the treatment of which constitutes surgical emergencies: arterial embolism and trauma. (The latter group will be dealt with separately at the end of the chapter.)

In this brief overview of certain problems of the treatment of arterial disease, consideration will be given only to reconstructive surgical procedures. The exposition, moreover, will be limited to the presentation of principles, with few specific details. This method of approach promises practical and theoretical advantages, since the general principles governing arterial surgery are quite widely accepted, whereas many idiosyncratic variations exist with regard to specific therapeutic details.

Arterial operations have many fundamental characteristics in common with other major operations but in addition have specific features resulting from the interference with blood flow and from the opening

444

and reconstructing of arterial structures. The systemic nature of atherosclerosis, moreover, lends to many arterial surgical procedures a physiologic gravity not usually seen with interventions of similar magnitude in non-atherosclerotic patients.

ATHEROSCLEROTIC ARTERIAL DISEASE

General Remarks. Atherosclerosis is a disease not necessarily of advanced age but certainly of aging. Aging in this context is not defined in terms of number of years but rather in terms of physiological changes. A patient relatively young in years will be physiologically aged if his atherosclerotic involvement is of a sufficiently advanced degree. In general, however, it is true that atherosclerosis is the disease of advanced years, the peak incidence of the surgically important clinical manifestations of occlusive arterial disease being in the sixth decade and that of aneurysmal disease in the seventh decade. Since this age distribution is similar to that of other degenerative diseases, the frequency of associated nonvascular degenerative lesions in patients with atherosclerotic arterial problems is high.[1] Particularly common are obstructive pulmonary diseases, malignant neoplasia, prostatism, and osteoarthritis. From the point of view of the surgeon, degenerative pulmonary disease is the most common nonvascular associated entity creating problems in the management of peripheral arterial disease. Indeed, chronic obstructive pulmonary insufficiency and the coronary, cerebral, and renal manifestations of atherosclerosis are the causes of the great bulk of postoperative problems in this field of surgery. The prevalence of degenerative lesions associated with arterial disease calling for surgical treatment creates two important tasks for the surgeon: he must very carefully search preoperatively for evidences of nonatherosclerotic as well as atherosclerotic associated disease, and he must be alert for complications that may result from the associated lesions. Needless to say, whenever the associated lesions are detected, he must take all curative steps possible.

In the presentation of therapeutic principles to be dealt with, the following scheme will be observed: In the main, occlusive and aneurysmal atherosclerotic lesions will be discussed together; the occasional differences will be dealt with in passing. (It may be pointed out at the outset, however, that, in general, aneurysmal lesions, because of the more severe atherosclerotic involvement and greater age of the patients, usually present problems of graver concern.) The main details of the therapeutic problems will be discussed in connection with aortoiliac and femoro-popliteal operations; necessary further remarks will be added for the consideration of visceral and carotid arterial operations. After the remarks on preoperative care, intraoperative and postoperative problems will be taken up in turn.

PREOPERATIVE CARE

Aorto-iliac and Femoro-popliteal Operations. GENERAL CONSIDERATIONS. As formerly stated, vascular operations combine the characteristics of major operations in any anatomical area with some special attributes related both to the direct attack on the blood vessels and to the unfailing presence of a systemic disease, atherosclerosis, of various degrees of severity. In general, this combination of characteristics foretells increased operative risk in terms of both mortality and morbidity for an operation of a given magnitude as defined by length of duration and extent of dissection. The portent of this fact is greater when one deals with operations of the abdominal aorta, especially when the operation is for an aneurysm.

USE OF ANGIOGRAPHY. Despite its being a diagnostic procedure, angiography is so closely allied to the decisions inherent in the management of arterial disease that its brief consideration is desirable as a part of the description of preoperative care.

In the preoperative planning for the treatment of occlusive arterial disease, angiography is indispensable. As regards aneurysmal disease, there is a division of views, and many surgeons do not routinely use preoperative angiographic investigation in the management of abdominal aortic aneurysms. This writer's experience has been that angiographic study of an abdominal aortic aneurysm is always useful for, and many times essential to, the evaluation of the technical difficulties to be expected and thus for the assessment of operative risk and for the formulation of an operative plan. Regarding the technique of angiography, practices vary, but this writer's method, which relies heavily on translumbar aortography for the visualization of the abdominal aorta and its branches, has proved safe, thrifty and reliable.[2] Percutaneous femoral arteriography is used when there is need for the visualization of the details of the femoropopliteal, and especially of the infrapopliteal, arterial tree. Selective angiography is only necessary in occasional cases of renal and mesenteric arterial disease. Aortography must be considered a major surgical procedure, and the patient has to be hospitalized for its performance. The same preoperative assessment is carried out as one would want for any major surgical procedure. Since in the very large majority of cases, the angiographic investigation is merely a step toward definitive surgical treatment, the pre-aortographic evaluation of the patient is usually also the work-up for the definitive surgical procedure, or at least forms the major part of it.

SYSTEMIC SURVEY. The preoperative systemic survey is carried out with particular care in cases of vascular disease. One must look with meticulous care for organ manifestations of systemic atherosclerosis other than the lesion involved in the clinical symptoms for which the patient is hospitalized. Electrocardiograms are routinely taken and cardiological consultation is advisable in most instances. Pulmonary function is evaluated clinically and by chest radiograms, and whenever necessary special pulmonary function tests are carried out. Blood urea nitrogen and creatinine determinations give information regarding renal function. The presence of abnormal lipid or carbohydrate metabolism and disturbances of liver function and blood clotting are searched for by appropriate laboratory tests. Blood serum potassium is measured because covert hypokalemia from potassium loss through diuretic medication, dietary restrictions, purging or diarrhea is a relatively common cause of intraoperative or postoperative arrhythmia in this class of patients.

A detailed and careful clinical history is directed at the detection of any possible associated nonvascular disease, and if a clue is obtained from the history further investigation is carried out (such as gastrointestinal x-ray studies or special hematological studies). If associated nonvascular surgical disease is discovered, often (in nearly 8 per cent of all the cases[1]) a question of priority of treatment arises. This problem becomes most vexing in the case of the association of malignant disease with an abdominal aortic aneurysm. It has been a satisfactory practice to rely on the size of the aneurysm as an important index of urgency for the treatment of the aneurysmal lesion. A number of complex situations may arise in this area, the discussion of which is beyond the scope of this survey.*

Physiological deficits revealed by the clinical and laboratory search are corrected whenever possible. It may be necessary to treat a recent (less than 3 months old) myocardial infarction and delay surgical procedure until cardiac function is properly restored. Congestive cardiac failure of even the mildest degree must be controlled. Angina, if readily responsive to medication, is not regarded as an absolute surgical contraindication but is a signal for especially critical review of the need for operation. On the eve of operation hydrating measures are probably useful for the improvement of renal blood flow. It is of great importance to instruct the patient to stop the use of tobacco, particularly cigarette smoking, at least two weeks before the surgical procedure is planned to be carried out. This is an important adjunct to preparation for the operation even if the patient will resume smoking when postoperative recovery is completed. If pulmonary emphysema or chronic bronchitis, or both, are present, inhalation therapy in instituted; proper preparation of the lungs for a major arterial operation may thus require 10 days or more. In cases that must have extensive intra-abdominal dissection for aortic occlusive or aneurysmal disease and who have had in the past intra-abdominal operations, it has been found a useful precautionary measure to insert a suction tube of the Miller-Abbott type. (Since adequate exposure of the abdominal aorta requires the temporary exte-

---

*Extensive consideration of the subject matter can be found in the reference cited above.[1]

riorization of the small bowel tract, the possibility of postoperative intestinal obstruction in the presence of adhesions is increased.)

If ischemic ulceration is present in the extremity, it is treated with cleansing measures to reduce the possibility of postoperative wound contamination. Debridement or local amputation must, of course, wait until adequate blood supply has been restored.

Operations on the Visceral Arteries. RENAL ARTERIAL AND SUPER-IOR MESENTERIC ARTERIAL OCCLUSIVE DISEASE; RENAL, SPLENIC AND HEPATIC ARTERIAL ANEURYSM. The recommendations listed in connection with aorto-iliac and femoropopliteal atherosclerotic arterial disease apply equally to these lesions. It should be noted, however, that the preoperative diagnostic work-up requires special procedures in cases of superior mesenteric artery and renal artery disease. In particular, selective angiographic visualization is essential.

Operations on the Carotid Artery. CAROTID ARTERIAL OCCLU-SIVE DISEASE. The principal concern of the preoperative diagnostic work-up of these cases relates to the exclusion of nonvascular central nervous system lesions, in particular neoplastic lesions of the brain. In addition to a careful and detailed clinical neurological analysis, angiographic visualization of the extracranial vascular arterial system is essential, usually through a four-artery arch aortogram. In some cases skull radiograms, electroencephalograms and radioisotope brain scan may be necessary.

INTRAOPERATIVE CARE

Certain principles of intraoperative management of the vascular patient, although not essentially different from those observed in all major surgical operations, must be given special emphasis.

An important detail of operative management is the preparation of the skin. As good an approximation of a sterile skin environment as possible is particularly important in vascular operations for which wound infection carries a special horror. In this writer's experience the use of plastic drapes glued to the appropriately prepared skin has been eminently effective.

The choice of anesthesia is of great importance, both because of the reduced respiratory capacity of the patient with obstructive pulmonary disease and because of the vulnerability of the myocardium in the presence of systemic atherosclerosis. Anesthetic agents allowing high oxygen saturation of the blood are preferred. Drugs that depress the respiratory center, particularly barbiturates, must be used with caution. Fluctuations in the blood pressure during the surgical procedure must be carefully avoided and blood loss replaced promptly and precisely; in aorto-iliac operations it is advisable to add 500 ml. of blood replacement to the actual loss for each limb to which preoperatively the blood flow has been completely obstructed. To this end continuous careful monitoring of the blood loss is most important. In operations in which the aorto-iliac segment is replaced or bypassed, it is a simple and effective maneuver, upon removal of the first distal clamp, to control the blood flow into the respective extremity by finger pressure on the open limb of the graft, increasing or reducing the flow according to the behavior of the blood pressure. Although the speed of the surgeon has lost much of its importance in the modern operating room, in the course of vascular operations on elderly patients prolongation of the anesthesia and of the recumbency of the patient are particularly harmful. Effort should be made to carry out the procedure with dispatch but without impairing gentleness.

In operations on the abdominal aorta, exposure requires exteriorization of the small bowel. A plastic bag has proved exceedingly useful as a protective cover for the exteriorized portion of the intestinal tract.

The use of heparin in the course of arterial operations is somewhat controversial. There are advocates of systemic heparinization for most major surgical interventions on the aorta, but this author's experience has been that heparinization is necessary only for those sections of the arterial tree that have been excluded from the general circulation by clamping. Systemic heparinization is reserved for cases with diffuse, disseminated atherosclerosis of advanced degree. (When systemic heparinization is used, careful neutralization of the circulating heparin is, of course, necessary at the end of the procedure.) In most hands the best approach for operations on the abdominal aorta is the long midline incision—an incision that does not always heal kindly. Careful closure of the midline anatomical structures in layers and the use of retention sutures are essential to guard against the danger of wound disruption. Throughout the operation, whenever clamping is resorted to, the limits of the tolerance of various organs for ischemia must be kept in mind. The normal kidneys will withstand 30 minutes of warm ischemia without permanent damage. The tolerance of the liver is somewhat higher, probably closer to 45 minutes. The small bowel has a tolerance similar to that of liver tissue.

One of the unique burdens of arterial surgery is that technical errors are often irretrievable. Unrelenting concentration on carrying out all technical steps with an intent for perfection must be the attitude of the surgeon.

POSTOPERATIVE CARE

Aorto-iliac and Femoro-popliteal Arterial Disease. The guiding principle is again the recognition of the complex character of surgical interventions on the arterial tree. In addition to the physiological disturbances attendant on major surgical procedures of any type, certain special consequences must be expected that derive from the operative manipulation of the arterial trunks themselves. The peripheral pulses must be carefully observed postoperatively and the clinical signs of ischemia constantly looked for in the parts that have been exposed to the dangers of thrombosis through the surgical intervention on the artery providing their blood supply. If the presence of thrombosis is strongly suspected or proved, the decision as to how to proceed is often complex and difficult. In the case of a visceral artery, if a vital organ is threatened and the time element is favorable, exploration and appropriate reoperation on the involved vessel are necessary. The time lapse between the original operation and the diagnosis of thrombosis is obviously of critical importance. If the period of tolerance of warm ischemia of the affected organ has been transgressed, reoperation for functional salvage will be futile. (In the case of the carotid artery, with the tolerance of the brain for ischemia under 5 minutes, such secondary intervention is obviously doomed to failure. In the aorto-iliac and femoropopliteal areas, early postoperative thrombosis of the site of reconstruction is often amenable to correction. Still, reoperation is not recommended as a routine procedure. After many trials with immediate and delayed correction of postoperative thrombosis, this writer has adopted a conservative approach and resorts to immediate intervention only if the life of the limb is at stake — a relatively rare occurrence. Allowing the patient to recover from the original operation whenever the limb is not in jeopardy and then planning a secondary procedure has proved safer and more fruitful.

Hemorrhage is a complication that occurs more frequently and with greater potential of disaster after arterial operations than it does after other types. Obviously, the treatment of hemorrhage requires immediate reoperation. Note should be made at this point, however, of a situation in which re-exploration is almost always useless. The reference is to the case in which, for reason of massive bleeding from a ruptured or injured artery (almost always in the abdomen) or of excessive intraoperative blood loss, large amounts of blood have to be transfused (in excess of 3000 to 4000 ml.). A profound disturbance of the coagulation mechanism often results, leading to widespread oozing of blood in the area of dissection, most notably in the retroperitoneal space. Surgical control of this type of bleeding is almost always unsuccessful, and resort must be made to medical means of correction of the clotting mechanism.

As previously mentioned, in this writer's experience systemic heparinization in vascular procedures is rarely necessary. The same statement can be made, in general, regarding the prophylactic use of antibiotics. As a rule, antibiotics are administered only for existing infection, preferably under specific indications determined by bacterial culture. Exceptions are made only in instances of secondary operations when wound contamination is feared. Antibiotic coverage for patients undergoing major vascular reconstruction is recommended by many but no convincing proof of the advantages of this practice has ever been presented.

The most common complications currently observed after major vascular operations are respiratory ones. The suctioning of the tracheo-bronchial tree at sufficiently frequent intervals through a nasal catheter is a most important measure to prevent serious bronchopulmonary infection. The encouragement of deep respiration and coughing and the periodic application of intermittent positive pressure respiration are most useful. Whenever secretions appear to collect at a rate faster than they can be removed, a tracheostomy is indicated. In questionable cases, the monitoring of blood gases is useful in determining whether the patient needs a tracheostomy or whether mechanically assisted respiration has to be instituted. Hypoxia, as a cause of cardiac arrhythmia, must be kept in mind.

If any evidence of instability of the blood pressure appears, a central venous catheter must be placed and the blood pressure carefully monitored. (Central venous pressure monitoring is, of course, an excellent tool also for gauging the speed and amount of the intravenous administration of fluids.) Consumption of alcohol among the elderly male of dimensions that may well be classified as chronic alcoholism is quite common, and, of course, a large majority of patients with arterial operations are elderly males. One must be on the alert not to mistake anoxia caused by pulmonary insufficiency for the symptoms of delirium tremens that are seen with fair frequency among patients of this class. The danger of hypotension, in addition to its generally acknowledged systemic ill effects, has the further unfavorable consequence of endangering the patency of the reconstructed arterial segment. When the patient has clinically manifest heart disease, or when cardiac arrhythmias appear postoperatively, continuous electrocardioscopic monitoring of the heart is obligatory.

The functional status of the kidneys can be satisfactorily checked with the observation of the hourly excretion and specific gravity. If excretion falls below 30 ml. per hour, the intravenous administration of an osmotic diuretic may be useful. If oliguria persists or anuria develops, they are treated promptly according to the methods described in Chapter 11.

In addition to the trivial gastrointestinal complications often seen after major abdominal operations, surgical procedures on the abdominal aorta may be followed by untoward events that are seldom if every seen after nonvascular interventions. The more common of these is ischemia of the left colon which occurs almost exclusively after operations for abdominal aortic aneurysm, with widely varying degrees of severity.[3] The rectosigmoid area is always deprived of its main blood supply for the duration of the clamping of the aortic inflow and outflow tracts during aneurysmectomy. This temporary interruption is usually entirely harmless, partly because of the tolerance of the colon and, more importantly, because of the presence of a satisfactory anastomotic arc between the inferior and left colic arteries on the one hand and the middle hemorrhoidal arteries on the other. Ischemia of relatively short duration supervenes whenever this collateral communication is inadequate. When, however, at the completion of the aorto-iliac reconstruction the patency of at least one internal iliac artery is not restored, lasting ischemia of the left colon of much greater severity will ensue. In fact, owing to this factor and to the fortuitous presence of other possible arterial anomalies, the entire left colon may become necrotic. The proper treatment of this potentially serious complication is prevention. This demands full attention during the operative procedure to the technical details that ensure adequate circulation to the distal left colon. Postoperatively, caution is required about abnormalities of bowel function. Diarrhea, especially when bloody, requires immediate, and if necessary repeated, investigation at the bedside with the sigmoidoscope. Depending on the severity of involvement, treatment may involve the use of oral antibiotics, diverting transverse colostomy for mucosal ulceration caused by mild temporary ischemia, or colectomy for bowel necrosis caused by permanent loss of blood supply.

The other serious alimentary tract complication is mesenteric arterial thrombosis. In patients with advanced diffuse atherosclerosis, the superior mesenteric artery or one of its branches may become occluded by thrombosis postoperatively, either because of operative manipulation or trauma, or, more commonly, because of episodic hypotension. In the immediately postoperative abdomen the physical signs of bowel necrosis are extremely difficult to detect and interpret. Diffuse, often ill-defined abdominal pain, persistent hypotension and adynamic ileus should be alerting signals for the possibility of this complication. Suspicion should be sharpened by the preoperative aortographic evidence of mesenteric arterial occlusive disease. Diagnosis calls for immediate laparotomy.

With these grave potential threats to his life, a patient immediately after a major vascular operation is obviously in need of a special nursing environment which can be afforded only in a properly organized and equipped intensive care ward.

The length of recumbency after arterial operations in the absence of significant complications depends partly on the magnitude of the surgical procedures, but even more importantly on the general preoperative physiological state of the patient. For aortic operation early mobilization (that is, getting out of bed, sitting up at the bedside) on the third to fifth postoperative day is desirable and usually possible, but the extent of ambulation is often limited by the general feebleness of the elderly patient. After femoro-popliteal operations very early mobilization (on the second or third day) is the rule unless some aspect of the arterial reconstruction demands special caution; ambulation for these patients is recommended as soon as wound comfort allows.

VASCULAR EMERGENCIES

Ruptured Abdominal Aortic Aneurysms. The first preoperative consideration in the management of ruptured abdominal aortic aneurysms[4] is the prevention of a second hemorrhage before the aneurysmal lesion can be repaired. In most instances, the patient is seen in a state of compensated hemorrhagic shock of varying but usually severe degree. In spite of the striking evidences of blood loss, at this stage active bleeding has stopped or has markedly slowed down owing to the tamponading effect of the lowered blood pressure and para-aortic hematoma. At this point the sole purpose of the surgeon must be to have the patient on the operating table with as little loss of time as possible, open the abdomen and control the rupture site by clamping the aorta at the appropriate level. It is wiser not to use blood transfusion at this phase unless the hemorrhage has been very severe. If blood is administered it should be given cautiously and as soon as the blood pressure responds the speed of infusion must be slowed. The obvious reason for this precaution is the fear of provoking a second hemorrhage. A sudden rise in the blood pressure, or agitation of the patient, or turbulent induction of anesthesia, all may cause dislodgment of the tamponading clot and the reactivation of severe bleeding. The second hemorrhage, though it may still be combated with massive transfusions, usually leads to irreparable myocardial damage; the patient, although capable of being carried through the surgical procedure of repair, will almost inevitably die of secondary irreversible shock. Once in the operating room, therefore, induction of anesthesia must be gentle, and the anesthesia proper, at first, need not be deep. To lessen the interval between the establishment of adequate anesthesia and the moment of access to the aorta, the operative area is prepared before induction is started. Upon opening the abdomen, the first concern of the surgeon must be to place the clamp on the aorta temporarily at any convenient site above the point of rupture, to remove the hematoma, to recognize the site of rupture, and then to replace the clamp at a level below the renal arteries. The physiologic effects of blood loss may now be corrected energetically, the anesthesia—if necessary—deepened, and the aneurysm resected at leisure. The postoperative care of patients with ruptured abdominal aortic aneurysms is different from that of other major vascular cases only in respect to the frequency and severity of complications, both of which are increased.

Arterial Embolization. When possessed of the characteristic features, arterial embolization is easy to diagnose and the level of lodgment of the clot is readily localized. If the clot is in a critical artery, the removal of the embolus constitutes an absolute emergency. Thus, there is little time or justification for preoperative preparations. The surgeon actually faces a categorical question: Is the patient capable of supporting the relatively minor intervention of embolectomy? If the answer to this question is affirmative, the operation must proceed without delay. If not, temporizing measures, such as the use of anticoagulants, will not change the fate to which the part is destined by the loss of its blood supply.

In preparing the limb for embolectomy—or, for that matter, for any surgical intervention aimed at correcting acute ischemia of the extremity—it is very helpful for the accuracy of the surgeon's judgment of the result of his efforts to prepare the skin with a colorless solution and to encase the foot in a transparent cover. With the recent introduction of Fogarty's balloon catheter, the approach to emboli can be standardized and greatly simplified. In the lower extremities all emboli can be successfully attacked, at least initially, through a groin incision and a superficial-femoral arteriotomy. The same type of incision can also be satisfactorily used for the removal of common iliac and aortic bifurcation emboli. In cases of popliteal embolization it is often necessary to add an anterolateral paratibial incision for complete removal of the secondary thrombi in the infrapopliteal arterial branches. Systemic heparinization is not necessary during embolectomy, and postoperative treatment from the purely surgical point of view is largely limited to the care of the wound. If excessive edema of a limb develops, appropriate fasciotomy is necessary. The principal task in postoperative care is the treatment of the pathological condition that originally led to the embolization.

Terminal Arterial Thrombosis. This is an expression that describes the formation of a thrombus in the lumen of an atherosclerotic artery at the site of a stenosing atheroma. An enlarging atheroma eventually causes a sufficient reduction of the arterial lumen to lead to stagnant flow and eventually to thrombosis. This is the end stage of all obstructive processes resulting from atherosclerosis. In about 90 per cent of cases of terminal thrombosis the gradual narrowing has elicited the formation of an ample collateral bed, and thus the final stage of occlusion will produce no dramatic ischemic change. When, however, thrombosis takes place in the presence of a relatively ample lumen, and when, therefore, the collateral bed is still meager, the final event of occlusion will lead to the appearance of symptoms of acute ischemia that resemble the clinical picture of arterial embolization. In most—over 80 per cent—of these cases the differential diagnostic problem can be resolved by clinical means, but in the remainder angiography is needed. This author's first approach to this type of sudden arterial occlusion is conservative management by means of an epidural block and careful observation of the extremity. If, in a viable limb, no worsening of the signs of ischemia occurs, and in particular if the ischemia improves, as happens in 90 per cent of the cases, the treatment is continued until the maximal improvement of the limb is reached. At this point appropriate angiographic studies are carried out and the patient is prepared for reconstructive surgical intervention according to the standard indications, or, if inoperable, treated medically. If, however, following the initial observation of 4 to 6 hours the condition of the limb deteriorates, angiograms are obtained and surgical intervention is carried out in a manner dictated by the angiographic findings. The general intraoperative and postoperative problems in these cases are not importantly different from those after the repair of other chronic vascular lesions. If, however, the ischemia has been severe and its duration over 6 hours, severe postoperative edema of the lower extremities can be expected. In this case appropriate fasciotomies are performed.

Arterial Trauma. The only significant preoperative problem of special interest in the management of arterial trauma is the determination, in some cases, of the need for exploration. In most instances, the answer to this question is obvious. In some cases of gunshot wound, however, in which a high-velocity bullet of relatively small size has passed through a limb, and in some instances of stab wounds, the evidence of hemorrhage is not convincing and there are no other *early* physical signs to confirm the presence of an injury to the wall of the artery. In these cases arteriographic visualization of the arterial tree is of great usefulness. Arteriography also helps in avoiding occasional false positive diagnoses by demonstrating an intact artery when the ischemic state of the limb caused by spasm may suggest injury to the arterial wall. One must bear in mind that radiologic visualization of the arteries has no bearing on the diagnosis of venous injuries. If the clinical findings suggest significant blood loss, and the arteriograms show intact arteries, the appropriate vein should be explored. The intra- and postoperative problems after the repair of arterial trauma, aside from the care required by the associated injuries, are similar to those encountered in other arterial vascular operations for acute lesions.

REFERENCES

1. Szilagyi, D. E., Smith, R. F., Elliott, J. P., Hageman, J. H., and Rodriguez, F. J.: Aortoiliac atherosclerotic and nonvascular intra-abdominal surgical lesions. Arch. Surg. *100*:470, 1970.
2. Szilagyi, D. E., Smith, R. F., Macksood, A. J., and Eyler, W. R.: Abdominal aortography: Its value and its hazards. Arch. Surg. *85*:25, 1962.
3. Smith, R. F., and Szilagyi, D. E.: Ischemia of the colon as a complication in the surgery of the abdominal aorta. A.M.A. Arch. Surg. *80*:806, 1960.
4. Smith, R. F., and Szilagyi, D. E.: Ruptured abdominal aortic aneurysms: Problems of diagnosis and management. Ann. Surg. *154* (Suppl.) 175, 1961.

CHAPTER 25

THE THYROID GLAND

OLIVER COPE, M.D., F.A.C.S.

Disturbance of Thyroid Function

INTRODUCTION

The capacity of the human organism to withstand an operation can be seriously jeopardized by disturbance of thyroid function, by either hyper- or hypothyroidism. Neglect to think of the possibility of concomitant thyroid disturbance when attention is focused on another disease can lead to unnecessary complications and even to disaster. It is essential, therefore, that the surgeon learn early to embody in his thinking an alertness to thyroid disturbance.

The problem of possible complicating thyroid disturbance is compounded by difficulties of diagnosis. It is not difficult to diagnose thyroid disease if the symptoms and signs are overt. The presence of a tremor, of exophthalmos and the other eye signs and of a rapid pulse unexplained by the other disease should register immediately in the physician's consciousness and a goiter should be searched for. If edema of the eyelids, shins and ankles is present it is not difficult to think of hypothyroidism, and the delay in recovery of the ankle tendon reflex will automatically come to mind.

The principal problem is found in patients in whom the disorder is masked. Hyperthyroidism, even severe hyperthyroidism, may exist in patients without obvious eye signs and this is particularly true in older people who are the least able to withstand the strain of the hyperthyroidism. Likewise hypothyroidism, particularly in its early phases, may not be associated with obvious edema, thickening of the tongue and a sluggish deep voice. These masked forms of thyroid disease require special awareness on the part of the physician and surgeon.

The physician who is able to make these diagnoses clinically, including the masked forms, and who observes the precautions outlined in this chapter, will have gone a long way in avoiding the troubles.

456

HYPERTHYROIDISM

THE PROBLEMS

From the practical clinical point of view the patient with hyperthyroidism presents the physician with two general sets of problems. First, the excess of thyroid hormone sensitizes the entire nervous system and may unbalance numerous organ systems. The second stems from the general effect of the hormone on metabolic rate. The oxygen consumption of tissues generally is increased, the demand for blood is raised and organs may become overloaded.

Central Nervous System Hypersensitivity. The excess of thyroid hormone keys up the entire central nervous system. Patients tend to be overly active physically and mentally. Responses are accelerated, exaggerated or inappropriate. Their emotional control is labile, sleep restless and fatigue common.

Autonomic Nervous System Imbalance. The increased nervous system sensitivity induced by the elevated concentration of thyroid hormone as a rule unbalances the autonomic nervous system. In general the responses mediated by adrenergic impulses are more highly sensitized than the cholinergic. Thus fright, pain, hunger and rage are poorly tolerated. Patients generally are acutely sensitive to even small doses of epinephrine, indeed so sensitive that in the 1920's epinephrine sensitivity was used as a test for the presence of hyperthyroidism (the so-called Goetsch test). The heart is especially sensitive and fibrillation of atrium and ventricle is readily induced. Because of its dangers in the severely hyperthyroid patient this test was but little employed. Other adrenergic drugs such as benzedrine also may induce physiologic turmoil. Drugs such as atropine, which reduce the cholinergic activity, may be followed by an undue release of the opposing force — a burst of unanticipated adrenergic activity.

The imbalance is sometimes the other way. Sweating may be profuse and diarrhea frequent; both are cholinergically transmitted mechanisms.

Cardiac Load. Hyperthyroidism induces an increase in cardiac output. The thyroid hormone is a principal regulator of the rate of metabolism of all tissues that have so far been tested. An increase in the concentration of the hormone increases the metabolic rate and the need for oxygen. The patient with hyperthyroidism therefore has a generalized need for a greater amount of oxygen, the basis of the measurement of the basal metabolic rate.

The increased need for oxygen is followed by an elevation of the blood flow and the heart is called upon to increase its output. The hyperthyroid patient lying comfortably at rest has the cardiac load, for example, of a normothyroid person constantly up and walking around.

The same patient, when walking at an average rate, has the cardiac load of a person who is jog trotting. The patient with hyperthyroidism who attempts to run or climb stairs quickly may easily place a demand upon the heart which cannot be met and deficit accumulates. The patient with hyperthyroidism who is to undergo an operation, therefore, faces an increased cardiac load throughout the induction of the anesthesia, the operation and the postoperative period, in addition to any increased load induced by the operation itself.

Thyroid Crisis.   Patients with severe hyperthyroidism are occasionally subject spontaneously to the development of a state of turmoil called thyroid crisis. The balance of the general nervous system as well as that of the cardiovascular system gives way under pressure and becomes severely disorganized. The patient becomes so keyed up that emotional restraint is lost, the temperature controlling mechanism fails and the patient develops a high fever. The fever compounds the metabolic load already placed upon the cardiovascular system, and the heart under the extreme pressure may pass into fibrillation and standstill.

Thyroid crisis is thus really an extension of the sensitivity and imbalance of the nervous system and excessive load upon a disorganized heart. Although it may develop spontaneously in the severely thyrotoxic, it is usually precipitated by some event which overtaxes the already overloaded nervous and cardiovascular systems. An inadvertent operation may serve as the overtaxing stimulus. Thus a patient who has only a moderate degree of hyperthyroidism and who under ordinary circumstances would not go into crisis may be thrown into crisis by anesthesia, operation and postoperative circumstances such as pain and anxiety.

MANAGEMENT

The general management of the patient with hyperthyroidism who needs to undergo an operation for a disease other than of the thyroid consists of decreasing as quickly as possible the secretion of additional thyroid hormone and of diminishing by every means possible the pathophysiologic effects of the excess of the hormone already in circulation. It is obvious that if the operation the patient faces is an elective one and ample time is available in order to correct the hyperthyroid situation, the problem from the point of view of management is relatively simple. If the condition is an urgent one, however, and the operation an emergency, the surgeon is faced with a more difficult problem with narrower margins of safety; the management is more critical. Because of this critical nature, the acute situation is considered first.

Acute Situation—The Patient Undergoing an Emergency Operation.   The first objective of the surgeon in managing the patient with hyperthyroidism is to assess the relative risks—that induced by the presence of hyperthyroidism, that of the disease if the patient is not operated upon, and that of the indicated operation itself. If hyperthyroidism is mild and the patient is otherwise a vigorous, healthy young adult, the patient may be able readily to absorb the increased load of anesthesia and operation without danger of inducing a crisis, particularly if it can be anticipated that the operation is not likely to be followed by a prolonged and difficult convalescence. If hyperthyroidism is severe, a crisis may develop in the patient exposed even to a minor surgical risk. Young children and older people tolerate hyperthyroidism poorly and the risk of undertaking an operation which could possibly be postponed may be prohibitive. Thus the severity of the hyperthyroidism, the age and general well-being of the patient, the condition for which an operation is indicated, the risk of not operating at all and finally the risk of the operation itself must all be taken into consideration.

PREOPERATIVE. If it is considered that operation is imperative in the patient who has hyperthyroidism, many precautions are to be undertaken and the entire surgical management of the patient should include consideration of those activators of the adrenergic nervous system—pain, hunger, fear and rage.

Reduction in amount of circulating hormone. Immediate attention should be given to reducing the amount of the hormone. Unfortunately there is at present no means of inactivating the thyroid hormone already in the tissues. It can be reduced in the circulation by plasmapheresis, to be resorted to in extreme cases. Two things that can be done generally, however, are to stop the new formation of hormone by an antithyroid drug and to lock up within the gland that hormone which is at the moment being made by the administration of iodine.

An antithyroid drug should be started immediately in maximal doses. The preferred drugs are propylthiouracil (at least 200 mg. every eight hours) and methimazole (20 mg. every eight hours). If the patient has previously had either of these two drugs and has been found sensitive to it, potassium perchlorate (100 mg. every eight hours) is a wise alternative.

For *iodine*, saturated solution of potassium iodide, 15 drops once a day, is adequate. Iodine is so promptly absorbed from the stomach and upper intestine that there is little advantage to giving the iodine intravenously, unless, of course, the patient is vomiting.

Fever. If the patient is running a fever it may be wise to reduce the body temperature by alcohol baths or by packing the patient in cold wet blankets during the operative procedure. At least the physician should watch closely for a rise in body temperature.

Medications. The beta-blocking agent, propranolol hydrochloride, is probably the most effective drug in controlling the overactive nervous system, but it is to be given with caution, because prolonged use and possible complications have not been studied. Reserpine may also be used but is less certain.

In the very young and the elderly, cardiac medications are advisable. It has been the practice to prescribe quinidine; it should be maintained through the operative period when cardiac arrhythmias might be precipitated by the extra load and irritation of anesthesia and operation. For the elderly, digitalis may also be advisable though the indications are less clear.

In general drugs relieving anxiety and depressing the adrenergic system are useful and those depressing the cholinergic system are dangerous and to be avoided. Epinephrine and norepinephrine are to be avoided at all costs. If a form of local anesthesia is to be used, the surgeon must be sure to use a solution free of epinephrine.

Fear alerts the adrenergic aspect of the autonomic nervous system. It is wise therefore to allay this as much as possible in the thyrotoxic patient by repeated reassurance and by such drugs as the barbiturates.

For *pain,* morphine continues to be as successful as any. The proprietary Demerol offers no established advantage. Codeine is useful.

Atropine is to be avoided because it has a generalized depressing effect upon the cholinergic responses, releasing the restraint of the cholinergic system and allowing a relative outburst of adrenergic activity. In the thyrotoxic patient atropine is followed by a rise in pulse rate. This poses a problem for the suppression of the bronchial and tracheal mucous secretions. It is believed that scopolamine has a more localized effect on the bronchial secretions with less upon the vagus nerves to the heart and is therefore preferred to atropine. It is perhaps wiser to avoid both drugs in the preoperative preparation of the patient and deal with the mucus by suction.

Hunger is poorly tolerated, partly because of the elevated metabolic need and possibly also in part because of the associated adrenergic response to hunger. The patient should be fed optimally in the preoperative phase up to the last reasonable moment. It is also wise to maintain the glucose level by intravenous glucose administration in the hours before starting the anesthetic. Although the patient with hyperthyroidism who has fasted does not ordinarily have a drop in blood sugar, this possibility is to be avoided because a drop in blood sugar to subnormal level induces an output of epinephrine. (This is a physiologic response of the normal individual to raise the blood sugar level back to normal.)

When it comes to *rage,* every opportunity should be taken to relieve the patient of irritations and frustrations. This is accomplished, of course, by repeated reassurance and attention in a number of ways to give the patient the feeling that matters are being taken care of.

Dehydration. Dehydration is sometimes encountered and this is particularly likely in a heavily medicated person. The excessive heat production of hyperthyroidism has to be dissipated in the periphery. This is frequently accompanied by sweating and therefore rapid loss of fluid.

Fever likewise increases the sweating and water of vaporization. The high metabolic rate elevates the respiratory exchange in the lungs and this is associated with an increased water of vaporization. Although this is partially compensated by the increased water of combustion, the greater loss needs to be taken into account.

INTRAOPERATIVE. The intraoperative management of the patient with uncontrolled hyperthyroidism follows the same principles as that of the management of the preoperative phase – namely, avoidance of adrenergic stimulants and cholinergic depressants, and maintenance of normal body temperature and a normal blood sugar level. Hydration should also be carefully watched.

Anesthesia. The anesthetic agent to be used should depend upon its effect on the heart and its relative cholinergic and adrenergic influences. The induction of anesthesia by the intravenous injection of Pentothal sodium, a quick acting barbiturate, is reasonable because it appears to affect both sides of the autonomic nervous system equally.

Cyclopropane has been shown to dispose to cardiac fibrillation and should not be used. The newer volatile anesthetics have not been tried sufficiently to permit a valid judgment at the present moment.

Ethyl ether is probably the definitive anesthesia of choice. It does not block completely action of the autonomic nervous system and leaves some control of the balance to the patient's own inner wisdom.

Hydration is to be maintained during the operation much as already stated. The fluid should presumably contain glucose. There is no known specific need for salts. Balanced electrolyte solutions containing glucose are presumably best. Lactated Ringer's is such a solution. There is no evidence that lactate metabolism is interfered with in hyperthyroidism.

The *body temperature* should be watched as described in the previous section and if it rises, cooling to normal should be induced. If the heart action remains adequate at a normal body temperature it is probably best to stop body cooling at the normal level. No studies or observations have as yet been made regarding cardiac sensitivity in the hyperthyroid patient under hypothermic conditions.

POSTOPERATIVE. In the postoperative care of the patient with hyperthyroidism undergoing an operation for another condition it is wise to continue the several recommendations that have been outlined above in the preoperative and the intraoperative care for at least three weeks. The rate of utilization and disappearance of the naturally secreted thyroid hormone is slow. Although the metabolic rate of the patient may fall rapidly in the first few days after complete cessation of thyroid hormone secretion, the half-life of the hormone is more nearly three weeks than one. Thus in a patient who has been severely thyrotoxic it will be three weeks before the thyroid hormone level approaches normal and it may be as long as six weeks before the patient begins to be significantly hypothyroid. Throughout the period of even slight hyperthyroidism, the sensitivity to epinephrine continues. At three weeks the patient may still be sensitive to epinephrine, norepinephrine, other adrenergic drugs and to the cholinergic depressants such as atropine.

Maintenance of thyroid suppression program. Since the patient with hyperthyroidism in this postoperative phase will continue to be exposed to conditions which might induce a thyroid crisis, it is essential to continue the antithyroid drugs and to institute iodine before operation. Once the metabolic rate is believed to have reached normal the iodine may be omitted but the antithyroid drugs are to be continued. The reason for this is that complete control of secretion at a normal level is possible with the antithyroid drugs, whereas with iodine there might be some resumption of hyperthyroidism. Iodine induces a partial remission of hyperthyroidism but as a rule there is smoldering continuing oversecretion from the gland.

Hypometabolism. As the drug-induced remission is taking place it is important to reduce the drug dosage as the normal metabolic rate is attained. Otherwise the continuation of the high dosages recommended in the preoperative section will result in untoward hypothyroidism, a state almost as undesirable from the point of view of the health of the patient as the hyperthyroidism. It may be possible in three to six weeks' time from the start of the drug to reduce the dosage to one third that used at the beginning.

Occasionally an event such as a surgical operation may induce a temporary remission of the thyrotoxic disease. This is the exact reverse of the induction of a crisis. This spontaneous resolution should be looked for and the antithyroid drugs omitted. The remission is usually only temporary and a recrudescence is to be anticipated.

Less Urgent Situation—The Patient Undergoing Operation of Election. The patient who requires an operation of election and who is found to have hyperthyroidism is in a much more favorable position than the patient whose disease requires an emergency procedure. The patient who has a simple inguinal hernia, for example, and whose hernia is causing minimal symptoms and is not obstructed, can have his hyperthyroidism controlled prior to the surgical repair of the hernia. The patient then will be freed of the possible complications and hazards of the hyperthyroidism.

The program in such a patient is obviously to reduce the thyroid function to normal and then to allow sufficient time to elapse for the autonomic nervous system to recover its balance and the heart to recover its strength. These two ordinarily require a minimum of three weeks. As soon as the hyperthyroidism is recognized the patient is to be put on an antithyroid drug. If there is no urgency it is better not to add the iodine medication because this complicates, somewhat, the subsequent care of the hyperthyroidism. The antithyroid drug may be started in high dosage (see the previous section) and then as the metabolic rate approaches normal the dose can well be reduced so that hypo-thyroidism will not be induced. Thus if 600 mg. of propylthiouracil were used at the beginning (in three divided doses, eight hours apart), it may well be possible to reduce the dose to 100 mg. or even 50 mg. every eight hours for the third to fifth weeks.

The drop in thyroid activity is often satisfactorily monitored by simple observation of the patient. The patient will report a return of a feeling of well-being, a loss of excitement and palpitation and a gain in strength as well as weight. The doctor will observe the pulse rate and the returning calm of the patient. It is well, however, to monitor the response by measuring either the fasting metabolic rate (the BMR) or chemical test of blood or both.

The uptake of radioactive iodine within the thyroid gland, most useful in measuring the intensity of the disease before the onset of therapy, is of no use in evaluating the effectiveness of the drug therapy. Because the antithyroid drug blocks the uptake of the iodine by the gland, the uptake may be well below normal even though the patient is still thyrotoxic. Used during therapy, it is a measure of the adequacy of the drug dosage. It is never a measure of the level of thyroid hormone within the body fluids.

There is some evidence that the adrenergic hypersensitivity so obvious during the active phase of hyperthyroidism may persist for one to three weeks after the hormone level and the metabolic rate have descended to normal. In other words it may take longer for the auto-nomic nervous system to regain its normal balance than for the oxygen consumption rate to return to normal. For this reason, if there is any doubt about when to undertake the operation, it is well to wait two to three weeks beyond the time when the patient feels better and the BMR has returned to normal.

The more prolonged wait is probably particularly advisable in the older patient whose heart may have been under severe strain during the period of active hyperthyroidism. A more prolonged wait at a nor-mal metabolic rate will allow recovery not only of the nerve balance but of the strength of the heart. During this phase of recovery any cardiac deficit and accumulation of excessive body fluid should have been eliminated. In the elderly patients, as suggested above under "Medications," it will have been wise to administer digitalis, and in those with cardiac arrhythmia, quinidine.

HYPOTHYROIDISM

From the point of view of oxygen consumption and metabolic rate, hypothyroidism is the reverse of hyperthyroidism. In terms of the com-plications and hazards of operating on a patient, they are by no means opposites. Indeed there are seeming paradoxic similarities, for the pa-tient with hypothyroidism is also sensitive to drugs. The sensitivity includes most drugs and probably most anesthetic agents, and the heart, though subjected to a lesser load quantitatively, is still the arbiter of fate.

THE PROBLEMS

The problems of the patient with hypothyroidism to keep in mind when planning an operation are of the same order as with hyperthyroidism, but to some extent reversed.

General Nervous System Depression. The nervous system is generally depressed by hypothyroidism. Cortical functions such as memory, perception and awareness are diminished; responses to questions are slowed. So too are the responses of many other parts of the nervous system. The slow recovery of the ankle jerk tendon reflex is an example. Such slowness is characteristic of all measurable reflexes, for the nervous system works at a slower rate. It is less agile and less active. It cannot be counted upon, therefore, to pick up harmful stimuli quickly and to make the necessary adjustments.

Decreased Cardiac Elasticity. With the lower metabolic rate of hypothyroidism, the cardiac output is actually decreased. The heart has less work to do. The hypothyroid heart, however, is less able to contract and tires more easily than when normal. Most important is that in the hypothyroid state it is less agile and has trouble picking up an added load.

Drug Hypersensitivity. The depression of the nervous system and the lower metabolic rate make patients with hypothyroidism generally sensitive to drugs and anesthetic agents. This hypersensitivity is a serious threat to the unaware physician.

MANAGEMENT

The patient who has hypothyroidism and is faced with an emergency operation poses a much more acute situation than one whose operation may be postponed until the hypothyroidism is corrected. Because the acute situation is more difficult and more detailed in its management it is considered first.

Acute Situation—The Patient Undergoing an Emergency Operation. The patient with hypothyroidism is a fragile patient physiologically and should be approached warily. Many a patient with hypothyroidism given a dose of morphine average for a normal individual has passed into a profound coma lasting 36 hours or longer. One of the most difficult of all the problems is that the patient is not only sensitive to drugs of various kinds but may also be sensitive to that very hormone, thyroid, which he lacks. Thus the administration of thyroid hormone has to be undertaken with deliberation and caution. The cardiovascular system and kidneys may fail to eliminate even a slight excess of fluid, resulting in water overloading and pulmonary edema.

PREOPERATIVE. The initial step is to start bringing the level of thyroid hormone and thus the metabolic rate to normal. This is is to be done with frequent small doses of the quickest-acting hormone, triiodothyronine. The patient should be carefully monitored with repeated, frequent electrocardiograms. A change in the electrocardiogram will take place as the level of the hormone rises and metabolic rate returns to normal. These are described in standard cardiac texts in detail.

If the thyroid hormone is given too rapidly, angina is often precipitated and cardiac standstill may occur. Therefore, great caution must be exercised in the thyroid administration. It is to be stressed that many severely hypothyroid patients have died suddenly during the early phase of thyroid therapy. Suggested dose schedules are given later.

If the surgical condition is urgent, it may be necessary to undertake the operation before the patient is more than just started on the return to normal thyroid function. If so, the following precautions must be followed. Minute or very small doses of drugs are to be given to begin with. Instead of 8 mg. of morphine, for example, 0.5 mg. should be tried first. This may prove ample to reduce pain and even to put the patient to sleep for three to four hours.

Because of sensitivity, other drugs such as atropine may well be omitted entirely.

Restraint must be used in the administration of fluids preoperatively. The renal output must be monitored and care taken not to exceed an output of 20 cc. per hour. As this limit is approached, the administration of fluids should be reduced until the urinary output falls off once again. In this manner pulmonary edema may be avoided.

INTRAOPERATIVE. The same considerations of drug sensitivity and limitation of cardiac function apply to intraoperative management. Intravenous Pentothal anesthesia is acceptable because it only slightly disturbs the autonomic balance. Here again a much smaller amount will suffice to put the patient to sleep and will also serve for a much more prolonged period without additional drugs. Start with tiny doses. Minimal doses of a volatile anesthetic will be needed to supplement the somnolent dosage of Pentothal.

Extensive operations have not been carried out on the fully hypothyroid or myxedematous patient and it is not really known whether they can tolerate extensive procedures. The minimum operative procedure sufficient to carry the patient over a hump is the one to be chosen. If the disease can be managed by multiple stage, relatively short, simple procedures, this should be the choice. For example, an ileostomy, colostomy or sidetracking operation should be done as the first stage for intestinal obstruction, leaving any resection of tumor to a second stage.

Regarding fluid management, minimal transfusions or fluid therapy are to be used during this phase as in the preoperative phase, for fear of overloading the heart and thus precipitating cardiac insufficiency.

POSTOPERATIVE. A principal therapy of this phase will be to bring the metabolic rate to normal. The same considerations as described above under "Preoperative" preparation apply here. The metabolic rate should be raised slowly and under careful monitoring. Otherwise angina and signs of coronary insufficiency may be precipitated.

It seems that the recovery of cardiac muscle from the state of hypothyroidism is slower than that of other tissue. The demands for oxygen, for more blood, and for a greater output by the heart gain in advance of the capacity of the heart muscle to pump the needed output. By slowing the pace of the restitution of thyroid function or thyroid hormone level, the heart muscle is allowed to retain its strength commensurate with the load imposed.

In the postoperative period also, drug sensitivity remains. Minimal doses of pain medication should suffice. Cautious fluid therapy continues as the rule.

Resumption of ambulation probably should also be gradual in order to avoid overloading the handicapped heart. Early ambulation, limited to having the patient stand at the bedside, is advised rather than having the patient walk along corridors. If the patient tolerates relatively large doses of thyroid, however, then he may be ambulated in accordance with the progress of the thyroid level and cardiac output.

Less Urgent Situation—The Patient Undergoing Operation of Election. It is obvious from the foregoing discussion that, if a patient faces an operation of election in the presence of hypothyroidism, the first objective should be to bring him into thyroid balance. It should again be stressed that this should be started slowly. It may be possible to raise the metabolic rate promptly within a matter of several days. On the other hand, if this is assumed at the beginning, severe angina may suddenly be precipitated and cardiac arrest may supervene. Although this is likely to occur only with severely hypothyroid patients who have frank myxedema, it may occur in elderly patients who are only moderately hypothyroid and who have no frank evidence of myxedema.

The procedure is the same, starting with small doses of triiodothyronine. These may be given intravenously if the patient is vomiting (5 μg. doses every four hours for the first 24 hours). The patient is to be monitored with each dose by electrocardiogram. If the patient remains symptom-free and electrocardiographic changes are acceptable, then the dose may be shifted to 50 μg. per day by mouth for the next three or four days. The total amount should be divided into three doses. If this dose is satisfactorily handled after a week, it may be wise to add thyroxine, the slower acting form of hormone; it too should be given by mouth. One hundred micrograms of thyroxine is equivalent to 25 μg. of triiodothyronine. An average full normal dose of thyroxine is 300 μg.

per day, and of triiodothyronine, 75 μg. A combination of the two is perhaps best. When the full dose is reached, perhaps two weeks since the start of the hormone therapy, the patient will be at the maintenance dosage and recovering rapidly from hypothyroidism.

In order to allow the patient to overcome drug sensitivity, to regain a balance in the central nervous system and recover strength in the heart, it will be wise to delay an elective operation longer. Presumably one to three weeks should be allowed after the recovery of the measurable euthyroid state, perhaps four to six weeks after the start of thyroid hormone therapy. Allowing ample time in this manner will insure success, for the patient should by now have returned to the normal thyroid state.

REFERENCES

Ashkar, F. S., Katims, R. B., Sudak, W. H., III, and Gilson, A. S.: Thyroid storm: Treatment with blood exchange and plasmapheresis. J.A.M.A., *214*:1275, 1970.
Lahey, F. H.: Apathetic thyroidism. Ann. Surg. 93:1026, 1931.
Lamberg, B. A.: The medical thyroid crisis. Acta Med. Scand. *164*:479, 1959.
Means, J. H., DeGroot, L. J., and Stanbury, J. B.: The Thyroid and Its Diseases. 3rd edition. New York, McGraw-Hill Book Co., Inc. 1963.
Sarnoff, S. J., and Cope, O.: The effect of atropine and scopolamine on the subsequent injection of epinephrine in thyrotoxic and euthyroid patients. Anesthesiology *15*:484, 1954.
Werner, S. C., ed.: The Thyroid. New York, Paul B. Hoeber, Inc., 1955.
Shanks, R. G., Lowe, D. C., Hadden, D. R., et al.: Controlled trial of propranolol in thyrotoxicosis. Lancet, *1*:993, 1969.

Thyroid Surgery

INTRODUCTION

The treatment of goiter is in transition from surgical to medical and preventive. Fifty years ago thyroidectomy was one of the commonest operations, and many a surgeon's reputation was built upon his capacity to carry out this operation with skill. Today the operation has become one of the less needed, and it can be foretold that the need will decrease further. The use of iodine to prevent endemic goiter, and the realization that thyroid therapy is a satisfactory treatment for many patients with sporadic nontoxic goiter, have gone a long way in eliminating nontoxic goiter as a surgical entity. Medical, radiologic and most recently psychologic therapies for Graves' disease are reducing the need of operation for hyperthyroidism, and mental health programs should eventually diminish its incidence. Still, the surgeon is needed for benign and malignant tumors and occasional thyroiditis, and until their etiology is understood, surgeons must continue to be educated in the refinements of thyroid surgery.

This account of the care of patients undergoing thyroid surgery includes patients with forms of hyperthyroidism, nontoxic nodular goiter, carcinoma and thyroiditis.

HYPERTHYROIDISM

Several alternatives are available for the treatment of the patient with hyperthyroidism. The surgeon should know the advantages and disadvantages of each, and so they are described in some detail.

The problems of diagnosis of hyperthyroidism have already been described in the first part of this chapter. Hyperthyroidism is usually overt and obvious. Hidden or masked hyperthyroidism occurs, however, and may present a considerable problem to the diagnostician, for it may be confused with other conditions, such as hyperadrenalism, essential hypertension and psychoneurosis. The difficulties in diagnosis are most often encountered when eye signs are absent and in the old and very young. The diagnosis of masked hyperthyroidism is made only when the physician keeps the possibility in mind.

CHOICE OF THERAPY

There are two types of therapy: the traditional, attacking the thyroid and the orbital contents, and the recently emerging therapy directed at one of the etiologic components—the emotional or central nervous system component. Those directed at the thyroid are the time-honored surgical subtotal thyroidectomy, radiation therapy and long-continued antithyroid drug therapy.

Initial Therapy. Just as soon as the diagnosis of hyperthyroidism has been established, antithyroid drug therapy should be started. The metabolic rate should be brought to normal as promptly as possible and maintained at a normal level for at least three weeks. The patient should be informed that this is the initial step and that until it has been accomplished the definitive therapy will not be decided upon.

There are three reasons for this initial step. First, the therapeutic response to the drug will have confirmed the diagnosis. The antithyroid drugs now available have a specific chemical action to block the formation of the thyroid hormone. Failure of the hypermetabolism to fall indicates that it is due to some other cause.

Second, the physician (this includes the surgeon) has the chance to come to know the patient. Extensive knowledge is essential to a wise choice of the ultimate therapy.

Third, the patient is returned to physical comfort and autonomic nervous system balance. The patient, relieved of the physical burden and emotional excitement induced by hyperthyroidism, gives the physician a truer picture of himself. The restoration of the balance of the autonomic nervous system eliminates the dangers, such as cardiac fibrillation, that are always pending in a patient with hyperthyroidism. An account of the autonomic system imbalance is given in detail earlier in this chapter.

Definitive Therapy. With surgery, radiation, drug and psychotherapy all available, how does one choose between them?

Surgery, the first approach to reach reasonable perfection, has been in large part surpassed by other methods, but it is still useful in the patient to whom one of the newer forms of therapy is not applicable. The advantage of surgical subtotal thyroidectomy is that it relieves hyperthyroidism most rapidly and perhaps most securely. Surgical therapy obviously means all the disagreeableness and threat of operation and it is expensive in physician time, requiring from 15 to 20 physician hours. There are also occasional operative accidents or complications. The surgeon has not as yet been trained who can remove sufficient thyroid tissue to cure the patient without damaging the parathyroids or a recurrent nerve and without postoperative hemorrhage, despite apparent meticulous technique. All of these can be major, even life-endangering, accidents. Because they may occur even in the best of hands, if a nonoperative therapy offers as good a promise as the surgical, the nonoperative is to be chosen.

Introduced in 1941, therapy using radioactive iodine eliminates hyperthyroidism successfully and with the greatest ease of all the methods. For the patient, it offers the least fuss and bother. Radiation therapy, however, is followed by a high incidence of progressive hypothyroidism. Thirty per cent or more of patients so treated thus far have developed hypothyroidism. This means that all patients receiving this therapy must be followed, and thyroid therapy must be given promptly in order to avoid dangerous levels of hypothyroidism. Present understanding suggests that this late failure of the gland to maintain a normal function is inevitable, because the continuing regeneration of thyroid cells in the normal gland is crippled by irradiation. This defect of irradiation therapy suggests in turn that this form of therapy will be but a passing phase in our treatment of patients with hyperthyroidism.

Antithyroid drug therapy is the simplest and least damaging of the measures that affect hyperthyroidism. Alone, however, it is not an adequate, definitive therapy. Something else has to happen. Either changes must take place within the patient or psychotherapy must be added. These changes are the spontaneously occurring social or emotional adjustments that enable the central nervous system balance to reestablish itself. Drug therapy will thus have tided the patient over the phase of overactive thyroid stimulation, and as such it is most useful.

Drug therapy has the disadvantage, however, of being associated occasionally with drug sensitivity. Reactions such as agranulocytosis or the Mikulicz syndrome are dangerous or disabling, and the physician must be constantly on the alert. Drug therapy, therefore, can also be expensive in physician time.

Psychotherapy is the most fundamental of the therapies. Long considered as a possibility, it has only recently been applied with success as a definitive therapy. Its use is based upon the concept that imbalance of the central nervous system is an important component in the etiology of Graves' disease.

Graves' disease, and hyperthyroidism in general, is caused almost certainly by multiple factors, components or contingencies. The sex of the patient is certainly one, and genetic susceptibility appears to be another in some patients. As far as the central nervous system component is concerned, there are two phases, and both are to be found in most patients. The first is an underlying emotional disquietude, a precarious emotional balance. The second is an acute, trying emotional episode immediately preceding the onset of the disease. Usually both of these phases are easily identifiable by relatively simple clinical questioning. If they can be offset, no other therapy may be needed. In other patients, either they are not identifiable or nothing effective can be done about them, and psychotherapy is therefore not available. Even if the circumstances can be only partially altered, psychotherapy should be pursued to preclude progressive exophthalmos.

Continuing Therapy—The Central Nervous System Hypothalamic Component. Graves' disease and hyperthyroidism in general is associated with a stubborn tendency to recur, in 15 per cent of patients following operation in some series and in 50 per cent even after two years of drug therapy. Its failure to reappear is perhaps an advantage of radiation therapy.

Reducing the tendency to recur is a theoretical advantage of psychotherapy. Even if it does not seem possible to use psychotherapy as the definitive therapy, it is to be kept in mind and used to its fullest extent as an adjunct to surgery, drug therapy or radiation. Not only will it theoretically reduce the incidence of recurrence but it should diminish the subsequent development of other psychosomatic disorders. (Patients with Graves' disease have had or will have, with greater than normal frequency, such disorders as Addison's disease, myasthenia gravis and ovarian and gastrointestinal disturbances.)

The Exophthalmos—Continuing or Progressive. For the majority of patients with hyperthyroidism, exophthalmos does not prove to be a clinically important problem. In a small minority the exophthalmos may be stubborn and disfiguring and will be the threatening issue. The majority of patients from early youth through middle age develop some exophthalmos associated with their hyperthyroidism—that is, they have true exophthalmic goiter or Graves' disease. Older patients are less likely to develop exophthalmos, but when they do, it may be particularly troublesome.

As a rule exophthalmos takes care of itself as the hyperthyroidism is treated. It was noted long ago that immediately following operation on the goiter, exophthalmos got a little worse for a few weeks and then began diminishing. It is quite clear that it is not the excess of thyroid hormone that creates exophthalmos, but rather it is an associated component of the basic disease. It is in those few patients in whom the exophthalmos persists, and particularly those in whom it increases (the progressive form), that the eye trouble is difficult. As it progresses, it may be associated with diplopia, loss of control of eye movements, severe conjunctivitis, ulceration of the cornea and finally, in extreme form, blindness. Long before these severe complications have occurred, indeed as soon as muscular lameness and double vision appear, surgical relief (orbital decompression) should be considered.

Almost nothing is known about the genesis of exophthalmos. The stimulus appears to be independent of that inducing the goiter; the exophthalmos may appear long before the goiter or long after. As there is no sound understanding, treatment is empirical. Clinical evidence suggests, however, that its etiology also has a central nervous system component, and it is therefore particularly important in patients with marked or progressive exophthalmos to pay attention to the possible psychologic components. It is only fair to say that evidence regarding the central nervous system component and etiology is much less persuasive than that in regard to the thyroid overactivity, where the physiologic steps involved between the hypothalamus and the thyroid gland have become well established.

MANAGEMENT

The management of the patient with hyperthyroidism is conveniently set forth in a series of steps.

Step 1. Reduction of Metabolic Rate to Normal. As soon as the diagnosis of hyperthyroidism is established, an antithyroid drug should be administered. The dose should be a large one at the beginning and gradually reduced as the metabolic rate reaches normal. In the northern hemisphere the thyroid mechanism in the patient with Graves' disease is stimulated to a greater degree during the winter months than during the summer and early fall. The dosage of drug needed, therefore, tends to be greater from January through April than from August to October. In general the antithyroid drugs should be given in divided doses, a dose every 8 hours. They are generally rapidly excreted by the kidney, and the 8 hour schedule helps maintain a chemically active level.

Propylthiouracil is the most commonly used antithyroid drug. In patients with severe hyperthyroidism the initial dose may well be 300 mg. every 8 hours. The maintenance dose in such a patient may be 100 mg. every 8 hours in winter and 50 mg. every 8 hours in late summer.

Methimazole (Tapazol) is an alternative drug, and the initial dose may be 15 mg. every 8 hours and the maintenance dose 5 mg. every 8 hours.

Both propylthiouracil and methimazole may become toxic in susceptible individuals. The commonest complication is agranulocytosis; the white count should therefore be followed periodically, probably once a month, and particular care should be taken if the patient develops an upper respiratory or other infection. Skin rashes and acute inflammation of the salivary glands are other forms of drug sensitivity. If sensitivity to propylthiouracil develops, the patient may be shifted to methimazole for a trial. If sensitivity also develops to this drug, a third alternative is potassium perchlorate, 100 mg. every 8 hours. Sensitivity may develop to this drug as well.

Step 2. Evaluation of Etiology and Choice of Definitive Therapy. As the patient is seen to observe the progress of the drug therapy and to check on possible complications, the opportunity is to be taken to look for possible psychogenic factors. Their nature and whether it is possible to deal with them in an effective manner will determine what part psychotherapy will play in the definitive treatment. For social and economic reasons it may be wise to combine it with one of the other therapies.

Step 3. Social and Psychologic Aid. As much as possible should be done to help the patient remedy both social and psychological situations.

If it proves advisable to elect surgical thyroidectomy as one part of the therapy of the patient, additional steps follow.

Step 4. Preparation for Operation. Because the patient will have been euthyroid for at least three weeks, long enough to have regained balance of the autonomic nervous system, there is less hazard to the operation and less of special nature in the preoperative management. It should in general follow those precepts outlined earlier in this chapter.

Step 5. Operative Management. The choice of drugs and anesthetic agents should in general follow the outline in the first part of this chapter.

Because the patient is euthyroid and should be in good balance, the operation need not be hurried. It should be carefully and meticulously carried out and the amount of thyroid tissue reduced to a remnant or remnants, whose output will be just normal.

In determining the size of the remnant it should be recalled that the same stimulus that gave rise to the hyperplasia originally will presumably continue, for psychotherapy will not have been effective. There will be therefore a tendency for the remnant to undergo continuing hyperplasia and increased output. To avoid recrudescence the remnant should be less than enough to produce a normal amount, anticipating that there will be some further hyperplasia. In the interval between operation and the time when this hyperplasia will have added sufficiently to the production of hormone, there will be a period of hypothyroidism. In order to keep the patient from being actually hypo-thyroid, thyroid medication should be planned. Fortunately in most patients there seems to be a limit to the degree of hyperplasia that thyroid tissue undergoes. (This is by no means always true, and full size goiters may eventually grow from small remnants.)

Step 6. Postoperative Program. The special care needed by the patient who has undergone a thyroidectomy relates to the complica-tions of the operation itself, namely recurrent laryngeal palsy, hemor-rhage and parathyroid gland damage. The ability of the patient to phonate immediately following anesthesia does not altogether exclude the possibility of bilateral vocal cord paralysis. The nerve may not have been severed at operation but only traumatized, and failure of the nerve may come hours later. At any rate, bilateral cord palsy is associated first with flaccid paralysis. Hours later the cords assume a fixed median position with virtually complete closure of the glottis. If this is not recognized promptly and a tracheostomy done, the patient will suffo-cate. The commonest time for this to occur is approximately 18 hours after the operation.

Hemorrhage in a thyroidectomy wound often does not occur imme-diately postoperatively but is delayed until the patient is swallowing. Again, the commonest time for a hemorrhage to be encountered is between 12 and 24 hours after operation. Because the hemorrhage is into an enclosed space and the internal jugular veins are pressed upon, edema of the larynx may develop rapidly. Again, if the blood is not evacuated promptly, there may be complete closure of the glottis and tracheostomy will be needed. Draining the operative wound is by no means a satisfactory method of recognizing the presence of a hemor-rhage. In many cases the blood clots promptly in the wound and does not seep out through the drain to a sufficient degree to warn the nurse or doctor. Regular breathing and the absence of swelling in the operative wound are more reliable signs that all is well.

Tetany also takes time to appear. The interval between operation and onset depends upon the degree to which the parathyroid glands have been molested. If only one parathyroid has been removed or disturbed, there may be no clinical tetany. If three have been disturbed and one unmolested, the tetany may be only mild and transient. If all four have been disturbed, even though not resected, tetany will have appeared by the twenty-fourth hour and may become severe in the next 24 hours. If the calcium level goes to as low as 6 mg./100 cc. (3 mEq.) by the forty-eighth hour, the tetany will be severe, and it is important to give calcium intravenously and intramuscularly. In severe tetany the feared complication is closure of the glottis and strangulation. The clini-cal sequence of developing tetany usually starts with a positive Chvostek sign. As tetany becomes stronger, the Trousseau sign will be positive. Then there will be spontaneous spasms, particularly of the fingers and toes. Next will come tingling of the fingers and toes and around the mouth and a general sense of apprehension, and finally, closure of the glottis.

The dosages of calcium to be given intravenously were outlined in the first part of this chapter. The most readily utilizable salt is calcium chloride. This should be administered in a 10 per cent solution intravenously. Care should be taken with the injection, because the solution is highly irritating. Two to five ml. of this solution is ordinarily sufficient to relieve severe tetany temporarily.

As indicated under "Operative Management," the patient is to be maintained on thyroid medication for some months, perhaps years. For the average patient, the dosage starts in the neighborhood of 120 mg. of desiccated thyroid daily. This is based on the assumption that the average normal requirement for thyroid hormone is 200 mg. of desiccated thyroid daily. Sixty to eighty mg. will presumably be secreted by the remnant, and the remainder will be supplied by pill. As the patient's wound heals, it may be possible to reduce this dosage slowly. It may be needed permanently, however, and it is even possible that the remnants will function very little over the following several years and a slightly larger dose of thyroid will be needed. It is not always possible to judge successfully the desired size of the remnants. It is presumed easier for the patient to have to take thyroid indefinitely than to need a second operation for recurrent hyperthyroidism.

NONTOXIC NODULAR (ADENOMATOUS) GOITER

In no other type of goiter is decision more difficult regarding the need for operation than in nontoxic nodular goiter.

Nodules in the thyroid are common, and increase in frequency with each decade of life. Malignancy is rare. The best estimate of the incidence of thyroid lumps is 40,000 per 1,000,000 people, of which in any one year only 25 will be cancerous. The problem, therefore, is to determine which of the many lumps are malignant. The treatment of those that are not malignant should preferably be by thyroid therapy and suppression of the pituitary's thyrotropic hormone.

If a lump is suspected of being cancerous on first examination, obviously a diagnosis should be established promptly and presumably the lump should be excised in appropriate fashion.

If no lump of a goiter is clearly suspected of being malignant, the patient should have a trial of thyroid medication. If the lumps diminish or resolve completely, then good enough. If they remain unchanged when the intervening tissue shrinks, they may be watched. If they continue to grow despite the suppression, then by physiologic definition they are outlaws and neoplastic, and they should be resected.

Prior to 1942, when there was no other therapy than operation, it was easier to decide whether to operate. Often the size and configuration of the goiter became the deciding issue. Since 1942, with the increasing understanding of the pituitary's role in the etiology of goiter, thyroid therapy has become an increasingly useful means of treating nodular goiter. The concept of the treatment is that thyroid medication suppresses the anterior pituitary's secreting of thyrotropic hormone and thus in turn quiets the thyroid. Hyperplasia, secretion and vascularity all are decreased. The colloid of the degenerative cystic areas is resorbed and the goiter shrinks. Frequently the original thyroid volume is reached, leaving no signs of the previously existing goiter. Even discrete nodules may resorb. How and when do you try thyroid, and for how long?

Index of Suspicion of Cancer. If the goiter seems to contain cancer, it is good judgment to proceed immediately to operation. If no one area is suspected of being malignant, a trial of thyroid is worthwhile. What leads one to suspect the presence of cancer?

Localized Versus Diffuse Goiter. By definition, cancer, a neoplasm, does not suddenly develop diffusely throughout an organ such as the thyroid. If the enlargement involves the gland proportionately and diffusely, malignant disease almost certainly is not the cause of the enlargement. Graves' disease, iodine deficiency, a goitrogen or thyroiditis is likely. If, on the other hand, one area of the gland is out of line with the rest, localized disease is present. The simplest example of this type is the single nodule. If that nodule is not a cyst, by definition it is a neoplasm, benign or malignant. In judging the presence of localized disease, the surgeon and physician should not be misled by the greater size of the right thyroid lobe. The thyroid gland is not symmetrical; the right lobe averages 25 per cent larger than the left. The disparity is reversed in patients with situs inversus.

Local Signs. Other important signs are the character of the localized disease process. Carcinoma is usually harder and more irregular; sometimes capsular irregularities can be felt. In contrast, benign adenomas and cysts are smoothly encapsulated. They often can be moved within the thyroid substance.

These two local signs, determined on physical examination, may be much more accurate if the patient has already had a trial of thyroid medication. The medication will have been followed by resolution and atrophy of the undiseased portion of the gland, whereas the neoplasm will have remained for the most part unaffected. The neoplasm will stand out like a sore thumb in the otherwise atrophic gland.

Similarly, at operation it will be easier for the surgeon to discriminate between that part of the thyroid gland obeying physiologic control and that which does not respond to physiologic control and is made up of outlaw cells. This will be referred to later under "Management."

Lymph Node Enlargement. The presence of enlarged lymph

nodes should immediately arouse the suspicion of the examiner. The Delphian lymph node group, in front of the cricoid cartilage immediately above the thyroid isthmus, is one of the easiest node groups to be felt. Normal nodes are very hard to palpate and when slightly enlarged are still difficult to identify in front of a soft organ, such as the internal jugular vein. Situated in front of the cricoid cartilage, however, the nodes are against a firm background and slight enlargement may be recognizable. The presence of enlarged nodes above or below the thyroid isthmus should immediately arouse suspicion of malignant disease. They are also commonly involved in Hashimoto's thyroiditis, a troublesome note in the differential diagnosis discussed later.

Needle Biopsy. A needle biopsy is helpful in the diagnosis of goiter. It is most reliable in differentiating Hashimoto's thyroiditis from other nodular goiters but may be misleading in identifying the character of various nodules in multinodular goiter. The presence of adenomatous tissue in one nodule of a multinodular goiter does not exclude the possible presence of carcinoma in another one of the nodules. In a well differentiated thyroid tumor, it is also difficult to exclude the possibility of adenocarcinoma of low malignancy. Many a solid thyroid tumor consisting of well differentiated tissue has been diagnosed as a benign follicular adenoma, only to later give rise to blood-borne metastases, usually to bone. The clue to this differentiation lies in careful search for capsular and venous invasion; a needle biopsy cannot be relied upon to give an adequate specimen for examination. This method, therefore, has strict limitations.

Roentgenograms. Roentgenograms are sometimes useful in the diagnosis of goiter. Pointlike calcifications indicate malignant disease. In contrast, larger plaques, particularly if arranged around the capsule of a nodule, suggest earlier necrosis with calcification of a benign lesion. The presence of incipient tracheal compression is useful knowledge, and the roentgenogram may show it before it has developed to a clinically recognizable state.

Radioactive Iodine Scan. The radioactive iodine scan yields much information regarding the secretory activity of the gland but disappointingly little about possible neoplasia. The vast majority of nodules are cold—the common degenerative cysts and benign adenomas, as well as the rare carcinomas. Hot nodules are uncommon, and an occasional one of these is a well-differentiated carcinoma of low-grade malignancy. The proportion of hot to malignancy is approximately the same as that of cold to malignancy. To operate upon a nodule because it is cold represents a misconception.

MANAGEMENT

If the clinical suspicion is firm that a nodular goiter, single or multinodular, harbors a carcinoma, proceed immediately to establish the diagnosis by either needle or open surgical biopsy. If the suspicion is slight and the nodule is single, do a needle biopsy. If there are multiple nodules, no one more suspicious than another, use a trial of thyroid medication and the passage of time to help make the diagnosis.

Trial of Thyroid Medication.   The trial of thyroid medication as a rule takes at least three or four months. Sometimes resolution of the goiter is already evident within the first four weeks. Occasionally, on the other hand, significant resolution of the goiter takes many months, and the goiter may not reach its point of final resolution for two or three years.

Once a patient has started on thyroid medication, he should be watched periodically, at first for tolerance of the medication and then subsequently to see whether any of the lumps left, as the main mass of the goiter resolves, are increasingly suspected of malignant disease.

If a patient tolerates the medication poorly, smoldering toxicity should be suspected. Occasionally a patient's tests for thyroid function are all within the accepted normal range and yet the patient is mildly hyperthyroid. Such a patient's indices would be in the upper normal range, and because toxicity is not evident clinically, the patient has masked Graves' disease. In such patients thyroid medication fails to suppress the pituitary stimulating mechanism; the medication becomes additive, and for the first time these patients develop symptoms of thyrotoxicosis. They are to be classified as having subclinical Graves' disease and are to be treated as patients with hyperthyroidism or a combination of nodular goiter with hyperthyroidism.

Thyroid medication is best started gradually. Many patients can take the full dose all at once, but the function in some cannot be suppressed in a few days and they may have mild symptoms in the first two or three weeks. It has become our custom, therefore, to place the average adult patient on 60 mg. of desiccated thyroid daily for one week, double the dose for the second week and from the beginning of the third week the fully suppressive dose of 180 mg. daily. Some doctors prefer the quick-acting triiodothyronine (T3), but for patients taking this type of hormone it is necessary to divide the daily dose into three parts, otherwise the level of administered hormone will fluctuate. For this reason either thyroxine or desiccated thyroid is better, because their action is much slower. The equivalents in thyroid effect are, for 60 mg. of desiccated thyroid, 100 μg. of L-thyroxine and 25 μg. of triiodothyronine.

Operation.   Even if the patient has been on a trial of thyroid medication and comes to operation, he is still euthyroid and there are therefore no special considerations. The program followed for the patient with hyperthyroidism rendered euthyroid is to be followed.

The intraoperative design is determined by the character of the goiter. The first objective is to make a diagnosis. In the order of exposure, first comes the thyroid isthmus, then the Delphian and pretracheal lymph nodes, and third the lateral thyroid lobes. As mentioned, if the patient has been on thyroid medication it will be relatively easy to differentiate between law-abiding atrophic thyroid tissue and neoplasia. The neoplasia will not have responded by undergoing atrophy and will stick out like a sore thumb, more easily seen and palpated. What has been law-abiding may be safely left behind. The outlaw cells are to be excised, usually with sufficient margin of uninvolved tissue to insure removing all of the capsule. The diagnosis of the outlaw tissue should be determined at the operating table. It can usually be established with certainty by gross appearance. Frozen section or permanent section is needed for confirmation only, rarely for the definitive diagnosis. If there is suspicion that the tumor may be malignant, the lymph node areas draining the site of the primary tumor should be documented by resection of at least one node from each area, so that when the diagnosis is firmly established, lymph nodes will be available to determine whether there has been any spread of the primary lesion via the lymphatic channels to the lymph nodes. The need for further operation will be clarified by this procedure. Similar lymph node identification is useful when the primary lesion is suspected of being papillary.

The exception is the well-differentiated adenocarcinoma, whose gross and microscopic appearance at first sight is benign (so-called metastasizing adenoma).

Postoperative Program. The need for special attention to the patient who has had a thyroidectomy has been discussed under "Hyperthyroidism." The program is to be followed here in the same careful manner.

Because it has been shown that thyroid medication is useful in the treatment of nodular goiter, it is logical to use thyroid medication as part of the postoperative program with the view of preventing recurrence of the goiter. An estimate is to be made of the secretory potential of the remaining thyroid tissue. Then, under the assumption that the total need of the average adult patient is 180 mg. of thyroid hormone per day, the amount that would have been secreted by the tissue resected is to be given in pill form by mouth. Thus the patient who has lost all of the right thyroid lobe but is left with a normal-appearing left thyroid lobe should receive approximately 60 to 70 per cent of the estimated normal need in pill form. The reasons for more than half the normal amount are that the right lobe is normally larger than the left and that it is wise to give a little more thyroid than needed in order to reduce the load on the remaining tissue. It is probably also wise to allow the remaining tissue to function and not to give a totally suppressive dose. The remaining tissue is thus allowed to follow the normal seasonal fluctuations in needs. The use of thyroid extract postoperatively, on the basis of prevention, has succeeded in reducing postoperative recurrence of goiter to a considerable extent.

CARCINOMA

The problems of carcinoma of the thyroid are of diagnosis, surgical judgment and technical needs in the therapy of each type. There are no special concerns regarding preoperative and postoperative care applying to carcinoma, beyond those applying to other thyroid operations. Carcinoma is a rare complication of hyperthyroidism. In the papillary form, it does sometimes appear in goiters of patients with long-standing Graves' disease. It is to be thought of when the form of definitive therapy is being considered. The presence in the overactive goiter of one area out of line with the rest of the goiter should arouse the suspicion of a probable neoplasm, possibly malignant.

The majority of thyroid carcinomas are of the papillary type. Twenty per cent of these are of mixed type, papillary and adenocarcinoma. The papillary carcinoma is ideal for surgical treatment. It is curable by surgery alone. It spreads via the lymphatics and lives for years in lymph nodes. It rarely gives rise to implants. Lymphatic channels can be cut across with impunity. Indeed the carcinoma itself can be cut into and the surgeon can then backtrack with safety.

This is also true with adenocarcinomas, most of which are very slow-growing. They only occasionally spread to the lymphatic nodes, their mode of spread being by the bloodstream. Occasionally there is a single metastasis in the bone. If such is found, radical excision of the bone may be indicated.

For the rapidly growing, undifferentiated carcinomas, surgery is an inadequate therapy. Operation, therefore, is used only to establish the diagnosis, and sometimes to get rid of a bulky mass of tumor. Radiation is the treatment of choice and the only hope. Usually by the time the diagnosis is made, however, it is too late. The blood has borne metastases to distant spots already, but radiation of the local masses in the neck is worthwhile, because an occasional patient is saved by this maneuver.

It is especially important in the surgical management of the more benign carcinomas, namely the papillary and well-differentiated adenocarcinomas, to be careful to spare both parathyroids and recurrent laryngeal nerves. For too long, surgeons have been rushing in with well intended but misguided therapeutic ambitions, carrying out radical removals of muscles, parathyroid glands and, indeed, recurrent laryngeal nerves. Rare is the occasion when the nerve has to be removed. Usually it can be teased out of the tumor-bearing lymph nodes or from the back of a primary carcinoma within the thyroid lobe. So, too, can parathyroids be found and left, either with a pedicle or free of the excision, or can be divided into small pieces and reimplanted subcutaneously between skin and platysma in the outer end of the thyroidectomy incision. It is not necessary to plant these little grafts into muscle. Indeed, the takes are probably better in areolar tissue than in muscle.

Then, too, muscles such as the sternocleidomastoid muscle do not need to be resected. Rare is the tumor that invades them. Fasciae can be cleared from them just as well as from the carotid artery, internal jugular vein and vagus nerve. The cosmetic result is incomparably better. The internal jugular veins also are rarely invaded, and they too are to be saved. If such invasion occurs, there will have been widespread dissemination, and because the carotid artery and vagus nerve may not be resected with impunity, cure by surgical excision is problematic. Radiation is to be tried.

THYROIDITIS

As with the carcinomas, there is little of special note regarding the preoperative and postoperative care of patients with the various forms of thyroiditis. The problems of thyroiditis again involve the intimate diagnosis and the application of the appropriate therapy. Rarely is surgical excision the therapy of choice for any one of the goiters due to thyroiditis. Acute thyroiditis runs its spontaneous course. Sometimes there are recurrences. What is important is to recognize the disease and restrain the surgical hand.

Similarly subacute thyroiditis rarely presents a surgical problem. Chronic thyroiditis, on the other hand, may slowly develop a goiter mass that is not restrained by either thyroid medication or a light dose of x-ray therapy. In this case removal of the thyroid isthmus, to relieve pressure, may be worthwhile.

For the most part, patients with thyroiditis should be put on thyroid medication. This is more to maintain a normal level of circulating thyroid hormone than to obtain any reduction in the process of thyroiditis by suppressing the thyrotropic secretion of the anterior pituitary. In some cases sufficient secreting thyroid cells are destroyed to produce severe hypothyroidism. Cortisone has been tried during the active inflammatory phase; relief has been reported. Until more is known of the nature of the genesis of these forms of thyroiditis, the treatment will remain empirical, using thyroid medication.

REFERENCES

Astwood, E. B.: Treatment of hyperthyroidism with thiourea and thiouracil. J.A.M.A. *122*:78, 1943.

Blizzard, R. M., Hung, W., Chandler, R. W., Aceto, T., Jr., Kyle, M., and Winship, T.: Hashimoto's thyroiditis: Clinical and laboratory response to prolonged cortisone therapy. N. Eng. J. Med. *267*:1015, 1962.

Davis, R. H., Fourman, P., and Smith, J. W. G.: Prevalence of parathyroid insufficiency after thyroidectomy. Lancet. 2:1432, 1961.

Dunn, J. T., and Chapman, E.: Rising incidence of hypothyroidism after radioactive iodine therapy in thyrotoxicosis. N. Eng. J. Med. *271*:1037, 1964.

Godley, A. F., and Stanbury, J. B.: Preliminary experience in treatment of hyperthyroidism with potassium perchlorate. J. Clin. Endocrinol. *14*:70, 1954.

Greer, M. A., and Astwood, E. B.: Treatment of simple goiter with thyroid. J. Clin.
Endocrinol. Metab. *13*:1312, 1953.

Harris, G. W., and Woods, J. W.: The effect of electrical stimulation of the hypothalamus
or pituitary gland on thyroid activity. J. Physiol. *143*:246, 1958.

Hazard, J. B.: Thyroiditis: A review. Am. J. Clin. Pathol. *25*:289, 399, 1955.

Hertz, S., and Roberts, A.: Radioactive iodine in the study of thyroid physiology. VIII.
The use of radioactive iodine therapy in hyperthyroidism. J.A.M.A. *131*:81, 1946.

Lidz, T., and Whitehorn, J. C.: Psychiatric problems in thyroid clinic. J.A.M.A. *139*:698,
1949.

McConahey, W. M., Keating, R. R., Jr., Beahrs, O. H., and Woolner, L. B.: On the
increasing occurrence of Hashimoto's thyroiditis. J. Clin. Endocrinol. Metab. *22*:542,
1962.

Rienhoff, W. F., Jr.: Microscopic changes induced in thyroid gland by oral administration
of desiccated thyroid. Arch. Surg. *41*:487, 1940.

Schlesinger, J. J., Gargill, G. L., and Saxe, I. H.: Studies in nodular goiter. I. Incidence of
thyroid nodules in routine necropsies in non-goitrous region. J.A.M.A. *110*:1638,
1938.

Sokal, J. E.: The incidence of thyroid cancer and the problem of malignancy in nodular
goiter. *In* Astwood, E. B., ed.: Clinical Endocrinology. New York, Grune & Stratton,
1960, Vol. 1, p. 168.

Taylor, G. W., and Painter, N. S.: Size of the thyroid remnant in partial thyroidectomy for
toxic goiter. Lancet *1*:287, 1962.

Warren, S., and Meissner, W. A.: Tumors of the thyroid gland. *In* Atlas of Tumor
Pathology. Washington, Armed Forces Institute of Pathology, 1953.

Werner, S. C.: The thyroid: Genetic and psychiatric relations. Dis. Nerv. Syst. *22*:Suppl.
33, 1961.

CHAPTER 26

THE PARATHYROID GLANDS

OLIVER COPE, M.D., F.A.C.S.

Disturbance of Parathyroid Function

INTRODUCTION

Disorders of the parathyroid glands, both hyper- and hypoparathyroidism, present special problems to the surgeon. Hyperparathyroidism is especially trying because it is so frequently blurred over by its complications, hard for the busy specialist to keep in mind and all too seldom diagnosed when the patient is first seen. Hypoparathyroidism, though more overt, presents a stubborn problem of management.

The primary glandular disorder of hyperparathyroidism has several separate complications, each of which may require an operation. The complications include not only those of the bones and kidneys, but also those of the upper gastrointestinal tract and pancreas. The emergency nature of the complication may require an operation which takes precedence over correction of the parathyroid disturbance. The patient with hyperparathyroidism may also, of course, suffer other emergency conditions unrelated to the glandular disturbance. For all of these conditions — the related and unrelated — the continued presence of the glandular disorder must be taken into account to insure smooth passage of the operation. Otherwise, continuing complications may occur.

Hypoparathyroidism, more overt, usually well known to the patient, and obvious to the physician, presents a more circumscribed type of complication. By its stubborn nature, however, it can be an annoying problem of management.

This discussion refers to problems of diagnosis of the glandular disorders and deals with the hazards of operation in their continuing active presence.

HYPERPARATHYROIDISM

Hyperparathyroidism presents special problems. First are those of diagnosis. Then there are the dangers of its presence — of the glandular disorder and of the complications which may occur even in the presence of a mild degree of the glandular disorder. These problems and dangers are considered first and the details of management second.

THE PROBLEMS AND THE DANGERS

The Problems of Diagnosis. The most trying matter about hyperparathyroidism is the difficulty of diagnosis. Rarely is this glandular disorder diagnosed on the basis of the primary disturbances. It is thought of and diagnosed only after a complication has taken place. This delay in diagnosis is regrettable because so often the complications become compounded and more difficult to remedy when the primary disorder is finally diagnosed. As will be recounted in the part of this chapter dealing with care of the primary disease, the difficulty of the diagnosis is not only that of keeping it in mind but in actually, definitively establishing the diagnosis.

So often a mild degree of the disease may result in severe complications and the mildness makes the chemical diagnostic signs equivocal. Thus it takes only a mild degree of hyperparathyroidism to produce kidney stones if the conditions are otherwise contributory. Renal calcification may also result from mild hyperparathyroidism, with severe impairment of renal function. The patient thus is ill, not from the primary disease, but from the renal damage. It is incumbent on the various specialists caring for the complications to keep the disorder in mind and to diagnose it as quickly as possible. The problems of diagnosis are also considered later in this chapter.

The Dangers of the Disease. The dangers which ensue from the presence of hyperparathyroidism are twofold: those from the primary disease and those from the complications. Those from the complications are also described later in this chapter under their separate entities in "Problems of Diagnosis."

The dangers of the disease itself stem from the rise in the level of the calcium ion in the plasma and body fluids. Of little consequence when the disease is mild and the calcium level is only slightly elevated, these dangers become of increasing importance as the disease worsens and the calcium level rises. The primary disturbances of the elevation of the calcium ion relate almost wholly to the nervous system, because the calcium ion is involved in the transmission of nervous impulses. There is also, apparently, an effect of calcium on the coagulating mechanism of the blood when the concentration of the total calcium reaches extraordinarily high levels (20 mg./100 cc. [10 mEq.] or over).

As the calcium level of the serum rises, muscular relaxation increases. Although patients may drop things from their hands or trip with their feet, this is of little consequence beyond the associated general fatigue until the calcium level rises to 16 mg./100 cc. or above. In the presence of the higher level, cardiac standstill may occur. This presumably arises from the change in sensitivity of the nerve-muscle transmission. Rare at 16 mg., it is considered imminent at 18 mg.

At these same high levels the mind is blurred and sometimes disturbed, and as the level of 18 mg. is reached coma may supervene. This blurring of mental acuity may be mistaken for cerebral vascular damage and, indeed, occasionally there are fleeting signs of strokes.

Thickening of the blood and spontaneous coagulation have been induced experimentally in animals given huge doses of parathormone, and these are believed to have occurred clinically in patients with severe degrees of hyperparathyroidism inadvertently fed large quantities of calcium. (A sign of the impending thickening of the blood may well be a preliminary renal shutdown.)

The Complications.   The complications by which the diagnosis is most often made and which lead to the commonest types of difficulties needing operation are those relating to the kidney, the upper gastrointestinal tract, the bones and the pancreas.

RENAL COLIC, CALCIFICATION AND SHUTDOWN.   The commonest complications thus far associated with hyperparathyroidism relate to the kidney and urinary tract. The simplest is the formation of renal stones. Stones may also form in the prostate. If the condition continues and particularly if the patient receives sufficient calcium in the diet, there may be calcification of the kidney parenchyma. When this is associated with the gastrointestinal complications for which milk and alkali are given in therapy, the kidney is faced with added difficulties and may become acutely impaired and shut down. This may happen even in the presence of a relatively mild degree of the glandular disorder.

The presence of hyperparathyroidism must be thought of when such complications are encountered in the urinary tract. The patient may present with a stone in the ureter, for example, with colic and possible reflex renal shutdown. Such a situation is an emergency and takes precedence. However, as soon as possible the primary glandular disorder must be attended to in order to prevent recurrence of stones.

UPPER GASTROINTESTINAL ULCERATION WITH HEMORRHAGE OR PERFORATION.   Ulceration of the upper gastrointestinal tract is an established complication of hyperparathyroidism and the possibility of hyperparathyroidism must be kept in mind when patients with ulcers are encountered. The ulcers may occur in the stomach, the duodenum and occasionally in the small intestine below. If the hyperparathyroidism is neglected, the ulcers may worsen with hemorrhage or perforation; the surgeon may be driven into an immediate emergency operation. The minimum should be done to the ulcer and resections and vagotomy avoided since healing will occur with correction of the hyperparathyroidism. As with the acute renal complications, correction of the hyperparathyroidism must follow to prevent continued ulcer formation, including a stomal ulcer if a resection has been carried out.

BONE DISEASE. Disease of the bones was the first complication of hyperparathyroidism to be described. Indeed, it was initially considered that the primary disease was one of the bone. It has subsequently been realized that the bone disease is a complication, for it is by no means always present. The parathyroid hormone, as one of its primary effects, increases the turnover of calcium and phosphorus and perhaps other minerals in bone. There is, therefore, an accelerated breakdown and compensatory regeneration of bone. If the degree of hyperparathyroidism is intense, the regeneration is inadequate and thinning of the bones occurs. This may be simple demineralization but there may also be associated brown tumors, cysts and fibrosis of the marrow. Fractures may occur through the brown tumors or cysts, rarely through simple thinning. Obviously when fractures occur, these need immediate attention. Curiously, these fractures usually heal despite the presence of continued hyperparathyroidism. Since troubles are going on in other parts of the body, care of the primary glandular disorder must follow immediately the setting of the fracture.

PANCREATITIS. Pancreatic calcification and pancreatitis are less frequent complications of hyperparathyroidism, but in patients with severe degrees of the disease, pancreatic calcification is common. It is found at autopsy in half the patients who die from the disease, while it is seen uncommonly by x-ray in patients with mild degrees of the disease. Acute pancreatitis may supervene occasionally in patients with moderate as well as severe degrees of hyperparathyroidism, and the reason for the onset of the attack is unexplained at the present time. Its possible occurrence is to be kept in mind, however, in patients with hyperparathyroidism and with abdominal pains of varying severity.

MANAGEMENT

There is nothing at present known to diminish the intensity of hyperparathyroidism, but much can be done to offset the possibility of impending complications by attention of hydration, avoidance of calcium and alkalis in the diet, and limiting the operative procedures whenever possible to permit early correction of the primary metabolic disorder.

Hyperparathyroidism is associated with some dehydration and the disease when severe and neglected is subject to so-called parathyroid poisoning. Care of the disease itself consists of the following:

Rehydration: It is to be assumed that the patient with hyperparathyroidism has some degree of dehydration, mild in mild disease, serious in severe disease. Attention to rehydration is an initial step in the care of the patient. Patients with hyperparathyroidism have polydipsia and polyuria. It is not clear which is cart and which is horse, but probably the polyuria is a necessary consequence of the effect of the hormone on the kidney and, therefore, polydipsia follows.

The patient is to be given enough fluid, by mouth, or intravenously if the patient is vomiting. The kind of fluid is important. Ordinarily water and glucose and physiologic electrolyte solutions are the ones indicated and in liberal quantities. Do not be led by the specific gravity of the urine into believing that low gravity means adequate hydration. If the kidney is calcified and its function damaged, the urine is of fixed low specific gravity and the BUN is generally elevated. The low gravity and need for a large volume of urine to excrete waste products accentuates the dehydration. If there is doubt regarding the dehydration and renal function, it may be important at some time to see whether the patient's kidneys are able to concentrate the urine. Failure to concentrate means renal damage.

A rising serum calcium level may indicate increasing dehydration and an impending crisis. The reverse, a falling calcium level, may indicate that dehydration did exist and that the program of rehydration is successful. Daily serum calcium and BUN determinations are therefore important.

The blood phosphate level should also be followed. It is normally depressed in hyperparathyroidism. A rise in the level generally indicates impairment of renal function. A rising level in the face of a low urinary output is an indication for increased fluid intake.

The calcium intake must be strictly limited and alkali therapy avoided. These are considered further in the following section.

Operations for Complications of Hyperparathyroidism. Emergency operations may be needed for the following complications of hyperparathyroidism.

RENAL COLIC, CALCIFICATION AND SHUTDOWN. The commonest complications of hyperparathyroidism currently encountered are stones in the urinary tract. The patient's first symptom of the primary disease may be a stone in the ureter with colic and blocking. If the stone does not pass spontaneously and is not dislodged by cystoscopic manipulation, surgical removal may be mandatory. Paradoxically, occasionally the passage of a stone in the ureter may be helped by giving a small dose of calcium intravenously. Obviously this maneuver should not be carried out in a patient who already has a worrisomely high calcium level. It may be feasible, however, to try it in a patient whose serum calcium is not above 12 to 13 mg./100 cc. Sometimes 2 to 4 cc. of a 10 per cent solution of calcium chloride intravenously suffices to relieve the spasm of the ureter and allow the passage of the stone into the bladder. Such a small amount of additional calcium ion does little to disturb the calcium balance.

Calcification of the renal parenchyma does not of itself cause symptoms. Its relation to renal impairment and dehydration have been discussed.

Until the problem of the primary hyperparathyroidism has been settled definitively, the patient must be on a low calcium intake and alkalis are to be avoided. This applies to the preoperative phase and postoperative care. The low intake and avoidance of alkali are necessary to avoid additional stone formation and renal calcification.

Care of infection in the urinary tract is also important. Infection may intensify stone formation and renal calcification. Appropriate antibiotics are to be used.

It is to be emphasized that as soon as the acute renal tract emergency has been settled, it is important to get on with the correction of the primary parathyroid condition to avoid new stone formation, further renal calcification and depletion of the skeleton of further calcium.

UPPER GASTROINTESTINAL ULCERATION WITH HEMORRHAGE OR PERFORATION. The traditional management of upper gastrointestinal ulceration is by milk, cream and alkalis. Milk and dilute cream contain large quantities of calcium (1 gm. per quart of milk). Alkali powders alkalinize the urine. Both tend to increase the precipitation of calcium within the urinary tract. These treatments for ulcer, therefore, are to be avoided at all costs if renal complications are to be minimized or prevented. It is doubly imperative, obviously, to make the diagnosis of hyperparathyroidism at the earliest possible moment in any patient who has upper intestinal ulceration. All patients with gastrointestinal ulceration should be screened for hyperparathyroidism, therefore, as an initial part of their care. This aspect of the diagnosis and subsequent care are dealt with at greater lengths in the latter part of this chapter.

Management of the ulceration until the hyperparathyroidism has been corrected should be by aluminum hydroxide and proteins other than those of milk.

If an acute massive hemorrhage occurs which does not stop on conservative measures, an operation for the hemorrhage may be required as the life saving measure. The simplest operation is to be chosen as a stopgap till the parathyroid disorder is rectified. Similarly, perforations may need to be sutured. It is to be recalled that the perforation may be below the duodenum; they have been encountered as low as the ileum. The possibility of concomitant Zollinger-Ellison syndrome is also to be kept in mind and if an operation is carried out for either hemorrhage or perforation, the possibility that the pancreas may harbor an islet cell tumor or hyperplasia is to be kept in mind. Insofar as the state of shock from hemorrhage or peritonitis from perforation permits, the pancreas is to carefully searched.

BONE FRACTURES.   Fractures are not uncommon in patients with severe hyperparathyroidism and the classic type of complication, von Recklinghausen's disease of bone. The most common fractures involve collapse of the vertebral bodies and fractures of the ribs. However, fractures may occur with minimal trauma in the long bones of the arms and legs. Usually such fractures occur through sites where the cortex of the bone is thinned by a brown tumor or cyst but occasionally fractures also occur in the long bones of patients who have only the osteoporotic type of bone disease. It is obvious that the patient is to be given the treatment needed for the specific fracture — support of hyperextension for vertebral body fractures, strapping for broken ribs and fixation of some sort for the long bones of the extremities.

For these patients with fractures there is one special thing to be kept in mind regarding the underlying hyperparathyroidism. When immobility of the skeleton is part of the treatment, demineralization may be accelerated and the concentration of calcium in the body fluids increased. This will place an extra load upon the kidney. Where the kidney is already under severe stress, the added burden of skeletal calcification from immobilization may bring shutdown. Particular attention, therefore, is needed to the continued hydration and thought must be given to reactivation of the skeleton at the earliest opportunity. The immobilization of long bone fractures by skeletal traction, therefore, is to be avoided if it is possible to fix the fracture by some form of plating or nail to permit walking ambulation. The skeleton is to be kept functioning as much as possible. The process of decalcification is already above normal owing to the hyperparathyroidism, and the lack of the counterposed recalcification stimulated by use may add quickly and significantly to the amount of decalcification.

Operations for Conditions Not Related to the Hyperparathyroidism.   The patient with hyperparathyroidism obviously may need an operation for some acute trouble unrelated to the hyperparathyroidism. The same considerations that apply to the complications of hyperparathyroidism apply to these cases. Rehydration, a low calcium intake and mobilization as early as possible should be parts of the treatment.

Complications Requiring Nonoperative Therapy — Pancreatitis.   Pancreatitis may occasionally be a complication of hyperparathyroidism. It occurs usually in a patient with moderate to severe hyperparathyroidism and is relatively rare in the person with the mild degree. There is nothing clinically to differentiate the type of pancreatitis from that of other and unknown causes. In the patient in whom hyperparathyroidism is apparently causally related, there are again those three special things to be kept in mind, which relate to the hyperparathyroidism — namely, rehydration, low milk diet and early mobilization.

Acute pancreatitis is associated with widespread irritation of the peritoneum and widespread edema. The loss of plasma fluid to form this edema is considerable and is much like that resulting from a burn in a patient already dehydrated from the glandular disturbance.

Fluid therapy must be even more prompt and full than in the usual or nonhyperparathyroid case of acute pancreatitis.

The choice of fluid in therapy is at the moment under reconsideration. Traditionally, high colloid therapy, principally plasma, has been the therapy of choice. Some whole blood may be needed. If the plasma is not available, much larger quantities of lactated Ringer's solution may be a reasonable alternative. Whichever is used or in whatever combination, kidney output is to be maintained at 20 to 30 cc. per hour, for this is the best test of the adequacy of fluid therapy available at present.

The effect of immobilization applies to the patient who has to be prone in bed suffering acute pancreatitis as well as (though perhaps not equally) to the patient with a bone fracture. The peritonitis, however, may delay the mobilization. Management requires a balance between care of the peritonitis and sparing skeleton and kidneys. Milk and milk products are to be avoided.

HYPOPARATHYROIDISM

THE PROBLEMS, THE DANGERS AND THEIR MANAGEMENT

The diagnosis of hypoparathyroidism is relatively simple. The patient usually is aware of the trouble and the physician can easily identify it. There are three parts needing attention: tetany, anxiety and possible complicating renal colic.

Tetany, Laryngeal Spasm and the Airway. The classic position of the hand and fingers and the muscular spasms of tetany are obvious if tetany is severe. Tetany, however, may only be latent and all the patient notices is tingling of fingers, toes and lips. The physician judges the intensity by both the Chvostek and Trousseau signs. If the Trousseau is negative and the Chvostek only slightly positive, it can be safely assumed that the calcium level is only slightly reduced; the hypoparathyroidism is of mild degree. There is little danger under this circumstance.

The dangers of tetany come when spontaneous tetany occurs, when the blood calcium level is reduced to low levels (7 mg./100 cc. or lower). The principal danger then is that laryngeal spasm may occur and the patient may suffocate before relief by calcium intravenously or by tracheostomy is available.

When tetany is diagnosed, the treatment is calcium in adequate quantities—intravenously if necessary. A syringe and ampule of a calcium solution should always be available at the bedside and go with the patient to the operating room. The most rapidly effective calcium solution is that of the ionized calcium chloride; a 10 per cent solution is usually available in ampules. This has to be administered slowly; it is highly irritating and burns, and it can cause thrombosis. A dose of 3 to 5 cc. intravenously is usually sufficient to relieve even severe tetany within two minutes.

Less active but also useful intravenously in a period of 10 to 20 munutes are the calcium carbohydrate combinations of either the gluco-nate or heptonate. These are also supplied in 10 per cent solutions in which the amount of calcium by weight is but one tenth that in the chloride solution. The carbohydrate salts, however, are not irritating and may be given rapidly intravenously. (They may also be given intramuscularly.)

In either situation, chloride or carbohydrate salt, the rate of intra-venous administration can be judged by the reaction of the patient. If the calcium chloride, particularly, is given too fast, not only does the vein burn, but the patient undergoes a disagreeable burning flush of the tongue and of the skin generally. The rate of injection should be reduced if this flush occurs.

A slow drip of an intravenous salt solution containing an ampule of the calcium gluconate should be maintained until the control of the tetany is assured, first by intramuscular injection of the carbohydrate salt solution and second by oral intake of both calcium and vitamin D.

The preparations of parathyroid hormone available at present are of little use in either immediate or long term therapy. Impurities arouse antibody formation with inactivation of subsequent injections.

Long term therapy depends upon a combination of a high calcium intake and a vitamin D preparation. The physiologic effect of large doses of vitamin D is the nearest known to that of the parathyroid hormone. The vitamin increases the absorption of calcium and also induces a high level of calcium in the bloodstream. The effect of an overdose of vitamin D is much like that of an excess of the parathyroid hormone. There may be a rise of calcium level to a degree of toxicity, and there may even be renal shutdown. Since the vitamin is slowly absorbed and remains for a long time in the intestinal tract, care must be taken in the long range therapy not to give an overdose of the vitamin. The effects of vitamin D toxicity may be as bad or dangerous as those of the hypoparathyroidism for which the vitamin is given.

Acute Anxiety. Acute anxiety may accompany hypoparathyroid-ism, and when it occurs it is very distressing. The patient has the feeling of impending disaster. Reassurance is of little help, but intra-venous calcium brings immediate relief. The presence of acute anxiety is of course alarming, for it indicates that the therapy of the hypoparathy-roidism is inadequate. The patients themselves may become acutely aware of the relationship and inform nurse and doctor that their calcium and vitamin D doses are not adequate.

Renal Colic. Renal colic may appear unexpectedly in the patient with hypoparathyroidism who has previously been troubled with renal stones. Uusally this is seen in patients who have had the renal stone complication of hyperparathyroidism and are hypocalcemic after the parathyroid operation. It may occur in such a patient perhaps weeks after the parathyroid operation. It may also appear in the patient suffering tetany after a thyroidectomy. The colic is believed due to stones which were present within the kidney before the appearance of the hypoparathyroidism. With partial dissolution of the stones and tightening of the musculature of the renal pelvis due to the tetany, these preexisting stones are freed and come tumbling down into the ureter. Treatment consists of correcting the hypoparathyroidism with intravenous calcium. This may aid the spontaneous passage of the smaller stones. It also will relieve the colic until the stone can be eased and passed by cystoscopic manipulation or, if need be, by surgical removal.

REFERENCES

Albright, F., Baird, P. C., Cope, O., and Bloomberg, E.: Studies on the physiology of the parathyroid glands. IV. Renal complications of hyperparathyroidism. Amer. J. Med. Sc. *187*:49, 1934.

Cope, O.: Hyperparathyroidism: Diagnosis and management. Amer. J. Surg. 99:394, 1960.

Cope, O., Culver, P. J., Mixter, C. G., Jr., and Nardi, G. L.: Pancreatitis, a diagnostis clue to hyperparathyroidism. Ann. Surg. *145*:857, 1957.

Frame, B., and Haubrich, W. S.: Peptic ulcer and hyperparathyroidism. Arch. Int. Med. *105*:536, 1960.

Norris, E. H.: Collective review: Carcinoma of the parathyroid glands with a preliminary report of three cases. Internat. Abstr. Surg. 86:1, 1048.

Rogers, H. M., and Keating, F. R., Jr.: Primary hypertrophy and hyperplasia of the parathyroid glands as a cause of hyperparathyroidism. Amer. J. Med. 3:384, 1947.

Woolner, L. B., Keating, F. R., Jr., and Black, B. M.: Tumors and hyperplasia of parathyroid glands. Cancer 5:1069, 1952.

Hyperparathyroidism

Hyperparathyroidism has gradually emerged as a disease of importance in surgery. In the first decade after its discovery in 1926, it was considered a disease of bone, and rare. As the complications of the disease have become appreciated, and it has been realized in how many clinical forms the disease appears, it is now established as one of the more common endocrine diseases to be treated by surgery. Unfortunately the diagnosis remains a problem. The variety of the disease is great and the symptomatology misleading to the untutored diagnostician. Missed over and over again, the diagnosis is made eventually only by the physician who has kept it in mind.

Hyperparathyroidism also presents problems of treatment to the surgeon. The care of many of the patients is relatively straightforward, but there are a stubborn few, difficult to manage. The knowledge and operative skill required are special and demanding.

Earlier in this chapter the dangers of hyperparathyroidism to the patient about to undergo an operation, the complications of the primary disease and their management are dealt with in detail. The present discussion describes how the diagnosis is established, and again alludes to the vagaries of the diagnosis. A reminder of the anatomic pathology of the parathyroid glands to be anticipated at operation follows, and the operative management and the needs of the recovery period are dealt with at length.

PARATHYROID HORMONE

The reason for the vagaries of the clinical manifestations of hyperparathyroidism lies in the diffuseness of the action of parathyroid hormone. The hormone has the dominant effect on the level of calcium in the blood serum and body fluids, and it also affects the concentration of the phosphate ion. It is not known how the hormone acts; it may do so directly or secondarily through its action on tissues, which include the bones, the kidneys, other glands and organs in which the calcium ion concentration is important (including the pancreas and the stomach) and nervous tissue generally. In the kidney the hormone controls the tubular reabsorption perhaps of both calcium and phosphorus. With increased activity, both are lost in the urine in greater concentration. There is a difference of opinion whether the primary action is on phosphate or calcium reabsorption. At any rate there are two effects: first, an increased obligatory excretion of water, causing some dehydration and increased thirst, and second, pathologic calcification. Because the disturbance involves the renal parenchyma, the calcification may be in the renal cells as well as in the form of stones in the urinary tract.

Similarly, where the calcium ion is excreted, or an important shift in pH takes place, there may be stone formation or calcification of the glandular parenchyma. Thus calculi are to be found in the pancreatic ducts, and there is calcification of pancreatic and gastric mucosae.

The hormone appears to influence the exchange of calcium and phosphorus in the bones, particularly the resorption of these ions from the bony matrix. Bones are thinned and the freed calcium plugs the kidneys.

Parathyroid hormone also influences the rate of absorption and excretion of calcium into and from the intestinal tract. The absorption is increased and the excretion into the large bowel is decreased by an increase of the hormone. Thus in a patient with hyperparathyroidism there is less calcium than normal in the feces. In the hyperparathyroid patient who has severe renal damage and who can no longer excrete the excess of calcium through the urine, the excess is found in the feces.

The calcium ion is an essential electrolyte in the transmission of the nervous impulse, both between nerves and between nerve and muscle. The increased concentration of calcium in hyperparathyroidism therefore widely influences nervous phenomena. The tone of the skeletal muscles is more relaxed, and this can be appreciated clinically as a spongy end point when the tendon and muscle are hyperextended (over-stretched). The thinking processes may be interfered with. When the calcium level is low, the patient is generally anxious and notices numbness and tinglings. When the calcium is elevated, there is sometimes a bizarre confusion and often somnolence and torpor when the level is as high as 18 mg. The transmission of the nervous impulse in the heart is also expedited in paradoxical fashion. An elevation of 14 mg. or more can ordinarily be picked up on the electrocardiogram. When this broad influence of the calcium ion concentration on tissues and body fluids is considered, it is not surprising that the clinical picture of hyperparathyroidism should be so widespread in its mimicry and confusing to the untutored.

DIAGNOSIS

Several special ways of establishing the diagnosis of hyperparathyroidism have been recommended, but the original measurement of the concentration of calcium and phosphorus in the serum remains the most secure and most dependable. Of the two the calcium level is the more important, because it is less affected by other conditions. Unless the serum calcium level is elevated above normal, the diagnosis is in doubt.

When the serum calcium is being measured, the serum protein should be measured simultaneously at least once; approximately half of the calcium in the serum is bound to protein, and the other half is free as the ionized form. If the protein concentration is depleted by a recent hemorrhage or inflammation, or the patient depleted by starvation and malnutrition, then the concentration of total calcium will have been lowered and is to be corrected. For every gram that the total protein level is below normal, one milligram is to be added to the measured level of calcium. Thus if the measured calcium level is 10 mg./100 ml. and the protein level is 5.5 gm., then the corrected calcium level is 11 mg., a level consistent with hyperparathyroidism.

The lowered phosphate concentration is the second most important determination in diagnosis. If the patient has no renal damage, the phosphate level is always depressed. If a normal phosphate is found and there is no impairment of renal functions, the patient probably does not have hyperparathyroidism. If there is impairment of renal function, then phosphate clearance is reduced, phosphate piles up in the body and the blood level rises. The level may be normal or above normal in hyperparathyroid patients with severely damaged kidneys.

The third test in order of usefulness is the urinary excretion of calcium. An excretion of a greater than normal amount of calcium in the urine is to be expected, but the variation in amount is so great that it is a less reliable, less exact diagnostic test. A satisfactory rule is that a normal adult person on an intake of calcium of 100 mg. per day should excrete less than that amount in the urine. Therefore an excretion of 120 mg. per day would favor the diagnosis of hyperparathyroidism. It is difficult, however, to achieve such a low calcium intake. The higher the calcium intake, the greater the variation in calcium excretion and the more difficult to use the excretion as a diagnostic test. Efforts to refine the calcium excretion as a diagnostic test have been made by reducing the calcium intake by special diet to as low as 20 mg. Still the normal and abnormal overlap in such a manner as to make this a less critical diagnostic test than the calcium blood level. A greatly increased excretion of calcium in the urine, however, is strongly in favor of hyperparathyroidism. Thus if a patient is taking in only 200 mg. of calcium per day by mouth, and is excreting 350 mg. in the urine, this is strong evidence in favor of hyperparathyroidism.

The other tests recommended include tubular resorption of phosphorus. This is positive in patients with obvious hyperparathyroidism, borderline in patients with boderline or mild disease. It is useful to have but is not quite as sharp and good as the calcium and phosphate levels. It is really an elegant way of measuring the depressed phosphate level in the blood.

What is needed, of course, is a direct measure of the concentration of the hormone in the blood. This has recently been achieved in three laboratories by immunoassay; better assay is not as yet generally available.

How is the patient with hyperparathyroidism ferreted out from among all those patients with the complexity of symptoms? The answer is, only by keeping the possibility of the diagnosis in mind; whenever patients with the various symptoms are encountered, they are to be painstakingly and repeatedly screened for possible hyperparathyroidism.

First to be considered are those patients with symptoms due to the primary changes of the metabolic disorder itself—namely, the changes of calcium in the serum and body fluids and the renal diabetes. The commonest symptom of the rise in calcium level and muscular relaxation is fatigue. Sometimes there is just plain backache. In extreme cases the patient shuffles along, drags his toes, trips on the rugs and wears down the fronts of the soles of his shoes. The fatigue and backache are the kind of thing all of us feel in the afternoon. The symptoms therefore are common and quite uncharacteristic. Still the disease must be kept in mind and some of the patients with these primary complaints screened by measuring the fasting blood serum calcium and phosphorus levels. Occasionally such a study pays off.

Screening. The screening of patients with complaints related to the kidneys, the gastrointestinal tract and the skeleton are statistically much more rewarding. In a patient with almost any symptom in the urinary tract, hyperparathyroidism is to be considered. The diabetes, dehydration and increased thirst of the patient with hyperparathyroidism are rarely sufficient to be noticed by the patient but still should be considered by the physician. The minimal symptoms of a little burning, or discomfort or transient hematuria should call the diagnosis to mind. When stones are formed, particularly those opaque to x-ray, which obviously contain calcium, then of course the diagnosis is even more likely. The presence of infection in the urinary tract, although it may contribute to stone formation, does not exclude the possibility of hyperparathyroidism. A wise step in the screening process is also to include screening for other causes of urinary tract pain, namely urates, cystinuria and porphyuria. Oxaluria does not exclude hyperparathyroidism, for 30 per cent of the calcium stones in hyperparathyroidism contain calcium oxalate.

The calcium level of the serum, and perhaps a primary effect of the hormone itself, influences the gastrointestinal tract virtually from top to bottom. There may be calculi in the salivary glands. Ulcers occur in the stomach, duodenum, jejunum and even ileum.* Hemorrhages occur from these ulcerations and occasional perforations also. Constipation is common and disappears spontaneously once the disease has been corrected. In contrast, sprue-like diarrhea is occasionally encountered, and patients with suspected sprue are also to be screened. The development of pancreatitis has already been described; stones in the pancreatic ducts are common in patients with a severe degree of the disease. The calcification in the ducts and parenchyma can be visualized by x-ray in severely disordered patients. So common are the abdominal and gastrointestinal symptoms that, even if a patient does not have a demonstrable ulcer or calcification in the pancreas, the symptoms may be the result of hyperparathyroidism and disappear after its correction. The diverse picture of abdominal symptoms means that a host of patients need to be screened. Can this screening be sharpened somewhat further?

The same considerations regarding the diagnostic tests apply to the screening for hyperparathyroidism. In the patients with peptic ulcers and pancreatitis, two additional points will be helpful. The first point has been included in the first part of this chapter—namely, that it may be particularly difficult to diagnose hyperparathyroidism in the days immediately following a hemorrhage, a perforation with widespread peritonitis or pancreatitis with its accompanying diffuse inflammation

---

*Hyperparathyroidism and the pancreatic tumors of the Zollinger-Ellison syndrome may occur together, so that in patients with the ulcer complication a pancreatic component is to be considered.

and edema. The dilution of the plasma proteins that occurs with rehydration has the effect of lowering the total calcium level, and it may be only as the proteins are replenished that the calcium level will rise to above normal and be diagnostic.

The second point is the sex difference. Hyperparathyroidism, like most endocrine diseases, is at least twice as common in the female as in the male, and ulceration in the intestinal tract, on the other hand, is far commoner in the male. From a statistical point of view, therefore, screening for hyperparathyroidism is more likely to be rewarding in a woman with a gastric or duodenal ulcer than in a male with a similar ulcer. This would be particularly true if the male were a skid row alcoholic—a patient with another plausible cause for ulceration. In other words, the possibility of the diagnosis should be pursued in a young woman, but another cause may be accepted in the skid row alcoholic.

The skeleton is the source of many complaints in patients with hyperparathyroidism. With the resorption of calcium and phosphorus from the bones, the periosteum becomes tender and the bones ache generally. With the development of cysts and brown tumors there may be localized pain. Tenderness of the shins is a prominent symptom. One patient was considered abnormal by his family when he complained if one of his children kicked him by accident under the table. This type of tenderness disappears within the first days following correction of the hyperparathyroidism.

The occurrence of a fracture through a cyst or tumor is obvious; often only slight trauma is needed. This form of the disease should be recognized immediately by the roentgenologist.

A recently identified skeletal complication of hyperparathyroidism is pseudo-gout. Although hyperparathyroidism plays no role in classic rheumatoid or degenerative arthritis, patients with unexplained arthritic symptoms should be screened for possible pseudo-gout.

The important thing about the decalcification of hyperparathyroidism is that it is generalized and affects the cold as well as the warm bones. Thus it is found in the fingers and toes, the coldest of the bones, as well as in the warm skull, spine, ribs and pelvis. The osteoporoses of other than parathyroid origin, such as the idiopathic and that of Cushing's disease, affect predominantly the warm bones; comparable thinning out is not seen in the hands. Cancers metastasize predominantly to the warm bones, and the metastases therefore are encountered with decreasing frequency from proximal to distal portions of the extremities.

Symptomless Hyperparathyroidism. The recent advent of the automatic analyzer for chemical entities in the blood plasma has posed a special problem in regard to hyperparathyroidism. In an occasional patient with no symptoms or signs apparently related to parathyroid disease, the routine analysis has revealed an elevated calcium and depressed phosphorus. It is evident that such patients do have chemical and, therefore, metabolic parathyroid overactivity. Should they be operated upon? Will they get into trouble if not operated upon? Of patients with kidney stones and established hyperparathyroidism, very few have peptic ulcers, pancreatitis or bone disease and many have noticed no fatigue. Of those with ulcers, few have had stones, pancreatitis or bone troubles. Thus, one complication, and only one, has been the rule, indicating that theoretically it is possible to have no complication and yet have metabolic hyperparathyroidism, perhaps for several years. Direct experience is lacking, and arbitrary rules become advisable. If the calcium level is less than 12 mg./100 cc., wait and see. If the calcium level falls, perhaps the patient has parathyroid hyperplasia and the stimulus is diminishing; that is, the patient is getting better spontaneously. If the calcium level rises, the disease is getting worse and the patient should be operated upon. If to begin with the calcium level is 13 mg. or higher despite no overt symptoms, it is wiser to operate forthwith. The patient will avoid complications and will presumably feel better with the calcium level down to normal.

Venous Catheterization and Blood Hormone Level. Measurement of the level of parathyroid hormone in the blood flowing from the parathyroid glands obtained by venous catheterization promises much in refining the diagnosis and in localizing the hyperactive parathyroid glands. By the immunoassay method already available, it has been possible to find as much as a tenfold increase in level in the blood obtained from one or another thyroid vein over that found in the general venous circulation. Such a concentration is well above that in blood flowing from normally functioning glands. When such a concentration has been found on one side and not on the other, it has pointed to the presence of a parathyroid neoplasm, rather than the diffuse hyperplasia. Further, it has directed the surgeon's attention to that spot as the first area to be exposed at operation. An additional refinement in localization has been the measurement of the level before and after planned spot palpation of either side of the neck.

PRECEDENCE IN OPERATIVE CARE

A problem in the management of patients with hyperparathyroidism is the question of which takes precedence, the care of the complication or the care of the primary hyperparathyroidism. The decision is simple enough when the patient breaks a bone. The fracture must be set. Unfortunately, care of the fracture may consume the attention of the physician and orthopedist so that the primary diagnosis may be delayed for several days. Not until further roentgenograms are taken or some other complication takes place is the disease thought of. The primary disease, however, should be recognized by the roentgenologist alone and without the aid of chemical analyses.

More difficult is the decision regarding precedence in the care of a renal stone. In general, only an acute renal emergency, such as a stone blocking the ureter, with pain and suppression of urinary function, or dilatation of the renal pelvis, should the renal situation be cared for first. Correct the hyperparathyroidism and then take care of whatever renal disease needs attention. Often by waiting the renal disease corrects itself. To have operated on ureteral or bladder stones first may have been unnecessary operating.

The same considerations apply to the complication of duodenal and gastric ulcers. Time and again, when surgeons have operated upon the ulcers, these operations would have been unnecessary had the hyperparathyroidism been corrected first. In general the ulcers heal promptly following correction of the hyperparathyroidism. Only in occasional instances do the ulcers continue or recur. The only question then comes when the patient has the acute emergency of a hemorrhage from the ulcer. In this event, if the hemorrhage does not stop, the simplest type of operative procedure is the one indicated—namely, suture of the bleeding vessel in the ulcer bed. Presumably nothing more is needed, not even a vagotomy. The next procedure should then be correction of the hyperparathyroidism, and as promptly as reasonable. As has been pointed out, the trouble with the bleeding ulcer situation is that it is often peculiarly difficult to make the diagnosis of hyperparathyroidism immediately following a hemorrhage.

THE PROBLEMS—THE DANGERS

The special problems of hyperparathyroidism, and the dangers that come from neglect of the disease, have already been covered in the first part of this chapter. Various of the important points are summarized in the next section. To be kept in mind are such problems as dehydration, renal shutdown, the danger of cardiac standstill, the mental disturbance and coma in the deteriorating acute situation, the hemorrhages and perforation of ulcers and pancreatitis.

MANAGEMENT

Once the diagnosis of hyperparathyroidism has been made, usually by repeated determinations of the blood level of calcium and phosphorus, plans should be laid for the early correction of the hyperparathyroidism. Otherwise unforeseen complications may intervene. Several aspects of the management have already been covered. The following deserve additional mention and emphasis.

PREOPERATIVE

The principal objectives of the preoperative preparation are rehydration and the avoidance of renal shutdown and parathyroid crisis.

Renal Problems. The obligatory loss of water with calcium and phosphorus through the kidney means that the patient generally is dehydrated. This is of little consequence in a patient with a mild degree of the disease but in a patient with moderate or severe degree, further dehydration may be impending unless care is taken. In such patients early emphasis should therefore be placed on rehydration.

The patient also must be on a low calcium diet. There is abundant evidence that a high calcium intake through the intestinal tract threatens renal shutdown by plugging the kidney. An adequate fluid intake with a low calcium content keeps the kidneys flushed. Move on to the parathyroid operation.

Gastrointestinal Problems. The presence of an ulcer in the duodenum or the stomach, or the diarrhea of sprue, invites preliminary care of these complications. To prolong this care may be unwise. In the first place, the usual care needed for an ulcer is the antithesis of what should be given the patient with hyperparathyroidism. Milk should be avoided at all costs and alkalis too, since they alkalinize the urine and increase the precipitation of calcium in the kidney. The milk-alkali syndrome is the result. It is to be stressed that a true milk-alkali syndrome apart from hyperparathyroidism is a rarity if it exists at all. The milk-alkali syndrome is usually a mild degree of hyperparathyroidism with a severe renal complication induced by milk and alkali. Rehydrate the patient intravenously if need be; give a protein diet low in calcium and, if necessary, an unabsorbable antacid such as aluminum hydroxide. Then get on with the correction of hyperparathyroidism as quickly as possible, for its correction is the best treatment for the ulcer.

Likewise about the diarrhea of the pseudo-sprue. Beyond rehydration with a low calcium intake, little will be accomplished until the hyperparathyroidism is corrected.

Parathyroid Crisis. Much has been written recently about parathyroid crisis. Usually it appears in a patient with an ulcer who has been treated inappropriately with milk and alkalis, but occasionally severe hyperparathyroidism gives rise to a high calcium level without the addition of a high calcium intake. Prompt rehydration and almost emergency operation is the treatment, as described earlier.

Informing the Patient Preoperatively Regarding Postoperative Events. The postoperative phase of the recovery from hyperparathyroidism may be stormy, and it has proved wise to warn the patient and family ahead of time regarding possible events. These do not need to be spelled out in detail or suggested too vividly, but a reminder, which may be referred to later, can be most helpful. The special events are tetany and renal colic. Severe tetany can be predicted if the patient has depleted bones and a preoperatively elevated level of alkaline phosphatase. The renal complication may be the sudden, unexpected passage of stones. This will be referred to in further detail under "Postoperative Program."

INTRAOPERATIVE MANAGEMENT

The intraoperative management is the surgery of hyperparathyroidism. There is nothing special about the drugs or anesthetics to be used. The operation may be long, and therefore the least toxic ethyl ether may be better than some of the more toxic but pleasanter and newer anesthetic agents. At operation it is essential that the surgeon identify with surety the type of parathyroid pathology with which he is dealing. The need for this is obvious in the case of carcinoma. It is also important to differentiate between hyperplasia and adenoma. If hyperplasia exists and is not identified, the surgeon will carry out an inadequate operation and will be on the wrong lead in his postoperative care of the patient. Chief-cell hyperplasia is particularly difficult to identify, yet it accounts for 20 to 25 per cent of the cases. The pathologist cannot differentiate it on microscopic section from adenoma. The clue to the differential is found by identifying at least one further gland beyond the enlargement. If the second gland found is normal and clearly normal, then the enlarged gland is an adenoma, since hyperplasia, if present, affects all glands and can be identified in whatever gland is found.

Although preoperative venous catheterization with measurement of the hormone level may, as indicated above, help in calling attention to the diffuse hyperplasia versus the localized neoplasia, still the final identification of the type of pathology will depend upon the surgeon at operation.

POSTOPERATIVE PROGRAM

The postoperative phase of hyperparathyroidism is conveniently considered under the early, acute phase and the later, longer, recovery phase. In the acute, attention is given to the continued need for rehydration, to tetany, psychological turmoil, the changing gastrointestinal picture and gout. In the later convalescence, attention is to be devoted to dissolution of kidney stones and the rebuilding of the skeleton.

Rehydration Phase. Immediately following correction of the hyperparathyroidism, most patients take on some fluid—a phase of rehydration. This phase is associated with a low urinary output. Unless the surgeon is mindful of this last, he may press intravenous fluids unduly.

A 24-hour urinary output as low as 500 ml. or even 300 ml. is not unusual for the first day or two. This phase ordinarily passes promptly.

Continued Low Calcium Intake. The low calcium intake mandatory before operation should be continued postoperatively for the first two days and perhaps longer and for three reasons. The first reason is to be sure that the operation is successful. The rate at which the calcium level falls and the level to which it falls give the clue regarding the adequacy of the resection of parathyroid tissue. If there was any doubt about whether the patient had a single adenoma or two adenomas, or hyperplasia, one of the best ways to be sure is to watch the calcium level after the operation. If the calcium level fails to fall, the operation was obviously inadequate and one can be reasonably sure that the tumor removed was not an adenoma but only one of several hyperplastic glands. If it falls slightly but not to normal and then promptly returns to a high level, even though below the preoperative level, one can again safely assume that the pathology was hyperplasia, or that, if the gland was malignant, metastases are already present. Calcium is not to be given postoperatively until the nature of the decline is established, for otherwise calcium might interfere and lead to false conclusions. There is an importance to the patient beyond the academic establishment of the type of pathology. At least one person has been killed by the thoughtless giving of a high calcium and vitamin D intake immediately after resecting a parathyroid incorrectly diagnosed. The huge tumor removed at operation was thought to have been an adenoma. Calcium and vitamin D were piled in. The calcium level failed to decline; indeed it went up. A full-blown parathyroid crisis was precipitated; the kidneys shut down, and the patient died on the sixth postoperative day. At autopsy, as could have been anticipated, three more hyperplastic parathyroids were found.

The second reason for withholding calcium in the first few postoperative days is again that the rate of fall of calcium and the level to which it falls are a barometer of the future need for calcium, namely the skeletal deficit. This is discussed under "Tetany."

The third reason for continuing the low calcium intake is to expedite the dissolution of residual renal stones. Not infrequently in the days and weeks immediately following correction of the hyperparathyroidism, a stone or two may break up, be dislodged and get impinged in the ureters. Sometimes the stones dissolve quietly over a period of many months. Since it is possible in some patients to obtain spontaneous dissolution of the stones, it is believed that a low calcium intake will help. If the patient's serum calcium level can tolerate it—that is, if the patient does not have a degree of tetany needing calcium therapy— then the low calcium intake is continued for months, at least until the renal status can be reviewed.

The warning to the patient preoperatively that a stone may be passed in the first days or weeks after operation has proved helpful in reassuring the patient when, indeed, stones do appear. The knowledge that they are old stones now coming out and not new stones is fine for morale.

Tetany. There are two types of tetany encountered following operative correction of hyperparathyroidism. The first is true hypoparathyroidism and is ordinarily transient, provided parathyroid tissue is left in the neck and is capable of normal function. Signs of subnormal calcium level, however, are frequently encountered. Usually they are symptomless and are due to true hypoparathyroidism. If a single adenoma was found and resected and the remaining three parathyroids were normal and were not disturbed by the operation, usually these glands are able to recover function within the first three days, and any hypoparathyroidism or tetany is transient. If the nonadenomatous parathyroids were damaged, or if an excessive amount of tissue was resected from hyperplastic glands, then the hypoparathyroidism may be more severe and more prolonged. If it is severe and prolonged, it will need therapy in the form of a high calcium and vitamin D intake.

The second form of tetany is that of the recalcification period. It may come on acutely, be dangerously severe and last for a long time, even three to four months. To foretell, like a storm warning, whether this type of tetany will be severe or not, is the second reason to observe the fall in calcium level uninterfered with by a high calcium intake. If the calcium level in the first days after operation goes well below normal, and the remaining parathyroids are known to be normal, and if the decline continues day by day past the first week, then obviously the bones are hungry and beginning to absorb calcium rapidly.

If there has been significant decalcification of the skeleton during the active phase of the disease, the skeleton needs calcium after operation in order to rebuild itself. If calcium is not available in the diet in an adequate amount, the calcium level in the blood will fall to tetanic levels. This is the commonest cause of the severe tetany encountered after hyperparathyroidism. It may be foretold by the preoperative alkaline phosphatase level. If elevated it means that already the recalcification process is trying to rebuild the bones. Correction of the hyperparathyroidism alters the adverse balance between destruction and construction, and recalcification gains rapidly. It reaches a peak at about three weeks after operation. It is at this time that there is the greatest need of calcium to assure comfort and safety.

The treatment of recalcification tetany is by feeding calcium in large quantities and by giving vitamin D to increase the rate of calcium absorption, not to act as a substitute for parathyroid hormone. If the operation has been correctly performed, there is a normal and adequate amount of hormone.

The calcium may be given as the lactate in huge doses (600 to 900 mg. four times a day), and the vitamin D in 50,000 or 100,000 units per day. In the acute phase, when the gastrointestinal tract cannot be counted upon to absorb a sufficient amount, calcium may be given intramuscularly as the gluconate or glucoheptonate. As described earlier in this chapter, acute tetany, if severe, may need to be treated by intravenous calcium in order to avoid spasm of the glottis. A patient with depleted bones and latent tetany should not be sent home until the program of calcium replenishment and close professional observation has been arranged. Two of our patients have died at home because of failure to make such arrangements.

Skeletal Recovery. The cysts, brown tumors and osteoporosis care for themselves. The fractures have not needed special attention, the usual orthopedic care being indicated. Bone pain for the most part diminishes quickly. A few patients who had a severe degree of osteoporosis have had long continuing pain, particularly of their ankles and feet. Reassurance in this regard is important. At least two patients have had gradually diminishing symptoms over a two-year period. Both of them became discouraged but eventually were reassured by disappearance of the pain and the return of the ability to walk.

Psychological Turmoil. Tetany is associated not only with tinglings and muscular cramps but also with an extraordinary feeling of apprehension, of impending doom. The psychological symptoms are apparently most disagreeable. The patient needs frequent reassurance and, of course, care of his calcium level. The preoperative mention of this possibility has proved helpful when reassuring the patient after operation.

The Peptic Ulcer Program. Those patients with active ulcers preoperatively need special consideration immediately after operation. Although it can be anticipated that eventually the ulcers will heal, healing obviously must require some time. The coordination of this program with the renal and bone programs is once again to be considered.

Pseudo-Sprue. No special attention is needed beyond the maintenance of nutrition. In those few patients thus far encountered, the intestinal symptoms and signs have disappeared quite quickly, in a matter of relatively few days. Not enough experience has been obtained as yet to be sure of the full clinical picture of this complication.

Gout and Pseudo-Gout. Several patients immediately after operation have had an attack of acute gout, usually in the toes but sometimes in the ankles and wrists. In many patients the uric acid level rises slightly in the first days after operation, during that phase of low urinary output, and it is probable that it is this rise that precipitates the acute attack. Eventually, however, there has been a drop in the uric acid level to normal and the patients can be reassured about this. Pseudo-gout, too, disappears promptly with the rebuilding of bone that follows the correction of the hyperparathyroidism.

REFERENCES

Anglem, T. J.: Acute hyperparathyroidism: A surgical emergency, *in* Marshall, S. F., and Nardi, G. L., eds.: The Management of Surgical Emergencies. Surg. Clin. N. Amer. *46*:727, 1966 (See Case 1).

Castleman, B.: Tumors of the parathyroid glands, *in* Atlas of Tumor Pathology. Washington, D.C., Armed Forces Inst. Path., 1952, p. 74.

Cope, O.: Surgery of hyperparathyroidism: The occurrence of parathyroids in the anterior mediastinum and the division of the operation into two stages. Ann. Surg. *114*:706, 1941.

Cope, O.: The story of hyperparathyroidism at the Massachusetts General Hospital. N. Eng. J. Med. *274*:1174, 1966.

Cope, O., Barnes, B. A., Castleman, B., Mueller, G. E. C., and Roth, S. I.: Vicissitudes of parathyroid surgery: Trials of diagnosis and management in 51 patients with a variety of disorders. Ann. Surg. *154*:491, 1961.

Cope, O., Keynes, W. M., Roth, S. I., and Castleman, B.: Primary chief-cell hyperplasia of the parathyroid glands: A new entity in the surgery of hyperparathyroidism. Ann. Surg. *148*:175, 1958.

Goldman, L., Gordan, G. S., and Chambers, E. L., Jr.: Changing diagnostic criteria for hyperparathyroidism. Ann. Surg. *146*:407, 1957.

Kyle, L. H., Mintz, D. H., Canary, J. J., and Carreon, G.: Hyperuricemia in hyperparathyroidism. N. Eng. J. Med. *265*:112, 1961.

McCarty, D. J., Jr., and Gatter, R. A.: Pseudogout syndrome (articular chondrocalcinosis). Bulletin on Rheumatic Diseases, *14*:No. 5, 1964.

Rogers, H. M., Keating, F. R., Jr., Morlock, C. G., and Barker, N. W.: Primary hypertrophy and hyperplasia of the parathyroid glands associated with duodenal ulcer. Report of an additional case, with special reference to metabolic, gastrointestinal and vascular manifestations. Arch. Int. Med. *79*:307, 1947.

CHAPTER 27

THE BREAST

David V. Habif, M.D.

The highest cure rate for mammary carcinoma is achieved in the treatment of very small cancers which are associated with no demonstrable lymph node metastases. Self-examination should increase the finding of very small lesions if the patient is instructed properly in the technique and she practices it on a regular monthly basis. The importance of treating benign lesions lies in the findings of these very small cancers and in the removal of certain benign diseases which are associated with a higher than usual incidence of malignancy.

Benign diseases of the breast include fibroadenoma, cystosarcoma phylloides, intraductal papilloma, papillary cystadenoma, multiple intraductal papilloma, fibrous disease, ectasia, lipoma, cystic disease, including simple cysts, adenosis, fibrosis and intraductal papillomatosis, lobular neoplasia in situ[8] and infections. The three benign diseases associated with a higher incidence of mammary carcinoma than that which develops in the population at large are multiple intraductal papilloma, 23 to 39 per cent;[8] lobular neoplasia in situ, 8 per cent after five years, to 35 per cent after 20 years;[11] and cystosarcoma phylloides, 3 per cent.[13] These diseases may be treated by subcutaneous or simple mastectomy in selected instances.

Cystic disease is the most common disease of the female breast. It is estimated to be present in the macroscopic form in approximately 19 per cent of adult women,[6] and it is bilateral in almost all these patients. It may be diagnosed clinically when a single (or multiple) cyst is aspirated of its characteristically greenish or bluish fluid. The patient requires no operation for biopsy or removal of the cyst unless the aspirated fluid contains fresh or old blood or there is a residual dominant lump or area which is suggestive of the presence of carcinoma. In the majority of patients who require an operation, using these criteria, the cyst from which bloody fluid is aspirated will be an inflamed one and the dominant lump or area will be composed of multiple small cysts, adenosis, fibrosis or intraductal papillomatosis. The surgeons at Presbyterian Hospital have treated simple cysts by aspiration alone over a period of more than 30 years and they continue to do so. Other surgeons have recently called attention to the use of this technique, and they have emphasized its many benefits.[2, 14]

The spontaneous discharge of serous or bloody fluid from the nipple occurs in the following diseases in a decreasing order of frequency: (1) intraductal papilloma, (2) cystic disease, (3) ectasia, and (4) carcinoma. Operation is indicated to remove the benign cause and to exclude the presence of carcinoma. Bloody discharge which occurs from multiple lactiferous ducts in one or both nipples during pregnancy and lactation is due to epithelial hyperplasia in the ducts and will subside spontaneously after lactation ceases. A biopsy is not required under these circumstances.

Infections develop in lactating breasts owing to microorganisms which gain entry through the nipple. Cellulitis will subside spontaneously in most patients if it is treated by stopping breast feeding and in others in conjunction with the use of an antibiotic. If the process goes on to abscess formation, incision and drainage at the earliest time is the best form of treatment.

The majority of abscesses that occur in nonlactating breasts are most probably associated with squamous metaplasia in a lactiferous duct.[7] The acute abscess should be treated by incision and drainage; definitive treatment requires the excision of the entire length of the diseased duct.

Sterile abscesses which occur in patients with ectasia may be treated by excision of the abscess and a 2 cm. segment of all lactiferous ducts, followed by primary closure of the skin.[3] Ectasia, papillary cystadenoma and traumatic fat necrosis with fibrosis are the three benign diseases which may produce true skin retraction.

MAMMOGRAPHY

Careful clinical examination of the breast is the most important method of detecting a dominant lump or area, and mammography is and will most probably always be an adjunctive diagnostic aid. The indications at the present time are (1) baseline films in patients with "normal" breasts and in those with cystic disease, (2) yearly examination starting at age 35 in those who have a strong family history of mammary carcinoma, and (3) preoperative study in those who have a unilateral dominant lump or area which is probably a carcinoma.[1, 9, 12, 15, 16, 17] During the past three years, new equipment has been introduced which improves the quality of the examination significantly, and there is a much better chance that an occult carcinoma may be found.

Primary carcinoma of the breast is treated with many different operations at present.[5] These operations are (1) excision of the carcinoma with a quadrant or half of the breast, (2) simple mastectomy, (3) modified radical mastectomy, (4) radical mastectomy, and (5) extended radical mastectomy. For a number of reasons, radical mastectomy has been performed most often, and the ten-year cure rate statistics are well known. The burden of proof lies with those who propose a different operation for the "cure" of primary carcinoma, and to date no one has provided this proof with any other of the operations cited above.

When a patient presents with a dominant lump which is or may be a carcinoma, a biopsy should always be performed. It is well to keep in mind that even a small carcinoma has probably been present for many months or a number of years before the biopsy is performed. Therefore, immediate hospital admission biopsy and mastectomy are difficult to justify on other than emotional grounds. Earle has suggested that biopsy of suspicious lesions be performed in the outpatient section and that admission to the hospital be reserved for those who have a proved carcinoma.[4] This suggestion has a great deal of merit.

In performing frozen sections the pathologist may encounter difficulty in distinguishing adenosis and intraductal papillary disease from carcinoma. When the diagnosis is in any doubt, the operation should be terminated until it is established from a review of paraffin block sections. We are not aware of any harm resulting from a delay of up to seven days between biopsy and a definitive operation.

The modern operation of radical mastectomy, as originally devised by W. S. Halsted in 1882 and improved upon by him up to 1910, continues to be the treatment of choice for the cure of early breast carcinoma in its early stages. This operation, although appearing reasonably simple, is in fact rather complex and should be performed with meticulous surgical technique in an unhurried fashion. All surgeons who undertake the procedure must strive for eradication of the carcinoma in the operative field and for perfect primary wound healing without any necrosis, infection or fluid accumulation. The majority of complications of wound healing which develop postoperatively are due to either poor technique or a violation of Halsted's surgical principles.

PREOPERATIVE CARE

A complete history of all previous illnesses is required, and the detailed account obtained of the present illness should include, in addition, any family history of mammary carcinoma, the status of menstruation, the number of children who were nursed and for what length of time, and any treatment with estrogen compounds which were taken by mouth, parenterally, vaginally or through the skin (creams).

The physical examination should include a very detailed description of the breast tumor, the breast itself, including the overlying skin, and the findings in the regional lymph nodes, both positive and negative. It is desirable to make a drawing of the physical findings related to the breast and regional lymph nodes and to use a clinical classification of the stage of the disease so that the data can be used for comparison with the results achieved in other institutions and with other operations.

The surgeon must spend the necessary time discussing with the patient the anticipated operation, not only from the physical aspect but from the mental aspect as well. He must establish the patient's confidence in him and try to allay her fears concerning mutilation and death.

Laboratory Tests. Routine: CBC, hematocrit, alkaline phosphatase, blood group and Rh, x-rays of chest and skeleton (skull, entire spine and pelvis). Additional tests when indicated because of age or history: bloods for clotting profile, sugar two hours after noon meal, urea nitrogen, EKG and bone scan.

Orders the Day Before Operation. Shave axilla. Clip periareolar hairs. Do not scrub the skin. Soapsuds enema. Nothing by mouth after midnight. Cross-match 500 ml. of whole blood on call for the operating room. Preoperative medication to be ordered by the anesthesiologist.

THE OPERATION

One of the essential features of the operative procedure is the removal of all mammary tissue. The plane of dissection of the skin and fat layers overlying the breast is immediately above the superficial layer of the superficial fascia. Skin flaps which are developed that thinly must not be wider than 10 cm. because of the very real possibility of necrosis; further, they should not be subjected to any tension or pressure. It is always better to close the wound with the aid of a skin graft if the possibility exists that the skin flaps with a marginal blood supply, brought together under tension, will not survive.

The skin closure, whether primary or with the use of a skin graft, should permit the axillary skin to mold in the axillary hollow without "bowstringing" across the concave space. This is the most important factor in forestalling the accumulation of serum or lymph in the axilla postoperatively.

Plastic catheter drains are used both for wounds that are sutured primarily and for those closed with a skin graft. The plastic catheters to which suction is applied should be brought out through the inferior aspect of the lateral flap in the posterior axillary line and never through the incision itself.

The gauze dressings which cover the wound are held in place with adhesive tape, and care must be exercised to avoid any pressure. The arm may be placed at the side or in a position of mild abduction, depending on which is better for molding the skin in the axilla.

During the operative procedure, 500 to 1000 ml. of lactated Ringer's solution and 500 to 1000 ml. of 5 per cent dextrose in water are given. A moderate blood loss of the order of 750 ml., associated with tachycardia or hypotension, should be treated by administering 500 to 1000 ml. of a 5 per cent albumin solution. If tachycardia or hypotension persists following the infusion of the albumin solution, an operative blood loss of more than 1000 ml. has usually occurred and whole blood should be given as required.

POSTOPERATIVE CARE

Postoperative orders are written as follows:

1. Clear liquids per os as tolerated.

2. Add 500 (or 1000) ml. of 5 per cent dextrose in water to the infusion (total for 24 hours 2000 to 2500 ml.).

3. Keep on back. Do not turn. May have head gatch to 30 degrees.

4. Specify dose and frequency of analgesic drug.

Position in Bed. When the wound is closed partially with a skin graft, it is desirable to keep the patient in bed in a supine position without turning for at least 48 hours, in order for the skin flaps and graft to adhere to the chest wall. Patients whose wounds are closed primarily and have suction catheters are allowed out of bed on the first postoperative day.

Dressings. The dressings are changed as indicated by the type of closure and the amount of soiling of the gauze. Wounds closed with a skin graft are dressed for the first time by the first or second postoperative day and thereafter as required. Incisions that are closed primarily usually require no dressings. If suction catheters are used and are effective in removing the fluid so that the flaps adhere, they may be removed when they are no longer functioning or by the fifth day. The skin sutures are removed between the seventh and twelfth postoperative days.

Axillary Fluids. Hemorrhage beneath the flaps or into the axilla occurs rarely, and it is apparent within 12 to 24 hours of operation. The source is usually an axillary venous or arterial branch or an intercostal artery overlying the internal mammary vessels. Serious or continuing bleeding is treated by returning the patient to the operating room, opening the incision, evacuating all the clots and ligating the bleeding vessel or vessels.

Accumulation of serum or lymph beneath the axillary flap is much more common and does occur at times in spite of the use of suction catheters. Such collections also appear for the first time after the catheters are removed, especially if the axillary skin flap is not molded well or if the arm is allowed to be abducted too early. Treatment consists of limiting abduction and flexion of the arm and daily aspirations of the fluid with an 18 gauge needle attached to a 50 ml. syringe. If the fluid persists in reaccumulating after four or five such aspirations, it should not be aspirated further but rather allowed to stabilize and absorb spontaneously over a period of one to three weeks. Continued aspirations or secondary surgical drainage is often followed by infection.

Regaining Arm Motion. The patient is permitted to use the arm for eating meals and so on, starting between the second and seventh postoperative days, depending upon the mold of skin in the axilla, the adherence of the flaps to the chest wall and the absence of fluid collections. Full abduction should be avoided at this time. Free use of the arm is allowed after the usual slight to moderately severe shoulder stiffness and pain have subsided.

In general, full arm motion is achieved sooner when early motion and subsequent exercises can be permitted. However, exercises undertaken when there is undue pain or shoulder spasm often result in decreased motion and an episode of myositis which can go on to a partially frozen shoulder. No patient should be encouraged to exercise the arm if excess pain in the shoulder or extreme nervous tension exists.

Lymphedema of the Arm. Lymphedema of moderate severity is one of the most common complications following operation, and it is distressing to the patient both mentally and physically. It is a preventable complication in the majority of patients. It develops following removal of the axillary lymph nodes, either because of an inadequate collateral pathway from the arm or because of superimposed infection in those channels.

The normal anatomy of the lymphatic drainage from the arm is well known. The vast majority of channels drain lymph directly into the axillary nodes, but there are a small number which run over the shoulder into the cervical nodes.

Lymphatic function studies of the arm both before and after operations performed at Columbia, using a 25μc. tracer dose of radioactive iodinated serum albumin (RISA), have added to our knowledge of the physiology of this system. Approximately 75 per cent of the tracer dose injected subcutaneously into the dorsal aspect of the web space will be absorbed within 48 hours from a normal arm. Following operation, for a period of four weeks, the amount of tracer absorbed in 48 hours varies between 40 and 60 per cent. Thereafter, if no edema develops, the absorption value returns to or near the normal figure. However, when edema occurs, the net absorption is found to be in the lower ranges and the degree of reduction is proportional to the severity of the edema.

Infrequently, particularly in the obese patient, lymphedema of slight to moderate severity develops in the postoperative period even though the wound heals perfectly without apparent infection or any fluid collection. The explanation is believed to be either that the patient has an inadequate collateral circulation or that there has been insufficient time for an adequate collateral system to become effective.

It is probable that the patients whose edema subsides spontaneously without any treatment fall into the latter category. Both categories of patients are treated with one of the chlorothiazides in moderate dosage. If the edema subsides within 72 hours, treatment is continued for a period of three to four weeks. If no improvement is apparent after the 72 hour period, the chlorothiazide is cancelled and the patient given Aldactone, 50 mg. at 8:00 A.M. and 2:00 P.M. daily for a one to three month period.

The most common cause of postoperative lymphedema is infection with or without an additional wound healing complication of flap necrosis and of axillary fluid collection. The most common microorganisms causing the infection in the flaps or lymphatics of the arm are hemolytic *Staphylococcus aureus,* coagulase positive, and beta hemolytic streptococcus Group A. The staphylococcus is found in 95 per cent of the patients who have had cultures taken. The infection may be so mild or slight that it may be overlooked clinically, for there may be no clinical signs of cellulitis or lymphangiitis. On the other hand, the infection may be obvious, as in the case of suture abscesses, infected necrotic flaps or infected axillary seroma.

TREATMENT OF EDEMA.   Edema of the arm which develops in the postoperative period should be treated promptly and vigorously. The assumption should be made that infection exists even though it may not be clinically apparent. When it is obvious, as in the case of suture abscesses, infected necrotic flaps or infected axillary fluid, local as well as systemic treatment is required.

Treatment consists of elevating the arm on one or more pillows so that it is higher than the heart. Chlorothiazide or Aldactone is ordered (as already mentioned) for as long as indicated. An appropriate antibiotic such as one of the synthetic penicillins is given parenterally or by mouth in moderately large doses for a period of seven days. When indicated, antibiotics may also be used topically or injected into the axilla. With this program of treatment, the edema usually subsides promptly and the arm returns to normal or almost normal size within a period of two weeks, providing that the infection is eradicated. No treatment is effective in reducing the size of an edematous arm in the presence of persistent infection.

INSTRUCTIONS TO THE PATIENT IN CARE OF THE ARM.   All patients who have had a radical mastectomy should receive detailed instructions in care of the arm in order to keep the arm a normal size or to prevent it from enlarging further. The surgeon should explain the normal anatomy and physiology of the lymphatic system and how these have been altered by the operation. It should be pointed out that the intact skin is an excellent barrier to bacteria but that they enter the lymphatic system readily when the skin is punctured, cut or burned. The bacteria may initiate a lymphangiitis which can produce or accentuate an existing edema.

Some patients apparently have a very effective collateral lymphatic system so that they may sustain a hundred or a thousand episodes of skin breaks and bacterial entry without ever developing edema. On the other hand, other patients may develop mild, moderate or severe edema following a single episode of puncturing, cutting or burning the skin of the hand or arm. Therefore, since there is no test for determining which patient has an effective collateral circulation, all patients should exercise the necessary caution and care. The instructions are as follows:

1. Avoid all cuts, punctures and burns of the hand and arm.

2. Do not permit injections of medicine into the arm or blood withdrawal from the arm or hand.

3. Do not manicure the cuticles or pick hangnails.

4. Use a potholder mitt when working at the stove.

5. Wear a long-sleeved dress or blouse and a leather glove for garden work.

6. Call the surgeon promptly if any infection or swelling occurs in the arm.

The infection should be treated with oral antibiotics. If swelling develops, oral diuretics should be used as well. Serious infection with moderate to severe edema is best treated on an in-hospital basis.

REPEATED EPISODES OF INFECTION. Some patients develop repeated episodes of slight lymphangiitis and cellulitis and even erysipeloid infections in the arm in spite of using due caution and instructions from the surgeon. Each attack can be traced to some form of break in the skin. Bicillin long-acting, 1,200,000 units intramuscularly once each month, has been found to be most effective in preventing attacks of infection and increase in size of the arm.

Other Complications. All patients complain during the postoperative period of a varying degree of numbness and hyperesthesia of the medial aspect of the arm from the axilla to the elbow. This results from severing the intercostal brachial nerve. The pain or abnormal feeling subsides spontaneously for the most part within a period of three to six months.

Many patients develop moderately severe pain in the medial arm from the axilla to the proximal forearm owing to skin cords which result from contraction of the axillary skin. The cords and pain subside spontaneously over a period of three to eight weeks as the axillary skin loosens.

Axillary vein phlebitis or thrombosis is an uncommon complication, and when it occurs it is practically always associated with severe trauma to the vein or its inadvertent ligation.

Phlebothrombosis of the leg veins and pulmonary embolus occur in a small percentage of patients and may be treated with appropriate anticoagulant therapy.

REFERENCES

1. Asch, T.: Mammography: A study of 500 patients. Amer. J. Roentgenol. *90*:366, 1963.
2. Bolton, J. P.: The breast cyst and the hospital bed. Arch. Surg. *101*:382, 1970.
3. Cooper, P.: Benign and malignant mammary lesions; *in* The Craft of Surgery, Vol. 1. Boston, Little, Brown & Company, 1964.
4. Earle, A. S.: Delayed operation for breast carcinoma—editorial. Surg. Gynec. & Obst. *131*:291, 1970.
5. Fisher, B.: The surgical dilemma in the primary therapy of invasive breast cancer: A critical appraisal. Curr. Probl. Surg. October, 1970.
6. Frantz, V. K., Pickren, J. W., Melcher, G. W., and Auchincloss, H., Jr.: Incidence of chronic cystic disease in so-called "normal breasts." Cancer *4*:762, 1951.
7. Habif, D. V., Perzin, K. H., Lipton, R., and Lattes, R.: Subareolar abscess associated with squamous metaplasia of lactiferous ducts. Amer. J. Surg. *119*:523, 1970.
8. Lattes, R.: Personal communications.
9. Lesnick, G. J.: Mammography: A word of caution. N.Y. State J. Med. *66*:2005, 1966.
10. Lewison, E. F.: Breast cancer and its diagnosis and treatment. Baltimore, Williams and Wilkins Company, 1955.
11. McDivitt, R. W., Hutter, R. V. P., Foote, R. W., Jr., and Stewart, F. W.: In-situ lobular carcinoma. J.A.M.A. *201*:82, 1967.
12. Missakian, M. M., Witten, D. M., and Harrison, E. G., Jr.: Mammography after mastectomy. Usefulness in search for recurrent carcinoma of breast. J.A.M.A. *191*:1045, 1965.
13. Presbyterian Hospital series.
14. Rosemond, G. P., Maier, W. P., and Brobyn, T. J.: Needle aspiration of breast cysts. Surg. Gynec. & Obst. *123*:351, 1969.
15. Stevens, G., and Weigen, J. F.: Mammography survey for breast cancer detection. A 2-year study of 1223 clinically negative asymptomatic women over 40. Cancer *19*:51, 1966.
16. Strax, P., Venet, L., Shapiro, S., and Gross, S.: Mammography and clinical examination in mass screening for cancer of the breast. Cancer *20*:2184, 1967.
17. Witten, D. M., and Thurber, D. L.: Mammography as a Routine Screening Examination for Detecting Breast Cancer. Presented at the 64th Annual Meeting of the American Roentgen Ray Society, Montreal, Quebec, Canada, October 8-11, 1963.

CHAPTER 28

THE ENDOCRINE PANCREAS

Stanley R. Friesen, M.D., Ph.D.

INTRODUCTION

The clinical conditions which arise because of abnormalities of the endocrine cells of the pancreas are the result of systemic manifestations of hypo- or hyperfunctioning cells. The abnormality within the endocrine cell may involve faulty hormonal production, storage, or liberation; in some clinical conditions there is faulty hormonal utilization at the target organ. The endocrine cells of the pancreas, described by Langerhans as being arranged in islets or clumps amid surrounding exocrine cells, are in immediate juxtaposition to capillaries into which humoral substances gain access to the circulation and ultimately to their end-organs. The islet cells may be affected simply by compression, restricted as it were by an encasement of fibrous and acinar tissue, as is seen in the diabetes mellitus of chronic pancreatitis. Hypofunction of the islet cells, particularly the beta cells, may also result from primary atrophy of those cells; or, on the other hand, dysfunction may not be attended by recognizable histologic changes, in which case faulty metabolism of insulin and carbohydrates results more from abnormalities in storage, secretion and utilization. Hyperfunction of the islet cells may be a result of de novo hyperplasia or neoplasia (benign or malignant).

Furthermore, clinical pictures of hyperfunction may, strangely, be extrapancreatic (ectopic) in origin, such as the hyperinsulinism associated with large mesodermal fibrous mesotheliomas found in retroperitoneal and extrapleural areas. The hyperplasias and neoplasias of the endocrine cells of the pancreas and duodenum may produce clinical pictures consistent with excessive secretion of hormones, i.e., hyperinsulinism (beta cells), hypergastrinism (delta cells), hyperglucagonism (alpha cells), or hypersecretinism (S-cells of the duodenum). The hyperplasias and multicentric adenomatoses of the islets, usually considered to be primary abnormalities, may actually be changes secondary

514

to pituitary stimulation. Even malignant islet cell tumors may be associated with pituitary abnormalities, as evidenced by the association of islet cell hyperfunction with pluriglandular endocrine tumors or hyperplasias. Furthermore, islet cell hyperfunction may be polyhormonal and may produce multiple superimposed clinical pictures owing to the liberation of several hormones. Such multiple hormonal secretions suggest that the endocrine cells of the islets are totipotential polypeptide-secreting cells. An awareness of the myriad of clinical pictures arising either at the same time or sequentially is necessary for their recognition. Diagnostic confirmation of the clinical pictures ideally involves bioassay and immunochemical assay of the excessive hormones.

DIABETES MELLITUS

Whether diabetes mellitus is due to hypofunction of the beta islet cells or to faulty metabolism of carbohydrate and insulin, the preoperative recognition of this disease is necessary for safe intra- and postoperative management of such patients. Diabetes, which may be in balance naturally preoperatively may be complicated by acidosis, ketosis and coma during the period postoperatively of uncontrolled glucose infusion and catabolism. Patients who are controlled by insulin administration preoperatively may easily slip over into hypoglycemic states during starvation postoperatively unless appropriate adjustments of insulin dosages are made.

Latent or undiagnosed diabetes mellitus is common; every prospective surgical patient should be screened for diabetes by examination of the urine for sugar and acetone and by fasting and controlled two-hour postprandial blood sugar determinations. The diabetes associated with a glucagon-secreting tumor of the islets should be kept in mind. Special diagnostic tests, such as the glucagon provocative test and serum assays for glucagon are indicated in such situations.

MANAGEMENT OF CONTROLLED DIABETES

Preoperative laboratory determinations are important in the known controlled diabetic patient. These tests include, in addition to the urinalysis and the fasting blood sugar determinations, analysis of the blood for serum sodium, chloride, potassium, bicarbonate, plasma protein and blood urea nitrogen. These being known and corrected preoperatively, the aim of management from that point on is to maintain a *mild* elevation of blood sugar levels (100 to 300 mg./100 ml.), with the attending 1 to 3+ glycosuria. This plan tends to protect against the dangerous hypoglycemia from too much insulin or against the acidosis from too little insulin. There is no harm in mild hyperglycemia or glycosuria, whereas striving for normal blood sugar values more easily results in imbalances caused by too much insulin.

The patient's diabetic status should be stabilized prior to a major operation. If the patient has been on an oral hypoglycemic agent, the drug should be discontinued and regular (soluble) insulin substituted. The patient who has been receiving long-acting insulin is changed to regular insulin given every six hours, or every four hours if he is very ill, in order to minimize the risk of hypoglycemia which may occur as a result of preoperative starvation. The total daily dose of regular insulin should be approximately equal to the dose of long-acting insulin which it replaces. If the patient has been on *large* doses of long-acting insulin, about one third of the daily dose may be continued as long-acting insulin and the remaining dosage divided up as regular insulin every six hours.

In order to minimize the period of preoperative fasting and keto-genesis, the operation should be done as early in the day as possible. On the day of operation, after a fasting blood sugar is drawn, an intravenous infusion containing 5 per cent glucose is begun, and approximately one third to one half of the usual morning dose of regular insulin is then given subcutaneously. If a *long* operation is anticipated, about half of the usual morning insulin dose may be given ahead of time as long-acting insulin. Some surgeons prefer to add regular insulin to the intravenous bottle at an approximate ratio of one unit of regular insulin to 5 grams of glucose (10 units per liter of 5 per cent glucose). The latter plan may result in erratic administration of insulin if the infusions are either accelerated or interrupted by the infusion of blood or colloids. Postoperatively, beginning immediately after operation, a sliding scale plan of insulin administration is begun, depending upon serial urine determinations of glucose and acetone, done every four hours or more often if necessary. Regular insulin is given subcutaneously, according to the following schedule:

Urinalysis	*Insulin Dosage**
++++ sugar	15 units
+++ "	10 "
++ "	5 "
+ "	no insulin

If the patient is receiving intravenous glucose solutions, the insulin dosage should not be regulated entirely on the basis of urine glucose, as this reflects the rate of intravenous administration; therefore, the sliding scale in such instances should be based primarily on urine acetone (plus urine glucose) determinations. Severe diabetics or those who have been on large doses of long-acting insulin should continue to receive one third of the total daily dose as long-acting insulin each

---

*Add 5 units for positive urine acetone.

morning in addition to the requirements as indicated by the sliding scale.

The blood sugar and bicarbonate should be checked on the morning of the first postoperative day and intermittently thereafter, in order to modify the the sliding scale if necessary. The sliding scale schedule is continued during the time the patient is receiving intravenous infusions approximating 3 liters of 5 per cent glucose in water daily. When oral intake is begun, the patient is placed on a 1000- to 1200-calorie diet and regular insulin is given before each meal and at midnight as indicated by the results of the urine tests. When the patient is able to resume his standard preoperative diabetic diet he is returned to an appropriate dose of long-acting insulin.

MANAGEMENT OF UNCONTROLLED DIABETES

Diabetic Acidosis or Coma. An acute surgical condition may precipitate the development of severe diabetic acidosis or coma with its attendant depletion of water and electrolytes, which obviously must be corrected prior to surgical treatment of the underlying urgent condition. The diagnosis of uncontrolled diabetes may not be obvious from the history of the patient, but the admitting urinalysis, blood sugar and electrolyte determinations should suggest the possibility. If there is doubt or if the urgency precludes waiting for these results, the possibility of diabetic acidosis can be confirmed by a determination of serum acetone (Acetest). A drop of serum is placed on sodium nitroprusside powder; if a dark purple color results, there is a high ketone level in the blood. Therapy should be instituted immediately when the diagnosis is confirmed, by beginning an infusion of normal saline and administering regular insulin (50 to 300 units, depending on the degree of ketosis and the age of the patient) with half the dose given intravenously and half subcutaneously. If the patient is in a state of vascular collapse, the entire dose of insulin should be given intravenously to avoid the delayed subcutaneous absorption. Further insulin administration is dependent on subsequent blood glucose levels determined at one-hour intervals.

An indwelling urinary catheter should be placed for monitoring hourly urine output. Plasmanate or dextran or blood should be administered as indicated by the type of loss, or if significant oliguria or hypotension is present. The saline infusion will initiate the correction of sodium losses, but a more rapid correction of the acidosis can be accomplished by administering sodium lactate (M/6 sodium lactate) or sodium bicarbonate solutions, which should be started when the blood chemistry results are known to be abnormal. The dosage of lactate or bicarbonate can be calculated as follows: Extracellular fluid volume (liters) × (25-plasma bicarbonate) = mEq. of lactate or bicarbonate.

Potassium replacement should not be started until an adequate urinary output (30 ml./ hour) is attained or until electrocardiograms show no evidence of hyperkalemia. Surgical treatment can be instituted if it is still indicated as soon as the acidosis appears to be corrected and the dehydration is on the way to an improved state. Since large volumes of infused solutions may be necessary, monitoring of the central venous pressure, of the plasma osmolarity and of the body weight is extremely valuable.

Hypoglycemic (Insulin) Reaction. If the diabetic patient is unconscious or severely disoriented, a decision must be made as to whether the patient is in acidotic coma or in a hypoglycemic reaction. A urine test for glycosuria, a blood sugar determination and the plasma acetone test usually clarify the situation. Insulin should never be given to an unconscious patient unless there is definite evidence of hyperglycemia; it is safer to give 50 ml. of 50 per cent glucose if it can be determined that plasma hyperosmolarity is not present. The glucose will do little harm if the patient is in acidosis, but will usually restore consciousness promptly in hypoglycemia unless the patient already has suffered serious brain damage. Following the resolution of the acute state, the sliding scale schedule of insulin administration should be instituted until normal maintenance can be resumed.

FUNCTIONING TUMORS OF THE ENDOCRINE PANCREAS

Insulinoma (Insulinogenic Betacytoma). The hyperinsulinism caused by hyperfunction of the beta islet cells in pancreatic tumors produces a hypoglycemia which in turn initiates clinical symptoms and signs not unlike those of hypoglycemia from any other cause. The predominant early symptoms associated with a rapid rate of fall in blood sugar consist of sweating, weakness, hunger, tachycardia and "inward trembling," and are produced by a compensatory hyperepinephrinemia. This mechanism represents an attempt to restore normal blood glucose levels by accelerating glycogenolysis. If the blood glucose falls slowly to low levels over a period of many hours, the manifestations are due to cerebral glucose deprivation and consist of headache, blurred vision, diplopia, mental confusion, incoherent speech, "blacking out," coma and convulsions. The two types of clinical picture may merge, and, if the hypoglycemia persists over long periods of time, serious psychiatric and neurologic sequelae occur, with permanent brain damage.

It is obvious that the alarming and serious clinical pictures produced by hypoglycemia require concerted diagnostic efforts in order to differentiate those patients who have recognizable anatomic lesions, most of which are amenable to surgical treatment. The most common organic cause of fasting hypoglycemia is the single beta islet cell adenoma. There may be multiple adenomas, or the lesion may be carcinomatous with metastases. The betacytoma may be associated with adenomas of other endocrine glands (familial multiple endocrine adenomatosis or pluriglandular involvement). The insulin-secreting tumor may be a mixed one, producing additional peptide hormones (polyhormonal). Moreover, a predominantly carcinoid tumor may produce insulin (heterotopic islet cell tumor). The latter two varieties represent peptide-secreting tumors derived embryologically from foregut anlage. The insulin-secreting tumors of the pancreas must also be differentiated from extrapancreatic neoplasms which produce hypoglycemia, such as the massive mesotheliomas and the carcinomas of the adrenal cortex, liver and gastrointestinal tract, which also may be treated surgically. Finally, it is necessary to further differentiate the tumors from the other causes of hypoglycemia which do not require surgical treatment, such as impaired hepatic function, pituitary and adrenocortical hypofunction, alimentary hyperinsulinism after gastric operations, reactive hypoglycemia in early diabetes mellitus, hypoglycemia caused by drugs such as aspirin, alcohol and hypoglycemic agents, and factitious hypoglycemia after insulin administration.

Spontaneous hypoglycemia caused by insulin-secreting tumors was not recognized as such until the clinical symptom complex was seen in overinsulinized diabetics after the isolation of insulin by Banting and Best in 1921. Wilder's demonstration of insulin in metastases confirmed the diagnostic triad, named after Whipple, in which gastrointestinal and neurologic symptoms occur in a fasting state, associated with a blood sugar level under 50 mg. per 100 ml., with clinical response after ingestion or administration of glucose. Attacks of hypoglycemia resulting from insulin-secreting tumors usually occur in a fasting state, before the next meal, particularly before breakfast. Prolonged fasting constitutes the most reliable diagnostic maneuver; at least a third of patients with insulinogenic betacytoma develop symptoms within 12 hours, and two thirds by 24 hours; occasionally 48 to 72 hours of food deprivation is necessary to bring out the symptoms if an adenoma is present. Symptoms are provoked with shorter fasting periods if the tumor is carcinomatous. Insulin assays of plasma, by either immunochemical or bioassay techniques, are inappropriately high in most patients with tumor after an overnight fast.

Further preoperative diagnostic testing may occasionally be indicated. The tolbutamide provocative test in patients with tumor shows a greater absolute reduction in blood glucose levels and a longer period of hypoglycemia than other causes of hypoglycemia. Abnormal hyperinsulinemia as measured by plasma insulin assays concomitant with prolonged hypoglycemia following the intravenous administration of tolbutamide is highly diagnostic of adenomas. Intravenous administration of L-leucine, glucagon or glucose is not as helpful as the prolonged fast or the tolbutamide provocative tests. The suspected pancreatic betacytoma may be located preoperatively in about half the patients by radio-logic selective arterial catheterization with injection of contrast media. Radioisotope techniques have yet to show promise of diagnostic confirmation.

Additional support of a diagnosis of insulin-secreting islet cell tumors is gained by ruling out (1) extrapancreatic insulin-secreting mesotheliomas by radiologic examination of the mediastinum and retroperitoneal areas for massive tumors, (2) factitious insulin administration by close observation of the patient and by testing for insulin antibodies, (3) alimentary "hyperinsulinism" by upper gastrointestinal x-rays for rapid emptying of the stomach, and (4) "functional" hypoglycemia by oral glucose tolerance testing for absence of fasting hypoglycemia and presence of a "reactive glucose tolerance curve."

Because some patients with betacytoma develop gastric hypersecretion of acid and duodenal ulcer caused supposedly by the frequent hypoglycemic stimulation of the vagi, a preoperative gastric analysis and radiologic upper gastrointestinal series are indicated.

Most patients with an insulinoma have learned that eating relieves the symptoms of hypoglycemia. Such frequent eating will lead to weight gain and obesity, adding to the surgeon's problem of finding the tumor at operation.

The surgical procedure requires very careful examination of the pancreas for the usually small, usually single, pinkish-tan nodule which may be located in any part of the pancreas. Usually the search may require only minimal dissection, including freeing up the second portion of the duodenum by a Kocher maneuver and inspection of the body and tail of the pancreas by entrance into the lesser omental bursa through the gastrohepatic membrane or the gastrocolic omentum. When the initial dissection does not reveal an obvious tumor, complete mobilization of the spleen and body and tail of the pancreas is mandatory for a thorough search by inspection and palpation. Extreme care must be taken to avoid injuring the surface of the pancreatic capsule. In the event that a nodule is not found and no retroperitoneal mesodermal tumor is found, some surgeons carry out distal pancreatectomy for serial section of the body and tail of the pancreas. Such "blind resections" as often as not fail to reveal the occult insulinoma. It is probably wiser to withhold "blind resection" and terminate the operation to wait for the tumor to become larger with time while controlling the symptoms medically by dietary management.

In those rare patients with a malignant beta islet cell carcinoma with metastases, surgical treatment has little to offer. It has been reported that one such patient, suffering from episodes of hypoglycemia with metastatic disease that was producing excessive insulin, gastrin and glucagon, was treated with streptozotocin with excellent symptomatic relief. Hepatic metastases were reduced in size, and the levels of hormones by assay were diminished.

Having found and excised the insulinoma, the postoperative management requires intermittent determinations of the blood glucose, particularly after intravenous feedings are eliminated. Because of the operative trauma to the pancreas, the gastrointestinal tract should be kept at rest by gastric suction, and the character and amount of the drainage from the pancreatic area (usually by sump-suction drainage tube) should be carefully observed.

Ulcerogenic Tumor (Gastrinogenic Deltacytoma). The hypergastrinism caused by hyperfunction of delta islet cells in pancreatic tumors produces a marked hypersecretion of gastric acids which in turn produces symptoms and signs of fulminating ulcer disease. It is generally believed that the gastrin-secreting islet cell tumors arise spontaneously, de novo, liberate excessive amounts of gastrin which humorally stimulates the end-organ, the gastric parietal cells, to become hyperplastic and hypersecretory. On the other hand, there is a definite possibility that the islet cell changes, including hyperplasia and benign and malignant tumors, are not the primary abnormality but are changes secondary to trophic stimulation from the pituitary. It is postulated that the pituitary feedback mechanism is caused by[7] a gastric antrum end-organ failure, i.e., acid-inhibition of the gastrin cells of the antrum, resulting from vagal gastric hypersecretion associated with duodenal ulcer which usually precedes the development of the Zollinger-Ellison syndrome.

Whatever the mechanism of the development of the hypergastrinism, it is the resulting marked gastric hypersecretion of acid which produces the fulminating ulcer disease and which must be differentiated from the ordinary duodenal ulcer diathesis. A high index of awareness of the possibility of the Zollinger-Ellison syndrome is paramount in patients with severe duodenal ulcer, recurrent stomal ulcer, unexplained diarrhea, or other endocrine disease. Failure to recognize the possibility of an ulcerogenic tumor or failure to control the excessive gastric acid secretion medically or surgically may result in catastrophe.

Several diagnostic features are usually present which lead to a high index of suspicion, including those described by Zollinger and Ellison in 1955: (1) Recurrent or ectopically situated (jejunal) acid peptic ulcers, (2) excessive hypersecretion of gastric acids, exceeding 1000 ml. or 100 mEq. in 12 hours, and (3) confirmation of the presence of a non-beta islet cell tumor of the pancreas. Other highly suggestive features include (1) unexplained diarrhea (steatorrhea caused by failure of activation of fat-splitting enzymes in the profuse acid media of the duodenum and jejunum); (2) a patient usually under 40 years of age, particularly in the "teens," with severe complications of duodenal ulcer; (3) a strong family history of peptic ulcer, diabetes, and endocrine tumors; (4) findings which suggest other endocrine abnormalities, particularly parathyroid, pituitary or carcinoid tumors; (5) radiologic findings of marked hyperrugosity of the gastric mucosa, duodenal nodularity, postbulbar ulcer, hypermotility of the small intestine with segmentation and rapid transit; and (6) the presence of gastrojejunal stomal ulceration after standard surgical operations for ulcer.

When the possibility of an ulcerogenic tumor is suspected in patients with recurrent ulcer after previous treatment, great care must be taken to rule out causes resulting from inadequate operations. To this end it is necessary to perform a Hollander insulin gastric analysis to confirm an incomplete vagotomy and to carry out radiologic surveys in search for inadequate gastrectomy or for retained excluded antrum; the latter may in itself produce hypergastrinism by either alkaline stimulation of the bypassed antrum or diversion of the acid-inhibition of the antrum. A recurrent ulcer may also be present as a complication of hepatic cirrhosis with natural or surgical portal-systemic shunting of intestinal histamine. Ulcers may be found also in association with chronic pancreatitis, pulmonary emphysema, parathyroid adenoma, or iatrogenically with cortisone or aspirin medication.

If these causes of recurrent ulcer are ruled out, the next step in preoperative management is to predict the possible presence of an ulcerogenic tumor before operation. Because the acid secretion levels in these patients may be inconsistent at different times, the volume and concentration of gastric acid secretion should be measured two or three times by means of 12-hour overnight aspirations. The position of the nasogastric tube should be checked fluoroscopically each time, and the initial aspirate should be discarded. A nine-hole No. 18 Wangensteen nasogastric tube usually is most efficient. The 12-hour aspirate should be measured for volume and HCl concentration (mEq./L.) and the output of HCl in 12 hours calculated. Before removing the gastric suction tube, a maximum stimulus to acid secretion should be done (Histalog gastric analysis). This test will allow the determination of the ratio of basal acid concentration to maximal acid concentration (BAC/MAC). If this ratio is higher than 0.7, the likelihood is present that basal gastrin stimulation of the gastric parietal cells by the tumor is already at a high (maximal) level. Water and electrolyte depletion may occur as a result of these tests and should be corrected. The confirmatory determination of the level of circulating gastrin in the serum, by bioassay and/or (preferably) by immunochemical assay should now be done. A venous sample (10 ml. without anticoagulant) from the fasting unmedicated patient is centrifuged and the serum is separated and frozen until the assay can be done.

The complex assay determinations of gastrin in serum and tissue may not be readily available. If arrangements with the few investigators doing such assays can be made, frozen tissues should be air-mailed to them; otherwise, the diagnosis must instead be based on firm clinical data such as profound acid hypersecretion, ectopic ulceration and, above all, histologic confirmation of islet cell abnormalities at the time of operation.

Accessible lymph node metastases, if palpably enlarged, such as a Virchow's left supraclavicular node, should be excised for microscopic study (stained for islet cell identification), for tissue assay of gastrin and for electron microscopic examination.

Having confirmed the definite possibility of a gastrin-secreting tumor of the pancreas, it is advisable now to screen the endocrine systems of the patient, because of the possibility that multiple systems may be involved (pluriglandular) or that multiple hormones may be elaborated from one tumor (polyhormonal). Because the association with parathyroid adenomas (or hyperplasias) is over 30 per cent, determinations of serum calcium and phosphorus are indicated (if abnormal, a tubular-reabsorption of phosphorus ratio should be determined), as well as radiologic surveys of the kidneys and bones. Furthermore, because the incidence of pituitary abnormalities, either as the primary or as the associated abnormality, may also be as frequent as 30 per cent, an x-ray of the sella turcica for enlargement should be done. The assay of human growth hormone (HGH) in this regard should be done at the time that a six-hour oral glucose tolerance test is done (serum is collected also for immunoreactive insulin [IRI]). Twenty-four hour collections of urine for 17-ketogenic steroid (17KGS) and 17-ketosteroid (17KS) determinations are done. Adrenal cortex monitoring is best done by testing the suppressibility of plasma corticoids with a single dose dexamethasone suppression (Forsham test). Determination of plasma follicular-stimulating hormone (FSH) and urine FSH are also obtained. A plasma thyroxine determination and a 5-HIAA urinary excretion test complete the endocrine screening tests. Any abnormality should be followed through with provocative or other confirmatory tests. Some islet cell tumors are polyhormonal in that the tumor may elaborate several hormones, with bizarre clinical pictures. Increases in serum cortisol, adrenocorticotrophic hormone (ACTH), melanocyte-stimulating hormone (MSH), immunoreactive insulin (IRI), glucagon, and human growth hormone (HGH) have been observed in a patient with a malignant islet cell tumor.

Before operation, a liver scan and chest x-ray for visualization of metastatic deposits should be done, but their presence should not deter operative treatment because metastases have been observed to disappear after total gastrectomy. These patients are usually partially depleted of blood, water and electrolytes, and this should be corrected as much as is possible prior to operation. It is particularly important to correct the metabolic alkalosis, if present, before operation, because of the tendency toward cardiac arrhythmias at the time of induction of anesthesia.

At operation, every effort should be made to absolutely confirm the diagnosis by a search for (1) the symptomatic ulceration, (2) the gastric hyperrugosity and (3) the islet cell tumor(s). The first requires visualization of the entire duodenum and jejunum; the ulcer(s) need not be dealt with unless there is active bleeding or free perforation. The gastric hyperrugosity is usually obvious from the thickness of the stomach wall. The islet cell tumor(s) or hyperplasia is not always as obvious. The two most likely sites where metastatic tumor is found are the liver, in which seed-like deposits should not be overlooked, and the enlarged pancreaticoduodenal lymph nodes posterior to the second portion of the duodenum. Biopsy of each of these areas should be done in any case for (1) frozen section histology, (2) permanent section, and (3) tissue assay for gastrin if islet cells are present. For the latter, the tissue is placed immediately on a small block of dry ice and kept frozen until the assay is done. The pancreas should not be dissected unless the diagnosis is still not obvious, in which case dissection often requires complete mobilization of the duodenal loop as well as the spleen and the body and tail of the pancreas. Amputation of the tail of the pancreas for biopsy is indicated if no other histologic confirmation has been obtained. If a single tumor is found, some surgeons advocate complete excision of the part of the pancreas bearing the tumor, either by distal pancreatectomy with splenectomy or by pancreaticoduodenectomy. Fewer than a dozen completely satisfactory results after tumor excision have been reported. More often total gastrectomy (after histologic confirmation has been obtained) yields better results than tumor excision because (1) the tumors may be multiple, (2) islet cell hyperplasia may be the only manifestation of islet cell abnormality (even if a tumor is found and removed, the remaining islets are usually hyperplastic), (3) the ulcer diathesis and marked gastric hypersecretion may be so fulminant that total gastrectomy is the only method of control, and (4) the metastatic and persistent tumors are likely to disappear after total gastrectomy.

The gastrectomy should be complete with positive identification of esophagus and duodenum at the lines of resection; a centimeter of gastric cardia is sufficient to negate good results. When the microscopic diagnosis is confirmed, no attempt at any procedure less than complete gastrectomy, with or without vagotomy, should be made. If the diagnosis is not confirmed microscopically or if the serum gastrin levels are under 250 pg./ml., a vagotomy with antrectomy is indicated, in which case the patient must be observed very cautiously postoperatively; most complications and deaths occur when the diagnosis of ulcerogenic tumor has been overlooked and some procedure short of total gastrectomy has been done, allowing the fulminant gastric hypersecretion to persist, causing stomal perforations and hemorrhage. The best results, when the syndrome is confirmed, follow total gastrectomy on the first surgical entry.

Postoperatively the patient is treated, as with any total gastrectomy, with nasogastric tube suction until intestinal function returns, and with water and electrolyte replacement. Serial serum gastrin levels are the best prognostic measures over the following months. Radiologic examinations of the chest and liver have been known to show reduction in size of and disappearance of metastatic deposits as early as 46 days, and second-look procedures at four and five years have shown complete absence of tumor and metastases. The well-being of patients treated by total gastrectomy is unusually good, i.e., much better than when the operation has been performed for gastric cancer. Six meals daily are required for a few months for adequate caloric intake.

When pluriglandular involvement is present, control of hyperparathyroidism, hyperadrenocorticism, etc., by surgical excision of the appropriate adenoma or hyperplasia is sometimes required. When metastases are not controlled by total gastrectomy or when polyhormonal manifestations continue, hypophysectomy may be the only effective recourse; in some patients the pituitary has been found to be histologically abnormal. Again, appropriate serum assays are of prognostic value in following these patients postoperatively. Subsequent endocrine abnormalities may appear at any time, and therefore long-term follow-up is advisable. Furthermore, because of the familial tendency in such patients, the members of the family should be studied and screened for endocrine and ulcer disease; even asymptomatic relatives have been found to harbor occult endocrinopathy.

Glucagonoma. The hyperglucagonism caused by hyperfunction of the alpha islet cells in pancreatic tumors produces a hyperglycemia not unlike that seen in diabetes mellitus. This similar feature in both the rare alpha cell tumor and the common diabetes mellitus adds to the difficulty in diagnosis of the former prior to the occurrence of metastases. Glucagon has been found by assay to be present in the serum of patients with alpha islet cell carcinoma, diabetes mellitus, pancreatitis, pheochromocytoma, hyperparathyroidism, associated with pancreatitis, bronchogenic carcinoma, and pluriglandular adenomatosis, including the ulcerogenic (delta cell) tumor of the pancreas. Glucagon also depresses the volume of gastric secretion (when a gastrin-secreting tumor is not also present), depresses intestinal motility, increases splanchnic blood flow, promotes tachycardia through a chronotropic action, increases cardiac output through its inotropic influence, induces hypocalcemia, and has been associated with resistant dermatitis. In a patient in whom hyperglucagonemia exists, an intravenous injection of glucagon may have no effect, although in a normal patient it should be expected to produce a rapid rise in serum insulin and plasma glucose. There will therefore be a blunted glucose curve after a glucagon injection in a patient with glucagonoma. When the glucagon-stimulating test shows no response, an assay of the serum for glucagon should be done. Assays for plasma glucagon in those rare instances when such tumors are suspected are available only in a few investigative laboratories by special arrangement. When arrangements for such confirmation are impractical, the diagnosis may have to await surgical exploration.

A celiac angiogram may demonstrate the tumor in the pancreas, but surgical exploration is more likely to lead to a diagnosis of this rare endocrine tumor. When metastases are not present, excision of the tumor is indicated. An assay of the tumor for glucagon should be done on the frozen tissue whenever possible. Since cobaltous chloride has been reported to have an affinity for alpha cells experimentally, it might be expected that isotopic cobaltous chloride would have an ameliorative effect on the tumor; however, in one study this isotope was not increased in the metastases of an alpha cell carcinoma. The preoperative and postoperative management of the hyperglycemia is similar to that of patients with diabetes mellitus.

Other Peptide-Secreting Tumors of the Pancreaticoduodenal Endocrine System.   Secreting adenomas are found in tissues which have developed embryologically from the endoderm of the primitive coelomic duct. Their humoral secretions are characterized as amino acid groups, polypeptides, which are physiologically active. Peptide-secreting cells in these adenomas are capable of hypersecreting one or more of these polypeptides. This totipotential hypersecretory capacity may have been stimulated by a pre-existing endocrine imbalance or by an altered feedback phenomenon or by pituitary stimulation. Neoplasia (DNA recoding) may modify a repressor activity built into normal cells which allows the unmasking of new coding instructions on the DNA molecule and may result in the production of new polypeptide hormones.

In addition to the peptide-secreting tumors already discussed (tumors secreting insulin, gastrin and glucagon), at least two other peptide-secreting adenomas of the pancreaticoduodenal system should be recognized: (1) tumors with secretin-like activity, and (2) carcinoid tumor.

TUMORS HAVING SECRETIN-LIKE ACTIVITY.   Such tumors produce "hypersecretinism," presumably from L- or S-cells of the pancreaticoduodenum. The resultant clinical picture has been termed pancreatic cholera, choleraic diarrhea, and potassium-losing diarrhea with achlorhydria. When the usual causes of diarrhea have been ruled out, choleraic diarrhea should be considered. Its presence is characterized by the large volume of virtually odorless stools, a profound myasthenia, the invariable electrolyte disturbance, intractable dyspepsia, and a family history of endocrine disorders. A Histalog gastric analysis will show an achlorhydria in spite of the presence of parietal cells in the gastric mucosa obtained by gastric mucosal biopsy. A palpably enlarged gallbladder in the absence of jaundice may be present also. After vigorous replacement of water and electrolytes, the resting output of the pancreatic exocrine discharge into the duodenum may be aspirated and measured. Until assays for the demonstration of circulating pancreatic secretagogue (secretin) are developed, the diagnosis may not be confirmed until at operation, at which time a distended gallbladder and a tumor of the pancreas or duodenum should be searched for, as with other adenomas. The tumor, if found, should be removed if possible; it should be frozen and extracted for bioassay (physiologic effect upon normal pancreatic exocrine secretion) and for immunochemical assay when available. Postoperatively, duodenal aspiration may show a reduced pancreatic exocrine secretion if the tumor has been completely removed.

CARCINOID TUMORS. Carcinoid tumors produce a hypersecretion of catecholamines from hyperfunctioning enterochromaffin (EC) cells. When hepatic metastases are present or when the secretions bypass the liver, a characteristic clinical picture results. The carcinoid picture of facial plethora with episodic flushing, abdominal colic and borborygmi should alert the clinician to disturbances of serotonin metabolism which may emanate from pancreatic and duodenal adenomas. The screening of the urine (5-HIAA) and blood may detect such breakdown products, and bioassay for bradykinin should also be considered. Upper gastrointestinal series for duodenal nodularity and intestinal hypermotility, hepatic scan for liver metastases, and a search for superimposed gastrin-secreting phenomena and hyperparathyroidism are indicated. The tumor, which should be searched for and removed at operation, has histologic characteristics similar to islet cell adenomas and is often confused with them until specific staining techniques for the EC cell and electron microscopic examinations are done. If hepatic metastases remain in the patient after the primary tumor is removed, some surgeons implant a small Silastic catheter through the gastroduodenal artery into the hepatic artery for subsequent continuous infusion (by a small portable pump) of chemotherapeutic drugs such as 5-fluorouracil.

SUMMARY

Hypofunctioning and hyperfunctioning endocrine cells of the pancreas produce characteristic clinical pictures. The many and unusual humoral substances which may be elaborated by the abnormal endocrine pancreas are being increasingly recognized and identified. These polypeptides may be present at the same time or sequentially in the same patient. The preoperative preparation of such patients includes diagnostic recognition, appropriate measurements of biochemical and physiologic aberrations, and the replacement of losses, for the safe surgical and medical interruption of the complex interactions within the endocrine system.

REFERENCES

Fajans, S. S., Schneider, J. M., Schteingart, D. E., and Conn, J. W.: The diagnostic value of sodium tolbutamide in hypoglycemic states. J. Clin. Endocrinol. 21:371, 1961.
Friesen, S. R., Bolinger, R. E., Pearse, A. G. E., and McGuigan, J. E.: Serum gastrin levels in malignant Zollinger-Ellison syndrome after total gastrectomy and hypophysectomy. Ann. Surg. 172:504, 1970.

Gregory, R. A., Grossman, M. I., Tracy, H. J., and Bentley, P. H.: Nature of the gastric secretagogue in Zollinger-Ellison tumors. Lancet 2:543, 1967.

Lipsett, M. B.: Hormonal syndromes associated with neoplasia. Adv. Metab. Dis. 3:111, 1968.

McGavran, M. H., Unger, R. H., Recant, L., Polk, H. C., Kilo, C., and Levin, M. D.: A glucagon-secreting alpha cell carcinoma of pancreas. N. Eng. J. Med. 274:1408, 1966.

McGuigan, J. E., and Trudeau, W. L.: Immunochemical measurement of elevated levels of gastrin in the serum of patients with pancreatic tumors of the Zollinger-Ellison variety. N. Eng. J. Med. 278:1308, 1968.

Murray-Lyon, I. M., Eddleston, A. L. W. F., Williams, R., Brown, M., Hogbin, B., Bennett, A., Edwards, J. C., and Taylor, K. W.: Treatment of multiple-hormone-producing malignant islet cell tumor with streptozotocin. Lancet 2:895, 1968.

Sircus, W.: Peptide-secreting tumours with special reference to the pancreas. Gut 10:506, 1969.

Wermer, P.: Genetic aspects of adenomatosis of endocrine glands. Am. J. Med. 16:363, 1954.

Yalow, R. S., and Berson, S.: Radioimmuno-assay of gastrin. Gastroenterology 58:1, 1970.

Zollinger, R. M., Elliott, D. W., Endahl, G. L., Grant, G. N., Goswitz, J. T., and Taft, D. A.: Origin of the ulcerogenic hormone in endocrine induced ulcer. Ann. Surg. 156:570, 1962.

SURGERY OF THE ADRENALS

DAVID M. HUME, M.D., F.A.C.S.

In this chapter consideration will be given to the various types of adrenal cortical and medullary disease with respect to symptoms and signs, special preoperative preparation, intraoperative and postoperative care, insufficiency, iatrogenic overadministration, and complications of surgery.

ADRENAL CORTICAL DISEASE OR ABLATION

TYPES OF DISEASE

Cushing's Syndrome. Cushing's syndrome arising spontaneously may result from any one of six different adrenal abnormalities, three of which are due to adrenal cortical hyperplasia from increased ACTH production, and three of which are due to cortisol-producing tumors of the adrenal cortex. The most common cause by far is bilateral adrenal cortical hyperplasia secondary to increased secretion of ACTH by the normal pituitary, presumably the result of an increased hypothalamic drive. The second most common is an adenoma of the adrenal cortex, the third is ACTH production from an ectopic extrapituitary source, the fourth is adrenal cortical carcinoma, the fifth is an ACTH-producing tumor of the pituitary, and the sixth is nodular dysplasia of the adrenal cortex. Ectopic ACTH production is sometimes seen in carcinoma of the lung (usually oat cell, or anaplastic bronchogenic), bronchial adenoma, thymoma, pancreatic carcinoma, ovarian tumors, thyroid carcinoma, parotid tumors, hepatic tumors, tumors of the esophagus and the adrenal medulla, and others.

Primary Aldosteronism. Primary aldosteronism usually results from an adenoma of the adrenal cortex, although it may also result from functional or anatomic hyperplasia of the adrenal cortex. The hyperplasia is autonomous and not related to increased secretions of ACTH, unlike that seen in Cushing's syndrome.

Adrenogenital Syndrome. The adrenogenital syndrome may appear at three different times in life—at birth, in childhood or in adult life. The congenital adrenogenital syndrome appearing at birth is by far the most common variety. The adrenogenital syndrome caused by congenital adrenal hyperplasia produces a pseudohermaphrodite in the female and sexual precocity in the male. The treatment is nonoperative, except for the occasional need to carry out plastic procedures on the genitalia of female pseudohermaphrodites.

The postnatal adrenogenital syndrome is usually the result of an adenoma or carcinoma of the adrenal cortex. In the female it produces masculinization, and in the male sexual precocity.

The adrenogenital syndrome appearing in adult life is usually due to a tumor and is much more common in women than in men. In women it produces virilism with male habitus, with or without signs of Cushing's disease. In the male it produces feminization or Cushing's syndrome without virilism. Mixed patterns are very common in both sexes.

The adrenogenital syndrome refers to any situation in which there is an overproduction of androgens resulting in virilization. For this reason the symptoms of the syndrome are much more marked and distressing in the female than in the male, with the solitary exception of the salt-losing form of the syndrome, which is often overlooked in males because of the apparent lack of physical stigmata, thus leading to fatal Addison's disease.

Estrogen-Secreting Tumors. Feminizing adrenogenital tumors are quite rare. They occur primarily in the male, are usually large, and about 90 per cent are carcinomas.

Nonfunctioning Adrenal Cortical Tumors. Some tumors of the adrenal cortex are nonfunctional and produce no endocrine change. At times they only appear nonfunctional because they produce sexual hormones of the same sex as the patient; thus virilizing tumors are difficult to detect in the male and feminizing tumors in the female. If the tumors are large when first discovered, they are apt to be carcinomatous.

Adrenal Ablation for Carcinoma of the Breast. Excision of normal adrenals is sometimes carried out in an attempt to ameliorate other diseases. This is particularly so for carcinoma of the breast with metastases, in which excision of the adrenals may decrease the hormonal stimulus to growth of the cancer.

Adrenal Insufficiency and Complications of Adrenal Steroid Therapy. Adrenal insufficiency may take the form of pre-existing Addison's disease which is unrecognized until the operative event, it may occur simultaneously with the operative event, or it may pre-exist as a consequence of adrenal atrophy secondary to the administration of adrenal steroids. In addition to producing secondary adrenal insufficiency, the administration of exogenous adrenal steroids may produce a series of other complications which require surgery.

SIGNS, SYMPTOMS AND LABORATORY FINDINGS

Cushing's Syndrome. The signs and symptoms of Cushing's syndrome are listed in Table 29-1. Cushing's syndrome is usually easily detected because of the characteristic appearance of the patient. There are, however, four circumstances in which more sophisticated laboratory tests may be required to make the diagnosis. The first of these is the differentiation between women with Cushing's syndrome and obese women with hirsutism who may show many of the physical signs of Cushing's syndrome. The second is the early phase of Cushing's syndrome when the development of the characteristic signs and symptoms may not have progressed sufficiently far to make them easily recognizable. The third is the mixed Cushing's syndrome in which an adrenal cortical tumor secretes excessive amounts of androgen as well as glucocorticoids, thus producing a combination of Cushing's syndrome with virilism, so that the patient does not have the typical habitus of Cushing's syndrome. The fourth is Cushing's syndrome resulting from ectopic ACTH production in which the electrolyte changes of hypokalemia and alkalosis are maximal and weakness may be the presenting symptom, with the physical appearances of Cushing's syndrome far less apparent than is ordinarily the case.

MEASUREMENTS OF BLOOD AND URINARY CORTICOSTEROIDS. Cushing's disease is characteristically accompanied by elevated plasma and urine 17-hydroxycorticosteroids. The normal plasma value is 3 to 24 μg. per cent, and the normal 24-hour urinary excretion is 3 to 10 mg. The urinary 17-ketosteroid excretion is often elevated as well. In men the normal value is 10 to 25 mg. for 24 hours, whereas in women it is 6 to 18 mg. There is a loss of cyclic daily variation in plasma 17-hydroxycorticosteroid levels, so that the 12 midnight and 8 A.M. values are

Table 29-1. SIGNS AND SYMPTOMS OF CUSHING'S SYNDROME

Moon facies	Buffalo hump
Truncal obesity	Acne
Hypertension	Back pain
Plethora	Headache
Amenorrhea or impotence	Emotional lability
Weakness and fatigue	Pathologic fractures
Hirsutism	Polyuria
Striae	Renal calculi
Bruisability and ecchymoses	IVP may show tumor
Osteoporosis	With malignant tumors, metastases may be detected by
Edema	x-ray

equal, whereas normally the former would be considerably lower. This is a particularly useful method for detecting early Cushing's disease.

STIMULATION AND SUPPRESSION TESTS.   These tests may be useful both in making the diagnosis of Cushing's syndrome and in differentiating between adrenal cortical tumor and hyperplasia.

The ACTH stimulation test is performed by infusing 25 units of ACTH intravenously over a six hour period and taking samples of plasma for the determination of 17-hydroxycorticosteroids at the beginning and at the end of infusion. The normal patient will show a rise in 17-hydroxycorticosteroids to values greater than 35 μg. per cent but usually less than 65 μg. per cent. The patient with Cushing's syndrome caused by hyperplasia will usually show a rise to a value greater than 65 μg. per cent. If the patient has a high initial 17-hydroxycorticosteroid value and fails to respond further to ACTH, this is highly suggestive of Cushing's disease caused by an autonomous tumor or an ectopic ACTH source.

The dexamethasone suppression test is done by administering 0.5 mg. of dexamethasone orally every six hours for 48 hours, followed by 2.0 mg. every six hours for 48 hours. Twenty-four hour urinary collections for the determination of 17-hydroxycorticosteroid excretion are carried out throughout the test. The normal patient shows a suppression of urinary 17-hydroxycorticosteroid secretion to low levels (3.0 μg./24 hours) on the smaller dose. The patient with Cushing's syndrome shows no suppression on the low dose, whereas suppression is noted with the larger dose if the syndrome is due to hyperplasia and not if it is due to tumor, extrapituitary ACTH source or nodular dysplasia. This is because the hyperplasia is under pituitary control and is therefore suppressible with exogenous corticosteroid, whereas the tumor is autonomous and not suppressible.

A rapid dexamethasone suppression test has recently been described which is better than the test outlined above. This can be carried out either with plasma cortisol measurements or with urinary corticosteroid and creatinine measurements. In the simplest form of the test, the patient receives 1 mg. of dexamethasone by mouth at 11 P.M. and after adequate sedation with barbiturate a plasma sample is drawn the next morning at 8 A.M. If the level of plasma 17-hydroxycorticosteroids is above 10 μg. per 100 ml., this suggests nonsuppressibility of ACTH secretion and is diagnostic of Cushing's syndrome. In the normal patient the level falls nearly to zero. In order to perform the test, the patient must not be taking birth control pills containing estrogen, because this raises the transcortin level and produces high levels of plasma hydroxycorticosteroids. It would be satisfactory to take two morning samples, one the day before and one the day after dexamethasone administration, because the normal patient, even on birth control pills, would be expected to show a very marked suppression of the cortisol level on the second day. The ratio of urinary corticosteroid/creatinine can be used in lieu of a plasmal cortisol level to indicate suppression by dexamethasone.

Nodular dysplasia is a rather peculiar disease in which the adrenal is hypertrophic but contains tiny nodules which respond to dexamethasone suppression as though they were autonomous. Why there is not an associated adrenal atrophy, as there is with other autonomous adenomas, instead of hypertrophy, is unknown.

PLASMA ACTH LEVELS. Now that plasma ACTH can be very conveniently measured by immunoassay, a wider application of this diagnostic test will come about. It is very helpful in differentiating between ectopic ACTH sources and adrenal adenoma, for example. The elevated plasma level of ACTH in the former circumstances can be easily detected.

The electrolyte changes in Cushing's disease are not consistent. About two thirds of the cases show alkalosis, whereas hypokalemia, hypochloremia and hypernatremia are occasionally present (15 to 30 per cent). In those cases caused by ectopic ACTH production, however, hypokalemia and alkalosis are frequently the most striking findings. The serum calcium is usally normal, and urinary calcium excretion is only occasionally increased. The alkaline phosphatase is elevated in one third of the cases. The laboratory findings in different types of Cushing's syndrome are shown in Table 29-2.

Impaired carbohydrate metabolism occurs in 80 to 90 per cent of the cases. This is manifested, in decreasing order of frequency, by a decreased glucose tolerance test, hyperglycemia, glycosuria, and insulin-resistant diabetes with polyuria and polydipsia.

X-rays of the sella turcica should be made in all patients with Cushing's syndrome, particularly those with pigmentation, because a pituitary tumor is more likely under these circumstances. X-ray of the bones will sometimes demonstrate pathologic fractures and osteoporosis which are characteristic of this syndrome. Recently arteriograms or venograms have been utilized to localize adrenal tumors. There is danger in the performance of venography, because bilateral adrenal hemorrhage and thrombosis have been observed when this technique was used. An increased secretion of adrenal steroids from one side suggests the localization of an adrenal tumor to that side.

Primary Aldosteronism. *The signs and symptoms* of classic aldosteronism are listed in Table 29-3. The entire spectrum may be seen from the full-blown case with muscle paralysis secondary to hypokalemia to the patient with no other symptom or sign than hypertension. The symptoms are typically made worse by the administration of the benzothiadiazine diuretics, such as Diuril and Hydrodiuril, because these drugs promote potassium loss in the urine and further accentuate the tendency to hypokalemia. The symptoms are made better by salt restriction and the administration of potassium. Although it was once suggested that primary aldosteronism might account for as much as 20

Table 29-2. LABORATORY DIAGNOSIS OF DIFFERENT TYPES OF CUSHING'S SYNDROME

	ADRENAL HYPERPLASIA	ADRENAL ADENOMA	ECTOPIC ACTH SOURCE	ADRENAL CARCINOMA	PITUITARY ACTH TUMOR	NODULAR DYSPLASIA	NORMAL
Plasma 17-OHCS 8 A.M. Midnight	Both up	Both up	Both up	Both up	Both up	Both up	6-26 µg./100 ml. 2-12 µg./100 ml.
Urine 17-OHCS	Moderately elevated	Moderately elevated	Very elevated	Elevated	Moderately elevated	Moderately elevated	3-11 mg./day
Urine 17-KS	Elevated	Elevated	Very elevated	Very elevated	Elevated	Elevated	M:10-20 mg./day F:5-15 mg./day
Plasma ACTH	Slightly elevated	Low	Very high	Low	Moderately elevated	Low	0-35 µg./100 ml.
Plasma 17-OHCS rise with ACTH infusion	Rise over 65 µg./100 ml.	No rise	No rise	No rise	May rise	May rise	Rise to 35-65 µg./100 ml.
Dexamethasone suppression 2 mg. 8 mg.	No Yes	No No	No No	No No	No No	No No	Yes Yes
Low serum K	±	±	4+	2+	±	±	3.5-5.0 mg./100 ml.

Table 29–3. SIGNS AND SYMPTOMS OF PRIMARY ALDOSTERONISM

Hypertension Headache Cardiac enlargement	Due to hypertension and Na retention
Muscle weakness and paralysis Tetany Paresthesias and muscle cramps	Due to hypokalemia and K deficit
Polyuria Polydipsia Nocturia	Due to hyperkaluria
Increased blood volume (edema rare)	Due to hypernatremia

per cent of all hypertensives, the figure now seems to be more in the range of 1 per cent.

LABORATORY FINDINGS. Laboratory tests for aldosteronism fall into two major categories, the first designed to distinguish increased secretion of aldosterone and the second to differentiate between primary and secondary aldosteronism. The most useful tests are summarized in Table 29-4. The patient is placed on a high sodium diet of 200 mEq./day for three days, during which time the urinary sodium and potassium are measured. The potassium intake is kept constant. The patient with primary or secondary aldosteronism will show a urinary potassium excretion ·that equals or exceeds the intake, whereas the normal patient will excrete less than the intake. For the next three days the patient is put on a low sodium diet of 10 mEq./day. With primary or secondary aldosteronism the urinary potassium excretion will fall sharply, whereas in the normal patient it will increase. The urinary aldosterone excretion will be increased in hyperaldosteronism, as will the aldosterone secretion rate. The secretion rate is determined by giving an intravenous infusion of radioactive aldosterone and measuring the urinary output of aldosterone or a metabolite.

The differentiation between primary and secondary aldosteronism is made on the basis of clinical grounds, on the demonstration that there is a cause for secondary aldosteronism, and by the plasma renin levels. The plasma renin levels are low or unmeasurable in primary aldosteronism, whereas they are generally high in secondary aldosteronism, particularly when the patient is on a low sodium diet. The administration of desoxycorticosterone acetate (DCA) produces no change in aldosterone excretion in primary aldosteronism, whereas it decreases the excretion in the secondary form. An infusion of angiotensin II produces a blood pressure rise in primary aldosteronism and no change in secondary aldosteronism. Adrenal vein blood aldosterone levels are high on the side of the tumor in primary aldosteronism, and high on both sides in secondary aldosteronism.

Table 29–4. LABORATORY DIAGNOSIS OF ALDOSTERONISM

TEST	PRIMARY ALDOSTERONISM	SECONDARY ALDOSTERONISM	NORMAL
To detect hyperaldosteronism:			
Serum K	Low	Low	3.5–5.0 mEq./L.
Serum Na	High normal or high	Normal or low	135–142 mEq./L.
Serum K high Na diet	Falls	May fall	No change
Urine K high Na diet	Equals or exceeds intake	Equals or exceeds intake	Less than intake
Urine K low Na diet	Falls	Falls	Increases
Urine aldosterone	Over 16 μg./day	Over 16 μg./day	16 μg./day or less
Aldosterone secretion	Over 180 μg./day	Over 180 μg./day	60–180 μg./day
To differentiate primary from secondary aldosteronism:			
Plasma renin high Na diet	Low or absent	High	Normal
Plasma renin low Na diet	Low or absent	Very high	High
Aldosterone response to DCA administration	No change	Falls	Falls
Angiotensin infusion	BP rises	No change in BP	BP rises
Adrenal vein blood aldosterone	High on side with tumor	High both sides	Normal

In the typical case of primary aldosteronism the serum electrolyte values are characteristic. There is a low serum potassium, a high normal or elevated sodium and an elevated CO_2. A low serum sodium argues against primary aldosteronism. The urine is usually of low specific gravity, a rather large volume, and alkaline pH. There is a reduced salivary Na:K ratio. The normal ratios very between 0.6 and 3.4, whereas in aldosteronism the ratios are between 0.2 and 0.6.

The EKG may show signs of hypokalemia in primary aldosteronism, and the diagnosis is sometimes suspected in this manner.

The Adrenogenital Syndrome. The signs and symptoms of the adrenogenital syndrome vary with the age of onset of the condition.

CONGENITAL. If the adrenogenital syndrome is present at birth, it is almost always due to congenital hyperplasia of the adrenal cortex.

In the female, congenital adrenal hyperplasia produces a pseudo-hermaphrodite. The internal genitalia are generally normal and the external genitalia abnormal. There is usually a partial fusion of the labial folds and hypertrophy of the clitoris. Pubic hair, acne and hirsutism appear early, somatic growth is accelerated at first, and bone age is advanced. The epiphyses close early, and ultimate stunting of growth results. Menses and breast development do not usually appear at puberty, if the patient is untreated.

In the male, congenital hyperplasia produces sexual precocity called macrogenitosomia praecox. There are well-developed musculature and short stature. The condition may not be recognized until the child is two or three years of age, when excessive penile growth, pubic hair, acne, and deepening of the voice are noted. The short stature results from early epiphyseal closure. The testes remain small.

In the salt-wasting variant of the disease the patients develop marked adrenal insufficiency. This is characterized by vomiting, apathy, weight loss, refusal to feed, dehydration, diarrhea, shock and death if untreated. This is more common in the female and more difficult to recognize in the male because penile changes may still be minimal at birth.

There are six recognized variants of congenital adrenal hyperplasia, although by far the most common type is that seen in patients with a block of C-21 hydroxylation. In the incomplete syndrome the female infants are pseudohermaphrodites and the males have macrogenitosomia praecox. In about one third of the cases the defect is more complete and subnormal amounts of aldosterone are formed, leading to a salt-losing syndrome with vascular collapse and death unless treatment with mineralocorticoids is promptly started. A C-11 hydroxylation block produces virulism with hypertension because of the production of 11-desoxycorticosterone and 11-desoxycortisol. The remaining four types of congenital adrenal hyperplasia do not produce virilism and are usually fatal.

The treatment is nonoperative, except for the occasional ultimate need to carry out plastic procedures on the genitalia of female pseudo-hermaphrodites.

POSTNATAL AND PREPUBERTAL.   The postnatal adrenogenital syndrome is usually the result of an adenoma or carcinoma of the adrenal cortex.

In the female, changes of masculinization occur without change in the genitalia except for enlargement of the clitoris. Hirsutism, usually with absence of menses, short stature and advanced bone age are characteristic.

In the male, pseudoprecocious puberty is seen, with pubic hair, phallic enlargement, short stature, advanced bone age and normal-sized testes.

If the adrenogenital syndrome is produced by a tumor of the adrenal cortex instead of hyperplasia, there is a much increased urinary 17-ketosteroid excretion, and this usually fails to be suppressed with corticoid administration. There is an excessive production of urinary dehydroepiandrosterone rather than α-pregnanetriol, which is typical of congenital adrenal hyperplasia.

ADULT ADRENOGENITAL SYNDROME.   The adult form of the adrenogenital syndrome is usually produced by a tumor, although on occasion it may result from acquired hyperplasia. It is much more common in women than in men.

In the female, virilism is seen with or without some of the changes of Cushing's syndrome. Hirsutism, scanty or absent menses, decreased libido, atrophy of the breasts, male habitus and hypertrophy of the clitoris are characteristic.

LABORATORY FINDINGS.   The hallmark of the adrenogenital syndrome is an increase in urinary excretion of 17-ketosteroids. The normal values for infants up to one year of age is 0.5 mg. for 24 hours, and in children from one to five years of age 1.0 mg. for 24 hours.

In congenital hyperplasia of the adrenal there is an excess secretion of pregnanetriolone and pregnanetriol in the urine. This results from a defect in C-11 or C-21 hydroxylation (or both), leading to excess production of 17-hydroxyprogesterone and decreased cortisol production. Pituitary ACTH release is thus unopposed, and this leads to overstimulation of the adrenal, which produces increased amounts of androgens. There is a decreased 17-hydroxycorticosteriod response to ACTH. The greater the defect of C-21 hydroxylation, the less cortisol is produced, and the greater is the likelihood that the salt-wasting syndrome will appear. If C-11 hydroxylation is impaired to a greater extent than C-21 hydroxylation, the hypertensive variant of the disease is likely to be present. The administration of cortisone produces a prompt decrease in urinary 17-ketosteroid excretion by its action in suppressing ACTH secretion. This is a diagnostic test for congenital adrenal hyperplasia.

If the adrenogenital syndrome is produced by a tumor of the adrenal cortex instead of hyperplasia, there is a much higher urinary 17-ketosteroid excretion, and suppression of 17-ketosteroid secretion with cortisone is minimal or absent. There is an excess production of urinary dehydroepiandrosterone, and no pregnanetriol excretion.

In the adult acquired hyperplasia, which is rare, there is an increase in urinary 17-ketosteroid excretion but pregnanetriol is not increased. ACTH produces a marked increase in 17-ketosteroid excretion in contrast to the findings when an adenoma or carcinoma is present, in which no further increase in 17-ketosteroid excretion is usually seen with ACTH.

When the diagnosis of virilism owing to an adrenal cortical tumor is suspected, the tumor should be localized by arteriography and the adrenal on that side removed.

Estrogen-Secreting Tumors. Feminizing adrenal cortical tumors are quite rare. In the male the presenting sign is usually gynecomastia, occasionally with lactation. In about half of the cases there are a palpable tumor, atrophy of the testes, diminished libido and potency, pain at the site of the tumor, and tenderness of the breast. In a smaller percentage of cases there may be obesity, feminizing hair change, atrophy of the penis, elevation of the blood pressure and increased skin pigmentation.

About 90 per cent of these tumors are malignant, and they are usually discovered late. They are most commonly seen between the ages of 25 and 45. When such tumors are seen in the female, they result in striking premature female sexual development. The signs of Cushing's syndrome are often present as well.

The laboratory findings reveal a marked increase in urinary estrogens and often in 17-hydroxycorticosteroids and 17-ketosteroids as well. The steroid excretion cannot be depressed by dexamethasone or stimulated by ACTH in most cases.

The patient is treated by surgical excision of the tumor as soon as the diagnosis is made, and this is followed by radiation therapy if the tumor is malignant. In most instances in men metastases are present by the time the patient is first seen, and the patient usually dies within a matter of two or three years. Almost all feminizing adrenal neoplasms in adult men have been malignant, whereas those in children have generally been benign. Because of the extreme malignancy of these tumors in the adult, a thoracoabdominal approach and concomitant lymphadenectomy are generally advocated.

Nonfunctioning Adrenal Cortical Tumor. If the tumor is large, there may be a palpable mass in the flank. The presence of a mass may be noted on intravenous pyelography, which characteristically shows tilting of the upper pole of the kidney laterally and down. Occasionally a sudden hemorrhage into the tumor will produce symptoms of pain and shock. There are no characteristic laboratory findings. The tumors may be either benign or malignant.

Adrenal Ablation for Carcinoma of the Breast. Adrenal ablation may be indicated for the treatment of metastatic carcinoma of the breast in patients who have had previous or simultaneous ovarian ablation. The response is most likely to be favorable when bony metastases are present and somewhat less so with lung metastases, whereas a relatively less good response can be expected if liver metastases are present, particularly when over 30 per cent of the liver is involved.

An elevated BSP retention and serum alkaline phosphatase with a positive liver scan suggest hepatic metastases and indicate the likelihood of failure of ablative therapy. An elevated plasma calcium responsive to cortisol and x-ray evidence of bony metastases indicate the likelihood of a more favorable response.

A series of steroid studies has been carried out which are said to be predictive of the likelihood of a favorable response to adrenalectomy or hypophysectomy. These "discriminant functions" are calculated by measuring the 24-hour urinary excretion of 17-hydroxycorticosteroids (17-OHCS) and etiocholanolone (ET), and substituting the values in the formula: $80 - 80$ (17-OHCS mg./24 hrs.) $+$ ET mg./24 hrs. If the answer is a positive number, the patient is said to have a positive discriminant. Patients with positive discriminants have a better remission rate with ablative therapy than those with negative discriminants, but the remission rate also improves as the "free period" between mastectomy and the first recurrence increases, and is less good the first six years after the menopause than either before or after this period. Response to androgen therapy was no guide to the outcome of ablative therapy, but a previous response to estrogen therapy was related to a favorable response to ablative therapy. If the patient has previously had mastectomy, the response to adrenalectomy and hypophysectomy was equivalent, but if mastectomy had not been carried out, adrenalectomy was far less effective than hypophysectomy. Patients with negative discriminants who fail to respond to estrogen, develop recurrences within six years after the menopause, and have a free period of under two years have almost no likelihood of responding to ablative therapy. With positive discriminants hypophysectomy is preferable to adrenalectomy if the patient has not previously had a mastectomy.

SPECIAL PREOPERATIVE PREPARATION FOR SURGERY

Cushing's Syndrome. If the patient with Cushing's syndrome has laboratory studies suggestive of an adrenal tumor, no preoperative preparation is necessary, except to localize the site of the tumor if possible, to reduce the blood pressure, and to correct the potassium deficiency if it exists. If the tests suggest hyperplasia rather than tumor, the operation is carried out without special preoperative preparation if the disease is very severe, rapid in onset or life threatening because of hypertension or some other complication.

If, however, hyperplasia is suspected and the disease is not immediately life threatening, it is best to give 4000 to 4500 r of irradiation to the pituitary and wait six months for an improvement of the disease. The irradiation may be repeated if necessary for further response. If the response has not been adequate after six months, or if the disease continues to get worse, operation should then be promptly carried out.

It is not necessary to carry out preoperative preparation with corticosteroids, because these patients already have excessive quantities of corticosteroids as a consequence of their disease. The corticosteroids are begun on the day of operation according to the schedule shown in Table 29-5.

If the patient has a functioning carcinoma with metastases demonstrated by previous biopsy, he may be treated with O-p'DDD. A dose of up to 10 gm. per day for two to four months may be given, depending upon the patient's tolerance. Side effects of nausea, vomiting, rash, somnolence and tremors may be a severe problem.

If the patient has Cushing's syndrome as a consequence of an extraadrenal ACTH-producing tumor, excision should be attempted if the tumor is accessible and particularly if the tumor is not malignant. If it is a malignant tumor which is inaccessible or unresectable, adrenalectomy may be carried out for palliative control of the Cushing's syndrome.

Primary Aldosteronism. Preoperative preparation for primary aldosteronism consists of the administration of potassium in doses of 100 to 150 mEq./day and utilization of a low sodium diet (10 to 20 mEq./day) to help correct hypokalemia and restore depleted body potassium stores. Chlorothiazide and related hypotensive-diuretic agents which compound potassium loss problems should be stopped.

Table 29–5. Schedule for Intraoperative and Postoperative Corticosteroid Administration after Adrenalectomy

	Intravenous Cortisol*	Intramuscular Cortisone†	Oral Cortisone‡
Day of operation	300 mg.	100 mg.	
First day	200 mg.	100 mg.	
Second day	100 mg.	100 mg.	
Third day	—	100 mg.	50 mg.
Fourth day	—	50 mg.	50 mg.
Fifth day	—	50 mg.	50 mg.
Sixth day	—	—	75 mg.
Thereafter	—	—	50–37.5 mg.

*Intravenous cortisol given by continuous infusion through plastic cannula. On the operative day, 100 mg. is given in the first four hours, 100 in the next eight hours and 100 in the next 12 hours.

†Intramuscular cortisone acetate given in two divided doses every 12 hours.

‡Oral cortisone given in divided doses every 12 hours. Reduction from 50 to 37.5 mg. should be done slowly and cautiously. Some patients have to be maintained on 50 or even 75 mg./day.

The Adrenogenital Syndrome. For congenital adrenal cortical hyperplasia, surgery is not indicated, except, occasionally, for plastic procedures on the genitalia. It is preferable not to amputate the clitoris, although this has been advocated by some. A better procedure is to relocate it while preserving its sensory nerve supply and at the same time burying most of its length in the tunnel so as to decrease its apparent size. Labioscrotal fusion is also corrected when present. No surgical procedure should be carried out until the patient has been adequately treated with cortisone (25 mg./day), or prednisone (5mg./day) if he is hypertensive, until the diagnosis is established and the 17-ketosteroids return to normal. At this time the dosage should be reduced to the lowest level that will keep urinary 17-ketosteroids in the normal range for the patient's age.

Salt losers should be given sodium chloride in addition, and may require salt-retaining hormones such as 9-α-fluorocortisol or desoxycorticosterone. Cortisone should be employed rather than prednisone in these cases because of its greater salt-retaining effect. Increased amounts of corticosteroids are needed just prior to and during operation or during intercurrent infections. Salt wasters are particularly likely to become dehydrated.

No special preoperative preparation is necessary for patients with adrenal tumors, because atrophy of the uninvolved adrenal does not occur in the adrenogenital syndrome as it does in Cushing's disease caused by tumor. If elements of Cushing's syndrome are present, however, excessive steroid secretion may lead to atrophy of the uninvolved adrenal, and intraoperative and postoperative corticosteroids will be necessary.

Estrogen-Secreting Tumors. No preoperative treatment is necessary except to attempt to establish whether metastases are present or not and to localize the site of the tumor with an intravenous pyelogram or arteriograms. Metastases generally occur in the liver, lungs, bone, brain and local lymph nodes.

Nonfunctioning Adrenal Cortical Tumor. No preoperative preparation is necessary for such a tumor, except to establish that some adrenal function is present by an ACTH test. An intravenous pyelogram, chest x-ray and liver scan are helpful to determine the presence or absence of metastases. If the tumor is extremely large, an inferior vena cavogram may be helpful in determining the extent of local spread of the growth.

Adrenal Ablation for Carcinoma of the Breast. Hypercalcemia, if present, should be corrected by cortisone administration preoperatively, and an oophorectomy should be done concomitantly with or prior to adrenal ablation.

Tests should be undertaken to determine the extent of pulmonary, bony, and hepatic metastases.

INTRAOPERATIVE AND POSTOPERATIVE CARE

Cushing's Syndrome.   In Cushing's syndrome the patients are generally explored from the flank or back because of the great amount of fat present in the abdominal wall. In most instances the tumor will probably have been localized to one side or the other, and the differentiation between adrenal hyperplasia and adrenal tumor will probably have been made. In those patients in whom it has not been possible to establish the differential diagnosis between tumor and hyperplasia, and who are explored from either the flank or the back, the left side is explored first. If an adrenal cortical tumor is found, the entire adrenal should be removed. If the gland appears normal or hypertrophic with rounded edges, both adrenals should be removed. If the gland appears atrophic with a very sharp, thin edge and no tumor is present on that side, the wound should be closed without disturbing the adrenal and the other side should be explored for the presence of a tumor. If the patient is explored abdominally, the tumor can usually be palpated if present, and the correct adrenal can be removed.

Corticosteroids are administered according to the schedule shown in Table 29-5.

If a tumor is found or a subtotal adrenalectomy is carried out, the dosage is gradually reduced over several days or weeks and finally stopped. An ACTH test will determine whether the remaining adrenal is functional. If the patient has had a bilateral total adrenalectomy for hyperplasia, he must be maintained on cortisone treatment indefinitely, in doses of 37.5 to 75 mg. daily. If salt loss becomes a problem, small amounts of 9-α-fluorocortisone may be needed in addition (0.05 to 0.10 mg./day).

The blood pressure should be carefully monitored postoperatively and additional intravenous cortisol administered if the patient becomes hypotensive without evidence of blood loss.

Irradiation should be given to the pituitary postoperatively if it has not been given preoperatively and the patient has been found to have adrenal hyperplasia. This is done to help prevent hypertrophy of the remaining fragment if subtotal adrenalectomy is done, or the development of a pituitary tumor if a total adrenalectomy has been done.

Primary Aldosteronism.   If a tumor is present, no special intra- or postoperative care is required except to maintain plasma potassium levels in the normal range. The preoperative hypokalemia is usually corrected fairly promptly postoperatively, and hyperkalemia may occur. Daily electrolyte determinations and electrocardiograms are obtained until stable.

If bilateral hyperplasia seems to be present, no tumor can be found, and the preoperative studies were unable to localize the excessive aldosterone secretion to one side or the other, samples of adrenal venous blood should again be obtained at the operating table and both glands should be carefully examined. Sometimes the adenomas producing excessive aldosterone secretion and hypertension are microscopic in size, being only 1 mm. or less in diameter. These patients respond well to adrenalectomy on the side of the microadenoma formation, whereas those patients who truly have bilateral hyperplasia with primary aldosteronism are apt to have poor responses to adrenalectomy. Therefore it is far preferable to localize the site of involvement preoperatively if possible.

Because both glands may have to be examined, the preferred operative approach is transabdominal, although some surgeons prefer the posterior route. The adenomas are usually relatively small, discrete and easily felt. The entire gland containing the adenoma is removed. In about 5 per cent of the cases the adenomas are bilateral. On rare occasions a heterotopic adrenocortical adenoma causing primary aldosteronism may be present.

If no adrenal tumor is found and preoperative studies including arteriograms and adrenal venous blood aldosterone measurements have failed to localize the tumor, one has the choice of taking out one adrenal and treating the patient with spironolactone, taking out both adrenals and treating the patient with corticosteroid replacement therapy, or leaving both adrenals in place and treating the patient with aldosterone inhibitors. It is probably preferable to obtain adrenal venous blood samples from each gland if this had not been possible prior to the operation, biopsy the adrenals and kidneys, and then close the incision. If subsequent analysis of the sample showed marked secretion of aldosterone from one side and not from the other, excision of the hyperfunctioning gland could be carried out later. If both glands were involved, the patient could be given a trial of treatment with aldosterone inhibitors, and if this were not well tolerated, bilateral adrenalectomy could then be carried out with the certainty that this was the only possible form of treatment.

If bilateral adrenalectomy is carried out, the patient is put on the maintenance schedule shown in Table 29-5, and potassium is administered as necessary postoperatively.

Adrenogenital Syndrome Due to Tumor.   No special intra- or postoperative treatment is necessary, unless elements of Cushing's syndrome are present in addition to the adrenogenital syndrome. Under these circumstances the normal adrenal may be atrophic, and 17-hydroxycorticosteroid response to ACTH may be reduced or absent. If this is the case, temporary supportive treatment with cortisone as outlined above (under Cushing's syndrome) should be utilized.

Estrogen-Secreting Tumor.   No special intra- or postoperative treatment is necessary except for the use of postoperative radiation if the tumor has been malignant.

Nonfunctioning Adrenal Cortical Tumor.   No special intra- or postoperative treatment is necessary.

Adrenal Ablation for Carcinoma of the Breast.   The patient should be given cortisone along the lines of the schedule outlined for

Cushing's disease. The maintenance dose of cortisone necessary for patients who have had bilateral adrenalectomy for carcinoma of the breast is usually less than that necessary for patients who have had bilateral adrenalectomy for Cushing's syndrome.

COMPLICATIONS OF SURGERY FOR ADRENAL CORTICAL DISEASE OR ABLATION

Pneumothorax is the most frequent complication of adrenal surgery, but is seen only with flank or back approaches. Although vena caval injury is relatively uncommon these days, it is seen more frequently with back or flank approaches than with abdominal approaches.

With the abdominal approach pancreatic or splenic injuries are much more common than with the flank and back approaches. Pancreatic injuries are sometimes associated with cyst formation, cutaneous fistulae, wound infection, and subdiaphragmatic abscesses.

Splenic injury occurs more commonly with the abdominal approach.

Postoperatively the patient with Cushing's disease is more apt to develop hematomas as a consequence of the tendency to easy bruisability, and hypertension. Wound infections are more common in patients with Cushing's disease than in other patients. The incidences of pulmonary embolism and wound infection are both significantly higher in abdominal approaches in Cushing's disease than in flank incisions. Occasionally pancreatitis may lead to death. The pancreatitis is related not only to the trauma to the pancreas on handling it, but also to the tendency of high levels of adrenal secretion to produce pancreatic lesions and lead to pancreatitis. There is an increased incidence of pancreatitis in patients without adrenal disease who are treated with exogenous corticosteroids.

Postoperative endocrine changes can sometimes produce serious complications. This is particularly true during the period of reduction of dosage of cortisone in Cushing's syndrome, in which depression, joint and muscle pains, fever, and sometimes adrenal insufficiency and even suicide may occur. The dose may be temporarily increased to overcome the complications, and subsequently be tapered slowly. There may be a transient postoperative hyperkalemia when the patient has been operated upon for primary aldosteronism.

PHEOCHROMOCYTOMA AND OTHER ADRENAL MEDULLARY TUMORS

TYPES OF DISEASE

Pheochromocytoma. A pheochromocytoma is a chromaffin tumor of the adrenal medulla which is usually functioning. It may exist as a benign tumor of the adrenal medulla, a benign tumor of extra-adrenal chromaffin cells (sometimes called a paraganglioma), a malignant tumor or a nonfunctioning tumor.

Nonchromaffin Tumor. Nonchromaffin tumors are usually non-functioning.

SYMPATHOGONIOMAS. These are highly malignant tumors occurring in the intrauterine period or in early infancy.

NEUROBLASTOMAS. These tumors usually occur in early childhood, are undifferentiated, sometimes functional, metastasize early and sometimes are cured even when metastases are present. In the adult these tumors are rare, but tend to be more differentiated than those occurring in early childhood.

GANGLIONEUROMA. These are rare tumors which are usually benign and occur in adults.

SIGNS, SYMPTOMS AND LABORATORY FINDINGS

Functioning Pheochromocytoma. The most common signs and symptoms of pheochromocytoma are listed in Table 29-6.

The hypertension in patients with pheochromocytomas is more often sustained than paroxysmal, particularly in children. Even when the hypertension is sustained, however, the patient may be subject to paroxysmal attacks in which the blood pressure rises even higher than usual. Less commonly the patient's blood pressure will be normal between attacks and rise to high levels only during paroxysms. Severe unpleasant headaches are also very common, and typically come on during an attack of hypertension. Attacks of some kind are very characteristic, although not all patients with pheochromocytoma have them. These attacks may vary from a typical one, consisting of hypertension, headaches, sweating, palpitation, weakness, pallor, anxiety and tachycardia, to transient pallor of the face. Usually, however, the patient regards the attacks as highly unpleasant.

Table 29–6. SIGNS AND SYMPTOMS OF PHEOCHROMOCYTOMA

Hypertension	Polydipsia
Headache	Convulsions
Sweating	Attacks of hypertension, sweating, tachycardia, etc.
Nausea or vomiting	Occasionally palpable tumor
Palpitation	IVP or abdominal x-ray may show tumor
Visual changes	Chest x-ray will show thoracic pheochromocytoma if
Dyspnea	present
Weakness, fatigue	More common on right
Vertigo	Multiple or extra-adrenal in 20% of adults, 55% of
Epigastric or substernal pain	children
Pallor	
Apprehension or anxiety	
Weight loss	

Table 29–7. SYMPTOM COMPLEXES OF PHEOCHROMOCYTOMA

Symptom-free patients, with pheochromocytoma an incidental or accidental finding
Symptom-free patients who die suddenly after minor trauma
Patients with typical attacks
Patients with sustained hypertension indistinguishable clinically from essential or renal
  vascular hypertension
"Diabetics," with or without hypertension
Patients who present with "hyperthyroidism," especially if BMR does not fall with treat-
  ment, RAI and PBI are normal, and patient has hypertension
Patients with unexplained shock during anesthesia or minor trauma
Patients with cardiac irregularities, tachycardia or arrest with induction of anesthesia or
  beginning of operation
Patients whose symptoms simulate an acute anxiety attack
Patients who have attacks when voiding—occasionally occurs with pheochromocytoma
  located in bladder

Pheochromocytomas are noted for the variety of clinical symptom complexes they may produce. The most common of these are listed in Table 29–7.

Patients who have hypertension should be suspected of having a possible pheochromocytoma if the hypertension is associated with any of the findings shown in Table 29–8.

Patients with pheochromocytomas are not always thin, but they usually are, particularly if they have sustained rather than paroxysmal hypertension.

The most characteristic laboratory finding in patients with pheochromocytomas is an elevation of the urinary catecholamine excretion. The normal values are 5 to 120 μg. per 24 hours. Patients with pheochromocytomas may have values of over 2500 μg. per 24 hours, although the values may be as low as 200 to 300 μg. per 24 hours. There is also an elevation of the urinary VMA excretion, the normal values of which are 1 to 10 mg. per 24 hours. VMA is a metabolic product of epinephrine and norepinephrine, and is present in the urine in greater amounts than are the free compounds themselves.

Table 29–8. FINDINGS SUGGESTIVE OF PHEOCHROMOCYTOMA
(IN THE PRESENCE OF HYPERTENSION)

Any sort of "attack"
Diabetes or elevated FBS, especially between the ages of 20 and 50
An elevated BMR (and normal RAI)
Childhood—in the absence of renal disease or coarctation
Postural hypotension, excessive sweating, an elevated temperature, frequent headaches
  or vasomotor phenomena
Pregnancy with sweating, vomiting and headaches; or shock or hypertension during
  delivery
Neurofibromatosis
Familial history of pheochromocytoma
A previously removed pheochromocytoma
Weight loss or failure to gain weight if already thin

The urinary catecholamine excretion is nearly always elevated in patients with pheochromocytoma. This is true even in patients who have paroxysmal hypertension, although a rare patient of this type may fail to show an elevated urinary catecholamine excretion during the periods of normal blood pressure between attacks. In these patients the diagnosis can be established by carrying out a standard histamine test and obtaining blood samples for catecholamine determinations just prior to the administration of the histamine and four and six minutes after its administration. The patient who has a pheochromocytoma will show an abrupt rise in blood catecholamine levels, whereas normal or hypertensive patients fail to show any change. This test should not be carried out in patients who have sustained hypertension, because it may be dangerous under these circumstances and because the diagnosis can always be made in these patients by a urinary catecholamine excretion measurement.

The blood sugar is elevated in 41 per cent of patients with pheochromocytomas, and this rises to 75 per cent if the value is obtained during an attack.

There is an elevated BMR in 50 per cent of patients with pheochromocytomas, and this is almost invariably accompanied by a normal RAI.

Nonfunctioning Pheochromocytoma. If the tumor is large, a mass can be felt in the flank. There is a lateral and downward displacement of the upper pole of the kidney on intravenous pyelography. Occasionally hemorrhage into the tumor may produce pain in the flank or shock. There are no characteristic laboratory findings.

Neuroblastoma and Sympathogonioma. These malignant tumors occur primarily in childhood, usually before the age of five. They commonly present with abdominal masses, often first noted by the mother or by the pediatrician on routine physical examination. There are five recognized symptom complexes, listed in Table 29–9.

Neuroblastomas metastasize to bone (30 per cent), regional lymph nodes (26 per cent), liver (20 per cent), skull or brain (11 per cent), lungs (9 per cent) or cervical lymph nodes (5 per cent). They are more common on the left, and, although usually arising from the adrenal, they can arise from the paraganglia or sympathetic chains, or rarely in the pelvis or neck.

Table 29–9. SYMPTOM COMPLEXES OF NEUROBLASTOMA

Abdominal mass and liver enlargement are the most common symptoms, with or without pallor, weight loss, diffuse adenopathy, leukocytosis, vomiting and abdominal pain

Swelling of head, exophthalmos with ecchymosis of eyelids, blindness, increased intracranial pressure and palpable abdominal tumor

Extensive bony metastases, pallor and severe anemia, without other findings

Abdominal distention and diarrhea with or without a mass

Hypertension may be an additional finding with any of the above

Liver function tests are usually not revealing, even with hepatic metastases. There is often anemia. The urinary excretion of catecholamines or the metabolites of the catecholamines (VMA, HVA) may be elevated. This is more apt to be the case when hypertension is present.

Ganglioneuroma. This is a rare tumor, almost always occurring in adults. It is benign and is usually discovered as an asymptomatic incidental finding. There are no laboratory findings.

SPECIAL PREOPERATIVE PREPARATION FOR SURGERY

Pheochromocytoma. Although many patients with pheochromocytoma have been operated upon successfully without preoperative preparation, it is advisable to use blocking agents if the patient has sustained hypertension, marked hypermetabolism or severe tachycardia. This is especially true for children and pregnant women, in whom the likelihood of mortality is greater. For α blockade either phentolamine (Regitine) or phenoxybenzamine (Dibenzyline) can be used, whereas in β blockade propranolol (Inderal) is used. Propranolol should never be used unless an α blocker is also given, because it causes hypertension. The prime indicator for β blockade is a tachycardia of 100 or more or arrhythmias. The usual dose of phentolamine is 50 mg. orally four to six times daily for four days preoperatively, and that of phenoxybenzamine is 10 to 30 mg. twice daily, gradually increasing the dose, for one week preoperatively. Propranolol is given in doses of 20 mg. three times daily for four days preoperatively. The dose must be adjusted to the individual patient. Regitine, given intravenously in 5 mg. increments, can be used to control blood pressure if necessary during a crisis, or to reduce it if it is sustained at a dangerously high level. It is usually advisable to give 5 mg. of regitine just prior to induction with anesthesia, whether or not preoperative blockade was used.

Although adrenal cortical function is essentially always normal, it is probably wise to perform an ACTH test if the patient has had a previous adrenalectomy for pheochromocytoma on the other side. Preoperative transfusion can be given if the blood pressure comes down with vasodilators.

Neuroblastoma. Anemia should be corrected by transfusion preoperatively.

INTRAOPERATIVE AND POSTOPERATIVE CARE

Pheochromocytoma. It is advisable to follow blood pressure electronically to avoid errors in sphygmomanometer reading and to note minute-to-minute values. Intravenous Regitine should be used to keep the pressure down prior to excision of the tumor.

It is important to absorb CO_2 well during the anesthesia, because this is a strong stimulus to catecholamine excretion. Cyclopropane, ether and spinal anesthesia are best avoided.

If relaxation is needed, succinylcholine should be used rather than curare. Atropine premedication should be avoided.

The operation should be carried out transabdominally so that both adrenals can be visualized, and so that the entire abdomen can be explored for extra-adrenal sites for location of the pheochromocytoma.

After excision of the tumor, it may be necessary to administer an intravenous norepinephrine drip to maintain the blood pressure. This is given in a solution containing at least 8 mg./1000 ml. of 5 per cent dextrose in water. It is continued until the pressure is maintained at normal levels without a drip. A low blood volume often occurs in patients with pheochromocytomas, owing to peripheral vasoconstriction. After excision of the tumor there is a sudden dilatation of peripheral vessels, producing hypotension. Patients often need blood transfusions at this time even if blood loss has not been great.

It is important to continue looking for a second pheochromocytoma if the blood pressure does not fall after excision of the first, especially in children. The entire abdomen should be explored in any case.

Corticosteroid administration is necessary only if bilateral adrenal pheochromocytomas require total adrenalectomy, which they usually do not.

Equipment should be available for cardiac resuscitation if cardiac arrest occurs.

Neuroblastoma.   The great problem in operations for neuroblastoma is hemorrhage. Fresh blood should be available to help counteract the bleeding.

Radiation may be useful postoperatively, and Cytoxan may be added for the treatment of metastases.

COMPLICATIONS OF SURGERY FOR PHEOCHROMOCYTOMA AND OTHER MEDULLARY TUMORS

Hypertension prior to the excision of a pheochromocytoma and hypotension afterward may both be severe problems.

Massive hemorrhage may occur, particularly with neuroblastomas.

Adrenal insufficiency is rare, but may occur if bilateral adrenal pheochromocytomas are excised.

Recurrence of the tumor may be a problem if the tumor is malignant. This especially applies to neuroblastomas.

A patient who has had a pheochromocytoma excised may subsequently develop a second pheochromocytoma, with a recurrence of all the symptoms.

Death may occur if a pheochromocytoma is removed from a patient and a second pheochromocytoma which was present remains undetected.

ADRENAL INSUFFICIENCY

While adrenal insufficiency is a relatively rare occurrence in the surgical patient, it is extremely important that it be recognized when present, because failure to do so usually leads to the death of the patient. Consideration will be given to the etiology of adrenal insufficiency, to a recognition of the four forms that it is likely to take, and to the administration of pharmacologic doses of corticosteroids in patients who do not have adrenal insufficiency per se but who may be benefited by temporary hypercorticism.

ETIOLOGY AND CLASSIFICATION OF ADRENAL INSUFFICIENCY

There are many different causes of adrenal insufficiency, and the symptoms and signs manifested by the patient will vary somewhat, depending upon the etiologic agent.

Classic Addison's Disease. The most common cause of Addison's disease is bilateral adrenal tuberculosis, but in recent years, with the decrease in tuberculosis generally, bilateral "atrophy" is probably a somewhat more common cause. The precise etiology of the atrophy is unknown, but in some cases the destruction may be due to an autoimmune mechanism. There are also a group of miscellaneous agents which can produce bilateral adrenal destruction, including fungus infection, amyloidosis, vascular lesions and others. Classic Addison's disease develops slowly and is usually not recognized until it is in the chronic state.

Addison's Disease Associated with Other Endocrine Disease. Addison's disease is sometimes associated with thyrotoxicosis, although the etiologic relationship between the two is far from clear. On occasion autoantibodies against both the adrenal cortex and the thyroid gland have been detected, although it is hard to explain the hyperthyroidism in the presence of antithyroid antibodies. There is also an association between myxedema and Addison's disease, particularly when the thyroid hypofunction is due to lymphocytic thyroiditis. In this latter case autoantibodies against both the thyroid and adrenal are postulated to be present. Hereditary Addison's disease is sometimes associated with hypoparathyroidism or diabetes.

Hereditary, Familial and Congenital Addison's Disease. Congenital familial adrenal hypoplasia has been reported in a number of cases, as has congenital absence or marked hypoplasia of the pituitary gland with secondary hypoplasia of the adrenal and insufficiency. Familial Addison's disease is sometimes associated with spastic paraplegia with or without gliosis of the cerebral hemispheres, and familial atrophy and fibrosis of the adrenal has also been associated with hypoparathyroidism, diabetes or moniliasis. Hereditary familial adrenal atrophy and fibrosis also occurs without other defects as an autosomal recessive. The adrenogenital syndrome is another congenital defect which may be associated with adrenal insufficiency.

Adrenogenital Syndrome Variant. The adrenogenital syndrome in the newborn infant is characterized by a congenital absence of certain enzymes in the adrenal cortex, which leads to a failure of hydroxylation at the C-11 or the C-21 position. The greater the defect of C-21 hydroxylation, the less cortisol is produced, and the greater the likelihood that the patient will be unable to retain salt adequately. These patients may die of adrenal insufficiency shortly after birth if the condition is unrecognized. The syndrome is much more difficult to recognize in the male infant, because the genitalia may appear relatively normal in the male, whereas in the female the characteristic changes of the genitalia suggest the diagnosis, and therapy is more rapidly instituted.

Cryptic Adrenocortical Insufficiency. There have been patients reported who show none of the usual stigmata of Addison's disease, and who may even have relatively normal urinary 17-hydroxycorticosteroid excretion, but who nonetheless demonstrate failure to respond normally to ACTH. The blood corticosteroids, which may be in the low normal range, fail to rise significantly in response to a four or six hour intravenous infusion of ACTH. Such patients would of course be poor operative risks.

Toxic Injury. Some chemical substances, such as O-p'DDD, are capable of interfering with adrenal production of corticosteroids and of producing insufficiency.

Infection. Infection can cause adrenal insufficiency by hemorrhage into the glands or by tubular degeneration of the adrenals. Bilateral adrenal hemorrhage as a consequence of infection, the so-called Waterhouse-Friderichsen syndrome, is usually produced by meningococcal septicemia, usually in children under the age of two. However, it has also been described in young adults.

There is some question as to whether the patients actually die of adrenal insufficiency or of the effects of the meningococcal septicemia, the adrenal hemorrhage being simply a terminal manifestation of the disease. It is likely that this latter circumstance is more often the case, the adrenal hemorrhage and consequent insufficiency developing so close to the terminal phase as to have little effect on the course of the patient.

Even without the presence of actual hemorrhage, infection can cause tubular degeneration of the adrenal. This is usually seen in the adult with severe septicemia, most commonly with the meningococcus, but also occasionally with pneumococcus, streptococcus and diphtheria. Adrenal insufficiency is occasionally seen in the severely burned patient with invasive sepsis.

Hemorrhage. In addition to adrenal destruction by hemorrhage secondary to infection, there are five other circumstances in which the adrenal can occasionally be destroyed by hemorrhage. Bilateral adrenal hemorrhage has been seen in the newborn infant as a consequence of asphyxia, syphilis or eclampsia of the mother. Occasionally hemorrhage and necrosis of the maternal adrenals will occur during pregnancy, the cause of this being unknown. There have been several reported cases in which bilateral adrenal hemorrhage has occurred as a consequence of anticoagulant therapy, with, in some instances, death of the patient owing to adrenal insufficiency. This has occurred both with dicumarol and heparin. Rarely hemorrhage into an adrenal tumor will produce destruction of the remaining adrenal. This can only produce adrenal insufficiency if the opposite adrenal has been removed or if it is likewise involved in some destructive process. Retrograde adrenal venography has produced bilateral adrenal hemorrhage.

Destruction by Cancer. Although it is not unusual for the adrenal to be the site of metastases from certain types of malignancies, it is very rare for destruction of the adrenal by such means to be sufficiently great to produce adrenal insufficiency. Bronchogenic carcinoma frequently metastasizes to the adrenal, whereas carcinoma of the breast and gastric carcinoma less frequently produce adrenal metastases. Metastases are usually incidental findings post mortem, and there is generally sufficient functional adrenal tissue left to maintain the patient. A nonfunctioning endogenous adrenal carcinoma may occasionally destroy both adrenal glands, but again this is very rare.

Surgical Excision of Pituitary or Adrenal. Patients undergoing pituitary or adrenal excision are always given corticosteroid therapy. However, adrenal insufficiency can occur if the patient forgets to take his medication, if the dose is too low, or if the patient is subjected to an intercurrent infection or trauma without an increase in the maintenance dose of steroid. In general, patients who have had bilateral adrenalectomy for Cushing's disease require more corticosteroid maintenance than those patients who have had adrenalectomy for cancer of the breast.

Nonfunctioning Remnant Left After Adrenal Surgery. There are three circumstances under which an adrenal remnant, left behind after surgery, may prove to be temporarily or permanently nonfunctioning, thus producing adrenal insufficiency. If the patient has had Cushing's disease caused by an adrenal tumor, there will be atrophy of the remaining adrenal tissue. If the tumor is removed and the patient is not given adequate hormone support until the atrophic adrenal can regain its functional capacity, he will be in a state of relative adrenal insufficiency.

Occasionally a subtotal adrenalectomy is done for Cushing's disease caused by bilateral adrenal hyperplasia. The remnant of adrenal left behind may become infarcted, thus leading to adrenal insufficiency unless the patient is maintained on corticosteroids. On rare occasions a patient who has had a unilateral adrenalectomy for pheochromocytoma will develop a second pheochromocytoma in the other adrenal. During excision of the second adrenal medullary tumor an inadequate blood supply may be left for the remnant of normal adrenal which is left behind, and adrenal insufficiency may eventuate.

Pituitary Insufficiency. Panhypopituitarism produces adrenal insufficiency through a lack of ACTH to maintain normal adrenal reactivity. This type of adrenal insufficiency is usually not quite as severe as that seen in classic Addison's disease with adrenal destruction. Since aldosterone secretion depends only partially upon ACTH stimulation, there is apt to be less urinary salt wasting in patients with pituitary insufficiency than in those with primary adrenal disease. Nevertheless, patients with hypopituitarism are brittle and usually hypoglycemic, and they withstand trauma poorly.

Relative Insufficiency in Operations upon Quadriplegics or Paraplegics. Operations carried out on paraplegic or quadriplegic patients in the denervated zone fail to elicit the increase in ACTH secretion normally seen in response to operative trauma. If the operation is one involving major trauma, the patient's adrenal response may be less than adequate.

Atrophy Due to Exogenous Adrenal Steroid Administration. This is by far the most common cause of adrenal insufficiency at present. Any patient who has been given adrenal steroids for a prolonged period will have adrenal atrophy as a consequence of the diminished ACTH output caused by the steroid administration. If the patient is operated upon without the knowledge that he has been on adrenal steroids, death may follow as a result of adrenal insufficiency. Although the adrenal will ultimately come back to normal size after the cessation of adrenal steroid therapy, this may take many months. It is therefore extremely important to ask all patients before operation whether they have received adrenal steroids within the previous year. If they have, adequate function of the adrenal should be established by an ACTH test, or the patients should be placed on adrenal steroid therapy prior to and during the operation and convalescence.

The symptoms and signs of Addison's disease will vary with the point of time at which adrenal insufficiency develops relative to the onset of trauma. In general there are four symptom complexes, described below.

Adrenal Insufficiency Appearing Shortly After Birth. This is most often a consequence of the salt-wasting variant of the adrenogenital syndrome. In female infants this may be suspected when there is enlargement of the clitoris with or without other abnormalities of the genitalia. In male infants this is much more difficult to detect, because enlargement of the penis may not be sufficiently striking to be easily recognizable, and is the only genital abnormality present. Adrenal insufficiency is of the salt-losing type and is manifested by fever, weight loss, vomiting, hyponatremia, shock and marked salt loss in the urine. Symptoms often appear within the first week after birth, but sometimes do not become apparent for five or six weeks.

Chronic Insufficiency Present Before Operation or Trauma. This is classic Addison's disease, which is recognized by the characteristic pigmentation, weakness, weight loss, orthostatic hypotension, easy fatigability, sometimes nausea, vomiting or abdominal pain, hypoglycemia, hyponatremia and hyperkalemia. An x-ray of the abdomen will often show adrenal calcification, particularly if the disease is caused by tuberculosis of the adrenals, and a chest x-ray will show reduced heart size. The diagnosis is confirmed by a demonstration of reduced urinary corticosteroid excretion and the failure of blood corticosteroids to increase in response to ACTH.

The Acute Addisonian Crisis. A crisis occurs when the patient with chronic adrenal insufficiency is inadvertently operated upon or subjected to an acute stress or infection. It is accompanied by fever, shock, lethargy, somnolence or coma, nausea and vomiting, abdominal pain and, if unrecognized and untreated, death in a few hours. The diagnosis is confirmed by low levels of blood corticosteroid and an absence of eosinopenia, in spite of the stimulus of trauma or infection. Hypoglycemia and the typical electrolyte changes of hyponatremia and hyperkalemia will usually be present if the patient is an unrecognized chronic addisonian. If the patient has adrenal insufficiency as a consequence of chronic steroid administration ending in the recent past, or if he has been a recognized addisonian on maintenance doses of corticosteroid without an increase to compensate for the infection, injury or operative trauma, the electrolyte changes and shock may not manifest themselves until the preterminal or terminal period.

Semiacute Adrenal Insufficiency. This is the type of adrenal insufficiency which is not present prior to the operation but which develops in the early postoperative period. It is seen, for example, when anticoagulants are begun in the immediate postoperative period and bilateral adrenal hemorrhages then develop, destroying the adrenals. It is also occasionally seen in the severely burned patient, in whom invasive infection sometimes leads to adrenal insufficiency, but here the symptoms and signs are usually masked by the infection and by other sequelae of the burn itself.

When the adrenal insufficiency begins with or immediately after the operative insult, the symptoms are much slower to develop than they are when a patient with pre-existing adrenal insufficiency is operated upon. The development of the symptoms takes place in a matter of days rather than hours, and is usually manifested in the convalescent period by weakness, decreased peristalsis, slight abdominal distention, anorexia, nausea and general lassitude out of proportion to that expected in the convalescent period.

If the injury to the adrenals begins at the time of the operation, the first symptoms usually appear about the third or fourth postoperative day. These gradually become worse during the next three or four days. If the condition is unrecognized or untreated, death is apt to ensue in about seven to ten days. The condition is recognized by a persistent hypoglycemia and hyponatremia. The hyponatremia continues in spite of the administration of large amounts of intravenous saline, and is accompanied by a massive urinary sodium loss. The urinary salt wasting is immediately corrected by desoxycorticosterone, and this is a diagnostic finding. The further demonstration that the patient is unresponsive to ACTH clinches the diagnosis. The adrenal insufficiency usually remains permanently, and the patient has to be maintained on corticosteroids.

PHARMACOLOGIC DOSES OF CORTICOSTEROIDS IN SURGICAL CASES

Under certain circumstances in which adrenal insufficiency is not present, the patient may benefit from the temporary use of large doses of corticosteroids.

Septic Shock. Most patients who die in septic shock have high blood corticosteroids, rather than low, and as a matter of fact in the severely burned septic patient the continued elevation of blood corticosteroid levels several days after the burn is usually a poor prognostic sign, suggesting fulminating sepsis. Corticosteroids are not, therefore, usually indicated to replace deficient adrenal function in the patient with septic shock. There is, however, some suggestion that pharmacologically high doses of corticosteroids may be of benefit in certain types of septic shock, particularly the gram-negative septic shock associated with urologic infection. Apart from the usual goal of attempting to combat shock, the large doses of corticosteroids may help prevent the rare occurrence of septic adrenal hemorrhage, which is facilitated by excessive ACTH output and endotoxin and is counteracted by exogenous corticosteroids.

Renal Homotransplant Rejection. Pharmacologic doses of corticosteroids are of unquestionable value in the treatment of renal homotransplant rejection. After the rejection episode has subsided, the dosage is gradually reduced.

Transfusion Reactions. Corticosteroids are of value in the treatment of transfusion reactions.

Some Bleeding Problems. Corticosteroids are of particular value when preparing patients with thrombocytopenic purpura for surgery, and may be of value in certain types of fibrinolytic reactions and other bleeding problems.

Various Disease States. Patients not infrequently come to surgery who have been maintained on corticosteroids or ACTH for various disease states. These include rheumatoid arthritis, ulcerative colitis, regional ileitis, hypersplenism, the nephrotic syndrome, various allergic conditions and others. The doses of corticosteroids should be increased during the operative and immediate postoperative periods.

Hypercalcemia. When hypercalcemia occurs as a consequence of metastatic carcinoma of the breast, it may be necessary to treat the patient acutely with pharmacologic doses of corticosteroids to prevent or correct a hypercalcemic crisis. Other adjuncts, such as EDTA, can also be used. These crises are sometimes precipitated by the administration of estrogens, either as a test or for therapy.

Cerebral Edema. Pharmacologic doses of corticosteroids seem to be of benefit in cerebral edema secondary to head trauma, intracranial operations or intracranial tumors.

REFERENCES

Atkins, H., Bulbrook, R. D., Falconer, M. A., Hayward, J. L., MacLean, K. S., and Schurr, P. H.: Ten years' experience of steroid assays in the management of breast cancer. A Review. Lancet 2:1255, 1968.

Baer, L., Sommers, S. C., Krakoff, L. R., Newton, M. A., and Laragh, J. H.: Pseudo-primary aldosteronism. An entity distinct from true primary aldosteronism. Suppl. I to Circ. Res. 26 and 27:I-203, 1970.

Biglieri, E. G., Schambelan, M., Slaton, P. E., and Stockigt, J. R.: The intercurrent hypertension of primary aldosteronism. Suppl. I to Circ. Res. 26 and 27:I-195, 1970.

Conn, J. W.: The evolution of primary aldosteronism, 1954-1967. Harvey Lectures 62:257, 1967.

Crago, R. M., Eckholdt, J. W., and Wiswell, J. G.: Pheochromocytoma. Treatment with α- and β- adrenergic blocking drugs. J.A.M.A. 202:104, 1967.

Egdahl, R. H., Kahn, P., and Melby, J. C.: Unilateral adrenalectomy for aldosteronomas, localized preoperatively by differential adrenal vein catheterization. Surgery 64:117, 1968.

Fortner, J., Nicastri, A., and Murphy, M. L.: Neuroblastoma: Natural history and results of treating 133 cases. Ann. Surg. 167:132, 1968.

Fracchia, A. A., Randall, H. T., and Farrow, J. H.: The results of adrenalectomy in advanced breast cancer in 500 consecutive patients. Surg. Gynec. & Obst. 15:747, 1967.

Gabrilove, J. L., Sharma, D. C., Wotiz, H. H., and Dorfman, R. I.: Feminizing adrenocortical tumors in the male: Review of 52 cases including case report. Medicine 44:37, 1965.

George, J. M., Wright, L., Bell, N. H., and Bartter, F. C.: The syndrome of primary aldosteronism. Amer. J. Med. 48:343, 1970.

Glen, F., and Grafe, W. B., Jr.: Surgical complications of adrenal steroid therapy. Ann. Surg. 165:1023, 1967.

Harrison, T., Bartlett, J. D., Jr., and Seaton, J. F.: Current evaluation and management of pheochromocytoma. Ann. Surg. 168:701, 1968.

Hume, D. M.: Pheochromocytoma; in Astwood, E. B., and Cassidy, C. E. (eds.): Clinical Endocrinology, II. New York, Grune and Stratton, Inc., 1968, p. 519.

Hume, D. M.: Pituitary and adrenal; in Schwartz, S. I., et al. (eds.): Principles of Surgery. New York, McGraw-Hill, 1969, p. 1217.

Kahn, P. C., and Nickrosz, L. V.: Selective angiography of the adrenal glands. Amer. J. Roentgenol. 101:732, 1967.

Koop, C. E.: The role of surgery in resectable, nonresectable, and metastatic neuroblastoma. J.A.M.A. 205:157, 1968.

Lauler, D. P.: Preoperative diagnosis of primary aldosteronism. Amer. J. Med. *41*:855, 1966.

Liddle, G. W., Island, D. P., Ney, R. L., Nicholson, W. E., and Shimizy, N.: Non-pituitary neoplasms and Cushing's syndrome. Arch. Int. Med. *111*:129, 1963.

Pezzullch, R. A., and Mannix, H., Jr.: Immediate complications of adrenal surgery. Ann. Surg. *172*:125, 1970.

Russ, E. J.: Conn's syndrome due to adrenal hyperplasia with hypertrophy of zona glomerulosa, relieved by unilateral adrenalectomy. Amer. J. Med. *39*:994, 1965.

Salti, I. S., Ruse, J. L., Stiefel, M., and Laidlaw, J. C.: Non-tumorous "primary" aldosteronism. I. Type relieved by glucocorticoid. Canad. M.A.J. *101*:1, 1969.

Scott, W. H., Jr., Foster, J. H., Liddle, G., and Davidson, E. T.: Cushing's syndrome due to adrenocortical tumor: 11-year review of 15 patients. Ann. Surg. *162*:505, 1969.

Segaloff, A., Meyers, K. K., and DeBakey, S.: Current Concepts in Breast Cancer. Baltimore, Williams and Wilkins, 1967.

Strott, C. A., Nugent, C. A., and Tyler, F. H.: Cushing's syndrome caused by bronchial adenomas. Amer. J. Med. *44*:97, 1968.

Tucci, J. R., Jagger, P. I., Lauler, D. P., and Thorn, G. W.: Rapid dexamethasone suppression test for Cushing's syndrome. J.A.M.A. *199*:379, 1967.

Tucker, H. St. G., Estep, H. L., Hume, D. M., Vinik, M., and Kay, S.: Cushing's syndrome with nodular adrenal hyperplasia. Tr. Amer. Clin. Climatol. Assn. *80*:37, 1968.

Chapter 30

THE PATIENT WITH MULTIPLE INJURIES

James D. Hardy, M.D.

The patient with multiple injuries now constitutes one of the most frequent admissions to hospitals in this country. Although some hospitals still receive relatively few trauma cases, more and more hospitals which previously admitted few such patients are finding themselves involved with victims of motor vehicle accidents and other types of blunt trauma, or with penetrating injuries from knife and bullet wounds. Many injuries are relatively simple, even those which occur from industrial accidents or falls, but other injuries involve multiple regions of the body and numerous organs. Injuries range from those easily treated, to complex and multiple injuries which may prove fatal on the spot. In contrast to elective surgery, operations for the management of trauma may occur at any time of the day or night, often when less experienced personnel are on duty. The patient may be under the influence of alcohol, which further complicates the management of shock and the conduct of anesthesia, and frequently several patients are injured in the same accident.

Transportation. The urgency of the injury frequently has to be faced at some point remote from an adequate medical facility, and the problem of transporting the patient from the scene of the injury to a hospital is extremely important. The quality of care provided during transport to the definitive hospital frequently determines whether or not the patient can be saved even when adequate medical facilities have been reached. For example, if the patient is losing blood internally at a given rate, he may well survive rapid transportation by helicopter, but he may well not survive a 4 or 5 hour trip by ambulance unattended. However, if a nurse or an adequately trained attendant can accompany the patient in the ambulance and give blood and other fluids intravenously en route, he may survive the trip and be cared for successfully. Much attention has been directed toward the quality of such transportation of injured individuals in recent years, and the value of the helicopter in rapid transportation cannot be overemphasized. Even here, however, adequate medical understanding on the part of the helicopter crewmen can be lacking, and patients' lives have been lost that might otherwise have been saved. Nevertheless, it is safe to predict that air transportation will be used on an increasing scale, and that appropriate medical indoctrination will be given to the pilots and other attendants who move the patients from the scene of the accident to the appropriate hospital. Fortunately, the patient is frequently seen by a physician before he is moved by ambulance or helicopter, and this often permits the administration of intravenous fluids and oxygen therapy and the splinting of fractures.

Trauma Team.   There is an increasing tendency to assign the management of injured patients to a trauma team or trauma service. In general, this is a sound procedure, for especially trained and specifically oriented surgeons and physicians can substantially reduce the morbidity and mortality associated with multiple injuries. To the uninitiated, the patient with massive trauma, involving multiple organs, may appear to represent an almost overwhelming problem, whereas to the surgeon experienced with such problems, the physiological and technical requirements are clear and can be dealt with in an orderly sequence. Furthermore, the uninitiated or less experienced physician may conclude prematurely and erroneously that the patient's injuries are such that he is beyond salvage. In fact, in few other types of surgical emergencies is a less than optimal result more likely to be assigned to the injury which the patient received, rather than (more accurately) to the quality of surgical treatment provided. Since the patient with multiple injuries is frequently a young person, most often a young man, many years of productive life lie ahead if rehabilitation can be achieved.

The team approach is especially valuable when several different areas of the body are involved. For example, the neurosurgeon may be preoccupied with the head injury while the patient goes into shock from a ruptured spleen. Likewise, the general surgeon or the orthopedist may be preoccupied with other problems and not fully appreciate the significance of increasing somnolence secondary to intracranial injury. However, one designated surgeon must be responsible for the whole patient and be captain of the team, with all other physicians acting as consultants. By and large, the general surgeon is probably the most appropriate captain of the team to care for the patient with complex multiple injuries, since the thorax and the abdomen are involved in perhaps a majority of such patients. Nevertheless, as soon as it is clear that the thoracic and abdominal viscera have escaped injury or have been adequately cared for, the patient can be transferred to a more specialized service such as orthopedics, urology, or neurosurgery for definitive management as indicated.

Legal Matters. Legal implications are involved in almost any type of trauma. Even if insurance or workmen's compensation is not involved, the assault with knife or gun will usually go to court, and appropriate records must be kept for all these purposes, not to mention the importance to the total care of the patient himself. It is mandatory to record the findings at the initial examination of the patient when he reaches the hospital, to obtain adequate roentgenograms of possibly injured portions of the body, and to solicit consultation in areas outside the usual practice of the primary surgeon in the case. Incidentally, x-ray studies, as for head injury, are best interpreted by an experienced radiologist. As regards the liability of a physician who happens to see the patient at the point of an accident, most states have now passed so-called "Good Samaritan laws" which limit the obligation of the physician who merely stops at the roadside and administers first aid, prior to the patient's being moved to some distant point by ambulance or police car. The passage of such laws has rendered such service by physicians more satisfactory for all concerned.

INITIAL EMERGENCY ASSESSMENT

The physician who first sees the severely injured person will seek to assess the gravity of the situation as quickly as possible. If the patient's condition appears to be stable and other factors permit, time will be available for an orderly sequence of procedures designed to disclose any and all significant defects or injuries which the patient may have sustained. On the other hand, if at a glance it is obvious that the patient is in dire peril, extremely rapid action may be required to save his life. Thus the initial emergency assessment is to determine the urgency of the total situation. The appearance of the individual, whether or not he is alert, or almost comatose, or unconscious; the quality of the air exchange and respiration in general; the pulse rate, its fullness, the blood pressure, and any apparent blood loss—all these factors will be considered. If the patient has sustained blunt trauma from an automobile accident, it may be readily apparent that he has various fractures, and he may show evidence of multiple rib fractures with a flail chest. On the other hand, if there was but a single bullet wound to the lower thorax, it may not be obvious that in addition to lung injury the missile has traversed the diaphragm and injured the liver, pancreas, aorta, or perhaps elements of the gastrointestinal tract. All these injuries within the abdomen must be discovered by appropriate examinations. On the other hand, if the patient is in shock and does not respond promptly to intravenous fluids, it may be essential to take him quickly and directly to the operating room in order to control intra-abdominal bleeding.

The patient with multiple injuries is often subjected to specific hazards. It has been noted that an effective airway must be preserved, and an adequate blood volume maintained. A large plastic catheter should be inserted into a suitable vein for measuring central venous pressure and for the administration of blood and other fluids as required. In fact, for the patient in shock it is well to establish two large and dependable intravenous routes for the administration of blood. A nasogastric tube should be passed to empty the stomach; it will be essential to have the stomach empty prior to the administration of anesthesia, and the mentally obtunded or drunk patient may vomit at any time and aspirate gastric contents into the lungs.

As soon as the initial evaluation of the probable degree of urgency has been made, time permitting, an orderly assessment of history and physical features should be established. The nature of the accident, whether the patient was unconscious at any time, whether any visible blood loss occurred, and any evidence of fractures or other injuries should be recorded. If family members have accompanied the patient, they should be questioned regarding antibiotic or drug sensitivities that he may have, and it should be learned whether or not he is a diabetic or has any other known systemic disease or organ failure such as renal or heart disease.

The patient with multiple injuries will usually have blood volume deficits, and a useful guide to effective fluid replacement is the hourly urine output. Therefore, a Foley catheter should be inserted, which also affords a urine specimen to examine for blood. From the outset a management flow sheet should be initiated and carefully kept up to date, so that all drugs and other substances administered to the patient are recorded to prevent excessive dosage of opiates or other therapy. In the rapid turmoil of salvaging a patient in severe shock with multiple injuries, it is easy to omit the recording of all blood transfusions and the types and amounts of drugs and other such items administered. All these considerations are important in treatment of the patient, and they may become critical later in court litigation.

It is essential for the primary surgeon to monitor the condition of the patient continuously. The patient may reach the hospital emergency room in reasonably good condition, certainly with the absence of severe shock, only to go abruptly into shock and be lost on the way to the operating room. If he is hypotensive on arrival at the hospital and then the blood pressure responds temporarily to the infusion of fluids but then falls again, the possibility of significant continuing internal hemorrhage must be considered, and the patient should be moved to an area from which emergency laparotomy or thoracotomy can be performed if necessary.

As soon as the patient with multiple injuries has reached the hospital, a crossmatch should be sent to the laboratory and adequate blood typed and crossed at once for possible need at operation. If the urgency of the situation does not permit typing and cross-matching, unmatched type O-negative blood should be used to preserve life.

Appropriate tetanus prophylaxis should be given, depending upon previous immunization.

After the initial evaluation has been made and the patient's condition appears to be reasonably stable, with little likelihood that significant internal hemorrhage has occurred and is continuing, a more orderly examination can be performed. Actually, all the above measures and those to follow will be made by the experienced surgeon almost simultaneously and in continuity, but it is important to emphasize that at least an initial impression of the probable urgency of the situation must be made promptly, for otherwise patients will die in the emergency room who should have been moved at once to the operating suite to permit operation for the control of severe hemorrhage, respiratory problems, or cardiac embarrassment.

The history and physical examination should be directed in an orderly sequence to the head and neck, the thorax, the abdomen and then the extremities and the body surface elsewhere. In the examination of the head and neck a search should be made for scalp injuries which may suggest underlying skull injuries. If a significant scalp abrasion exists, or even the history of possible head injury, skull films should be taken when the patient's condition permits. Furthermore, these films should be analyzed by experts as soon as feasible, for fractures at the base of the skull may be missed on the wet film or even on the dry film by personnel not especially trained to detect linear fractures, which may be associated with serious intracranial injuries. Soft tissue wounds about the face and mouth are particularly hazardous from the point of view of airway obstruction by either tissue swelling or bleeding. The patient with serious facial and mandibular injuries should have tracheostomy performed, in many instances. Actually, the main cause of death from face and neck injuries is either hemorrhage or respiratory obstruction. The possibility of injury to the esophagus and trachea must be considered. Severe injuries to the posterior pharynx may not be visible unless careful endoscopic examination is performed. The adequacy of the examination must be appropriate to the apparent or possible nature of the injury.

Thoracic injuries involve many possibilities. Blunt trauma frequently causes rib fractures and, if several adjacent ribs are fractured in two places, serious flail chest with paradoxical motion of the defective thoracic cage may markedly diminish pulmonary ventilation. Single rib injuries may cause puncture of the lung by sharp fragments and produce simple or tension pneumothorax or pneumohemothorax. Other results of blunt trauma are rupture of the aorta, rupture of a ventricle or of the interventricular septum, or coronary thrombosis. The body is often unable to resist the enormous stress imposed by severe deceleration accidents, such as those imposed by cars traveling at high speed or by airplane crashes. Almost any possible injury may occur under such circumstances. Traumatic rupture of the aorta is likely to occur just above the heart or, more often, just distal to the ligamentum arteriosum in the upper part of the descending aorta. Such a rupture, with false aneurysm, may be reflected in a widening of the mediastinum on a plain chest x-ray, confirmed with an arch aortogram. Widening of the mediastinum alone is considered by many to be an adequate indication for exploratory thoracotomy, without the added risk of performing an aortogram in the x-ray department. Nevertheless, it has been our experience that such patients are usually in serious condition from multiple injuries, and an unnecessary thoracotomy is almost too much of a risk to take, in the event the patient proves not to have a rupture of the aorta.

Penetrating injuries of the thorax are very common, whether caused by bullet wound or stabbing. It is well to realize that, no matter where the bullet entered the thorax, it may have traveled in any direction and may actually have entered the abdomen to cause injury to several of the abdominal viscera. Even if there is a wound of entrance and a wound of exit, the bullet may have struck the spine and changed course, and it may have injured organs which one would not ordinarily suspect had been in its path. Therefore, continued vigilance should be exercised in managing the patient with a gunshot wound. In contrast, stabbings usually result in relatively simple injuries, though a stab wound in the lower chest may involve viscera beneath the diaphragm.

A penetrating injury of the thorax most often produces pneumothorax or hemopneumothorax. Most of these injuries respond readily to the insertion of a chest drainage tube placed under water—the so-called closed thoracostomy. If bleeding is from a pulmonary artery or vein, certainly if of small or intermediate size, it will usually cease spontaneously. Underwater seal drainage, plus adequate blood transfusion, will usually suffice without formal thoracotomy. It is important, however, to keep the hemithorax well drained of blood, to prevent its clotting with subsequent embarrassment of lung expansion and the possible need for later decortication. Plastic or siliconized tubes are preferable to rubber, because they are less likely to become blocked with clots. Frequent stripping of the chest tube will facilitate drainage and render more accurate the estimation of rate of blood loss. If the bleeding is from a systemic artery, such as an intercostal or internal mammary, the vessel will usually have to be exposed and ligated. Any wound which penetrates the thorax in the region of the heart can produce cardiac injury, and this may result in the loss of blood into the pericardial sac with pericardial tamponade. The injuring agent may also enter the heart and produce intracardiac defects such as interatrial or interventricular septal defects or valve injuries. If the patient develops a murmur following the injury, he should be properly studied at an appropriate time to determine the nature of the intracardiac lesion.

Esophageal lesions are not rare, and the aorta may also be perforated. Thoracic duct injuries are not common, but they do occur. Lesions of the spinal cord will usually be obvious from the neurologic deficits that are found.

Chest injuries lend themselves particularly well to diagnosis and further observation by appropriate roentgenograms. This is in marked contrast to the plain films of the abdomen, where large volumes of blood may be lost into the peritoneal cavity without remarkable changes in the appearance of the roentgenogram.

Abdominal injuries may take many forms. It was noted previously that most or at least many penetrating thoracic injuries can be managed without thoracotomy. This is not true of penetrating abdominal injuries from knife wounds, although there is an increasing tendency to observe such patients carefully, and not to perform routine laparotomy in every patient who has sustained penetrating injury of the abdomen. Other clinics take a middle ground: they perform a sinugram through the skin laceration, using a purse string suture to fix a catheter in place and then inject radiopaque medium. If this material does not enter the peritoneal cavity, the skin laceration is loosely sutured and no laparotomy is performed. On the other hand, if the radiopaque medium does enter the peritoneal cavity, a formal laparotomy is performed. Still others would continue to observe the patient, even if the sinugram discloses that the radiopaque medium enters the peritoneal cavity, unless the patient gives evidence of intra-abdominal injury which has resulted in significant blood loss or in peritoneal irritation suggesting frank peritonitis. Groups who employ the watchful waiting type of management claim that they have had no greater mortality or morbidity than they had previously when every patient was routinely operated upon. Certainly these changes in philosophy regarding the management of penetrating abdominal injuries will be watched with much interest. At present we continue to explore most patients who exhibit evidence of penetrating wounds of the abdomen. Gunshot wounds should all be explored, and should not be treated by sinugram or by selective management as described above.

Penetrating injuries may of course injure any organ within the abdomen, including the liver and biliary tract, the spleen, pancreas, kidney, ureter and bladder, and all elements of the gastrointestinal tract, as well as major blood vessels.

The patient who sustains blunt trauma to the abdomen is most likely to have injuries of the liver and spleen, followed by fixed portions of the alimentary tract, the kidney and the pancreas. Particularly likely to be overlooked is the acute or delayed rupture of the spleen, because this may occur without any penetration of the abdomen, as may of course injuries to other intra-abdominal viscera caused by blunt trauma. Serial measurements of the hemoglobin and hematocrit levels, over a period of up to 10 days, are frequently indicated.

Extremity injuries consist principally of fractures, soft tissue contusions or deficits, vascular disorders, and nerve trauma. Fat embolism may result from long bone fractures. Since the extremities are readily accessible to at least reasonably adequate physical examination, it is far less likely that a serious extremity injury will be overlooked than will injuries within the chest and especially within the abdomen. Furthermore, since changes in the extremities are readily observed by both the patient and the physician, death from extremity injuries is far less common than is death from intracranial, intrathoracic, or intra-abdominal injuries. Nevertheless, severe extremity injuries can result in great blood and fluid loss, and adequate transfusion of blood and other fluids is essential in many of these patients. Furthermore, the extremities are often involved with massive soft tissue deficits, as well as thermal burns, and the extremities represent over approximately one half of the total body surface area.

DEFINITIVE DIAGNOSIS AND MANAGEMENT

EMERGENCY RESUSCITATION

Respiration. The need for adequate respiration supersedes all other considerations in the physiological priorities of the patient with multiple injuries. Although the patient may often survive a markedly diminished cardiac output for a moderate period of time, he can survive grossly inadequate respiration for only several minutes, following which irreversible brain damage and other physiological onslaughts will have occurred, among these being cardiac arrest. Therefore, when the patient is seen by a physician, the first requirement is to make certain that there exists an adequate airway and that pulmonary ventilation and blood-gas exchange are adequate. This requirement takes on particular urgency if there are injuries around the face or mouth. If the patient is conscious, it is usually an easy matter to determine whether or not reasonably satisfactory ventilation is being achieved. However, in the comatose patient it is not always readily possible to make certain that adequate ventilation exists. If the tongue has fallen back into the pharynx it should be drawn forward, and this can be done either by manually holding the tongue or, preferably, by the insertion of an oral airway. However, if the patient is comatose and is not moving sufficient air, it may be wise to insert an endotracheal tube temporarily, following later if necessary with a tracheostomy. If difficulty is met in passing an endotracheal tube, tracheostomy should be performed without delay. A major hazard in the comatose or severely obtunded patient is that he may vomit at any time, with resulting aspiration of liquid and often semi-solid food particles into the tracheobronchial tree. If this occurs, it is usually extremely difficult to clear the air passages of this food sufficiently to permit satisfactory resuscitation. Therefore, in such patients an endotracheal tube should be inserted and the balloon cuff fully inflated, where indicated. Incidentally, hemorrhage from the face, mouth or neck can result in actual drowning of the patient by a relatively small amount of blood. Immediate steps must be taken to halt blood loss, and blood should be administered to maintain an adequate circulating blood volume.

In order of preference to maintain a dependable airway, we prefer to insert a nasotracheal tube and inflate the cuff, if the patient is sufficiently cooperative to be able to participate in the insertion of the tube through the nose and into the trachea. Although the nasotracheal tube has the disadvantage of making it difficult to suction the tracheobronchial tree as well as can be accomplished through the usual orally inserted endotracheal tube, it does not continually stimulate the tongue, and thus it is much better tolerated by the patient over a period of several days. Furthermore, it can be more easily inserted into the awake patient than can the oral endotracheal tube, because the latter causes much more stimulation of the gag reflex, and the patient finds it difficult to cooperate.

If an endotracheal tube can be passed quickly, the physician is afforded a secure airway, by means of which blood can be aspirated from the tracheobronchial tree as necessary. Subsequently, if required, tracheostomy can be safely performed directly over this tube, the endotracheal tube then being withdrawn from the trachea completely as soon as the tracheostomy tube is in place. However, it is unwise to remove the endotracheal tube completely until the tracheostomy tube has been securely inserted just below it.

Once the airway is secure, thoracic auscultation should be employed to confirm bilateral ventilation of the lungs. If the patient has aspirated vomitus or blood, bronchoscopy may be required. However, a considerable amount of material may be removed from the lungs by placing the patient in a very steep Trendelenburg position and using intermittent catheter suctioning. If each lung is not being satisfactorily ventilated, as determined by auscultation, the chest x-ray will further identify impediments to satisfactory respiratory gas exchange. These may include pneumothorax, hemothorax, severe lung contusion, or pulmonary edema from one cause or another. Massive blunt trauma may produce complete separation of one or the other main stem bronchi, or rupture of the trachea. The presence of subcutaneous emphysema in the neck or mediastinum should also suggest the possibility of rupture of one of the major tracheobronchial structures (Fig. 30-1). The presence of a first rib fracture indicates trauma of a severe nature, and an especially careful search for associated arterial or bronchial injuries is thus indicated.

These various measures aimed toward making certain that ade-

PATHOPHYSIOLOGY OF TRAUMA

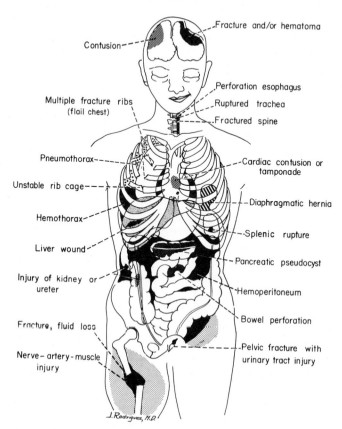

Figure 30–1. The patient with multiple injuries can be subjected to a wide variety of life-threatening complications. (From Hardy, J. D.: Pathophysiology in Surgery. Baltimore, Williams and Wilkins Company, 1968.)

quate respiration is present should take only a few moments, and thereafter the adequacy of respiration should be immediately determined by measurement of the arterial blood gas values. The patient can be attached to a simple ventilator or to a volume controlled ventilator, if these are necessary, to make certain that respiration is adequate to prevent brain damage or cardiac arrest.

Restoration of Adequate Blood Volume. Once reasonably satisfactory respiration has been established and if necessary maintained by a ventilator or other means at hand, immediate attention should be turned to the maintenance of an adequate circulating blood volume. This is probably the most common requirement in the patient with multiple injuries, and it still remains the requirement which is most often misjudged. To begin with, it is often difficult to know just how much blood the patient has lost externally en route to the hospital from some distant point where he was injured, and it may be impossible to know how much blood is still being lost internally or even from visible external oozing. Unfortunately, the measurement of circulating blood volume with various methods has never proved to be very helpful in the acute emergency situation. However, there are a number of measurements which can be extremely valuable in permitting one to judge the adequacy of the effective circulating blood volume at a given time. Several of these factors were mentioned previously, and they include the general appearance of the patient (does he appear "bled out"?), is the pulse rapid and thready?, what is the brachial or cuff blood pressure?, what is the central venous pressure through the previously inserted large bore plastic catheter?, and is the adult patient secreting urine at a rate of at least 30 cc. per hour? If the blood volume is adequate, to permit an adequate cardiac output and if renal damage has not already occurred (it will usually not have occurred if the injury was sustained only a brief time previously), the patient should form urine at a satisfactory rate. If he does excrete urine at a satisfactory rate, this in itself affords much reassurance that the cardiovascular system, including blood volume, is reasonably stable at the moment. It does not imply that continuing blood loss, if unreplaced and unchecked, may not later precipitate disaster unless effective measures are taken. Nevertheless, the blood pressure, the central venous pressure, the pulse rate and pulse volume, the appearance of the patient and the urine output per hour or per half hour are very helpful guides to the requirement for whole blood transfusion. They should be used in an orderly fashion in any patient who has sustained multiple injuries.

If the patient has sustained thermal burns in addition to other injuries, considerable fluid will be lost under the burn wounds in due course, as it will be lost around major fractures of long bones and in patients with peritonitis. Accordingly the fluid requirements must be adjusted to meet such anticipated third space losses.

The patient who exhibits severe vasoconstriction can at times be more effectively managed if a catheter is inserted into a femoral artery for pressure measurements. The intra-arterial pressure may be found to be normal or even elevated, when no pressure is obtainable with a blood pressure cuff on the arm. Such patients have at times been remarkably benefited by the administration of Thorazine, though this drug should be used judiciously and only in such special circumstances. In by far the majority of patients the severe arteriospasm reflects increased peripheral resistance secondary to reduced cardiac output caused by hypovolemia. The dosage of Thorazine used is 25 mg. given slowly intravenously and repeated as indicated over the next hour or so. As the severe vasoconstriction is relieved, the skin and internal organs are better perfused; additional blood can be transferred without excessive elevation of the central venous pressure, respiration is improved and urine output increases.

The patient who has lost blood from massive or multiple trauma will usually require blood transfusion. We have been conservative in adopting a policy of massive intravenous infusion of Ringer's lactate solution in patients in whom the actual deficit is whole blood from actual blood loss. The reasons for this policy are multiple, but the primary one is that there remains no adequate substitute for whole blood when whole blood has been lost. In addition, the patient may eventually go into renal failure, perhaps because of severe hypotension which existed for several hours before he reached the hospital, where definitive resuscitation was administered. If the patient does develop severe oliguria, it is highly desirable that a fluid overload be avoided. Therefore, we would approach the potentially oliguric patient, who may develop acute tubular necrosis, by replacing blood and giving a limited amount of fluid such as Ringer's lactate to replace third space losses beneath burns, around fractures and soft tissue injuries, and perhaps in peritonitis with ileus. Beyond this, we would be conservative in the administration of fluids which were not being readily excreted by the kidneys. The patient should be weighed on admission and then daily. We would give sufficient quantities of blood to maintain an adequate central venous pressure (above 10 cm. saline and below 20), to maintain an adequate systemic blood pressure level and to afford a pulse of good volume and preferably of modest rate, and to achieve urine output if the kidneys are capable of producing an adequate urine output. Oliguria can of course be due to many factors, the most serious in this instance usually being the renal damage resulting from underperfusion of the kidneys following the injury. However, in older patients there is often the possibility that borderline renal, hepatic, cardiac or pulmonary insufficiency existed prior to the accident. All these possibilities must be considered in judging the most appropriate therapy for the given patient.

Assuming that blood transfusion is required, it is frequently impossible to determine at the outset the exact volume of blood which will be necessary for the given patient. If the patient is in shock owing to blood loss, an adult will require at least 1 liter of blood, having lost perhaps a third of his total blood volume if he is hypotensive in the supine position. The response to blood transfusion must be carefully monitored, both by physical examination and by the response of the pulse rate and volume, the blood pressure, the central venous pressure and the urine output. If the blood pressure and the central venous pressure have risen satisfactorily but the urine output remains low, one must tentatively assume that the oliguria is due to renal damage, and blood transfused thereafter must be administered with caution.

Meanwhile, the urgency of the situation will have been assessed. If it is apparent on a clinical basis that a large amount of blood has been lost and that blood loss is probably continuing, the patient should be moved promptly to an area for intensive care adjacent to the operating suite. A quickly performed chest x-ray will exclude massive hemor-rhage into the thorax in most instances. Therefore, blood loss which is continuing will frequently be due to ruptured spleen or ruptured liver or to trauma to other organs within the abdomen, depending upon the nature of the injury. If the patient has been in shock or is clearly losing blood, a physician should monitor his condition continuously, to pre-vent sudden shock and cardiac arrest.

If it is not possible to get sufficient cross-matched blood promptly, many lives will be saved by using adequate volumes of O-negative blood. However, it is now possible to get a rapid cross-match on an emergency basis. These rapid cross-matches are not as dependable as are the longer methods, but they do suffice in most instances without significant danger, and it is frequently impossible to wait for definitive blood crossing in a major catastrophic emergency. Furthermore, even if some unknown minor blood incompatibility exists, it is far better to have a living patient who can be treated if necessary by renal hemodial-ysis than it is to have a patient who has died for lack of adequate blood volume. It must be stressed that in the patient with multiple injuries, at least two secure routes in satisfactory veins should be available for the rapid administration of blood. For example, if the patient proves to have an aortic injury, which suddenly begins bleeding again after he has reached the hospital and been resuscitated, it will at times be impossible to pump enough blood through a single venous line to achieve a life-maintaining blood volume while the aortic bleeding is being controlled. Also, we cannot overemphasize the importance of having such a patient in the general area of the operating suite for emergency laparotomy or thoracotomy, to control blood loss, often giving the anesthesiologist time to restore blood volume before more definitive technical maneuvers are embarked upon.

Thus far attention has been directed to the restoration of adequate respiration (determined by physical examination and arterial blood gas values) as soon as possible, and to the restoration of an adequate circulating blood volume. These are the two primary requirements, in the order of physiological urgency, that are most often met in the patient with multiple injuries. However, there remain a number of other considerations which should be touched upon in discussing the emergency resuscitation of the patient with multiple injuries, prior to more definitive measures to complete diagnosis and management.

At the time the arterial blood gas values are determined, the arte-rial blood pH should also be determined. If the patient is acidotic, which often happens when the blood pressure has been low or when the blood volume has been barely adequate to permit perfusion of the tissues at a less than optimal level, adequate amounts of sodium bicar-bonate should be given intravenously to correct the acidosis and to achieve an arterial blood pH of approximately 7.4. If the patient is acidotic, usually at least 2 ampules of sodium bicarbonate (44 mEq. of sodium per ampule) will be required. This base should be placed in a drip or injected slowly into the intravenous tubing over a period of several minutes. In the given patient it is not possible to estimate exactly how much bicarbonate will be required or how often it will need to be given, while resuscitative measures are being carried forward, and the dosage should be governed by repeated measurements of the arterial blood pH. Sodium bicarbonate should be continued intermittently until a pH of approximately 7.4 has been achieved and has stabilized.

If the well-ventilated patient has not responded to blood transfusion and correction of acidosis, digitalization should be considered. Actually, at times so much blood has been administered so rapidly, in the extreme emergency in which the central venous pressure measurements may not be reliable, that the patient is actually overloaded with blood and the blood volume becomes so great as to precipitate pulmonary edema. This must be avoided. Furthermore, the heart that has been hypoxic from severe shock, or has actually arrested, may not be able initially to tolerate the normal blood volume, particularly in the presence of intense vasoconstriction. Later, however, when the heart has been well perfused with oxygenated blood and has improved the strength of its contractions, it may be able to move the blood forward in such a manner as to disclose the need for additional blood transfusion. In other words, the total efficiency of the circulation will vary from time to time, depending upon the effective blood volume, the quality of myocardial function, the quality of respiration, and the state of the peripheral resistance. These complex and exquisitely interrelated physiological processes must be clearly understood and each component considered in the replacement of blood, the correction of acidosis, the possible administration of digitalis, the possible use of vasopressor drugs as a temporary expedient to maintain a blood pressure which will keep the heart beating, and the very occasional patient in whom the use of sympathetic ganglionic blocking agents may be indicated.

Having mentioned these general guides, one should emphasize the fact that the patient with multiple injuries should be cared for by the most experienced surgeon available to him. To achieve the best possible results in these critically ill patients, a great deal of experience, wisdom and expeditious action is frequently required.

In the critically ill patient who may exhibit arrhythmia or actually go into cardiac arrest, it is well to use an electrocardiographic monitor, which is of considerable assistance to the nursing staff in detecting arrhythmia or actual cardiac arrest. Although it may be somewhat disturbing to other patients, equipment which makes a noise with each heart beat is preferable to one which merely exhibits the electrocardiogram on a screen, since with the "beeping" equipment the nurse can go about other duties and simply be listening for the regular beating of the heart of the patient with multiple injuries in the critical care unit.

HEAD AND NECK INJURIES

Diagnosis. It is important to ascertain whether or not the patient was at any time unconscious, whether there was any respiratory difficulty, and whether he now has any difficulty with swallowing. A careful neurological examination, immediately recorded on the chart, is essential. If there is no obvious bleeding and if there is adequate respiration and swallowing function, then the next steps include roentgen examinations. However, the patient with multiple injuries should not be sent to the x-ray department unattended. In fact, at times it may be wise to take the patient directly to the operating suite and to perform what roentgen studies are available in that location, since immediate operation may be required for lesions which could otherwise prove fatal.

The patient who has a laceration of the scalp should usually have skull x-rays for possible fractures. The presence of a skull fracture at least indicates the possibility that significant brain damage may have occurred, or perhaps hemorrhage which may later result in an epidural hematoma or a subdural hematoma, or in actual bleeding into the brain substance itself. Adequate films of the facial bones and mandible are essential both for therapy and for legal purposes, and it is wise to perform a barium swallow in any patient who may have sustained injury to the pharynx or the esophagus. Endoscopy should be employed if there is the possibility of injury in the posterior pharnyx or to the trachea or the esophagus. An occasional patient will have a serious laceration in the posterior pharnyx which may not be identified and which can cause serious cervical infection. Adequate drainage is essential for the proper management of pharyngeal or esophageal perforations.

Management of Head and Neck Injuries. It is beyond the scope of this discussion to present in any detail the management of head and neck injuries. Suffice it to say that the surgeon must recognize such injuries when they are present, and either initiate the proper measures or request consultation of those particularly experienced in the management of specific problems. In general, intracranial injuries must be viewed as lesions with very serious potentialities, and neurological and neurosurgical consultation should be requested and the results recorded. Fractures of the upper face and the mandible should be managed by specialists in this field, usually with elevation of fractures of the zygoma and the maxilla, and with wiring of lesions of the mandible. The possibility of esophageal perforation or tracheal injury should always be considered. The tracheal injury may be disclosed by bronchoscopy, and the esophageal injury by appropriate studies with a radiopaque medium. Tracheal injuries should be repaired by direct suture, as should esophageal injuries. Again, the esophageal injuries should be drained, in addition to suture of the laceration. Even severe lacerations of the face may be repaired with excellent cosmetic results. Lacerations of the scalp generally heal satisfactorily when sutured. The scalp has an excellent blood supply, and the hair will usually cover the scar.

If there is serious question regarding injury to the larynx or to the vocal cords or trachea, a tracheostomy may be required. Blunt trauma to the larynx may result in displacement or actual avulsion of cartilaginous elements of this structure, with severe embarrassment of respiration. We know of one patient who was in an automobile accident in which several persons were injured. The patient readily assisted the others in reaching the hospital, whereupon he suddenly became cyanotic and sustained respiratory and cardiac arrest. The physician present was able to perform tracheostomy and to resuscitate the patient, with complete absence of apparent neurological deficits. Subsequent examination of the larynx revealed that one chord and a major portion of its cartilaginous supporting structure were completely absent. The patient either had swallowed the structures or had spat them out at the time of the accident. The family had noticed that his voice was abnormal at the time he was marshaling the group into the ambulance to go to the hospital, but only after he reached the hospital had there been evidence of severe respiratory difficulty. Apparently submucosal hemorrhage and clotted blood had resulted in abrupt occlusion of the air passage at the level of the larynx after he reached the hospital.

THORACIC INJURIES

Diagnosis. The types of thoracic injury most often encountered were discussed previously.

The presence of rib fractures can usually be made fairly accurately on a clinical basis, by pressing with one hand placed on the posterior thorax and the other hand on the anterior thorax. Pain will be experienced by the patient over the fractured rib. Of course, if multiple adjacent ribs are fractured in at least two places, there will usually be paradoxical motion which is visible to the naked eye, certainly in patients who are not obese. The patient who has had a rupture of a bronchus may show subcutaneous emphysema over the thorax, or in the neck, or even extending all the way up to the face with such severity that the eyes are closed by the subcutaneous air. The quality of pulmonary ventilation can be determined by brief examination of the volume of air being exchanged through the nose or mouth, and by auscultation of the hemithorax on each side. Simple observation of the thorax may disclose that neither lung is being well ventilated or that one hemithorax exhibits much greater excursion with respiration than does the other. Percussion may suggest the presence of fluid in the chest, which must be presumed to be blood in the patient in shock who has not previously had an illness that might have caused hydrothorax. Rupture of a bronchus may produce pneumothorax, or subcutaneous emphysema, or simply atelectasis of the lung. After the initial examination has been made and the patient's condition is judged to be sufficiently stable to permit movement to the adjacent x-ray department, a chest x-ray should always be performed to aid in the diagnosis of significant intrathoracic changes. A portable film may be necessary, but the best possible roentgenograms should be achieved whenever feasible. Most injuries with pneumothorax or hemothorax will respond to underwater tube drainage, and it is essential to be certain that neither air nor blood is accumulating in the thorax, prior to any induction of anesthesia for possible exploratory laparotomy. It is equally important to exclude pericardial tamponade. To re-emphasize, chest x-rays are very helpful in the diagnosis of intrathoracic pathology, far more so than are plain films of the abdomen. Serial chest x-rays will go far toward excluding the development of tension pneumothorax, hemothorax, mediastinal widening caused by traumatic aneurysm, and other types of lesions.

If there is widening of the mediastinum following a severe deceleration accident or even a penetrating injury, the possibility of hemorrhage into the mediastinum from aortic injury must be considered. Sound judgment is required to determine whether or not a patient who has other injuries such as serious brain concussion or possible intra-abdominal hemorrhage should be subjected to an aortogram in the x-ray department. Frequently, the patient is comatose, and the most delicate types of decisions are required in order to conclude whether or not thoracotomy or laparotomy is to be undertaken. By and large, the patient with a head injury serious enough to produce coma should not have thoracotomy if it can possibly be avoided. In contrast, if there is also a penetrating wound of the abdomen which may have perforated a hollow viscus, or if there is evidence that blunt trauma has produced rupture of the liver or the spleen or kidney, laparotomy may be unavoidable to save the patient's life.

Management. Certain comments have already been made relative to the management of particular thoracic injuries. The flail chest which is interfering seriously with respiratory gas exchange must be managed either by external splinting or, preferably, by internal splinting, using an endotracheal tube or cuffed tracheostomy tube, with a ventilator. The use of internal fixation by positive pressure assisted ventilation has been widely adopted and, in our institution, is now the method of choice. When internal stabilization with a ventilator is employed, it is well to use a volume respirator, because the pressure requirements may be such that the pressure level set on the gauge may be reached before an adequate volume of gas has been delivered to achieve adequate pulmonary ventilation. On the other hand, there are certain risks with volume ventilators, because the machine will automatically deliver the volume for which it is set and may occasionally cause rupture of the lung. If there is any question of an accompanying pneumothorax, chest catheters should be inserted to prevent development of tension pneumothorax.

Pneumothorax or hemothorax, often in combination, can usually be managed successfully by underwater tube drainage. If the chief problem is pneumothorax, the tube should be inserted anteriorly in approximately the second intercostal space. If drainage is required for hemothorax, the tube should be inserted in the lower portion of the thorax, in the posterior axillary line. To insert the tube higher or anteriorly will not achieve the most dependent possible drainage, and to insert the tube more posteriorly will cause the patient discomfort from lying on the tube when he is in the supine position. If blood clots in the hemithorax, it may be preferable to make a small incision, even under local anesthesia, and to remove the clots that are accessible by a so-called "mini-thoracotomy." However, effective stripping of the plastic or siliconized tubes inserted at the time of injury will usually remove most of the blood from the chest, and no further measures are required. As indicated previously, however, if the bleeding is massive, or if it continues with multiple blood transfusions being required, a thoracotomy should be performed.

Heart injuries constitute a particular problem, and there has long existed a difference of opinion regarding how they should be managed. There are those, including ourselves, who believe that it is not possible in all instances to determine whether or not the heart has actually been injured, and that routine thoracotomy for all possible heart injuries in the essentially asymptomatic patient is not justified. On the other hand, we have become more and more liberal in our early use of thoracotomy for possible pericardial tamponade in trauma, though by individualization of cases we have not thus far had a fatality in patients who had no other serious injuries. We do move the patient to the Recovery Ward just adjacent to the operating suite, and the patient is carefully observed by experienced personnel. Pericardiocentesis may be employed once or even twice. If it is required more than once, however, we usually proceed with a thoracotomy. Incidentally, there is always the hazard of injuring a coronary artery, and we are aware of one instance in which death rapidly ensued following puncture of a major coronary vessel in the process of performing pericardiocentesis. If the patient with a penetrating wound of the thorax develops a murmur postoperatively when he had not had a murmur previously, especially if hemopericardium was present, an intracardiac injury should be suspected and the patient should be studied by appropriate heart catheterization and angiocardiography. Obviously, adequate blood for transfusion must be present when the possibility of injury to the heart or great vessels exists. Hemorrhage from aortic injury may cease during shock, only to recur with catastrophic consequences just when the patient appears to have stabilized.

Esophageal perforation should be suspected when there is pain from the mediastinum or evidence of pneumomediastinum, or when the patient exhibits evidence of mediastinitis with fever and the other usual signs of sepsis. An esophageal perforation should be exposed by thoracotomy, sutured, and drained well by underwater seal. Esophageal lacerations represent very serious injuries, for serious mediastinal infection may proceed to a fatal issue. Antibiotic coverage should accompany suture of the esophageal laceration and drainage of the mediastinum and the hemithorax.

A full survey of the wide variety and combinations of intrathoracic injuries and the complications that may occur is not within the scope of this chapter. Attention has been drawn to some of the more common injuries and their initial management. Any serious injury to the lung can result in atelectasis, lung abscess, empyema, and other chronic and severely disabling complications. These complications will often have to be treated in the presence of injuries elsewhere such as long bone fractures, intraperitoneal sepsis and even skull fractures with brain damage and coma.

ABDOMINAL INJURIES

Diagnosis. The nature and the extent of intra-abdominal injuries can be difficult to determine by history and physical examination alone, or even by roentgen examinations; diagnostic laparotomy may be required. However, much can be learned short of operation. Peritoneal contamination, even by blood, may produce abdominal pain and tenderness, rigidity and quiet or absent peristaltic sounds. There may be blood in the gastric aspirate, the rectum or the bladder. Clinical evidence may suggest internal hemorrhage. Pain referred to the left shoulder may indicate rupture of the spleen. A four quadrant peritoneal tap may disclose free blood, but a negative tap is not significant.

The injection of the abdominal wound with radiopaque medium, the "sinugram," may decide whether the injury did or did not penetrate into the free peritoneal cavity. The plain film may disclose free air in the peritoneal cavity, and various pyelograms, alimentary tract studies or arteriograms may demonstrate injury to specific organs. Pelvic fractures, especially in the region of the symphysis pubis, may be associated with urethral injury.

Frequently, exploratory laparotomy must be performed to permit certain diagnosis and the correction of pathology.

If it is elected to try a period of nonoperative management, following blunt or penetrating abdominal trauma, the symptoms, vital signs, physical examination and serial white blood cell counts and red cell data should all be utilized to monitor the total clinical situation. A falling hematocrit or hemoglobin level will suggest continued blood loss as from a ruptured spleen, liver or pancreas, or injury to kidney, veins or arteries. A rising body temperature, with a rising white cell count and pulse rate and other collateral evidence of intraperitoneal contamination, should suggest leakage from a hollow viscus. If nonoperative management is elected initially, the patient must be carefully followed and operation performed without further delay once the indications for surgery are clearly present. To delay further is to risk serious peritonitis, abscess formation, perhaps septicemia, prolonged paralytic ileus with probable fibrinous-to-fibrous adhesions, late small bowel obstruction, inanition, pulmonary complications, hepatic and renal dysfunction, and other sequelae.

Management. The management of various injuries is implicit in the foregoing discussion. Nevertheless, a few specific comments are in order regarding damage to specific organs.

First, before placing the patient under anesthesia for exploratory laparotomy, the condition of the sensorium should be ascertained, and certainly the possibility of serious embarrassment of cardiac function or respiration should have been excluded by appropriate clinical studies and roentgenograms. The patient can withstand intra-abdominal pathology for considerable periods of time, unless massive hemorrhage is occurring, but serious embarrassment to cardiac and respiratory function can prove rapidly fatal. It is often difficult to detect these deficits after the patient has been placed under general anesthesia.

MANAGEMENT OF SPECIFIC INJURIES. Assuming that laparotomy has been performed, the presence of substantial blood in the peritoneal cavity should at once suggest injury to an intraperitoneal organ, in contrast to a retroperitoneal organ such as the aorta or vena cava. The first site to inspect is the spleen, because it is frequently injured and is readily excised. If the spleen is seen to be fractured and bleeding substantially, it should be delivered into the wound and clamps placed rapidly across the hilum to stop blood loss. In the more elective splenectomy, it is preferable to isolate the splenic artery in the lesser sac and to ligate it initially, followed by an orderly dissection of the structures of the hilum before or after delivering the organ into the wound. After having taken care of the ruptured spleen, if such were found, attention should be turned to the liver, if some other obvious and rapidly bleeding site of injury is not noted. The liver may be crushed, fractured, or simply lacerated by objects such as a bullet or knife. A crushing injury of the liver, frequently to the right lobe, may be so extensive that a limited right lobectomy may be required. Under other circumstances, however, blunt trauma produces a stellate laceration in the right lobe of the liver, and frequently this can be repaired by suitable use of mattress sutures of catgut swedged on to large needles. Some type of backing to prevent these sutures from cutting into the liver tissue may be useful.

Hepatic lobectomy is rarely required for stellate lacerations. However, a common error made by the inexperienced surgeon, upon encountering a severe crushing injury of the right lobe of the liver, may be an attempt to manage bleeding by ligating or cauterizing various small vessels in a disorganized mass of tissue, without realizing that only a right hepatic lobectomy will provide the hemostasis and removal of devitalized tissue that will achieve a successful outcome. Furthermore, such a lobectomy should be performed at the first operation, when the patient is in the best possible physical condition, rather than at a second operation when continuing hemorrhage has produced a state of shock with severe metabolic depletion. It has been frequently suggested that a T-tube be placed in the common bile duct following repair of liver injuries, to decompress the biliary tract and reduce the chance that bile leakage will occur from the site of liver injury above. We have used a T-tube under these circumstances, but we do not employ it routinely. Preoperative use of selective arteriography may demonstrate fracture of the spleen, liver, or kidney, and we have used this modality increasingly in recent years. Furthermore, if late liver necrosis and abscess formation lead to blood vessel erosion and hemobilia, the site of bleeding may occasionally be identified with selective arteriography through the gastrohepatic artery. Finally, packing to control liver hemorrhage has been abandoned by virtually all clinics. The bleeding must be controlled by ligatures or cautery, and packing will rarely achieve adequate hemostasis. If introduced firmly enough, packing will cause additional liver necrosis which can result in infection and secondary hemorrhage later in the clinical course.

Injuries to the alimentary tract must be managed as the findings dictate. Massive injury to the mesentery of a segment of bowel will require resection of this portion of the bowel, either with end-to-end anastomosis or, in the case of the colon and occasionally even the small bowel, with exteriorization of elements of the intestinal tract. Injuries to the stomach are sutured, and minor perforations of the small bowel are also closed with sutures. In civilian life, there is an increasing tendency to close colon injuries primarily, if produced by knife or low velocity missile and if only 2 or 3 hours have elapsed since injury. The safest course in most instances, however, is to treat colon injuries by closure of the perforation, drainage of the site of this portion of the abdomen, and performance of a proximal colostomy. If indicated, it may be possible to exteriorize the injured portion of the colon, and this will permit simple resection of this portion and restoration of gut continuity at a second operation. Although there is a great temptation to attempt to avoid the need for a future operation, by closing colon perforations and not performing a colostomy or exteriorization of the injured portion of the colon, it should never be forgotten that the bacterial flora of the colon represents a sinister source of peritonitis, and many patients will die if the perforation of the colon is not dealt with definitively at the initial operation. It is far better to be safe than to risk extensive soiling of the peritoneal cavity with the fecal contents from the unprepared colon — and the colon is always unprepared in the patient with multiple injuries. Furthermore, it is to be remembered at all times that the colon injury may represent only one of perhaps numerous other serious lesions which the patient with multiple injuries has sustained, and any further metabolic assault during his postoperative course is to be avoided if possible, to preserve metabolic strength to permit him to survive the various other injuries and the complications of these injuries which may ensue.

To avoid overlooking a perforation of the alimentary tract, an orderly and systematic search from the terminal esophagus to the pelvic floor should be employed, as indicated by the circumstances. Particular attention should be devoted to the retroperitoneal portions of the bowel, such as the duodenum, and the splenic flexure of the colon. We have seen tremendous contamination from a tangential posterior wound of the splenic flexure of the colon, with no blood or other contamination present in the peritoneal cavity itself; only after mobilization of the splenic flexure, done because blood was found in the rectum, was the extensive fecal soiling of the retroperitoneal space discovered. Similarly, we treated a child whose abdomen had been run over by an automobile. Although the patient appeared to be doing well for several days, peritonitis then developed, and at laparotomy it was found that the fourth portion of the duodenum had been severed completely, just proximal to the ligament of Treitz. Since this gut was retroperitoneal in location, the peritoneal cavity had not become contaminated initially and no abdominal tenderness or rigidity had been present on admission.

Pancreatic injuries can be difficult to manage. If the injury is to the tail or body of the pancreas, this portion of the organ can be excised, along with the spleen if necessary, and the stump of the pancreas oversewn with silk or monofilament synthetic sutures. However, if there is extensive damage to the head of the pancreas, the difficult decision must be made regarding whether or not to perform a pancreaticoduodenectomy, in the face of perhaps multiple other injuries elsewhere, or whether to place a T-tube in the common bile duct and to drain the area extensively and await results. Actually, it is often surprising how extensive the apparent damage to the pancreas can be without the serious consequences of pancreatic fistula, sepsis, delayed hemorrhage, pseudocyst formation or other complications of pancreatic trauma. In general, we take the conservative course and simply drain, because to embark upon a pancreaticoduodenectomy in the presence of extensive other trauma entails a considerable metabolic assault and a time-consuming operation in itself. Obviously, hemorrhage from the pancreas must be satisfactorily controlled, and because of the digestive capacity of activated pancreatic juice, a nonabsorbable type of suture material should be employed. If there is no obstruction of the pancreatic duct, most well-drained pancreatic fistulas will close in due course. There is always the risk that sepsis and secondary hemorrhage will occur, which represent serious complications indeed. However, these need not occur, and in a gratifying percentage of cases they do not. Certainly the risk of conservative management of pancreatic injuries is probably no greater than is the risk of extensive pancreatic surgery in the presence of other injuries elsewhere in the body. Once again, however, measures to be employed will be decided by the pathology found at operation, the general condition of the patient, and the experience of the surgeon in charge.

Kidney injuries should be managed with all the conservatism that is possible, compatible with the injuries found. If the kidney has been fractured but still has adequate blood supply, the organ should be repaired with chromic catgut sutures and the area well drained through the flank. If hemorrhage can be satisfactorily controlled and the general structure of the organ restored with appropriate sutures, healing will often occur and the kidney can be preserved. Or perhaps only a portion of the crushed or fractured kidney need be removed. In the patient who has sustained significant abdominal trauma, whether blunt or penetrating, an intravenous pyelogram is frequently useful to demonstrate the quality of renal function on both sides as well as the condition of the ureters and of the bladder. This can be done quickly and it gives much information relative to whether or not the kidneys and ureters need to be explored at the time of laparotomy. A considerable dissection in the retroperitoneal space is required for adequate exposure of the kidneys and the ureters, not to mention the oozing which is often initiated by this extensive dissection in an area which frequently contains much fat and areolar tissue. Therefore, unless there is serious bleeding and evidence of gross extravasation of the radiopaque medium on intravenous pyelogram, the kidneys and ureters need not be explored at operation. A severed ureter should be anastomosed over a catheter that is led into the bladder. The ureteral anastomosis should be of an oblique nature, with a single layer of interrupted chromic catgut sutures. In contrast to the results achieved several decades ago, most such anastomoses of the ureter prove successful at the present time.

It is not necessary to review the various operative maneuvers which are now available to salvage renal function in the presence of ureteral injury which does not respond to simple anastomosis. Obviously, one kidney should never be sacrificed without knowledge of the presence and function of the opposite kidney, to the extent feasible under the circumstances.

Arterial injuries continue to represent a common cause of death in the traumatized patient. Although such injuries may be caused by blunt trauma, with severe injury to the elements of the vena cava or the aorta or mesenteric vessels, it is gunshot injuries which most often result in injury to the structures which are placed well back in the abdominal cavity. A common feature is that the patient may have bled massively into the abdomen and reached the hospital, whereupon the blood pressure responds promptly to the intravenous infusion of electrolyte solution, plasma expander, or whole blood. At this point the physicians in charge may be lulled into a sense of complacency, with the belief that hemorrhage is no longer continuing, and the inadequately attended patient may be sent to the x-ray department for roentgenograms. Unfortunately, the temporary stabilization of the blood pressure at a reasonably satisfactory level may be abruptly followed by a second episode of profound hypotension, which is often due to resumption of hemorrhage that had stopped when the blood pressure was low and clot formation had been permitted to occur. If there is the serious possibility of massive and continuing intra-abdominal bleeding, the patient should be taken immediately to the operating room and any available blood, either cross-matched or O-negative blood, should be employed to permit rapid laparotomy. If the liver and spleen are normal and other obvious areas are not involved, and especially if there is a large hematoma in the retroperitoneal space, it should be tentatively assumed that the bleeding is from either the vena cava or the aorta. The small bowel should be eviscerated and the peritoneum overlying the aorta incised to permit removal of the clot and inspection of the aorta and vena cava. As soon as the general area of hemorrhage has been noted, firm point pressure should be placed over this area, while vascular clamps are applied above and below this level. It is not necessary to expose the aorta completely in order to place clamps so that hemorrhage can be at least reduced if not controlled: the aorta lies along the anterior surface of the vertebrae, and a clamp placed down over the spine and then closed progressively will include the aorta, as the jaws of the clamp are allowed to come up over the vertebral column and close completely just anterior to the spine. Multiple clamps can be applied if necessary to control bleeding, until adequate blood volume has been restored. Once the blood volume is adequate and the circulation is stable, the clamps can be carefully removed, in successive fashion, and the precise site of bleeding identified and appropriately sutured. Many patients who are lost on the operating table under these circumstances are lost because of failure to occlude the aorta appropriately with clamps, to reduce massive hemorrhage until the anesthesiologist can restore an adequate circulating blood volume; cardiac arrest occurs and then the situation rapidly becomes irretrievable. What may initially appear to be an impossible situation can actually prove to be readily managed with proper handling by an experienced vascular surgeon.

EXTREMITY INJURIES

Diagnosis. The detection of significant extremity injuries is usually not difficult. At least, it is not difficult to perceive that some type of damage has occurred. First, the patient will usually complain of pain, which is often well localized to the area of injury, in the case of blunt trauma. For example, the fracture is painful at the fracture site, abnormal bone mobility can be detected, and there may be gross deformity of the extremity owing to the fracture, as well as similar changes. It is occasionally difficult to determine whether the numbness and lack of motor power are due to ischemia from an arterial injury or due to a nerve injury. Nonetheless, the possibility of arterial injury can usually be excluded by palpation of the pulses in the feet, supplemented by arteriograms as necessary. Of course, the presence of distal pulses does not exclude injury to an artery. Venous occlusion will produce swelling of the leg, usually accompanied by cyanosis. Neurological deficit is determined by a careful neurological examination. However, high velocity missiles may produce extensive muscle damage even when the wounds of entrance and exit are small and nerve, blood vessel and bone injuries are absent. The wound should be explored and the injured muscle excised until bleeding is encountered and free drainage provided. Tetanus prophylaxis and antibiotic coverage should be instituted.

If there is marked swelling in one region of the leg, perhaps in the thigh, in the general region at which the bullet entered the extremity, a large hematoma may have developed in the muscle planes of the thigh, perhaps resulting from a tangential injury or partial division of the artery even though a good distal pulse may be present. A femoral arteriogram is easily performed and often diagnostic.

The findings at the time the initial examination is performed should be recorded immediately. It may be difficult later to recall just what the extent of the vascular or neurological deficit was at the time of the initial examination, and the significance of a progressing lesion, perhaps caused by spinal cord injury, may not be fully appreciated unless progress notes are kept meticulously. If there is a progression in the lesion, it often signifies increasing pressure, edema, or other considerations which may require careful evaluation by a neurologist or neurosurgeon.

Blunt trauma often produces fractures, and there is no substitute for adequate and sufficiently extensive roentgen studies to document the fractures and to permit effective temporary and permanent immobilization of the fragments. If the fracture is properly immobilized and a satisfactory pulse is not present in the foot, in a person of the age group who would normally have a dorsalis pedis or posterior tibial pulse, a femoral arteriogram should be performed to determine the status of the artery. Severe spasm of the vessel may exist and no actual exploration of the vessel may be indicated. On the other hand, if there is extravasation of the contrast medium, indicating either partial division or loss of arterial substance or thrombosis of the vessel, immediate operation will almost invariably permit restoration of arterial continuity with adequate arterial perfusion of the distal extremity, whether in the arm or the leg.

Soft tissue injury can present a wide variety of damage. First, a considerable segment of the overlying skin and subcutaneous fat and deeper muscle may have been devitalized and require excision. It is fortunate that a very considerable amount of muscle can be excised without precluding a rather satisfactory use of the extremity, especially of the leg. However, a common error is to underestimate the extent of the muscle damage, especially when the skin remains intact, and thus to have a large amount of necrotic muscle which can become infected and may produce a very serious type of sepsis, even gas gangrene. Second, large amounts of skin may be devitalized or completely avulsed, as in industrial accidents in which an arm or leg is caught in a conveyor belt, and these sites will ultimately require skin grafting. Occasionally the swelling in the tight vascular compartments of the lower leg or forearm is such that blood flow is inadequate, and distal gangrene may occur unless fasciotomy is performed. However, the indications for fasciotomy should be definite, for this procedure leaves a very considerable anatomic and cosmetic defect which often has to be skin grafted. In summary, fractures should be appropriately immobilized. Injured arteries are almost routinely treated successfully either with excision of damaged portions with end-to-end anastomosis, or with a vein graft or, less satisfactorily, a fabric prosthesis. Nerve deficits require neurological consultation and preferably neurosurgical or specialized care, because better results will be achieved by surgeons commonly caring for these injuries and because most accidents are accompanied by the high probability of litigation. If a specialist in the field fails to achieve an optimal result with nerve suture, this is likely to be more readily accepted than if a person less experienced with such nerve suturing achieves the same result. Finally, considerable conservatism should be exercised before amputating traumatized extremities. There is one school of thought which emphasizes that the badly damaged extremity would best be amputated early, to prevent a long period of disability and to permit prompt fitting of an artificial prosthesis. Nevertheless, many extremities can be salvaged and made much more useful than an artificial prosthesis, and certainly in general the patient's psychological welfare is better served by preserving even a somewhat deformed extremity.

COMMON COMPLICATIONS IN THE PATIENT WITH MULTIPLE INJURIES

The foregoing discussion has been directed principally toward the emergency and intermediate care of the patient with multiple injuries. It has frequently been emphasized that the cardiovascular function and adequate respiration must be preserved in the emergency situation, to permit an orderly and more definitive management of the multiple injuries which may be present. It is appropriate here to indicate some of the very serious complications, of a more general nature, which may be expected to develop in the severely traumatized patient who survives the immediate period of shock and possible blood loss and enters a more chronic phase of his hospitalization. Many patients are able to survive for several days, with a stable cardiorespiratory system and a clear sensorium. Unfortunately, complications may then develop which, even in husky young men, are never satisfactorily controlled and lead to a fatal issue.

Almost every system of the body is subject to late complications peculiar to the given organ, and these are well known. Intracranial injury may have appeared to have been minor initially, with the unfortunate late result that an expanding subdural hematoma is not fully appreciated, and the patient may suffer considerable brain damage before the condition is fully realized and corrected by operation. Similarly, fractures of the skull which produce a loss of cerebral spinal fluid through the ear or the nose may permit the entrance of bacteria and produce a fatal meningitis.

Pulmonary complications are among the most serious which may involve the patient with multiple injuries. If brain damage or some other aspect of the initial injury permits the aspiration of pulmonary contents, or requires prolonged use of the mechanical ventilator for days or weeks, pulmonary secretions may not be adequately removed and the patient may gradually develop a hypostatic pneumonia, often with an overgrowth of pseudomonas or other organisms.

Pneumonitis and pulmonary sepsis may become extremely debilitating and may eventually result in the death of the patient. Furthermore, the so-called "traumatic lung" may result in serious hypoxia and hypercarbia, which of themselves may produce cardiac arrest and death. The elements of this pulmonary respiratory deficit are discussed elsewhere in this volume, but suffice it to say that the problem is complex and can be extremely difficult to manage successfully.

Late hemorrhage is an ever present possibility in patients who have sustained gunshot wounds of the abdomen which resulted in arterial injury, especially when associated with bacterial contamination as might follow gut perforation. The escape of pancreatic enzymes in and around a ligated artery or sutured aorta, perhaps aggravated by organisms which escaped from an injury to the lower ileum or colon, will continue to pose a threat of late secondary hemorrhage until the patient has completely recovered, which may take weeks or months. If massive late hemorrhage does occur from infection in the region of an intra-abdominal arterial injury, it is frequently difficult if not impossible to extricate the patient successfully from this dire complication because additional hemorrhage may occur again and again, regardless of management. The possibility of late hemorrhage should always be considered in a patient who goes into shock unexpectedly many days after his initial injury. The possibility of a delayed rupture of the spleen, or of bleeding from the liver, must also be considered.

Sepsis has been accorded relatively little space in the discussion in this chapter, because sepsis is not an immediate problem in most patients with multiple injuries. Of course, if the injury resulted in a significant injury to the colon, peritoneal contamination will have occurred, but even here prompt operation, within a matter of hours, will usually prevent massive peritonitis and blood vessel invasion by bacteria, at least in the first several days, Nonetheless, peritonitis will frequently develop when there has been injury to gut. Many patients with injury to the abdomen, especially penetrating wounds and above all gunshot injuries, do eventually have extensive morbidity and frequently mortality from peritonitis, abscesses, ileus, adhesions, inanition, and even invasion of the bloodstream with septicemia. Furthermore, massive intraperitoneal sepsis is frequently followed by pneumonitis, jaundice, or renal failure. Therefore, potential sepsis is an extremely important element of many multiple injury problems. The management of sepsis is considered elsewhere in this volume. Suffice it to say here that the possibility of the development of infection should always be considered at the time the patient is first seen, and all possible steps taken to close injuries of the alimentary tract that may lead to additional contamination of the region involved, to afford adequate drainage, and to cover the patient with broad-spectrum antibiotics if contamination has occurred.

Renal failure commonly develops in the patient who has sustained massive trauma. The causes are often complex, quite aside from potential injury to the urinary tract itself. First, the patient may have been in shock or with a profound reduction in circulating blood volume for hours prior to his arrival at the hospital where definitive management was initiated. Second, even if the shock to which the kidney was exposed was relatively brief, the elderly patient with advanced nephrosclerosis or the younger patient with pre-existing renal disease may not be able to tolerate even a relatively short period of severe renal ischemia. The administration of massive volumes of blood may produce minor reactions which may further impair renal function, and the as yet poorly understood mechanisms by which sepsis and liver failure produce renal failure must also be taken into consideration. Frequently, it is difficult to determine whether the patient actually has prerenal azotemia or renal azotemia. This differential diagnosis is covered elsewhere in this volume. We would stress the fact that it is very difficult to control sepsis in the uremic patient. Therefore, we urge the early use of hemodialysis or of peritoneal dialysis if the peritoneal cavity was not involved in the injury, to prevent the ravages of uremia which lower the capacity of the body to defend itself against the invasion of bacteria. In the septic patient, daily consideration must be given to every possible means of draining purulent collections and of providing the patient with every possible capacity to survive the serious infection. The adequate management of dialysis represents a very important aspect of this total program. We strongly disagree with the practice of 20 or 30 years ago, in which no serious consideration of hemodialysis or peritoneal dialysis was made until the BUN had risen to almost 200 mg. per 100 ml. and the serum creatinine level to perhaps 16 to 18 mg. per 100 ml. Such patients are subject to a variety of very serious hazards, including cardiac arrhythmia, coma, poor defense against invading bacterial organisms, inanition, abnormal blood coagulation, and stress ulceration with hemorrhage. If sufficient renal function is provided, either by the patient's own kidneys or by artificial means, extremely important time is secured during which the other problems which the patient has can often be effectively managed.

Stress ulceration in the upper gastrointestinal tract remains an unsolved problem, and the causes are not clearly understood. Stress ulceration with massive hemorrhage, occasionally with perforation of the stomach or duodenum, is common in severely injured patients, and it appears to be particularly common in patients with sepsis or burns. This stress ulceration often occurs in patients who are extremely ill, and there is always a reluctance to perform an operation for control of the hemorrhage. Nevertheless, if conservative measures, including the introduction of antacids and cold solutions into the stomach, do not halt the bleeding, it will often be necessary to operate. There has been a difference of opinion as to what operation should be performed for stress ulcer bleeding, and many observers prefer vagotomy-pyloroplasty, with oversewing of the bleeding point. Our preference is to perform vagotomy, with a fairly radical distal subtotal gastrectomy, and either a Billroth I or a Billroth II anastomosis, depending on the circumstances. Any bleeding points in the residual gastric pouch are oversewn.

Starvation often presents a major problem in the patient with multiple injuries. As the days go by with a low intake of calories and protein, many deleterious effects upon almost all organs can be expected, and in fact have been clearly documented in various observations during periods of experimental starvation or famine. Therefore, when it is clear that the patient will have an extended period during which he may not be able to ingest nutrients in a normal manner, possibly because of brain injury or intraperitoneal injury or esophageal injury, every consideration should be given immediately to the prevention of serious inanition. This can be done in a variety of ways, preferably by use of the alimentary tract itself, either by insisting that the patient take food or by the use of a small feeding tube introduced through the nose. By using a blender, the whole food materials can be converted to a liquid state and injected through the small feeding tube. However, if intraperitoneal sepsis and ileus prevent the use of the alimentary tract, then the calories should be introduced by the intravenous route to the extent possible. It is possible by routine means to introduce 800 to 1200 calories per day, with amino acid solutions to provide the elements for protein fabrication. Nevertheless, the recent widespread application of intravenous hyperalimentation has added an additional and very valuable dimension to the nutritional therapy of patients who are unable to take food by mouth over an extended period of time. Several thousand calories can be introduced in the 24 hour period, and, although intravenous hyperalimentation is associated with certain complications, the advantages of the method in carefully selected patients far outweigh the occasional complications of hemorrhage, vein thrombosis, and infection which have been observed and reported.

To recapitulate, the provision of adequate blood volume, adequate respiration, adequate renal function, and adequate nutrition will go far toward preserving the vitality of the patient with multiple injuries while the various life-threatening problems are being dealt with systematically.

CHAPTER 31

CARE OF THE BURNED PATIENT

Curtis P. Artz, M.D., F.A.C.S.

A burn is a very complex injury and there are many acceptable methods of care. There are differences in types of burns, in configuration, in patients and in facilities that should influence the selection of technique of management. This chapter presents basic principles of pre- and postoperative care and mentions some accepted methods of treatment.

FIRST AID

A person whose clothes are on fire should not run as this only fans the flames. He should not remain standing since this position may cause him to inhale flames or cause his hair to be ignited. He should be placed in a horizontal position and then rolled in a blanket to smother the flames.

The objectives of first aid are to prevent further wound contamination and injury, to alleviate pain and to transport the patient safely to a location where professional care is available. Application of towels soaked in ice water brings almost immediate pain relief. This amount of cold may have some value in arresting the effect of heat on the tissues. The application of cold by any convenient method immediately after the burn is the best known first aid measure. Any burn involving more than 10 per cent of the body surface should be seen by a physician; medication or home remedies should not be applied. The wound should be covered; this minimizes contamination and inhibits pain by preventing the air from coming in contact with the injured surface. A clean sheet makes a useful emergency dressing. The patient with an extensive burn should not be given water because of the danger from vomiting. Stimulants are unnecessary and should be avoided. The patient suffering from respiratory arrest due to smoke inhalation should receive artificial respiration by the mouth-to-mouth technique.

Table 31–1.   POPULAR BURN FLUID FORMULAS

Brooke
>   First 24 hours:
>   Colloids (plasma, dextran): 0.5 ml./kg./per cent of body surface burned
>   Lactated Ringer's solution: 1.5 ml./kg./per cent of body surface burned
>   Water requirement (dextrose in water): 2000 ml. for adults, children correspondingly less
>   Second 24 hours:
>   Colloid and lactated Ringer's solution requirements are about one-half those of the first 24 hours

Parkland
>   First 24 hours:
>   Lactated Ringer's solution in the amount of 4 ml./kg./per cent of body surface burned

TRANSPORTATION

Burn shock is insidious in its onset; therefore, burned patients usually tolerate transportation well during the immediate postburn period. If transportation to a hospital requires less than half an hour, the only treatment required is a small dose of morphine intravenously. However, if transportation is expected to require a prolonged period, a cannula should be well anchored in a vein, lactated Ringer's started and an adequate airway assured. Occasionally it may be necessary to do a tracheotomy.

Patients may be transported several hundred miles by air during the first 24 hours provided fluid and electrolyte requirements are fulfilled in transit. Physiologic derangements grow progressively worse after injury and the patient does not tolerate prolonged transportation as well after 24 hours as he does before that time. In critical burns a medical escort is essential.

MINOR BURNS

Minor burns include those partial-thickness burns of less than 10 per cent of the body surface and full-thickness burns of less than 2 per cent of the body surface. These do not usually require fluid replacement and should be treated with local cleansing and the appropriate type of wound care. Usually victims of such burns are treated on an outpatient basis. Minor burns, like other burns, should be cared for as aseptically as possible by attendants who wear masks. Debris and loose devitalized tissue should be gently removed and the burn wound cleansed with warm water and bland soap. The wound may be treated by the intermittent application of cold. The best way to apply cold is by the use of compresses soaked in ice water. As soon as the pain has been relieved, the cold application may be discontinued until the pain recurs.

The chief aim of local care of minor burns is to make the patient as comfortable as possible. Although exposure is a good method of local care, most patients treated on an outpatient basis for minor burns should have the burn dressed. Sterile, nonadherent fine-mesh gauze is placed over the burn and fixed in place with a large bulky dressing. The patient should return for a dressing change in two to five days. Antibiotics are rarely necessary.

EARLY HOSPITAL MANAGEMENT

The emergency department care of a patient with a major burn should be an orderly execution of several established routine procedures.

As soon as the patient arrives, the responsible attending physician should be contacted. Arrangements should be made for adequate assistance. Several nurses, technicians, medical students, house officers or other physicians may be profitably utilized in expeditious emergency department care. All attendants must put on a cap and mask. The patient's clothing or emergency dressing must be removed and all burned areas completely exposed for initial evaluation.

A brief history should be obtained—when, where and how the injury occurred, the age of the patient, any allergies, status of tetanus immunization and previous health. It is important to determine immediately if there are any associated injuries. Later, a more thorough examination is performed.

Intravenous fluid therapy is indicated in burns of 20 per cent or more (15 per cent in children) and when clinical shock is present. A large bore needle should be inserted into any available vein and blood obtained for cross matching, hemoglobin, hematocrit, blood urea nitrogen and base line electrolyte determinations. Through the same needle, replacement therapy may be started. Morphine sulfate, 0.1 mg./pound for children and 10 mg. total for adults, allays apprehension and is an excellent analgesic. When such medication is required in acutely burned patients, it must be given intravenously; subcutaneous medications are not absorbed because of circulatory derangements. Morphine sulfate is usually diluted in 3 to 5 ml. of saline and injected into the vein over a period of one to two minutes.

Because the life of the burned patient frequently depends on the infusion of replacement solutions, it is wise to plan for various routes of administration. A cutdown cannula should be inserted in adult patients with greater than 20 per cent burn injury and in children with greater than 15 per cent. Intravenous fluids may be required for as long as 12 days. Before the site for the intravenous portal is selected, considerable thought should be given to the best utilization of available veins. Veins in burned patients are used primarily for two purposes: intravenous infusions and procurement of blood samples for laboratory determinations. It is desirable to insert the cutdown in the most distal vein of an available extremity, because if thrombosis occurs the same vein may be used in its more proximal part. In adults it is preferable to use veins of the upper extremities if available, because intravenous catheters in the lower extremities lead to more extensive and troublesome thrombotic complications. The best vein, if available, is an antecubital one. It is usually wise to insert a long plastic catheter, large enough to accept a 16- or 18-gauge needle. In patients with very extensive burns it may be desirable to monitor the venous pressure. A catheter inserted through the antecubital vein and put into the superior vena cava attached to a venous manometer is an excellent method of determining venous pressure along with its use as an infusion site for replacement therapy. Care should be taken to make sure that the tip of the catheter does not go into the auricle. Occasionally, catheters erode the wall of the auricle and fluids are infused into the pericardial sac causing cardiac tamponade. As soon as the infusion site is established, lactated Ringer's solution or dextran may be started; detailed fluid therapy can be planned later.

On all major burns the hourly measurement of urinary output by means of an indwelling catheter in the bladder is the most reliable method for determining the adequacy of replacement therapy. As soon as the catheter is not absolutely necessary, it should be removed—in most instances after 48 to 72 hours. A urine specimen should be sent to the laboratory.

Estimation of the Severity of the Burn. A number of factors must be taken into consideration in evaluating the severity of the burn in an individual patient. These include the extent of surface areas burned, the depth of the burn, the age of the patient and the anatomic location of the burn. Other factors of importance are pre-existing diseases and any associated fractures or soft tissue injury.

EXTENT OF BURN. A simple and rapid method of estimating the amount of body surface involved is the use of the Rule of Nines (Table 31–2).

The most accurate method for determining the percentage of

Table 31–2. RULE OF NINES

REGION	PER CENT
Head and neck	9
Upper extremities	18 (9 × 2)
Lower extremities	36 (18 × 2)
Anterior surface of trunk	18
Posterior surface of trunk	18
Perineum	1
Total	100

body surface burned is to map out the areas of injury on a Lund and Browder chart (Fig. 31-1). The best time to plot the burn surface is immediately after cleansing the wound. At this time the burned area can be clearly seen and the difference between second- and third-degree injury can be best evaluated.

DEPTH OF BURN.   A first-degree burn involves only the epidermis and requires only symptomatic therapy for relief of pain. Most burns characterized by simple blisters are partial thickness but some blistered areas may be third degree.

The most difficult burn to evaluate is the one with a mottled red and white appearance with loss of the superficial layers of the skin. The redness is not affected by pressure and is due to the diapedesis of red blood cells through the damaged dermal capillaries. This appearance is sometimes associated with a partial-thickness burn and sometimes with

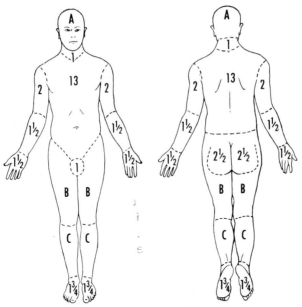

Relative Percentage of Areas Affected by Growth

Age	Age in Years					
	0	1	5	10	15	Adult
A—½ of head	9½	8½	6½	5½	4½	3½
B—½ of one thigh	2¾	3¼	4	4¼	4½	4¾
C—½ of one leg	2½	2½	2¾	3	3¼	3½

Figure 31-1. Lund and Browder charts. These charts permit a rather accurate method for determining percentage of body surface involved. (Artz, C. P., and Reiss, E.: Treatment of Burns, W. B. Saunders Co., 1957.)

one which proves to be of full thickness. In general, the thicker the skin showing this appearance, the more likely it is that some viable epithelium remains. Because sensory end organs are concentrated in the skin, evidence of sensation indicates that part of the skin is still viable. Absence of sensation suggests full-thickness loss. The presence of pain on pricking with a pin denotes the existence of a viable layer of the skin and a partial-thickness injury. Absence of pain usually means full-thickness skin loss. A useful guide to severity is the presence or absence of tissue resistance to extracting the remains of hair and the degree of related pain. In third-degree burns a hair is easily removed with no pain.

AGE OF THE PATIENT.   The age of the patient is important. Although a 30 per cent third-degree burn in a 60-year-old individual usually results in death, a younger person with the same lesion may be expected to recover without unusual complications. In burns involving up to 30 per cent of the body surface and patients under the age of 50, the mortality is low. As the extent of body surface involved increases beyond 30 per cent, the mortality rises in all age groups. Infants tolerate burning poorly and the mortality for those younger than one year is quite high even with moderate burns.

ANATOMIC LOCATION OF INJURY.   In certain parts of the body, third-degree burns produce defects resulting in increased losses of function and disfigurement although the total percentage of body surface involvement is small. The critical anatomic locations are hands, feet, face, neck and joint surfaces. The possibility of respiratory tract injury must be kept in mind in any burn involving the face or neck or in patients who have inhaled smoke or noxious gases. Patients tolerate burns of the upper part of the body and head less well than burns of the trunk and lower extremities.

PRE-EXISTING DISEASE AND CONCOMITANT INJURIES.   Other factors influencing the severity of burns are obesity, alcoholism, pre-existing cardiac or renal disease, concomitant metabolic disease such as diabetes or arthritis, and associated injuries like fractures or major soft tissue trauma.

Replacement Therapy.   A burned patient loses fluid to the exterior and into the burn wound and adjacent areas. The accumulation of fluid in and around the burn wound is secondary to the increase in capillary permeability as well as to vasodilatation, both being a direct result of capillary injury caused by the heat. Significant loss of fluid is also seen from the burned surface.

During the first 48 hours, calculation of fluid replacement can be aided by the use of a burn fluid formula. Because of the complexity of the burn wound and its associated variables, it is impossible to state the fluids required in simple arithmetic terms. A burn formula expresses the fluid needs of the patient about as well as the average digitalizing dose expresses digitalis requirements. Just as the internist is guided in the administration of digitalis by certain signs and symptoms, the surgeon treating a burn varies the fluid requirements predicted by the formula in accordance with the clinical response of the patient.

The popular Brooke formula for estimating fluids in the first 24 hours is shown in Table 31-1. In the second 24 hours about half the colloid and electrolyte requirements of the first 24 hours are needed, in addition to the water requirement. Because the rate of edema formation is maximal in the first 8 hours after injury, half of the estimated amount of replacement solution for the first day is administered in this period. The remaining half is divided equally in the second and third 8-hour intervals. Fluid requirements are needed and are met on the basis of time elapsed since burning—*not* since the patient was admitted to the hospital.

Another formula is the Parkland regimen, which estimates replacement *in the first 24 hours as 4 ml. of lactated Ringer's/kg./per cent of burn.*

Having estimated the needs, a number of factors must be considered before proceeding with therapy. Young children and elderly adults will not tolerate excessive fluids and should receive minimal amounts. Patients with pre-existing cardiovascular or renal disease must be similarly treated.

When it is anticipated that there may be difficulty from overloading of fluids, as in elderly patients or patients with pre-existing cardiovascular disease, the cutdown cannula should be put in a large vein and the central venous pressure monitored. One can continue to give fluids without fear of overloading as long as the venous pressure does not rise above normal.

Most of the calculated colloid requirements should be given early. Plasmanate, virus-free plasma and dextran are all acceptable colloid solutions. Patients with flame burns rarely need blood in the first six days. Some patients with electrical injuries require blood for resuscitation in the first 24 hours. Thereafter, the blood requirements should be determined by the hematocrit. When the hematocrit falls below 36, blood should be given.

Because of the tendency of metabolic acidosis to develop in the early postburn period, lactated Ringer's, a balanced salt solution, is preferred to normal saline for filling the electrolyte requirements.

Oral fluids should be withheld for two days in patients treated by intravenous infusion because of the fear of gastric distention and dilatation followed by vomiting and aspiration.

APPRAISAL OF THERAPY. Undoubtedly the most valuable single index for fluid replacement in the first 48 hours is the urinary output. In adults, fluid should be given so that the output is maintained in the range of 30 to 50 ml./hour. A decreasing blood pressure and a decreasing urinary output mean that more colloids should be given. A decreasing urinary output with normal blood pressure indicates that an electrolyte solution or water is required.

After 48 hours most of the fluid should be electrolyte-free water and blood. The most useful laboratory determination is the serum sodium concentration. The insensible water loss after the first 48 hours may be as much as 3 to 6 liters/day in an adult. After the acute stress of the injury, the body tends to conserve sodium. Little is excreted by the kidneys, so that the loss of water by the insensible route and by the urine will be relatively greater than the loss of sodium. Since the water load diminishes more rapidly than the sodium load, a rise in serum sodium usually occurs. A serum sodium concentration of 135 to 140 mEq./liter is usually ideal in the first few days after injury. When the serum sodium rises to 140 mEq. or more, additional electrolyte-free water must be given. By the third day many patients will take oral fluids and regulate their own intake. When food cannot be taken after 72 hours, it may be necessary to give 40 to 80 mEq. of potassium each day.

ACUTE RENAL INSUFFICIENCY. Many physicians fear acute renal insufficiency in burns, and there is little doubt that renal function is considerably diminished after severe thermal trauma when no treatment is instituted. With adequate replacement, however, diminution of renal function is minimal. The clinician's dilemma usually arises when the patient, who has seemingly received adequate fluid replacement, fails to excrete urine. An infusion test may be given to determine whether the oliguria is due to decreased plasma volume or to acute renal failure. Approximately 1 liter of plasma or dextran is given in 30 minutes as a test load. If no increase in urine excretion occurs, renal insufficiency is likely. Laboratory determinations of urine osmolarity and sodium content may be of diagnostic value. A low urine osmolarity suggests renal insufficiency, and a high osmolarity is evidence that insufficient replacement therapy has been given. If the urinary sodium is above 40 mEq./liter there is evidence that the kidney is failing to reabsorb sodium, and acute renal insufficiency is suspected. If the urinary sodium is less than 20 mEq., tubular reabsorption appears to be adequate and additional fluids should be given.

Tracheostomy. Tracheostomy is indicated in all patients with respiratory tract injury from the inhalation of noxious gases and in some very deep burns of the face and neck. Most patients with burns involving the head and neck do not require tracheostomy. Furthermore, if a tracheotomy is performed through burned tissue, purulent drainage from the wound will carry organisms into the lower respiratory tree. There is also the possibility of mechanical injury to the trachea from the cannula. Nevertheless, when respiratory distress develops tracheostomy is indicated.

The initial effect of inhalation of flames and noxious irritants associated with flame burns of the face and upper chest is laryngeal edema. This may appear early but in most cases symptoms of respiratory distress are delayed for hours. Cough, labored breathing and sometimes stridor develop. Tracheostomy relieves respiratory obstruction and improves tracheobronchial toilet. When respiratory tract damage is present the best therapy in addition to tracheostomy is antibiotics and adrenocorticosteroids.

Tetanus Immunization. All patients with severe burns should receive prophylaxis against tetanus. If the patient has maintained appropriate basic immunization, prophylaxis consists of a booster dose of alum-precipitated toxoid. Passive immunity is best achieved with human immune globulin.

Antibiotics. Because of the frequent infection of burn wounds with beta hemolytic streptococci, penicillin should be given to patients with major burns for five days. Thereafter, it should be discontinued or changed in accordance with the degree and type of infection present. Cultures of the burn wound should be taken at regular intervals throughout the course of therapy.

Narcotics. One of the greatest deterrents to an adequate nutritional intake is the use of narcotics in burned patients. Few narcotics should be necessary. Soon after the burn one or two doses of a narcotic may be used intravenously. After this time, to prevent addiction, anorexia and constipation, narcotics should not be used except in connection with operative procedures. Most burned patients require the judicious use of hypnotics and tranquilizing drugs.

WOUND CARE

After replacement therapy has been instituted, attention may be directed to the care of the burn wound. Every effort should be made to minimize further contamination and achieve a clean wound. The patient should be taken to a dressing room or operating room for cleansing of the burned areas with bland soap and water. All debris and detached epidermis should be removed.

There are many accepted methods of caring for the burn wound. They include initial excision, dressings with or without antibacterial creams and exposure with or without antibacterial agents. In minor burns antibacterial agents are probably unnecessary. In more extensive burns these medicaments considerably diminish infection. Most surgeons use all methods. The type selected varies with each patient. In many instances some areas may be treated by one method and other areas by another in the same patient. At times treatment of a burn may be started by one method of local care and then changed to another during the course of therapy. It is up to the physician to select the method most desirable for a particular patient at a particular time. The choice of the method is determined by the location of the burn, size of the injury, depth of the burn, type of patient, facilities available and the patient's response. Small full-thickness burns lend themselves to initial excision. Most patients treated on an outpatient basis do better when the wounds are dressed. Exposure and the use of antibacterial agents are preferred for extensive burns.

Initial Excision and Grafting. This method has one great advantage in that all the burned area can be excised soon after injury and a graft applied two days later. This permits the patient to be discharged from the hospital much earlier than by other methods of management. The technique is particularly indicated in small full-thickness burns with clearly defined edges. It is also preferred in some types of electrical injury. Excision is usually accomplished in the first 48 hours under general anesthesia. The burned skin and underlying subcutaneous tissue down to the fascia are completely excised and careful hemostasis is achieved. A large bulky dressing is applied and skin grafting is performed three or four days later.

In patients with burns not exceeding 15 per cent of the body surface and when there is definite evidence that the injury is third degree, initial excision followed by grafting is desirable. Treatment of more extensive wounds by initial excision is contraindicated.

Dressing Method. The aim of a good dressing is to cover the open wound to protect it from infection. The material placed next to the wound may be commercially prepared nylon fabric (Adaptic), lightly impregnated petrolatum gauze, Carbowax gauze or plain dry fine-mesh gauze. When antibacterial agents such as Gentamicin cream or silver sulfadiazine cream are used, the ointment is spread on dry fine-mesh gauze and placed next to the wound.

The dressing should be occlusive to prevent the invasion of bacteria; it should be absorptive to keep the wound surface dry; and it should be applied with even resilient compression. A burn dressing should be changed every two to five days. If it is a large dressing, and changing may cause considerable pain, use of ketamine analgesia is to be recommended.

With some of the antibacterial creams a very light dressing is placed over the cream which is changed daily. This is not an occlusive method technique for the management of the burn wound.

Exposure Method. The exposure method is preferred for most burns. Usually the burn wound is exposed and some type of antibacterial cream, such as Sulfamylon or silver sulfadiazine, is applied daily.

The usual technique of exposure is to apply the antibacterial cream immediately after thorough cleansing. Each 24 hours the patient is bathed and all the cream removed or the patient is placed in a Hubbard tank. After the wounds are thoroughly cleansed another application of the antibacterial cream is made. This offers the best control of infection. In addition, it allows for motion of joints and is very comfortable for the patient.

Burns of the hands have always presented special problems. Like other areas, there are many ways to manage burns of the hands. At the present time, the best technique seems to be the use of an antibacterial agent removed and replaced daily and an abundant amount of active motion.

Antibacterial creams have the real advantage of reducing the magnitude of the bacterial population in and around the burn wound. They have one disadvantage in that the eschar remains firmly attached to the underlying tissue for a much longer period of time than when other methods are used. When antibacterial creams are used one should be particularly careful to evaluate the eschar at about the twenty-eighth day. If healing beneath it is not almost complete, it probably should be removed surgically and a skin graft applied.

Use of Escharotomy. The formation of a dry, leathery eschar will on occasion result in ischemia of the extremity distal to the constriction. A circumferential eschar of the chest may inhibit respiratory excursion. When there is a very deep circumferential burn of the extremity, there may be avascular necrosis of the deeper tissue. Such a tragic circumstance occurs when burn wound edema progressively accumulates beneath the unyielding eschar, the resulting pressure occluding first the venous and then the arterial blood supply. At the first sign of vascular insufficiency, escharotomy down to or including the fascia should be done.

GRAFTING

Prevention of serious complications and ensuring a satisfactory recovery depend upon an aggressive approach to early wound closure. The surgeon should establish a timetable for the application of grafts. All well treated burned patients should be completely covered by three months post injury unless homografts have been required as a life-saving measure. The first grafting procedure should be performed at least by the thirtieth day. In small wounds it may be possible to have the area ready for grafting at the end of two weeks.

Preparation of the Recipient Site. Several methods may be employed to prepare the recipient site for grafting. Frequent changes of dry dressing will achieve the desired result in most cases. An excellent method for cleansing a wound is the application of wet dressings which are changed every four hours. They afford good drainage for the wound and decrease the bacterial inoculum. Sometimes immersing the patient in a Hubbard tank is helpful in cleansing the wound and preparing the area for grafting.

Removal of Skin for Grafting. In extensive burns, flat surfaces should be covered with skin approximately 0.010 to 0.012 of an inch in thickness. Skin for areas over joints should be somewhat thicker—about 0.015 of an inch.

The donor site should be the most accessible area from which skin can be taken and the site then properly exposed.

A variety of instruments is available for obtaining a split-thickness graft. The instrument used varies with the experience of the operator and the type of skin required. The Brown and Howmet air-driven dermatomes are both very excellent instruments for obtaining skin in burned patients. They are easy to use and skin can be obtained rapidly.

On uneven surfaces a Pitkin syringe may be used to inject saline into the subcutaneous tissue to provide a smooth surface. This technique is of particular value on the feet, over the rib cage, and on the arms and lower legs.

The Padgett and Reese dermatomes are drum type instruments useful for obtaining grafts from uneven surfaces. A wider piece of skin can be excised with these instruments than with an air-driven dermatome and better skin for coverage of critical areas. A recent advance in the use of the Padgett dermatome is the availability of a special type of cellophane tape with adhesive surfaces on both sides. This tape is made to fit the drum. With this tape on the drum and cement on the skin, the drum adheres extremely well.

Treatment of Donor Sites. Donor sites are best treated by exposure. Fine-mesh gauze is placed over the donor area as soon as the skin is excised. A moist gauze pad is then applied to achieve hemostasis. At the end of the operative procedure, the pad is removed and the donor site is exposed to the air. A firm coagulum forms from the blood that is caught in the interlacing fibers of the gauze. This coagulum dries within 48 hours and serves as a protective covering for the wound. In about two weeks epithelization takes place. This crust loosens at the edges and falls off.

Application of Grafts. The best method of applying grafts to burned patients is by the lay-on technique. Occasionally a few sutures may be necessary where the skin is placed over irregular surfaces and points of motion. Sheets of skin are placed on the wound and pushed into position so that there is little space between them. In some instances where there are extensive areas to be covered and a minimal amount of skin is available, postage stamp grafts cut about 1 × 2 inches in size may be placed in brick layer fashion not more than half an inch apart.

When skin is applied by the lay-on technique, grafts may be exposed. This is the best technique for management of grafts, as it permits them to be observed carefully. As serum or purulent material collects beneath the graft it should be rolled out with an applicator.

When it is not possible to expose grafts, a large bulky dressing should be applied and must be changed in five days.

Homografts. Undoubtedly the best dressing for a burn wound is a homograft or heterograft. Postmortem homografts taken from a recently deceased body, homografts taken from a live donor and porcine heterografts all work extremely well.

Homografts as biological skin dressings may be used in a number of ways. They are extremely valuable in the critically burned patient who has a large open wound but is too ill to withstand an autografting procedure. Homografts changed every three days for a week or so will diminish fluid and protein losses from the wound while the patient's general condition is improving.

In some very extensively burned patients where there is not enough autograft skin to cover a recipient site, the remainder of the area may be treated with homografts until another crop of autograft skin can be taken.

Acceleration of the healing process of partial-thickness burns occurs beneath the homograft. A good method of preparing recipient sites for grafting is by the use of homografts. These may be applied every three days until the wound is ready for grafting.

Postgraft Care. When patients have been virtually covered with skin with only small granulating areas remaining, daily tubbing in the Hubbard tank for cleanliness and exercise is useful. Following soaking and exercise in the tank, small granulating areas are covered with fine-mesh gauze.

After the acute phase of the burn, ambulation is encouraged. If there has been injury to the lower limbs, elastic supportive dressings must be applied. They are worn until complete restoration of circulatory equilibrium has been established, which usually takes about three months.

NUTRITIONAL SUPPORT

The amount of nitrogen per square meter of body surface per day necessary for equilibrium in the first three weeks following injury is about 20 to 25 gm.; later this diminishes to 12 to 16 gm. The aim is to achieve a daily protein intake of 2 to 3 gm./kg. of body weight with a caloric intake of 50 to 70 calories/kg.

Burned patients should receive two multiple vitamin tablets and additional ascorbic acid each day.

Unfortunately, the burned patient will rarely maintain an oral intake to meet his requirements. It is almost always necessary to administer supplementary high protein between-meal feedings. A liter of this supplementary preparation each day in addition to a high protein, high calorie diet is desirable.

When the patient does not maintain an adequate intake voluntarily, it may be necessary to insert a nasogastric feeding tube for the administration of a high protein formula on an hourly basis. Extreme care must be used with feeding tubes in children and in seriously ill patients to avoid acute gastric dilatation.

SPECIAL PROBLEMS

Electrical Injury. Electrical injuries are usually deeper than ordinary flame burns. Because there is usually damage to the deeper tissues by the electricity, an electrical injury more nearly simulates crush injury than it does a thermal burn. Damage associated with electricity may be divided into three categories. *Electrical contact injury* caused by an electric current passing through the skin produces damage to the skin, subcutaneous tissue, muscle and other deeper structures. It is well known that the current follows blood vessels and that thrombosis, even at some distance from the original injury, is common. Thrombosis is partly responsible for the fact that more tissue is always destroyed by an electrical injury than is apparent at first inspection. Necrosis of blood vessel walls frequently leads to secondary hemorrhage. *Electrical thermal burns,* which result from electrical generation of heat outside the skin such as flash or arc burns, occur by the leaping of an electric arc from the conductor to the skin. These are mainly associated with high intensity current which results in severe burns of the skin caused by the high intensity heat of short duration. *Flame burns* resulting from the ignition of clothing by electrical sparks or arcing are sometimes associated with electrical injury. Many times all three types of injury are evident in the same patient.

The treatment of electrical thermal burns and flame burns associated with ignition of clothing is the same as for any similar thermal injury. The management of a true electrical injury, however, is entirely different. Such an injury must be recognized early. There is usually dead and devitalized muscle beneath the charred skin. If dead muscle is present, it must be excised. Failure to remove the extensively damaged muscle may lead to clostridial myositis and death. After excision a dressing should be applied and the wound reinspected with possible further debridement three or four days later.

Renal damage is more common and therefore massive replacement therapy is essential. In many instances the use of an osmotic diuretic is indicated. An electrical injury with associated thermal injury does not conform to the usual requirements for replacement therapy. Electrical injury always requires more fluid therapy than a thermal burn of similar extent.

Burns of the Eyes. Burn of the tissue of the eye rarely occurs in the absence of deep incineration of surrounding tissue, electrical or chemical injury. The lids and surrounding skin of the forehead, however, are frequently burned. The resultant contracture which occurs not only in full-thickness burns but also in deep second-degree burns frequently results in ectropion. If there is a burn around the eye it should be repeatedly irrigated and a bland ointment instilled daily. The chief problem with burns about the eye is the drying of the cornea. This may result in chronic conjunctivitis and corneal ulceration.

If an ectropion is mild and the secondary conjunctivitis easily controlled, correction should be delayed until maturation of the involved tissue has occurred. Should the ectropion become rapidly progressive, tarsorrhaphy should be accomplished. It should be performed at the first indication that the lids are not closing sufficiently to protect the cornea from drying.

Burns of the Ears. Except in very deep burns it is impossible to predict how much of the substance of the ear will ultimately be lost. The cause of the difficulty is not the immediate burn injury but the chrondritis that may follow. A slow, painful, red, suppurative chondritis may occur beneath a superficial second-degree burn of the ear or in deeper burns. Once the chondritis has developed, surgical evacuation of the necrotic cartilage must be performed. This is best achieved through a linear incision along the curved margin of the helix of the ear with sharp and blunt dissection of the necrotic cartilage. Following this, a fine-mesh gauze pack is inserted and wet saline compresses are used.

Curling's Ulcer. The exact incidence of gastroduodenal ulceration associated with burns is difficult to evaluate; it may be as high as 20 per cent. Ulcers may occur in the stomach or in the duodenum or other parts of the small intestine. They are most common in the stomach and a high percentage in this area are multiple. Many ulcers give few if any symptoms unless there is hemorrhage or perforation. Not infrequently ulcers develop and are completely unrecognized until noted as an incidental finding at autopsy. Frequently, there are no signs or symptoms of ulcer formation. Patients may complain of some abdominal discomfort and if a nasogastric tube is in place, small amounts of blood may be seen. The first sign is usually related to acute hemorrhage or perforation. Ulcers may develop as early as the first or second postburn day, but the usual time for manifestation of hemorrhage is near the end of the first week.

When perforation occurs, it should be surgically closed. When bleeding occurs a nasogastric tube should be inserted and the stomach irrigated frequently with iced saline. If the hemorrhage does not stop, operation will be necessary. One should not delay an inordinate period before operation if hemorrhage is continuing. The main indications for severe hemorrhage apply to Curling's ulcers as to any type of bleeding gastrointestinal ulcer. There is a common belief that gastrointestinal bleeding in burned patients may be coming from multiple small ulcers in the stomach and jejunum. This is not true. Practically all ulcers associated with burns that produce massive hemorrhage are located in the stomach or the duodenum. Usually there is one large ulcer overlying a good sized blood vessel. The operative procedure of choice is a resection of about two thirds of the stomach performed as rapidly and expeditiously as possible.

Septicemia. Septicemia or overwhelming sepsis appears to be the terminal and causative complication in a high proportion of fatal burn cases. The coagulase-positive *Staphylococcus aureus* and *Pseudomonas* are the most common offending organisms. *S. aureus* invades the blood stream rather early and may give rise to small abscesses in the viscera. Pseudomonas sepsis presents an entirely different picture. Pseudomonas infection seems to spread by way of the lymph channels and outside the blood vessels. Rarely is there any evidence of abscesses in the abdominal organs.

Ideally, therapy for septicemia should commence as soon as clinical suspicion is aroused and before the full blown pattern becomes manifest. At the first signs that the disease might be developing, a patient should be given large doses of sodium oxacillin and gentamicin. For pseudomonas sepsis, gentamicin and carbenicillin are recommended.

Blood cultures should be drawn two or three times a day. When a positive blood culture is obtained, antibiotic therapy should be given according to the sensitivity of the organisms involved. Infections with gram-positive organisms usually respond to sodium oxacillin. Cephalothin may be of value also. In well established gram-negative septicemia, colistimethate sodium and kanamycin may be combined.

One of the more important aspects in the treatment of septicemia is the management of the wound. Care of the wound depends upon its status at the time septicemia is recognized. Every effort should be made to debride the eschar progressively and to cover the wound with autografts or homografts. Wet soaks will provide good drainage and at the same time assist in the removal of the slough.

Supportive therapy in the form of whole blood transfusions should be combined with massive antibiotic therapy. Because the insensible water loss in septicemia is quite high, a good intake of water is mandatory.

REFERENCES

Artz, C. P., and Moncrief, J. A.: The Treatment of Burns. 2nd Ed. Philadelphia, W. B. Saunders Co., 1969.

Moncrief, J. A.: Complications of burns and burn treatment; *In* Artz, C. P., and Hardy, J. D. (eds.): Complications in Surgery and Their Management. 2nd Ed. Philadelphia, W. B. Saunders Co., 1967.

Order, S. E., and Moncrief, J. A.: The Burn Wound. Springfield, Ill., Charles C Thomas, 1965.

Stone, N. H., and Boswick, J. A., Jr.: Profiles of Burn Management. Miami, Industrial Medicine Publishing Company, Inc., 1969.

APPENDIX

NORMAL BLOOD, PLASMA AND SERUM VALUES

For some procedures, the values may vary depending on the method of analysis used. The range of normal includes both normal biologic variation and the error inherent in the laboratory method of determining a particular value. In many instances, the ranges will be the mean (average) value in man, ± two standard deviations of the mean, and thus will encompass 95 per cent of the total distribution of values found in groups of presumably well persons of various ages and of both sexes.

Good biochemistry and clinical pathological laboratory procedure should include not only frequent checking of methods against meticulously prepared standards, including serum pools, but also the routine of repeating the determination on any blood or other specimen in which an abnormal value has been found. Additional specimens should be obtained for analysis whenever needed to check an abnormal value. Serious deviation from normal should be reported at once as an emergency to permit immediate action in treatment. Emergency reporting levels are suggested in the tables for a number of procedures.

It is wise for the surgeon to determine, from each laboratory to which he may send specimens, what the normal range is *for that laboratory* for each commonly used test. It is also important to consult with the clinical pathologist or clinical biochemist in charge of the laboratory when wide fluctuation in reported values, or abnormal values that do not apparently fit the clinical picture, are found. Repeating the determinations and re-examining the patient will usually solve the problem. Additional tests may be recommended that will assist in clarifying more obscure difficulties.

FUNCTION TESTS FOR EVALUATION OF ORGANS AND SYSTEMS

Several of the following tests are related to body surface area in square meters, and Figure 3 will be found useful (DuBois, 1936). Note that height is in centimeters and weight in kilograms.

(Text continued on page 613)

605

Normal Blood, Plasma and Serum Values*
For some procedures the normal values may vary depending upon the methods used.

Acetone, serum	
Qualitative	Negative
Quantitative	0.3–2.0 mg./100 ml.
Aldolase, serum	0.8–3.0 mI. U./ml. (30°) (Sibley-Lehninger)
Alpha amino nitrogen (serum)	4–6 mg./100 ml.
Amino acid nitrogen, serum	4–6 mg./100 ml.
Ammonia nitrogen, blood	75–196 mcg./100 ml.
plasma	56–122 mcg./100 ml.
Amylase, serum	80–160 Somogyi units/100 ml.
Ascorbic acid	See Vitamin C
Base, total, serum	145–160 mEq./liter
Bilirubin, serum	
Direct	0.1–0.4 mg./100 ml.
Indirect	0.2–0.7 mg./100 ml.
	(Total minus direct)
Total	0.3–1.1 mg./100 ml.
Calcium, serum	4.5–5.5 mEq./liter
	(9.0–11.0 mg./100 ml.)
	(Slightly higher in children)
	(Varies with protein concentration)
Calcium, serum, ionized	2.1–2.6 mEq./liter
	(4.25–5.25 mg./100 ml.)
Carbon dioxide content, serum	24–30 mEq./liter
	Infants: 20–28 mEq./liter
Carbon dioxide tension (P_{CO_2}), blood	35–45 mm. Hg
Carotene, serum	50–300 mcg./100 ml.
Ceruloplasmin, serum	23–44 mg./100 ml.
Chloride, serum	96–106 mEq./liter
Cholesterol, serum	
Total	150–250 mg./100 ml.
Esters	68–76% of total cholesterol
Cholinesterase, serum	0.5–1.3 pH units
RBC	0.5–1.0 pH units
Copper, serum	
Male	70–140 mcg./100 ml.
Female	85–155 mcg./100 ml.
Cortisol, plasma	6–16 mcg./100 ml.
Creatine, serum	0.2–0.8 mg./100 ml.
Creatine phosphokinase, serum	
Male	0–50 mI. U./ml. (30°) (Oliver-Rosalki)
Female	0–30 mI. U./ml. (30°) (Oliver-Rosalki)
Creatinine, serum	0.7–1.5 mg./100 ml.
Cryoglobulins, serum	0
Fatty acids, total, serum	190–420 mg./100 ml.
Fibrinogen, plasma	200–400 mg./100 ml.
Folic acid, serum	7–16 nanogm./ml.
Glucose (fasting)	
blood, true	60–100 mg./100 ml.
Folin	80–120 mg./100 ml.
plasma or serum, true	70–115 mg./100 ml.
Haptoglobin, serum	40–170 mg./100 ml.
Hydroxybutyric dehydrogenase, serum	0–180 mI. U./ml. (30°) (Rosalki-Wilkinson)
	114–290 units/ml. (Wroblewski)

*From Conn, R. B., *in* Current Therapy – 1972 (H. F. Conn, ed.).

Normal Blood, Plasma and Serum Values *(Continued)*

17-Hydroxycorticosteroids, plasma	8–18 mcg./100 ml.
Icterus index, serum	4–7
Immunoglobulins, serum	
IgG	800–1500 mg./100 ml.
IgA	50–200 mg./100 ml.
IgM	40–120 mg./100 ml.
Iodine, butanol extractable, serum	3.2–6.4 mcg./100 ml.
Iodine, protein bound, serum	3.5–8.0 mcg./100 ml.
	(May be slightly higher in infants)
Iron, serum	75–175 mcg./100 ml.
Iron binding capacity, total, serum	250–410 mcg./100 ml.
% saturation	20–55%
17-Ketosteroids, plasma	25–125 mcg./100 ml.
Lactic acid, blood	6–16 mcg./100 ml.
Lactic dehydrogenase, serum	0–300 mI.U./ml. (30°) (Wroblewski modified)
	150–450 units/ml. (Wroblewski)
	80–120 units/ml. (Wacker)
	0–1.5 units (Cherry-Crandall)
Lipase, serum	450–850 mg./100 ml.
Lipids, total, serum	1.5–2.5 mEq./liter
Magnesium, serum	(1.8–3.0 mg./100 ml.)
Nitrogen, nonprotein, serum	15–35 mg./100 ml.
Osmolality, serum	285–295 mOsm./liter
Oxygen, blood	
Capacity	16–24 vol. % (varies with Hb)
Content Arterial	15–23 vol. %
Venous	10–16 vol. %
Saturation Arterial	94–100% of capacity
Venous	60–85% of capacity
Tension, PO_2 Arterial	75–100 mm. Hg
pH, arterial, blood	7.35–7.45
Phenylalanine, serum	Less than 3 mg./100 ml.
Phosphatase, acid, serum	1.0–5.0 units (King-Armstrong)
	0.5–2.0 units (Bodansky)
	0.5–2.0 units (Gutman)
	0.0–1.1 units (Shinowara)
	0.1–0.63 units (Bessey-Lowry)
Phosphatase, alkaline, serum	5.0–13.0 units (King-Armstrong)
	2.0–4.5 units (Bodansky)
	3.0–10.0 units (Gutman)
	2.2–8.6 units (Shinowara)
	0.8–2.3 units (Bassey-Lowry)
	30–85 milliunits/ml. (I.U.)
	(Values are higher in children)
Phosphate, inorganic, serum	3.0–4.5 mg./100 ml.
	(Children: 4.0–7.0 mg./100 ml.)
Phospholipids, serum	6–12 mg./100 ml. as lipid phosphorus
Potassium, serum	3.5–5.0 mEq./liter
Proteins, serum	
Total	6.0–8.0 grams/100 ml.
Albumin	3.5–5.5 grams/100 ml.
Globulin	2.5–3.5 grams/100 ml.

NORMAL BLOOD, PLASMA AND SERUM VALUES *(Continued)*

Electrophoresis	
Albumin	3.5–5.5 grams/100 ml.
	52–68% of total
Globulin	
Alpha$_1$	0.2–0.4 gram/100 ml.
	2–5% of total
Alpha$_2$	0.5–0.9 gram/100 ml.
	7–14% of total
Beta	0.6–1.1 grams/100 ml.
	9–15% of total
Gamma	0.7–1.7 grams/100 ml.
	11–21% of total
Pyruvic acid, plasma	1.0–2.0 mg./100 ml.
Serotonin, platelet suspension	0.1–0.3 mcg./ml. blood
serum	0.10–0.32 mcg./ml.
Sodium, serum	136–145 mEq./liter
Sulfates, inorganic, serum	0.8–1.2 mg./100 ml. (as S)
Thyroxine, free, serum	1.0–2.1 nanogm./100 ml.
Thyroxine binding globulin (TBG), serum	10–26 mcg./100 ml.
Thyroxine iodine (T$_4$), serum	2.9–6.4 mcg./100 ml.
Transaminase, serum: SGOT	0–19 mI.U./ml. (30°) (Karmen modified)
	15–40 units/ml. (Karmen)
	18–40 units/ml. (Reitman-Frankel)
SGPT	0–17 mI.U./ml. (30°) (Karmen modified)
	6–35 units/ml. (Karmen)
	5–35 units/ml. (Reitman-Frankel)
Triglycerides, serum	0–150 mg./100 ml.
Urea, blood	21–43 mg./100 ml.
plasma or serum	24–49 mg./100 ml.
Urea nitrogen, blood (BUN)	10–20 mg./100 ml.
plasma or serum	11–23 mg./100 ml.
Uric acid, serum	
Male	2.5–8.0 mg./100 ml.
Female	1.5–6.0 mg./100 ml.
Vitamin A, serum	20–80 mcg./100 ml.
Vitamin B$_{12}$, serum	200–800 picogm./ml.
Vitamin C, blood	0.4–1.5 mg./100 ml.

NORMAL URINE VALUES

		SUGGESTED EMERGENCY REPORT VALUES
Acetone and acetoacetate	0	>2+ >1+ with positive glucose
Aldosterone	6 to 16 μg./24 hours	
Ammonia	20 to 70 mEq./liter	
Amylase (Somogyi)	Up to 4000 units/24 hours	
Calcium		
Low intake (300 mg./day)	Less than 150 mg./24 hours	
Normal diet	Less than 250 mg./24 hours	
Catecholamines	0 to 0.08 mg./gm. creatinine 0.07 to 0.19 mg./gm. creatinine (children)	
Chorionic gonadotropins	0	
Creatine		
(male)	5.1 to 8.8% of creatinine	
(female)	4.8 to 18% of creatinine (Higher in children & in pregnancy)	
Creatinine	15 to 25 mg./kg./24 hours	
Cystine or cysteine	0	
5-hydroxy-indoleacetic acid	< 16 mg./24 hours	
17-hydroxycorticoids		
male	5 to 15 mg./24 hours	
female	4 to 10 mg./24 hours (Depends on method used)	
17-ketosteroids		
Male	10 to 20 mg./24 hours	
Female	5 to 15 mg./24 hours	
Child <8	0 to 2 mg./24 hours	
Magnesium	24 to 36% of dietary intake	
pH	4.6 to 8.0, average 6.0 (Depends on diet)	
Phosphorus	53 to 61% of dietary intake	
Pituitary gonadotropins		
Male	6.5 to 13 mouse units	
Female	6.5 to 52 mouse units	
Postmenopausal	> 104 mouse units	
Child	0 to 6.5 mouse units	
Potassium	66 to 90% of dietary intake	
Protein	0 (Quantitative < 30 mg./24 hours)	
Specific gravity	1.003 to 1.030	
Sodium	88 to 100% of dietary intake	
Sugar	0	3+ or 4+ with acetone 1+ or more
Titratable acidity	20 to 40 mEq./24 hours	
Urobilinogen	0.1 to 1.5 E units/2 hours	
Vanilmandelic acid (VMA)	11 to 25 mg./gm. creatinine	

Normal Values for Cerebrospinal Fluid

		Suggested Emergency Report Values
Cells	0 to 5, all mononuclear	>25 cells
Chloride	116 to 132 mEq./liter	
Glucose	38 to 82 mg./100 ml.	<20 mg./100 ml.
Pressure	70 to 180 mm. of fluid	
Protein	21 to 38 mg./100 ml.	>60 mg./100 ml.

Normal Values for Gastric Analysis

Acidity	
Fasting	Free, 0 to 30 degrees/100 ml.
	Total, 10 to 50 degrees/100 ml.
1 hour after histamine	Free, 30 to 85 degrees/100 ml.
Volume, fasting	50 to 100 ml.
Color	Opalescent to colorless
Specific gravity	1.006 to 1.009
pH (adults)	0.8 to 1.5

NORMAL HEMATOLOGIC VALUES

		SUGGESTED EMERGENCY REPORT VALUES
Bleeding time		
Ivy	Less than 4 min.	>6 min.
Duke	1 to 4 min.	>6 min.
Cell counts		
Erythrocytes		
Male	5.4 ± 0.8 million/cu. mm.	
Female	4.8 ± 0.6 million/cu. mm.	
Children	4.5 to 5.1 million/cu. mm. (Varies with age)	
Leukocytes	5000 to 10,000/cu. mm.	>15,000 or <3000 + all abnormal forms
Myelocytes or earlier forms	0	All early forms
Juvenile neutrophils	3 to 5%	
Segmented neutrophils	54 to 62%	
Lymphocytes	25 to 33%	
Monocytes	3 to 7%	
Eosinophils	1 to 3%	
Basophils	0 to 0.75% (Infants and children have a higher percentage of lymphocytes and monocytes)	
Platelets	150,000 to 450,000/cu. mm.	<100,000
Reticulocytes	0.5 to 1.5% of RBC	
Coagulation time	Glass tubes, 6 to 17 min. Silicone tubes, 19 to 60 min.	>125% normal unless under anticoagulant therapy
Hematocrit		
Male	47.0 ± 7.0 ml./100 ml.	<30 or >60
Female	42.0 ± 5.0 ml./100 ml.	<30 or >55
Newborn	49.0 to 54.0 ml./100 ml.	<30 or >55
Children	35 to 49 ml./100 ml.	<30 or >55
Prothrombin time	Same as control	
Prothrombin content	100%	<50% unless under anticoagulant therapy when <10%

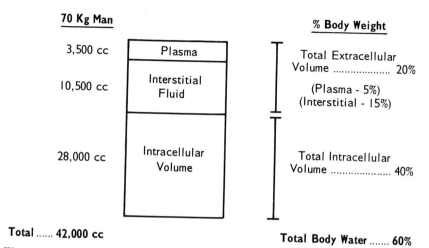

70 Kg Man

3,500 cc	Plasma
10,500 cc	Interstitial Fluid
28,000 cc	Intracellular Volume

Total ...... 42,000 cc

% Body Weight

Total Extracellular Volume 20%

(Plasma - 5%)
(Interstitial - 15%)

Total Intracellular Volume 40%

Total Body Water 60%

Figure 1. Functional compartments of body units. (Supplied by G. Tom Shires, M.D.)

PLASMA

154 mEq/l		154 mEq/l	
CATIONS		**ANIONS**	
Na⁺	142	Cl⁻	103
		HCO₃⁻	27
		SO₄⁻⁻ PO₄⁻⁻⁻	3
K⁺	4		
Ca⁺⁺	5	Organic Acids	5
Mg⁺⁺	3	Protein	16

PLASMA

INTERSTITIAL FLUID

153 mEq/l		153 mEq/l	
CATIONS		**ANIONS**	
Na⁺	144	Cl⁻	114
		HCO₃⁻	30
K⁺	4	SO₄⁻⁻ PO₄⁻⁻⁻	3
Ca⁺⁺	3	Organic Acids	5
Mg⁺⁺	2	Proteins	1

INTERSTITIAL FLUID

INTRACELLULAR FLUID

200 mEq/l		200 mEq/l	
CATIONS		**ANIONS**	
K⁺	150	HPO₄⁼ SO₄⁻⁻	150
		HCO₃⁻	10
Mg⁺⁺	40	Protein	40
Na⁺	10		

INTRACELLULAR FLUID

Figure 2. Chemical composition of body fluid compartments. (Suppled by G. Tom Shires, M.D.)

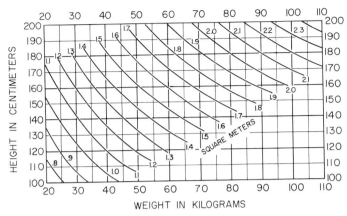

Figure 3.

PULMONARY FUNCTION TESTS

Comroe and associates divide tests of pulmonary function into those useful in office, clinic or small hospital, those useful in cardiopulmonary laboratory in a medical center, and those for a research cardiopulmonary laboratory.*

Vital Capacity. Two formulas give vital capacity in cubic centimeters of air.

Male: $(-38 \times \text{age}) + (121 \times \text{height in inches}) - 2100. \pm 970$ cc.
Female: $(-22 \times \text{age}) + (110 \times \text{height in inches}) - 2980. \pm 790$ cc.

Alternate formula:

Male: $[27.63 - (0.122 \times \text{age in years})] \times \text{height in cm.}$
Female: $[21.78 - (0.101 \times \text{age in years})] \times \text{height in cm.}$

Pulmonary Ventilation. Clinical and fluoroscopic evaluation of reasons for hypoventilation consists of measurements of rate, tidal volume and minute volume, plus basal oxygen consumption.

Rate (basal conditions): 11 to 14/minute (adult).

Tidal volume (basal conditions): 450 to 600 ml. (adult).

Minute volume (basal conditions): SA = surface area in square meters. SD = standard deviation. The result is expressed in liters/minute.

Age range	Males	Females
16–34	$3.6 \times \text{SA}$ (SD $0.3 \times \text{SA}$)	$3.2 \times \text{SA}$ (SD $0.4 \times \text{SA}$)
35–49	$3.1 \times \text{SA}$ (SD $0.5 \times \text{SA}$)	$3.2 \times \text{SA}$ (SD $0.4 \times \text{SA}$)
50–69	$3.9 \times \text{SA}$ (SD $0.45 \times \text{SA}$)	$3.4 \times \text{SA}$ (SD $0.4 \times \text{SA}$)

Basal oxygen consumption: 135 to 145 ml./min./square meter $\pm 10\%$.

---

*Comroe, J. H., et al.: *The Lung: Clinical Physiology and Pulmonary Function Tests.* 2nd edition. Chicago, Year Book Medical Publishers, Inc., 1963. Only those values for office, clinic or small hospital are summarized here, and the reader is referred to Comroe and to other publications for more extensive detail.

DISTRIBUTION. Clinical and radiologic evidence of uneven expansion of lungs, changes in breath sounds, percussion notes and radiolucent areas.

Pulmonary Circulation. Clinical, electrocardiographic and radiologic means provide evidence of pulmonary hypertension or congestion, circulation times and venous pressure.

Abnormalities of pulmonary vascular markings can be determined by x-ray. Pulmonary bruits and lung scanning with albumin microaggregates may indicate abnormalities.

Alveolar-Capillary Diffusion. There are no specific tests. See Comroe for discussion.

Arterial O_2, CO_2 and pH. Look for cyanosis and for increased RBC mass and hemoglobin; measure changes in respiration rate and pulse on breathing oxygen. Measure blood gases and pH (normal values for blood oxygen, arterial pH and serum carbon dioxide are given on pages 606 and 607).

Mechanical Factors in Breathing. All tests are to be performed before and after administration of bronchodilator drugs.

Maximum expiratory and inspiratory flow rates (normal, > 200 liters/minute at peak).

Maximum voluntary ventilation (maximum breathing capacity), which depends highly on patient cooperation. Normal values:

Males: $[86.5 - (0.522 \times age\ in\ years)] \times SA$ in square meters
Females: $[71.3 - (0.474 \times age\ in\ years)] \times SA$ in square meters

Forced expiratory volume (timed vital capacity): Normal values are 75 to 83 per cent of vital capacity in 1 second; 97 per cent of vital capacity in 3 seconds.

Analysis of spirogram: A high speed record of single maximum inspiration and expiration and pattern during maximum voluntary ventilation test may show significant changes.

CIRCULATORY FUNCTION TESTS

Blood Volume. "Normal" blood volume depends upon the method of determination, and also on patient age, sex, body habitus and history of recent change in body weight. Blood volume determinations are most useful in comparing sequential changes in the same patient. Plasma volume determinations using either I^{131} labeled albumin (RISA) or Evans Blue dye with multiple sampling points on the dilution curve are more accurate than single sample determinations, and are considerably more accurate than whole blood counting of an isotope, which is large vessel hematocrit dependent. Cr^{51} tagged red blood cell dilution measurements with timed samples are quite accurate when utilized with hematocrit determinations. Tourniquets *seriously* alter measurement accuracy by concentrating both red blood cells and plasma protein, with its label, in the vein distal to the occlusion. A false low value for blood volume and high value for hematocrit results.

The mixing time of radioactively labeled albumin or red blood cells, and of dyes, is prolonged in shock, and caution must be used in interpreting results obtained.

For a discussion of blood volume measurements, and nomograms for predicting normal values, see Dagher et al.: *Advances in Surgery* (Chicago, Year Book Medical Publishers, Inc., 1965), Vol. 1, pp. 69–108.

Approximate values for normal blood volumes* are as shown in the following table:

AGE	BLOOD VOLUME AS % OF BODY WEIGHT	AGE	BLOOD VOLUME AS % OF BODY WEIGHT
Female: 20–40	7.0%	Male: 20–40	8.0%
40–60	6.5%	40–60	7.5%
Over 60	6.0%	Over 60	7.0%

Obese patients will have a smaller blood volume, in terms of body weight, and thin or very muscular patients a somewhat higher value.

Cardiac Output. Cardiac output is measured either by the direct Fick method, measuring oxygen consumption in ml./minute and dividing by the arterial mixed central venous oxygen difference in ml./liter, or by the dilution method, using a rapid central venous injection of an indicator dye and measuring of changes in concentration of the dye during its initial circulation by continuous sampling of arterial blood. Cardiac output in the normal-sized, resting, healthy male averages almost exactly 6.0 liters/minute. Cardiac output falls slowly with age and may be 7 to 10 per cent lower in females. Cardiac output is increased by exercise, mild anoxia, fever, anxiety, pulmonary disease, anemia, hyperthyroidism and arteriovenous shunts. It usually rises significantly following trauma and with infection. It is low in myocardial infarction, severe valvular disease, and in traumatic, hemorrhagic and sometimes septic shock. A failure to respond by increasing cardiac output following major surgery and with infection may herald a fatal outcome; a fall in output is often followed by death.

Cardiac output is usually expressed as the *cardiac index,* which is the cardiac output in liters per minute divided by the body surface area (M²). The cardiac index of healthy young adults averages 3.52; that of 45 year old healthy patients averages 3.0. A cardiac index of 2.8 has been

---

*As measured by the sum of Cr^{51} tagged RBC and I^{131} RISA. Single isotope determinations and Evans Blue dye plasma volume determinations usually yield slightly higher values for total blood volume.

used as a baseline in surgical studies, relating cardiac index to response to surgery.

Central Venous Pressure. Central venous pressure measurements are determined at the level of the right atrium by the insertion of a venous catheter through a peripheral vein, either arm or external jugular, in the superior vena cava. The required catheter length from the point of insertion should be measured on the body surface, following the known course of the veins, prior to insertion of the catheter. The catheter is then attached to a simple water manometer, or to a strain gauge transducer. The level of the right atrium is approximated externally at the mid-axillary line. An infusion set is connected to permit flushing the catheter and filling the manometer with saline or other intravenous fluids, but this must be excluded when pressures are measured. Intrathoracic position of the catheter tip is indicated by changes of several millimeters of water pressure with each respiration, and by a sharp and immediate rise with the Valsalva maneuver.

Excessive catheter length is to be avoided to prevent the catheter tip's entering the heart or passing below the diaphragm. Catheters may be filled with a dilute heparin solution in saline between measurements if a slow infusion is contraindicated. It is better to use other venous channels for blood replacement and other parenteral fluids to avoid interruption of therapy with each venous pressure measurement.

Normal central venous pressure is from 6 to 16 cm. of saline or 5 to 12 mm. of Hg. If the central venous pressure is less than 6 or 7 cm. of saline, hypotension is likely to be due to decreased blood volume, whereas if the pressure is 15 cm. or more of saline, hypotension is unlikely to be due to a volume defect, and blood and fluid replacement are not ordinarily indicated.

See Chapters 9, 10 and 15 of this manual and A. C. Guyton: *Circulatory Physiology: Cardiac Output and Its Regulation* (Philadelphia, W. B. Saunders Co., 1963).

RENAL FUNCTION TESTS

Clearance Tests. The values shown have been corrected to 1.73 square meters of body surface area.

Glomerular filtration (GFR):

Inulin clearance	
Mannitol clearance	Males, 110 to 150 ml./minute
Endogenous creatinine clearance	Females, 105 to 132 ml./minute

Renal plasma flow (RPF):

Para amino hippurate (PAH)	Males, 560 to 830 ml./minute
Diodrast	Females, 490 to 700 ml./minute

Filtration fraction (FF)

$$\left.\frac{\text{GFR}}{\text{RPF}}\right\}$$

Males, 17 to 21%

Females, 17 to 23%

Maximal PAH excretory capacity (Tm_{PAH})   80 to 90 mg./minute

Phenolsulfonphthalein excretion (PSP): Urine excretion following intravenous injection:

> 25 per cent in 15 minutes
> 40 per cent in 30 minutes
> 55 per cent in 2 hours

Concentration in 24 hours: dry day, specific gravity 1.025; wet day, specific gravity 1.003.

GASTROINTESTINAL ABSORPTION TESTS

d-Xylose Absorption Test.   After an 8 hour fast, 10 ml./kg. body weight of 5 per cent d-xylose is given by mouth. Nothing further is given by mouth until the test is completed. All urine voided in the next 5 hours is pooled, and blood samples are taken at 0, 60 and 120 minutes. Normal urinary excretion is 16 to 33 per cent of ingested xylose, average 26 per cent, and normal blood levels of 25 to 40 mg./100 ml. are found at one and two hours.

Fat Absorption Tests. I^{131} triolein, 2 to 5 microcuries, by mouth, with neutral fat carrier. Normally, 90 to 95 per cent of the radioactivity is absorbed from the intestine, 10 per cent of the total dose is present in the total blood volume at 4 to 6 hours after ingestion.

TOTAL FAT.   Normally, 90 to 95 per cent of total ingested fat is absorbed, and stool contains less than 10 per cent of dietary fat with intake of from 50 to 200 gm. of fat a day.

Vitamin A Absorption Test.   A fasting blood specimen is obtained, and then 200,000 units of vitamin A is given by mouth. Serum vitamin A levels should rise to twice fasting levels in 3 to 5 hours.

Vitamin B_{12} Absorption Test.   One microcurie of Co^{57} labeled vitamin B_{12} is given in 5 μg. vitamin B_{12}, by mouth. Plasma activity is 1% of total dose per liter of plasma at 8 hours. Following 1 mg. vitamin B_{12} intramuscularly (flushing dose), 15 to 20 per cent of the administered dose appears in the urine in 24 hours.

LIVER FUNCTION TESTS

BROMSULFALEIN.   Less than 5 per cent remaining in serum at 45 minutes after intravenous injection of 5 mg./kg. body weight. Not valid in the presence of jaundice.

CEPHALIN CHOLESTEROL FLOCCULATION.   0 to 2+ in 48 hours.

GALACTOSE TOLERANCE.   Excretion in the urine of not more than 3.0 gm. galactose during 5 hours after ingestion of 40 gm.

HIPPURIC ACID.   Excretion of 3.0 to 3.5 gm. hippuric acid in the urine in 4 hours after ingestion of 6.0 gm. sodium benzoate; *or* excretion of 0.7 gm. hippuric acid in the urine in 1 hour after intravenous administration of 1.77 gm. sodium benzoate.

THYMOL TURBIDITY.   0 to 5 units.

Other tests of importance (q.v.) include direct and total serum bilirubin, alkaline phosphatase and serum glutamic-oxaloacetic transaminase.

GLUCOSE TOLERANCE TESTS

The patient should be on a 300 gm./day carbohydrate diet for 3 days preceding a glucose tolerance test. Values are given for true glucose.

Oral: after 100 gm. glucose, or 1.75 gm./kg., blood glucose level not above 160 mg. % at 1 hour, 140 mg. % at 90 minutes, and 120 mg. % after 120 minutes.

Intravenous: Blood glucose does not exceed 200 mg. % after infusion of 0.5 gm. glucose/kg. in 30 minutes. Blood glucose falls below initial level by 2 hours and returns to preinfusion levels by 3 to 4 hours.

THYROID FUNCTION TESTS

Radioactive iodine uptake, 20 to 50 per cent of dose in 24 hours. Radioactive iodine excretion, 30 to 70 per cent of administered dose in 24 hours.

ADRENAL FUNCTION TESTS

Adrenocortical inhibition test: 0.5 mg. of either Δ-1,9-α-fluorocortisone or 16-methyl-α-hydrocortisone every 6 hours reduces the excretion of 17-OH corticoids from 4 to 20 mg./24 hours to less than 2.0 mg./24 hours.

Corticotropin (ACTH) response test (eosinophil response test— Thorn): 4 hours after 25 USP units of ACTH intramuscularly, the decrease in eosinophil count should be more than 50 per cent of the original count.

Plasma 17-hydroxycorticoids: After an 8 hour infusion of 25 USP units of ACTH, plasma 17-hydroxycorticoids rise from a normal level of 5 to 25 μg/100 ml. to 35 to 55 μg./100 ml.

Urinary steroids: After an 8 hour infusion of 25 USP units of ACTH, urinary 17-hydroxycorticoids rise 200 to 400 per cent and urinary 17-ketosteroids by 50 to 100 per cent above control level.

NOMENCLATURE AND EQUIVALENT VALUES IN
ACID-BASE BALANCE

Equivalents and Milliequivalents (Eq. and mEq.). An equivalent is the amount (in gm.) of an ion that will react with or be equivalent to 1 gm. of hydrogen ions, and a milliequivalent is 1/1000 of an equivalent. An equivalent of an ion is equal to its gram molecular weight, divided by its valence. Thus sodium has a molecular weight of 23, and a valence of 1,

so 1 Eq. of $Na^+ = \dfrac{23}{1} = 23$ gm. The gram molecular weight of calcium is

40 and its valence is 2. 1 Eq. of $Ca^{++} = \dfrac{40}{2} = 20$ gm. 1 mEq. $= \dfrac{40}{2} = 20$

mg. Some molecules behave as ions under biological conditions. For example, bicarbonate (HCO_3) accepts one electron and has a single negative charge. The molecular weight is 61 $(1 + 12 + 3(16))$. 1 Eq. of

$(HCO_3)^- = \dfrac{61}{1} = 61$ gm. 1 mEq. of $(HCO_3)^- = 61$ mg.

The table indicates the gram molecular weight, valence and equivalent weight of common ions in human plasma.

Symbol	Gram molecular weight	Valence	Equivalent weight
H^+	1	1	1
Na^+	23	1	23
K^+	39	1	39
Ca^{++}	40	2	20
Mg^{++}	24	2	12
Cl^-	35.5	1	35.5
$(HCO_3)^-$	61	1	61
$(SO_4)^=$	96	2	48
$(HPO_4)^=$	96	2	48

Salts that dissociate virtually completely in water, as do those containing sodium or potassium, ionize into positively charged cations $(^+)$ and negatively charged anions $(^-)$. For example, 1 Eq. of NaCl will dissociate into 1 Eq. of Na^+ and 1 Eq. of Cl^-. In the same fashion 58.5 mg. of NaCl will dissociate into 1 mEq. of Na^+ and 1 mEq. of Cl^-.

How many mEq. of Na^+ and Cl^- are there in 1 liter of 0.9 per cent NaCl?

$$0.9\% = 9.0 \text{ gm./liter}$$

The molecular weight of 1 Eq. of NaCl is 58.5.

$$\frac{9}{58.5} = 0.154 \text{ Eq.}$$

Therefore there are 154 mEq. of Na$^+$ and 154 mEq. of Cl$^-$ in 1 liter of 0.9 per cent NaCl.

How much KCl must be added to 1 liter of 5 per cent glucose in water to have 40 mEq. of potassium?

$$1 \text{ mEq. of KCl} = 39 + 35.5 = 74.5 \text{ mg.}$$
$$40 \text{ mEq.} \times 74.5 = 2980 \text{ mg. or } 2.98 \text{ gm. KCl}$$

CONVERSION OF CO_2 IN VOLUMES % TO MILLIEQUIVALENTS. 1 molecular weight of a gas is contained in 22.4 liters at 760 mm. Hg barometric pressure and 0° C.

$$\frac{CO_2 \text{ in volumes } \%}{2.24} = \text{mEq. of } HCO_3/\text{liter}$$

Moles and Millimoles (M. and mM.). A mole is 1 gram molecular weight of an ion *without regard to valence,* and a millimole (mM) is 1/1000 of a mole. For univalent ions, mole and equivalent are the same; however, with divalent ions, an equivalent is 1/2 of a mole.

$$1 \text{ mEq. Na}^+ = 23 \text{ mg.}$$
$$1 \text{ mM. of Na}^+ = 23 \text{ mg.}$$
$$1 \text{ mEq. of Ca}^{++} = 20 \text{ mg.}$$
$$1 \text{ mM. of Ca}^{++} = 40 \text{ mg.}$$

Osmoles and Milliosmoles (O. and mO.). Each substance in solution, whether it be extracellular or intracellular, exerts an osmotic effect in proportion to its concentration. Each of several ions produces an independent effect. As in calculating moles, valence is not considered in computing milliosmoles. Hence, 1 millimole of NaCl in solution in water to make 1 liter has a milliosmolar effect of 2 milliosmoles, one each for Na$^+$ and Cl$^-$. Sugar, urea and other undissociated substances have an osmotic effect equal to their molecular weight and concentration only, as they do not dissociate into ions. A milliosmole, therefore, equals

$$\frac{\text{mg. of substance or ion per liter of solution}}{\text{atomic weight of substance (or ion if dissociated)}}$$

Thus:

$$23 \text{ mg. Na per liter} = 1 \text{ mO. per liter}$$
$$35.5 \text{ mg. Cl per liter} = 1 \text{ mO. per liter}$$
$$58.5 \text{ mg. NaCl per liter} = 2 \text{ mO. per liter}$$
$$60 \text{ mg. urea per liter} = 1 \text{ mO. per liter}$$
$$180 \text{ mg. of glucose per liter} = 1 \text{ mO. per liter}$$

The normal milliosmolar tension of extracellular fluid is about 285 mO., which includes both ionizable and nonionizable substances. The milliosmolar concentration of 0.9 per cent NaCl is determined as follows:

$$9 \text{ gm. NaCl per liter} = \frac{9}{58.5} = 0.154 \text{ Eq.} =$$

$$\begin{array}{r} 154 \text{ mEq. Na}^+ \\ +154 \text{ mEq. Cl}^- \\ \hline 308 \text{ mO.} \end{array}$$

A 5 per cent glucose in water solution contains 50 gm. of glucose per liter, whereas an osmolar solution contains 180 gm.

$$\frac{50}{180} = 0.278 \text{ O.} = 278 \text{ mO.}$$

The 5 per cent glucose solution is therefore hypotonic to plasma.

A 5 per cent solution of glucose in 0.9 per cent NaCl contains 308 mO. for Na$^+$ and Cl$^-$ plus 278 mO. for glucose. The total milliosmolar concentration is 586 mO., and this solution is hypertonic to plasma.

Osmolarity and Osmolality. The preceding discussion pertains to the common method of making solutions, that of weight-volume, in which a specific amount in weight of a substance, for example 9 gm. of NaCl, is dissolved in distilled water to make a volume of 1 liter. This produces a 0.9 per cent solution of NaCl with an osmolarity of 308 milliosmoles. However, the common method of determining osmotic activity depends on the effect of dissolved substances in depressing the freezing point of water. Such determinations are expressed in terms of the effect on *1 liter of water,* rather than 1 liter of solution. This is more important biologically, and therefore *osmolality* rather than osmolarity is discussed and used in this manual.

This differences are quite small at biologic concentrations, because the amounts of electrolytes, urea, glucose, etc., necessary to produce normal concentrations, when added to 1 liter of water, would increase the volume only very slightly. Much more important is the permeability of cell membranes to various substances in solution, and the effect of these substances on the balance between intracellular and extracellular water. Urea, for example, is distributed evenly in cellular and extracellular water; it adds to total osmolality by 16.7 mO. for each 100 mg. % increase in concentration, but does not affect the hydration of cells except as it acts as an osmotic diuretic and reduces ECF volume. Glucose is relatively slowly permeable through cell membranes, and sodium is normally largely excluded by cells. A rapid infusion of a hypertonic solution, such as 5 per cent glucose in 0.9 per cent saline, will result in a shift of water from cells to extracellular fluid. Excessive water administration, usually as 5 per cent glucose solution, in a patient with reduced renal free water clearance will result in reducing the extracellular osmolality as the glucose is metabolized and results in dilutional over-hydration of cells and ECF.

Serum sodium, under most circumstances, is an accurate measure of osmolality. Twice the serum sodium will closely approximate plasma osmolality if excessive amounts of glucose or urea are not present.

ACID-BASE TERMINOLOGY

The traditional method of determining the state of acid-base balance was to determine the pH of arterial or arteriolized venous blood and the total CO_2 content of the plasma. Now the partial pressure of CO_2 is most commonly measured directly in whole blood or calculated from pH and CO_2 content.

From these data, H_2CO_3 can easily be determined, as can bicarbonate, and the $\frac{BHCO_3}{HHCO_3}$ ratio directly evaluated. Pure states of respiratory acidosis or alkalosis, and metabolic acidosis and alkalosis, rarely exist except transiently in an acute form, because compensation takes place quite rapidly. Most patients will have a pattern that consists of the effect of the primary alteration and of the compensations that have been made in response to it.

For these reasons, a careful study of all the clinical problems and physiologic mechanisms present is essential to a complete under-standing of any clinical problem involving acid-base derangements.

Several different methods of approaching an understanding of acid-base balance have been developed and are in use today. Unfortunately, each has its own specific terminology, and it is necessary to understand not only the terms but the methods used in arriving at a conclusion in order to interpret the values for clinical use.

Whole Blood Buffer Base. Introduced by Singer and Hastings in 1948, whole blood buffer base represents the sum of the red cell and plasma buffers, including bicarbonate in both plasma and red cells, hemoglobin, plasma proteins and phosphate in both red cells and plasma. The total quantity of buffer anions in normal blood with normal hematocrit is about 45 to 50 mEq./liter, almost all of it in bicarbonate and hemoglobin.

Whole blood buffer base is not altered by changes in P_{CO_2} in vitro. It may be calculated from any two of the three components of the Henderson-Hasselbalch equation (pH, P_{CO_2}, bicarbonate concentration) *with the hematocrit or hemoglobin concentration of blood* by using a nomogram constructed by Singer and Hastings and a clinical inter-pretation diagram described by Singer, which indicates variations both in buffer base, due to changes in fixed acid, and in P_{CO_2}.

One of the popular ways of visualizing acid-base changes has been to plot the plasma bicarbonate concentration against the value for pH. The development of this approach to visualizing acid base chemistry has been presented by Davenport in successive editions, over 25 years, of a small monograph entitled *The ABC of Acid Base Chemistry*. A slight modification of this pH-bicarbonate diagram is taken from Moore (p. 333 in *The Metabolic Care of the Surgical Patient*) and reproduced in Figure 4.

    Standard Bicarbonate and Base Excess. In the past five years, an ingenious apparatus developed by Astrup and his associates has come into extensive use in the United States. This apparatus permits the measurement of the pH of blood as drawn from the patient, and also the pH of the blood when saturated with oxygen and equilibrated with CO_2 at two known partial pressures.

    Standard bicarbonate is defined as the concentration of bicarbonate in plasma when whole blood, fully saturated with oxygen is equilibrated with carbon dioxide at a P_{CO_2} of 40 mm. Hg at 38° C. Normal values (95 per cent range) are given as 21.3 to 24.8 mEq./liter.

    Standard bicarbonate does not directly show the amount of fixed acid or base causing a change in the base content of whole blood, because bicarbonate is responsible for only about 75 per cent of buffering at a fixed P_{CO_2}. So this is approximated in the Astrup system by multiplying variation in standard bicarbonate by 1.20. An exact correction requires knowledge of the hemoglobin concentration of whole blood, as is also the case with whole blood buffer base.

    Base excess is the actual buffer base minus the normal buffer base. It may have either a positive or a negative sign. Thus a negative base excess is a base deficit, representing an increase in fixed acid. The 95 per cent range for normal base excess is stated to be −2.3 to +2.3 mEq./liter.

    The Siggaard Andersen nomogram is used with the Astrup apparatus in determining standard bicarbonate, buffer base, base excess and P_{CO_2}. It assumes that the blood is at least 90 per cent saturated with oxygen, and correction factors must be used if this is not so either because venous blood is used or because of arterial blood unsaturation.

    The pH of the blood is measured in oxygen at 38° C. at two known P_{CO_2} values, one higher and one lower than P_{CO_2} of 40 mm. pH values at these P_{CO_2} values are plotted on the nomogram and connected by a straight line. The P_{CO_2} of the blood sample is then read at its actual pH. Standard bicarbonate, buffer base and base excess are read at the points where the line crosses the appropriate scales.

    The problems inherent in the use of either the Singer-Hastings, the Davenport, or the Astrup method of interpretation of acid-base derangements are discussed in detail by Schwartz and Relman. This article should be read carefully by any surgeon who wishes to understand the limitations, as well as the advantages, of some of the newer methods of approach to problems in acid-base balance. In particular, the nature of

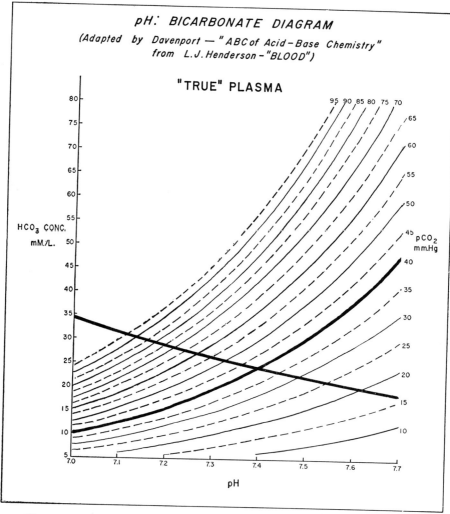

Figure 4. Acid-base balance. The pH-bicarbonate diagram. (From Moore, F. D.: Metabolic Care of the Surgical Patient. Philadelphia, W. B. Saunders Company, 1959.)

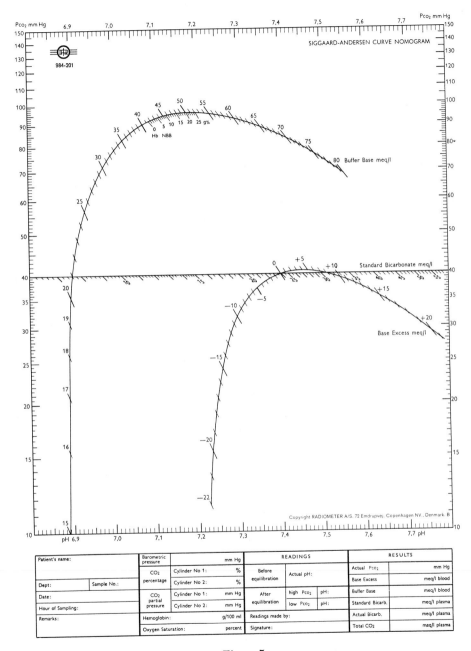

Figure 5.

normal compensation for respiratory acidosis and for respiratory alkalosis must be understood, if acid-base changes of an acute nature superimposed on a chronic and compensated respiratory alteration are to be understood and properly treated.

REFERENCES

1. Davenport, H. W.: The ABC of Acid-Base Chemistry. 5th ed. Chicago, University of Chicago Press, 1969.
2. Siggaard Andersen, O.: The Acid-Base Status of the Blood. 3rd ed. Baltimore, Williams and Wilkins Company, 1966.
3. Schwartz, W. B., and Relman, A. S.: A critique of the parameters used in the evaluation of acid-base disorders. New Eng. J. Med. 268:225, 1963.
4. Singer, R. B.: A new diagram for the visualization and interpretation of acid-base changes. Am. J. Med. Sci. 221:199, 1951.
5. Singer, R. B., and Hastings, A. B.: An improved clinical method for the estimation of disturbances of the acid-base balance of human blood. Medicine 27:223, 1948.

Index

627